Cardiovascular Emergencies

Amal Mattu, MD, FACEP, Editor-in-Chief
Professor and Vice Chair
Director, Emergency Cardiology Fellowship
Department of Emergency Medicine
University of Maryland School of Medicine
Baltimore, Maryland

William J. Brady, MD, FACEP, Associate Editor
Professor of Emergency Medicine and Medicine
Chair, Medical Emergency Response Committee
Medical Director, Emergency Management
University of Virginia
Charlottesville, Virginia

Michael Jay Bresler, MD, FACEP, Associate Editor
Clinical Professor
Division of Emergency Medicine
Stanford University School of Medicine
Stanford, California

Scott M. Silvers, MD, FACEP, Associate Editor
Chair, Department of Emergency Medicine
Assistant Professor of Emergency Medicine
Mayo Clinic College of Medicine
Jacksonville, Florida

Sarah A. Stahmer, MD, Associate Editor
Associate Professor Emergency Medicine
Department of Emergency Medicine
University of North Carolina at Chapel Hill

Jeffrey A. Tabas, MD, FACEP, Associate Editor
Professor, Department of Emergency Medicine
University of California, San Francisco
San Francisco, California

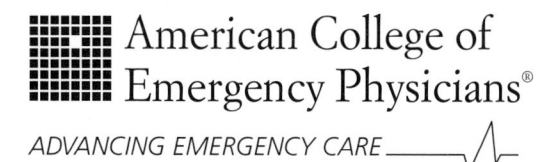

American College of Emergency Physicians®
ADVANCING EMERGENCY CARE

PUBLISHER'S NOTICE

The American College of Emergency Physicians (ACEP) makes every effort to ensure that contributors to its publications are knowledgeable subject matter experts. Readers are nevertheless advised that the statements and opinions expressed in this publication are provided as the contributors' recommendations at the time of publication and should not be construed as official College policy. ACEP recognizes the complexity of emergency medicine and makes no representation that this publication serves as an authoritative resource for the prevention, diagnosis, treatment, or intervention for any medical condition, nor should it be the basis for the definition of or standard of care that should be practiced by all health care providers at any particular time or place. Drugs are generally referred to by generic names. In some instances, brand names might be added for easier recognition. Device manufacturer information, if provided, is listed according to style conventions of the American Medical Association. ACEP received no commercial support for this publication. To the fullest extent permitted by law, and without limitation, ACEP expressly disclaims all liability for errors or omissions contained within this publication, and for damages of any kind or nature, arising out of use, reference to, reliance on, or performance of such information. To contact ACEP, write to PO Box 619911, Dallas TX 75261-9911; or call toll-free 800-798-1822, or 972-550-0911.

Copyright 2015, American College of Emergency Physicians, Dallas, Texas. All rights reserved. Except as permitted under the US Copyright Act of 1976, no part of this publication may be reproduced, stored, or transmitted in any form or by any means, electronic or mechanical, including storage and retrieval systems, without permission in writing from the publisher. Printed in the USA.

Additional copies of this publication can be ordered from the ACEP Bookstore, PO Box 619911, Dallas TX 75261-9911; toll-free 800-798-1822, or 972-550-0911; www.acep.org/bookstore.

First printing October 2014

ISBN 978-0-9889973-0-1

Mary Anne Mitchell, ELS, Managing Editor
Jessica Hamilton, Educational Products Assistant
Mike C. Goodwin, Creative Services Manager
Nicole Tidwell, Publications Sales and Marketing Manager
Marta Foster, Director, Educational Products
Robert Heard, MBA, CAE, Associate Executive Director, Membership and Education Division

Indexing: Hughes Analytics, Chicago, Illinois

Printing: The Covington Group, Kansas City, Missouri

About the Editors

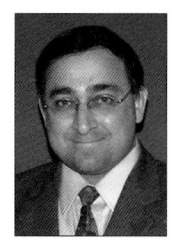

Amal Mattu, MD, FACEP. Since joining the faculty at the University of Maryland School of Medicine in 1996, Dr. Mattu has had a passion for teaching and writing about emergency cardiology. His commitment to teaching has earned him more than twenty teaching awards, including national awards from the American College of Emergency Physicians (ACEP) and local honors including the Teacher of the Year for the University of Maryland at Baltimore campus and the Maryland State Emergency Physician of the Year Award. He is a regular speaker at national and international conferences on topics pertaining to emergency cardiology. Dr. Mattu has authored or edited 16 textbooks in emergency medicine, including seven focused on emergency cardiology and electrocardiography. He is also the only emergency physician to serve as primary Guest Editor for *Cardiology Clinics*, which he has done twice. Dr. Mattu is currently a tenured professor, Vice Chair, and director of the Emergency Cardiology Fellowship for the Department of Emergency Medicine at the University of Maryland School of Medicine.

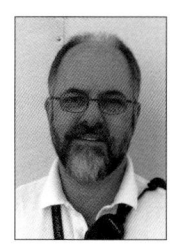

William J. Brady, MD, FACEP. Dr. Brady is a tenured professor of emergency medicine and internal medicine at the University of Virginia School of Medicine and is a senator in the Faculty Senate of the University of Virginia. He is the chief medical officer and medical director of Allianz Global Assistance (United States and Canada). He lectures locally, regionally, nationally, and internationally on many topics, including the electrocardiogram, cardiac arrest resuscitation, acute coronary syndrome, and emergency preparedness and response. He is a member of the Academy of Distinguished Educators at the University of Virginia and has received numerous teaching awards, including ACEP's National Faculty Teaching Award, the University of Virginia School of Medicine Dean's Award for Excellence in Teaching, and the David A. Harrison Distinguished Educator Award. He has also published numerous scholarly works, written or edited multiple textbooks, and contributed to clinical policy guidelines for both ACEP and the American Heart Association.

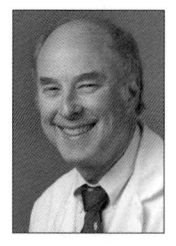

Michael Jay Bresler, MD, FACEP. Dr. Bresler is a clinical professor in the Division of Emergency Medicine of the Stanford University School of Medicine. Well known as an educator, he is frequently invited to lecture throughout the United States and internationally. His publications in the medical literature include a number of textbooks, textbook chapters, and peer reviewed journal articles. Dr. Bresler has been quite active in the legislative process at both the state and federal levels. He has written portions of both Federal and California anti-dumping laws, as well as legislation that generates over $200 million annually in California for the emergency care of indigent patients. Dr. Bresler has won the highest awards for leadership from both ACEP and the California chapter of ACEP. He served for a number of years as Speaker of the National Council of ACEP, and before that as President of the California chapter. ACEP has honored Dr. Bresler as a Life Fellow of the College, an Honorary Member, and a Hero of Emergency Medicine.

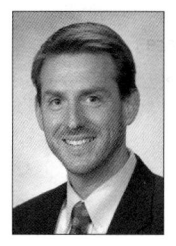

Scott Silvers, MD, FACEP. Dr. Silvers attended medical school at the University of Rochester School of Medicine in Rochester, New York, and received his training in emergency medicine at the Harvard Affiliated Emergency Residency in Boston, Massachusetts. Currently, he is chair of the Department of Emergency Medicine at Mayo Clinic in Jacksonville, Florida, where he also serves as co-director of the Mayo Clinic Comprehensive Stroke Center and Chest Pain Center. Dr. Silvers is a member of both the ACEP Clinical Policies Committee as well as the American Heart Association's Emergency Cardiovascular Care Committee where he contributes to the development of national, evidence-based guidelines. He was a co-author of the first Blueprints in Emergency Medicine study guide, and a co-editor of the *Textbook of Emergency Cardiovascular Care and CPR*. In coordination with the University of Miami's Center for Research in Medical Education, Dr. Silvers contributed to the development of the national advanced stroke life support curriculum. He is a reviewer for several journals and a member of the editorial board of *Emergency Medicine Practice*.

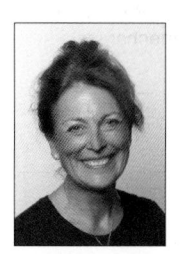

Sarah A. Stahmer, MD. Dr. Stahmer is an associate professor of emergency medicine at the University of North Carolina, Chapel Hill. She has been a program training director in emergency medicine for 15 years, building the academic training programs at Hospital of the University of Pennsylvania, Cooper/RWJ University Hospital, and Duke University Hospital. Her academic interests are ultrasound in emergency medicine, cardiovascular emergencies, and medical education. She has lectured extensively on these and other topics regionally, nationally, and internationally. She has received numerous awards for leadership and teaching in medical education that include the 2013 Council of Residency Directors Michael Wainscott Award for leadership and teaching in residency education, the Socrates Teaching Award UNC Emergency Medicine Residency, and the Council of Residency Directors Impact Award. Her publications are numerous in the fields of medical education, ultrasound, and cardiac emergencies.

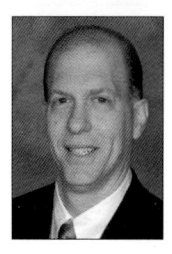

Jeffrey A. Tabas, MD, FACEP. Dr. Tabas is a professor of emergency medicine at the University of California San Francisco School of Medicine and practices at San Francisco General Hospital. He received degrees from Brown University and University of Pennsylvania School of Medicine and completed both internal medicine and emergency medicine residencies at University of California Los Angeles Medical Center. Dr. Tabas has worked with ACEP to teach emergency medicine, advanced procedural skills, and cardiovascular emergencies to a generation of students, residents, and physicians. He has been an active lecturer, author, and editor as well as course chair for ACEP Scientific Assembly and other popular emergency medicine conferences. When not pursuing clinical or academic activities, he is busy spending time with his wife and three children as well as pursuing his interest in sports, especially throwing hip checks in his ice hockey league for minimally skilled adult players.

Dedications

I would like to thank my wife, Sejal, for her constant support and encouragement; I thank my children, Nikhil, Eleena, and Kamran, for always reminding me of my proper priorities in life; I thank the residents and students at the University of Maryland School of Medicine for providing me the inspiration for the work I do every day; and finally, thanks to my colleagues and mentors, who continue to exemplify what I hope one day to become.

—Amal Mattu

I am most fortunate and am appreciative of many people—my parents, William and Joann Brady, for providing the opportunities; my wife, King Brady, for her support, patience, and love; my children, Lauren, Anne, Chip, and Katherine, for their love and inspiration; my chair, Robert O'Connor, MD, for his mentorship and leadership; and my colleagues in emergency medical care, both hospital- and prehospital-based, for their partnership in healthcare and dedication to the patient.

—William J. Brady

I would like to dedicate this work to my family, Adrienne, Ben, and Aaron, and to the thousands of emergency physicians whose efforts day and night provide care and comfort for our fellow human beings.

—Michael Jay Bresler

This book is dedicated to my parents for showing me how to live a life of integrity and devotion; to the love of my life, Avery, who is my greatest support and best friend; to my boys, Levi and Austin, who are my best buds and who motivate me to be the best that I can be; and to all of my many mentors in medicine who have challenged me to understand more about why we do what we do.

—Scott Silvers

For all those who let me teach the subtleties of ECG interpretation, medication effects on transmembrane potentials, and the evidence behind ACS risk stratification protocols…at 2 AM and feign to appear interested! I thank you for that gift.

—Sarah A. Stahmer

This text is dedicated to my wife, children, and parents for their support, love, and faith. I thank my colleagues at University of California San Francisco and at the American College of Emergency Physicians for their brilliance, fantastic attitude, and great friendship. I also thank the amazing staff at ACEP who made this all possible and finally, the amazing Amal Mattu, who continues to lead and inspire a generation of physicians.

—Jeffrey A. Tabas

Contributors

Benjamin S. Abella, MD, MPhil, FACEP
Center for Resuscitation Science
Department of Emergency Medicine
University of Pennsylvania
Philadelphia, Pennsylvania
Chapter 13, Post–Cardiac Arrest Syndrome

Tyler W. Barrett, MD, MSci, FACEP, FHRS
Associate Professor
Department of Emergency Medicine
Vanderbilt University Medical Center
Nashville, Tennessee
Chapter 8, Bradyarrhythmias

Christopher W. Baugh MD, MBA, FACEP
Director of Observation Medicine
Department of Emergency Medicine
Brigham and Women's Hospital
Assistant Professor of Medicine
Harvard Medical School
Boston, Massachusetts
Chapter 20, Use of Emergency Department Observation Units for Cardiac Patients

J. Stephen Bohan, MS, MD, FACP, FACEP
Executive Vice Chair
Department of Emergency Medicine
Brigham and Women's Hospital
Associate Professor
Harvard Medical School
Boston, Massachusetts
Chapter 20, Use of Emergency Department Observation Units for Cardiac Patients

William J. Brady, MD, FACEP, Associate Editor
Professor of Emergency Medicine and Medicine
Chair, Medical Emergency Response Committee
Medical Director, Emergency Management
University of Virginia
Charlottesville, Virginia
Operational Medical Director, Albemarle County Fire Rescue & Madison County EMS
Charlottesville, Virginia
Chief Medical Officer & Medical Director, Allianz Global Assistance
United States & Canada
Chapter 2, The Electrocardiogram in the Evaluation and Management of Acute Coronary Syndrome
Chapter 9, Narrow Complex Tachycardia: Diagnosis and Management in the Emergency Department

Michael Jay Bresler, MD, FACEP, Associate Editor
Clinical Professor
Division of Emergency Medicine
Stanford University School of Medicine
Stanford, California
Chapter 15, Hypertensive Emergencies and Elevated Blood Pressure
Chapter 21, Reducing the Risk of Malpractice

David F. M. Brown, MD, FACEP
Chair and Associate Professor
Department of Emergency Medicine
Massachusetts General Hospital
Harvard Medical School
Boston, Massachusetts
Chapter 10, Wide Complex Tachycardia

Theodore C. Chan, MD, FAAEM, FACEP
Professor and Chair
Department of Emergency Medicine
University of California, San Diego Health Sciences
San Diego, California
Chapter 19, Complications of Implanted Cardiac Devices

Emily K. Damuth, MD
Attending Physician
Division of Critical Care Medicine
Department of Emergency Medicine
Cooper University Hospital
Camden, New Jersey
Chapter 8, Bradyarrhythmias

Gail Delfin, MSN, RN
Clinical Research
Center for Resuscitation Science
University of Pennsylvania
Philadelphia, Pennsylvania
Chapter 13, Post–Cardiac Arrest Syndrome

Deborah B. Diercks, MD, MSc, FACEP
Professor and Vice Chair of Research
Department of Emergency Medicine
University of California, Davis Medical Center
Sacramento, California
Chapter 1, Approach to Acute Chest Pain

Laleh Gharahbaghian, MD, FACEP
Clinical Assistant Professor
Director, Emergency Ultrasound Program and Fellowship
Division of Emergency Medicine
Stanford University School of Medicine
Stanford, California
Chapter 4, Bedside Ultrasound for Emergency Cardiovascular Disorders

John C. Greenwood, MD
Department of Pulmonary & Critical Care Medicine
University of Maryland Medical Center
Baltimore, Maryland
Chapter 17, Special Populations: Pulmonary Hypertension and Cardiac Transplant

Tarlan Hedayati, MD, FACEP
Associate Program Director
Emergency Medicine Residency Program
Assistant Professor
Department of Emergency Medicine
Cook County (Stroger) Hospital
Rush University Medical Center
Chicago, Illinois
Chapter 5, Acute Coronary Syndrome: Modern Treatment of STEMI and NSTEMI

Korin B. Hudson, MD, FACEP
Associate Professor
Department of Emergency Medicine
MedStar Georgetown University Hospital
Washington, District of Columbia
Chapter 2, The Electrocardiogram in the Evaluation and Management of Acute Coronary Syndrome

Keith A. Marill, MD
Research Faculty
Department of Emergency Medicine
University of Pittsburgh
Pittsburgh, Pennsylvania
Chapter 10, Wide Complex Tachycardia

Amal Mattu, MD, FACEP, Editor-in-Chief
Professor and Vice Chair
Director, Emergency Cardiology Fellowship
Department of Emergency Medicine
University of Maryland School of Medicine
Baltimore, Maryland

Norine A. McGrath, MD, FACEP
Attending Physician
Department of Emergency Medicine
Chair, Bioethics Committee
Medstar Washington Hospital Center
Medstar Georgetown University Hospital
Washington, DC
Chapter 2, The Electrocardiogram in the Evaluation and Management of Acute Coronary Syndrome

Abhi Mehrotra, MD, FACEP
Associate Professor
Chief, Division of Quality and Performance
Department of Emergency Medicine
University of North Carolina School of Medicine
Chapel Hill, North Carolina
Chapter 14, Pericarditis, Myocarditis, and Endocarditis

Chadwick D. Miller, MD, MS, FACEP
Associate Professor
Executive Vice Chair and Director of Clinical Research
Department of Emergency Medicine
Wake Forest University School of Medicine
Winston-Salem, North Carolina
Chapter 3, Acute Coronary Syndrome: Biomarkers and Imaging

Siamak Moayedi, MD
Assistant Professor
Department of Emergency Medicine
University of Maryland School of Medicine
Baltimore, Maryland
Chapter 16, Cardiac Disease in Special Populations: HIV, Pregnancy, and Cancer

James V. Quinn, MD, MS, FACEP
Professor of Surgery/Emergency Medicine
Stanford University
Stanford, California
Chapter 11, Syncope

Peter S. Pang, MD, MSc, FACEP, FAAEM, FACC, FAHA
Associate Professor
Indiana University School of Medicine
Indianapolis, Indiana
Chapter 7, Acute Heart Failure

Nathan Parker, MD
Department of Emergency Medicine
University of California, Davis Medical Center
Sacramento, California
Chapter 1, Approach to Acute Chest Pain

Phillips Perera, MD, RDMS, FACEP
Clinical Associate Professor
Director, Emergency Ultrasound Research
Associate Director, Emergency Ultrasound Division
Division of Emergency Medicine
Department of Surgery
Stanford University Medical Center
Stanford, California
Chapter 4, Bedside Ultrasound for Emergency Cardiovascular Disorders

Joshua C. Reynolds, MD, MS
Assistant Professor
Department of Emergency Medicine
College of Human Medicine
Michigan State University
Grand Rapids, Michigan
Chapter 12, Modern Management of Cardiac Arrest

Matthew Salzman, MD
Assistant Professor
Medical Toxicologist
Department of Emergency Medicine
Cooper Medical School of Rowan University
Camden, New Jersey
Chapter 18, Pharmacologic Approach to the Emergency Cardiac Patient

Atman P. Shah, MD, FACC, FSCAI
Co-Director, Hans Hecht Cardiac Catheterization Laboratory
Director, Coronary Care Unit
Assistant Professor of Medicine
The University of Chicago
Chicago, Illinois
Chapter 5, Acute Coronary Syndrome: Modern Treatment of STEMI and NSTEMI

Scott M. Silvers, MD, FACEP, Associate Editor
Chair, Department of Emergency Medicine
Assistant Professor of Emergency Medicine
Mayo Clinic College of Medicine
Jacksonville, Florida

Sarah A. Stahmer, MD, Associate Editor
Associate Professor Emergency Medicine
Department of Emergency Medicine
University of North Carolina at Chapel Hill

Amita Sudhir, MD
Assistant Professor
Department of Emergency Medicine
University of Virginia
Charlottesville, Virginia
Chapter 9, Narrow Complex Tachycardia: Diagnosis and Management in the Emergency Department

Jeffrey A. Tabas, MD, FACEP, Associate Editor
Professor, Department of Emergency Medicine
University of California, San Francisco
San Francisco, California

Semhar Z. Tewelde, MD
Instructor
Department of Emergency Medicine
University of Maryland School of Medicine
Baltimore, Maryland
Chapter 6, Cardiogenic Shock

Vaishal M. Tolia, MD, MPH, FACEP
Assistant Clinical Professor
Associate Medical Director, Division of Observation Medicine
Department of Emergency Medicine
University of California San Diego Health System
San Diego, California
Chapter 19, Complications of Implanted Cardiac Devices

Mercedes Torres, MD
Clinical Assistant Professor
Department of Emergency Medicine
University of Maryland School of Medicine
Baltimore, Maryland
Chapter 16, Cardiac Disease in Special Populations: HIV, Pregnancy, and Cancer

Nikki B. Waller, MD
Assistant Residency Program Director
Department of Emergency Medicine
University of North Carolina School of Medicine
Chapel Hill, North Carolina
Chapter 14, Pericarditis, Myocarditis, and Endocarditis

Natasha B. Wheaton, MD
Assistant Residency Program Director and Clinical Assistant Professor
Department of Emergency Medicine
University of Iowa Carver College of Medicine
Iowa City, Iowa
Chapter 7, Acute Heart Failure

Sarah R. Williams, MD, FACEP, FAAEM
Clinical Associate Professor
Associate Program Director, Stanford/Kaiser Emergency Medicine Residency
Founder & Director Emeritus, Stanford EM Ultrasound Program and Fellowship
Stanford University School of Medicine
Stanford, California
Chapter 4, Bedside Ultrasound for Emergency Cardiovascular Disorders

Michael E. Winters, MD, FACEP, FAAEM
Associate Professor of Emergency Medicine and Medicine
University of Maryland School of Medicine
Co-Director, Combined EM/IM/Critical Care Program
Medical Director, Adult Emergency Department
University of Maryland Medical Center
Baltimore, Maryland
Chapter 17, Special Populations: Pulmonary Hypertension and Cardiac Transplant

Maame Yaa A. B. Yiadom, MD, MPH
Assistant Professor
Cooper University Hospital
Camden, New Jersey
Chapter 3, Acute Coronary Syndrome: Biomarkers and Imaging

Foreword

Emergency physicians serve as front-line clinicians who are expected to evaluate, stabilize, and begin treatment whenever an emergency patient presents to the emergency department (ED). As the specialty of emergency medicine has evolved and matured, so have the expectations for the expertise of the emergency physician. This creates a very exciting but also a very challenging work environment.

Gone are the days when all patients with chest pain get admitted for observation, every patient who is critically ill is whisked to an ICU before the initiation of critical care or a cardiologist is routinely called to the ED for patients with an unusual or unstable rhythm. Physicians working in an ED are now expected to have a high level of sophisticated knowledge in all areas of emergency care, with cardiovascular emergencies being one of the most important.

Cardiovascular Emergencies by Mattu, Brady, Bresler, Silvers, Stahmer, and Tabas brings together experts in our specialty to create an authoritative text for emergency providers. It is a book by emergency physicians *for* emergency physicians. It is also an excellent resource for physicians training in any specialty who will see cardiovascular emergencies. Each of the editors is a renowned educator and they have carefully selected authors for each topic. The text's value is maximized by extremely clear ECGs and very high quality graphics and illustrations.

The best textbooks are broad enough to include all relevant information, but are focused on the core topics readers will need to develop expertise or to serve as a reference. The editors and authors drew on their many years of experience educating students, residents, and fellow physicians to create a comprehensive textbook of cardiovascular emergencies. They begin with a chapter on how to approach chest pain and follow with a chapter on the overt and subtle ECG signs of ischemia and infarction. The evolution of biomarkers as well as the "best" imaging study to evaluate patients for ischemia follows in separate chapters devoted to each. Up until a few years ago, only cardiologists performed cardiovascular ultrasound. Now emergency physicians are increasingly using ultrasound to evaluate the heart and great vessels for evidence of heart failure, tamponade, contractility, RV strain, and volume status; thus, a chapter is devoted to the ultrasound findings needed for acute diagnosis and treatment of cardiovascular emergencies. Finally, there is no emergency that is more central to emergency care than the treatment of an acute myocardial infarction. This text covers all facets of the acute therapy of both STEMI and NSTEMI.

Chapters are also devoted to the management of arrhythmias seen near daily in the ED, including wide and narrow complex tachycardias along with bradycardias and heart block. Critical care medicine and cardiology share a number of emergencies, and this text provides up-to-date management of acute decompensated heart failure, cardiogenic shock, cardiac arrest, and post-cardiac arrest care, covering each with a detailed but succinct chapter. *Key Point* sections throughout all chapters highlight the most important concepts and clinical insights of the authors.

Other topics also covered in *Cardiovascular Emergencies* are syncope and hypertension, two very common entities, as well as less common but important conditions such as pulmonary hypertension, myocarditis, and pericarditis; complications due to implanted devices including pacemakers, AICDs, and LVADs; and cardiovascular emergencies in pregnant patients. Cardiac pharmacology, as it applies to emergent patients, and the use of the ED for observation are also presented. Because missing a cardiovascular emergency such as a myocardial infarction leads all other causes in dollars lost to malpractice claims paid, the final chapter is devoted to reducing malpractice risks.

Cardiovascular Emergencies is a book for anyone who will see a cardiovascular emergency. It is written and edited by expert emergency physicians and is a superb resource. All of us should be indebted to its editors and authors.

Corey M. Slovis, MD, FACEP, FACP, FAAEM
Professor of Emergency Medicine and Medicine
Chairman, Department of Emergency Medicine
Vanderbilt University Medical Center
Medical Director, Metro Nashville Fire Department and International Airport
Nashville, Tennessee
May 2014

Preface

Cardiovascular disease accounts for more deaths in the United States and most other first-world countries than any other cause. This number-one ranking has persisted for many years despite marked advances in preventive medicine, diagnostics, and therapeutics. Not only has this rank remained immobile, but the absolute number of deaths due to cardiac disease continues to rise. Most "experts" predict that this is not going to change in the near future. Therefore, if we in the health care field have any hope of changing these statistics, we must be optimally prepared to diagnose and treat patients when they present with acute cardiovascular conditions or complications.

The specialty of Emergency Medicine bears a great responsibility for the acute care of these patients. We must diagnose and initiate stabilizing treatment for patients with acute coronary syndromes, acute heart failure, pericarditis, myocarditis, arrhythmias, and many other conditions, and we are frequently the key providers who determine the prognosis of patients presenting with cardiac arrest. We are required to carry out these duties while working under significant time constraints; we are forced to make life-and-death decisions, often with minimal objective data; and we are often held to impossible standards of care by society and the legal profession.

The goal of this textbook is to facilitate the efficient and cutting-edge delivery of care to patients who present with acute cardiovascular conditions. To accomplish this goal, we brought together many of the brightest minds in Emergency Medicine from various institutions to collaborate and create best practices for emergency cardiovascular conditions. We believe we have formulated approaches to the workup and management that will optimize patient care.

In the pages that follow, we address many of the most common emergency cardiovascular conditions we face in Emergency Medicine as well as some conditions that are rising in import around the world. Initial chapters focus on the complicated evaluation and differential diagnosis of chest pain and modern approaches to "low-risk" chest pain. Acute coronary syndromes are covered in depth, and subsequent chapters address many of the complications associated with coronary artery disease, including acute heart failure, arrhythmias, and cardiogenic shock. Recent "hot topics" in the Emergency Medicine literature are addressed, including bedside echocardiography, observation units, cardiac arrest, and post-arrest care. Special populations are also discussed: oncologic patients, pregnant patients, transplant patients, patients with HIV, patients with pulmonary hypertension, and patients with implanted devices. A special chapter is devoted to issues related to malpractice.

In overseeing the development of this text, our goal has been to provide an easily understood, highly visual resource that is readable from cover to cover. Although this text might be considered a "bookshelf reference," that designation is at odds with our goal of cover-to-cover readability. We have tried to format the chapters for quick reference during everyday patient care.

We hope you enjoy reading this book and welcome any and all of your feedback. We would like to thank Linda Kesselring, copyeditor at University of Maryland, and Mary Anne Mitchell, copyeditor at ACEP, whose persistence and insight saw this project through to completion and excellence. We would also like to thank our families for their patience and understanding while we worked on this project, and we thank our colleagues, students, and residents, who have been a constant source of inspiration for our work. We would especially like to thank you, the readers, for your unwavering dedication and commitment to patient care.

Amal Mattu
William J. Brady
Michael J. Bresler
Scott M. Silvers
Sarah A. Stahmer
Jeffrey A. Tabas

Contents

Foreword ix

Preface xi

1. Approach to Acute Chest Pain 1
2. The Electrocardiogram in the Evaluation and Management of Acute Coronary Syndrome 11
3. Acute Coronary Syndrome: Biomarkers and Imaging 37
4. Bedside Ultrasound for Emergency Cardiovascular Disorders 53
5. Acute Coronary Syndrome: Modern Treatment of STEMI and NSTEMI 91
6. Cardiogenic Shock 103
7. Acute Heart Failure 111
8. Bradyarrhythmias 129
9. Narrow Complex Tachycardia: Diagnosis and Management in the Emergency Department 143
10. Wide Complex Tachycardia 161
11. Syncope 177
12. Modern Management of Cardiac Arrest 187
13. Post–Cardiac Arrest Syndrome 201
14. Pericarditis, Myocarditis, and Endocarditis 209
15. Hypertensive Emergencies and Elevated Blood Pressure 227
16. Cardiac Disease in Special Populations: HIV, Pregnancy, and Cancer 243
17. Special Populations: Pulmonary Hypertension and Cardiac Transplant 255
18. Pharmacologic Approach to Cardiac Emergencies 269
19. Complications of Implanted Cardiac Devices 283
20. Use of Emergency Department Observation Units for Cardiac Patients 293
21. Reducing the Risk of Malpractice 301

Index 311

CHAPTER 1

Approach to Acute Chest Pain

Deborah B. Diercks and Nathan Parker

IN THIS CHAPTER

Initial approach
Acute coronary syndrome
Pulmonary embolism
Esophageal rupture
Tension pneumothorax
Aortic dissection
Cardiac tamponade
Ancillary tests
Advanced imaging
Clinical decision rules

More than 6 million Americans present to emergency departments every year with the chief complaint of acute chest pain.[1] The differential diagnosis is extremely broad (Table 1-1). Emergency physicians have the difficult task of differentiating life-threatening causes requiring immediate intervention from more benign causes. In this chapter, we focus on the presentation of the most common critical diagnoses, their initial workup, and the strategies employed to ensure a safe and successful disposition.

Initial Approach

All patients without an obviously benign cause of chest pain should have their vital signs assessed immediately, be connected to a monitor, and have intravenous access established. Ideally, an electrocardiogram (ECG) should be obtained in the prehospital setting. Recent data have shown that paramedics and nurses, given adequate training, can reliably diagnose ST-elevation myocardial infarction (STEMI) and subsequently alert destination hospitals.[2] Since it has been well established that early reperfusion reduces mortality and morbidity, a system should be in place to facilitate rapid percutaneous intervention or fibrinolysis once STEMI has been confirmed.[3] A focused history and physical examination should be performed promptly by the emergency care provider because successful management of conditions such as tension pneumothorax depends on the provider's acting within minutes of a patient's presentation.

KEY POINT

Patients with chest pain should have an ECG obtained on arrival.

Acute Coronary Syndrome

Of the common presenting causes of chest pain, acute coronary syndrome (ACS) presents a particular challenge to emergency physicians. Defined as the syndrome resulting from acute cardiac ischemia, ACS encompasses stable angina, unstable angina, STEMI, and non-STEMI (NSTEMI).

Missed acute myocardial infarctions (AMIs) are frequent causes of litigation against medical providers. Emergency physicians disagree over the acceptable rate of missed acute MI; most accept a rate between 0.01% and 2%.[4] Care providers in emergency departments with low patient volumes and limited resources face particularly difficult challenges in making the diagnosis; miss rates tend to be higher in these facilities.[5]

In the "classic" presentation of ACS, the patient usually describes the pain as pressure, squeezing, or crushing. The pain is located substernally or on the left, and it can radiate to the jaw, neck, or arms. Associated symptoms usually include diaphoresis, nausea, vomiting, weakness, and syncope.[6] However, none of these signs and symptoms is sensitive or specific enough on its own to rule in or out ACS independent of an ECG, cardiac biomarkers, and other diagnostic tests.[7] Similarly, the presence of traditional risk factors such as hypertension, hyperlipidemia, diabetes mellitus, family history of coronary artery disease (CAD), and history of smoking, although positively correlating with adverse events within 6 months, does not correlate with the incidence of acute MI in the emergency department.[8] However, emergency care providers should be cautious about an initial impression of "noncardiac chest pain" if traditional risk factors are present because 3% of patients with those factors will experience an adverse cardiac event within 30 days.[9]

To further complicate the establishment of a diagnosis, many patients with an eventual diagnosis of acute MI present without chest pain at all.[10] This presentation is more common among women than men (42% and 31%, respectively), but the difference decreases with increasing age.[11] Atypical presentation of acute MI is also associated with diabetes, heart failure, advanced age, and nonwhite races.[12]

TABLE 1-1.
Causes of Chest Pain

Cardiovascular
- Acute MI
- Aortic dissection
- Cardiac tamponade
- Coronary spasm
- Pericarditis
- Stable angina
- Unstable angina

Pulmonary
- Bronchitis
- Pneumonia
- Pneumothorax
- Pulmonary embolus

Gastrointestinal
- Cholecystitis
- Esophageal reflux
- Esophageal rupture
- Esophageal spasm
- Esophageal tear
- Gastritis
- Hepatitis
- Pancreatitis
- Peptic ulcer disease

Musculoskeletal
- Costochondritis
- Muscle strain
- Rib fracture

KEY POINT
Many patients with ACS present without chest pain.

Pulmonary Embolism

Pulmonary embolism (PE) accounts for up to 200,000 deaths in the United States annually.[13] Like ACS, PE represents a broad range of disease, from asymptomatic incidental findings to saddle embolus causing shock and sudden death. Among patients presenting in shock, the short-term mortality rate can reach as high as 50%.[14]

Reflecting this broad spectrum of disease, the clinical signs and symptoms are especially difficult to interpret. In a large, prospective study, the following symptoms were present in patients diagnosed with PE: dyspnea (79%), pleuritic pain (49%), cough (43%), wheezing (31%), calf or thigh swelling (39%), and calf or thigh pain (16%). On physical examination, the following signs were present: tachypnea (57%), tachycardia (26%), rales (21%), and signs of deep vein thrombosis (DVT) in the calf or thigh (47%).[15]

Risk factors for acute PE include recent surgery, trauma, immobility, cancer, neurologic disease with lower extremity paresis, oral contraceptive use, hormone therapy, and pregnancy.[12] Given the difficulty in diagnosing PE, multiple clinical decision rules have been devised to aid in the workup. These rules are discussed later in this chapter.

Esophageal Rupture

Esophageal rupture is a relatively rare cause of acute chest pain among emergency department patients. Although its true incidence is unknown, the diagnosis carries a high mortality rate—approximately 20% despite modern therapies.[16] The mean age of patients with esophageal rupture is the early 60s, and more than two thirds of patients are male.[17] Esophageal perforations are most commonly iatrogenic, usually caused by endoscopic procedures, with a minority of ruptures resulting spontaneously from increased intraabdominal pressures typically associated with vomiting (eg, Boerhaave syndrome).[18] Other causes include caustic ingestions and blunt or penetrating trauma.

The classic features of esophageal rupture include the sudden onset of chest pain precipitated by severe vomiting or retching. The Mackler triad of esophageal rupture—chest pain, vomiting, and subcutaneous emphysema—was first described in 1952; this triad is absent in most patients.[12] Associated symptoms include shortness of breath, dysphonia, dysphagia, abdominal pain, hematemesis, and melena. On physical examination, tachycardia is frequently noted, with fever presenting later. Crepitus in the neck or chest wall is indicative of subcutaneous emphysema. Rapidly progressing pleural effusions can be a late sign.[19]

Tension Pneumothorax

Nontraumatic spontaneous tension pneumothorax is also a relatively uncommon cause of acute chest pain. Approximately 1% to 2% of all spontaneous pneumothoraxes present under tension.[20] Clinically, a pneumothorax is considered to be under tension when it causes significant respiratory or hemodynamic compromise as a result of positive intrapleural pressure. In an awake patient being ventilated without positive pressure, this process can develop only if the intrapleural pressure is less than the atmospheric pressure during some period of the respiratory cycle. Therefore, the spectrum of tension pneumothorax can range from intrapleural pressure that is positive only at the end expiratory phase to pressure that is positive throughout the entire respiratory cycle.[21]

Spontaneous pneumothorax can be divided into the following two classifications: primary spontaneous pneumothorax, which occurs in the absence of apparent underlying lung disease, and secondary spontaneous pneumothorax, which develops as a result of underlying lung pathology. Risk factors for primary spontaneous pneumothorax include male sex (6:1 relative risk compared with females), tall stature, smoking, low body mass index, sudden changes in environmental pressure, genetic predisposition, inhalant use, and even exposure to loud music.[22,23] Risk factors for secondary spontaneous pneumothorax include chronic obstructive pulmonary disease, interstitial lung disease, infection, neoplasm, and connective tissue disease.[22]

Symptoms of tension pneumothorax typically include the rapid onset of pleuritic chest pain and shortness of breath. In addition to unilateral reduced breath sounds and hyperresonance, tension pneumothorax also can present with tachycardia, tachypnea, hypotension, and tracheal deviation away from the affected side.[24] If a tension pneumothorax is highly suspected based on the history and physical examination alone, steps should be taken immediately to relieve the pressure via needle or tube thoracostomy. A recent review showed tube thoracostomy to be superior to percutaneous aspiration; the reason was initially thought to be that the chest wall thickness exceeded the length of the catheter in percutaneous aspiration, but this does not appear to be the case.[25,26] Therefore, in patients with tension pneumothorax, immediate tube thoracostomy is indicated.

KEY POINT

Immediate decompression of a suspected tension pneumothorax with tube thoracostomy is indicated before confirmation with chest radiography.

Aortic Dissection

Few critical diagnoses are as feared by emergency care providers as acute aortic dissection, which is notoriously difficult to diagnose. Some studies suggest that up to one-third of all aortic dissections are initially misdiagnosed. The difficulty is compounded by its relatively low prevalence (1 case per every 10,000 emergency department visits).[27,28] Acute aortic dissection is often mistaken for myocardial infarction. The mortality rate associated with untreated dissection reaches 1% to 2% per hour during the first 48 hours.[29,30]

KEY POINT

Up to one-third of all aortic dissections are misdiagnosed.

Both the DeBakey and Stanford classifications systems have been widely used for describing aortic dissections. DeBakey type I begins in the ascending aorta and extends beyond the arch. Type II involves the ascending aorta only, while type III involves only the descending aorta. Stanford type A is any dissection that involves the ascending aorta, and type B dissections do not. Although both classifications can be used, it is most important to identify if the ascending arch is involved, as dissections involving the ascending arch usually require emergent surgical intervention.[31]

Recent guidelines published by the American Heart Association, in conjunction with other professional societies, describe important clinical risk factors for assessing the pretest probability of acute aortic dissection in patients with chest pain. These factors include Marfan or Ehlers-Danlos syndrome, a family history of aortic disease, aortic valve disease, recent aortic manipulation, thoracic aortic aneurysm, abrupt onset of pain, pain that is severe, pain that is ripping or tearing, pulse deficit in the upper limbs, focal neurologic deficit, hypotension or shock, and new aortic regurgitation murmur.[32] When these features were applied to the International Registry of Acute Aortic Dissection, over 95% of patients with confirmed aortic dissection had at least one of them.[28]

Research has been done to determine the factors that delay the time from presentation to diagnosis. Female patients, patients transferred from a non-tertiary care facility, and patients who have had previous cardiac surgery all had longer delays in diagnosis. The same is true for patients with mild or no pain, patients with atypical features such as fever, those with heart failure, and those with an initial ECG suggestive of myocardial ischemia.[33] A Japanese study suggested that patients who walk into the emergency department are also more likely to have a delay in diagnosis.[34] Given the high mortality rate associated with missed diagnosis and the relatively low incidence of this dangerous condition, high suspicion must be maintained to prevent complications.

Cardiac Tamponade

Cardiac tamponade, another relatively rare diagnosis, refers to hemodynamic compromise caused by increased pericardial pressure. The spectrum of this disease ranges from mild and asymptomatic (pericardial pressure <10 mm Hg) to severe, causing shock (pericardial pressure >20 mm Hg).[35] Other than trauma and recent cardiac surgery, medical causes of pericardial effusion include acute pericarditis, malignancy, acute MI causing wall rupture, aortic dissection, uremia, heart failure, bacterial or viral infection, and collagen vascular disease.[12]

The Beck triad of low arterial blood pressure, distended neck veins, and muffled heart sounds has been used to describe the signs of cardiac tamponade, but these are probably late findings. Increased sympathetic drive usually causes hypertension before the physiologic reserve is exhausted.[36] A recent review of studies involving patients with pericardial effusion delineated the following signs and symptoms associated with the disease and their related sensitivities: dyspnea (87%–88%), pulsus paradoxus greater than 10 mm Hg (82%), tachycardia (77%), hypotension (26%), diminished heart sounds (28%), and elevated jugular venous pressure (76%).[37]

Ancillary Tests

Electrocardiography

The 12-lead ECG is one of the cornerstones in chest pain evaluation. This chapter reviews common ECG changes that, in general, suggest important diagnoses; subtleties of ECG interpretation are discussed in depth elsewhere in this book. ECGs provide a "snapshot" of the heart's electrophysiology. To fully capture a dynamic process, including an evolving myocardial infarction, serial ECGs repeated 30 to 60 minutes after the initial study are recommended when the initial tracing is nondiagnostic and suspicion remains for ongoing ischemia.[38] It is important to remember that a normal ECG does not rule out acute ischemia; more than 50% of patients with missed AMI had a normal initial ECG.[12]

ST-segment elevation has a variety of causes (Table 1-2). ST-segment elevation should raise suspicion for acute ischemia/infarct when it exists in two or more contiguous leads.[39] When reciprocal ST-segment depression is present, the diagnosis of STEMI becomes more likely.[40] When an inferior STEMI is suspected (elevation in lead II, III, or aVF), tracings from leads V_4R through V_6R can be obtained to evaluate for right ventricular infarction, as these patients are often preload dependent.[41]

Although diffuse ST elevation and PR depression (ST depression and PR elevation in aVR) constitute the classic ECG finding in acute pericarditis, once the condition has progressed to a significant pericardial effusion, electrical alternans can be seen.[42,43] For PE, the ECG is usually of little diagnostic utility. In PE, the classic finding of $S_1Q_3T_3$ is rarely seen. The most common ECG findings are sinus tachycardia or nonspecific ST-segment or T-wave changes.[44]

A recent study of 159 patients with type A aortic dissection showed that almost half of them had acute changes on the ECG. ST depression (34%) was the most common, but ST elevation (8%) was present as well. Finding these ST changes increases the risk of misdiagnosis.[45] ST elevation in acute dissection is also associated with involvement of the coronary ostia, the right coronary artery being most commonly involved.[46]

Chest Radiograph

The chest radiograph (CXR) is another important diagnostic tool in patients with acute chest pain. Although the CXR rarely provides the diagnosis in isolation, it can rapidly change a treatment algorithm. For example, although a CXR can provide important information in a stable patient, delaying treatment for imaging in a patient with clinically suspected tension pneumothorax is not optimal. Still, tube thoracostomy is not indicated in other diagnoses such as diaphragm rupture, which can mimic the presentation of tension pneumothorax, so the decision to image or not must be individualized for each patient.

The CXR is commonly used to evaluate patients with suspected aortic dissection, but it is neither sensitive nor specific for this disease. In one study, only 73% of patients with known type A aortic dissection had signs suggesting dissection, most commonly widened mediastinum, while 16% of normal CXRs were thought to be suspicious for dissection.[47] Up to 90% of patients with esophageal rupture have abnormal findings on CXR, most commonly pneumomediastinum, hydropneumothorax, and isolated pleural effusion.[48] Interestingly, the esophagus ruptures most often on the left, with subsequent development of a pleural effusion on that side.[49]

KEY POINT

A normal chest radiograph does not rule out aortic dissection.

FIGURE 1-1.

Right heart strain; note dilated right ventricle. Photo courtesy of K. Kelley.

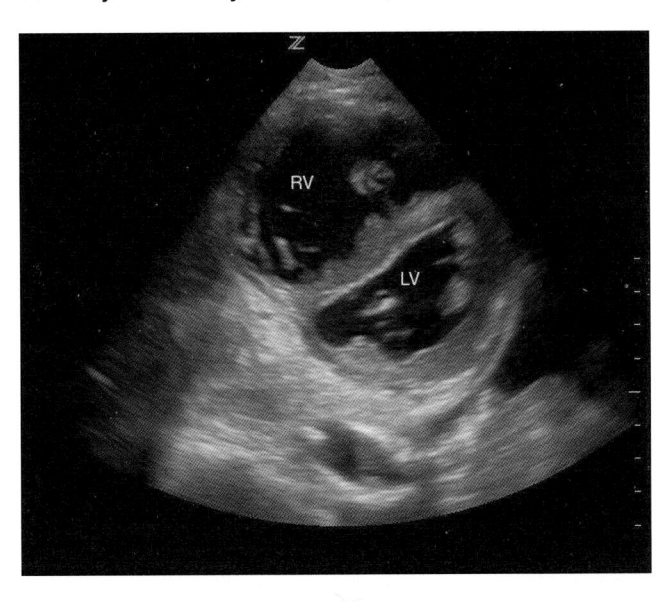

TABLE 1-2.

Causes of ST Elevation on ECG

Acute MI
Pericarditis
Left ventricular hypertrophy
Benign early repolarization
Prinzmetal angina
Brugada syndrome
Left ventricular aneurysm

In one large study of patients known to have PE, cardiomegaly (27%) was the abnormality most frequently seen on CXR; 24% of patients had a normal CXR.[50] The classic Hampton hump is rarely seen. The CXR can provide useful information when the physician is deciding whether to perform ventilation-perfusion scintigraphy or CT angiography, as patients with known chronic lung disease have a higher incidence of nondiagnostic ventilation-perfusion scans.[51]

Ultrasonography

Ultrasonography has become an integral diagnostic tool in the provision of emergency care. In patients who come to the emergency department in shock, a two-dimensional transthoracic echocardiogram (2D-TTE) that shows no signs of right ventricular strain (Figure 1-1) can practically exclude PE as the cause of hypotension.[52] However, a negative ultrasound scan does not rule out PE as a cause of chest pain.[53] Two-dimensional transthoracic echocardiography is the gold standard for diagnosing pericardial effusion in the emergency department, and all patients with suspected pericarditis and any high-risk features should have bedside echocardiography to aid in diagnosis and rule out pericardial tamponade (Figure 1-2).[54]

When ACS is suspected, early 2D-TTE can contribute information to the prognosis by identifying wall motion abnormalities.[55] In a study of patients presenting to an emergency department with acute chest pain and a nondiagnostic ECG, those with a normal 2D-TTE (performed by a cardiologist) had no major cardiac events at 30 days.[56] Structural abnormalities that might change therapeutic management, such as papillary muscle rupture or ventricular septum rupture, can also be identified; images suggesting such abnormalities should be interpreted only by experienced cardiac sonographers.[57]

Limited data exist on the role of ultrasonography in the diagnosis of aortic dissection. In evaluating for an intimal flap, 2D-TTE can be combined with abdominal ultrasonography. The sensitivity of 2D-TTE in detecting acute aortic dissection has been reported to be 67% to 80%, while its specificity is 99% to 100%.[58] When dissection is identified in an unstable patient, emergent cardiothoracic surgery should be expedited.[59]

Bedside ultrasonography performed by emergency physicians has a sensitivity approaching 100% for pneumothorax, compared with a 75% sensitivity for an upright CXR.[60] This degree of sensitivity, as well as ultrasound's portability, has fostered the use of ultrasonography in military operations and in remote locations where other imaging modalities are unavailable.[61] The detection of occult pneumothorax that was not seen on a CXR might not prove to be clinically significant, but it should prompt the care provider to monitor the patient closely for pneumothorax expansion.[62]

KEY POINT

Bedside emergency ultrasonography is a valuable tool in the workup of chest pain.

Troponins

Cardiac troponins (T and I) are the preferred markers of myocardial injury in patients presenting with chest pain. They are more sensitive and specific than the biomarkers used in the past.[63] It is important to remember, however, that myocardial necrosis can result from pathologies other than MI or ACS.[64] With the introduction of new highly sensitive troponin (hs-cTn) assays, which are 1,000- to 10,000-fold more sensitive than the original first-generation troponin assays, differentiating the causes of myocardial necrosis (including MI and ACS) will be more important as medical care providers are challenged with interpreting an increasing number of positive tests.[65]

Given our increased ability to measure very low concentrations of cardiac troponins, an upper limit of normal at the population-adjusted 99th percentile has been defined.[66] With the application of this newly defined cutoff, more patients with signs and symptoms suggesting acute MI have an elevated hs-cTn level when they come to the emergency department; a recent study showed an almost 200% increase in the number of hs-cTn–positive patients who were eventually diagnosed with chest pain unrelated to coronary occlusion. Troponin is released during tachyarrhythmia in young healthy people as well as in those undergoing sustained strenuous exercise.[67] However, even small increases in hs-cTn levels in patients presenting with chest pain have been associated with adverse short- and long-term prognoses.[68]

The definition of AMI, which includes the "rise and/or fall of cardiac biomarkers," may have to be refined with the advent of hs-cTn assays.[69] An acute change in the hs-cTn level of more than 20% has been suggested as representing either new or resolving myocardial injury. However, healthy study subjects have demonstrated a baseline variability of more than 50%.[70,71] It is important to note that simply changing the diagnostic criterion of AMI to include a hs-cTn change of more than 50% decreases the sensitivity of the test to less than 70%.[64]

It is likely that the introduction of hs-cTn assays will provide several benefits to emergency medicine practice, but its place in our diagnostic algorithm has not been fully defined. It has

FIGURE 1-2.

Echocardiographic image of a patient with a pericardial effusion. Photo courtesy of K. Kelley.

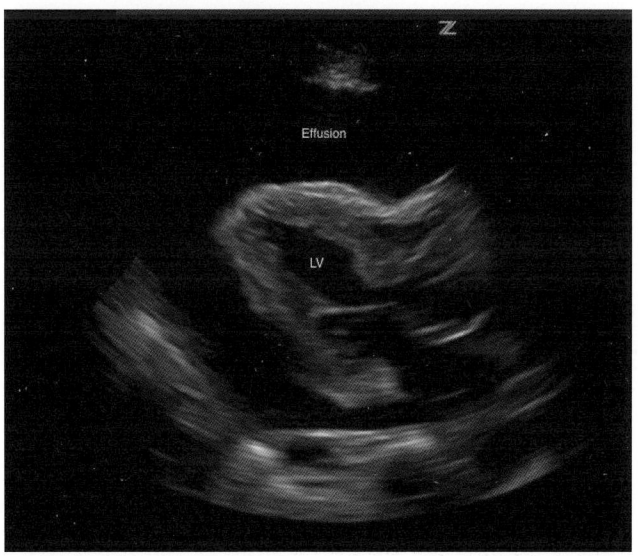

been suggested that, given the fact that hs-cTn levels elevate earlier, the timing of our serial cardiac marker testing could be shortened to less than 3 hours after initial presentation.[72] The assay might take a role analogous to the D-dimer test, given its relatively high negative predictive value.[73] It will also be important to reevaluate our chest pain clinical decision rules, as most of them were developed before hs-cTn assays became available.

> **KEY POINT**
>
> The role of the new highly sensitive troponin assays remains unclear in the evaluation of patients with chest pain.

D-Dimer

The D-dimer assay has been used in the evaluation of patients for PE for more than 20 years. Although many assays exist, most used in emergency practice have a high sensitivity (typically in the mid 90% range) but low specificity for venous thromboembolism (VTE).[74] In the contemporary diagnostic algorithm, a highly sensitive D-dimer assay that is below the designated cutoff in a non–high-risk population can be used to exclude VTE because of its negative predictive value of more than 99% in this population.[75] In fact, the highly sensitive quantitative D-dimer test has one of the highest sensitivities of any test used in the screening of patients for VTE.

The D-dimer assay has been studied for both prognostic purposes and for evaluation of the burden of disease in PE. High D-dimer levels are associated with increased 15-day and 3-month mortality rates as well as a more central location of clots on CT angiogram.[76,77] High levels are also associated with a higher pulmonary artery obstruction index.[78]

> **KEY POINT**
>
> A negative D-dimer does not rule out pulmonary embolus in a population at high risk for the disease.

Recently, the use of the D-dimer assay was studied in the context of aortic dissection. A metaanalysis found a pooled sensitivity of 94%, but specificity remained poor.[79] Concern exists regarding the proposed use of the test to rule out aortic dissection in low-risk populations, as isolated intramural hematomas or thromboses have been associated with false-negative tests.[80] Given the low incidence of acute aortic dissection in the general population presenting with chest pain, it has been suggested that routine screening with D-dimer assays would increase CT scan utilization by approximately 40% and would not necessarily aid in timely diagnosis.[81]

Other Biomarkers

New research has focused on addressing methods for shortening the time needed to rule out MI in the emergency department. In low-risk populations, adding either N-terminal pro-B type natriuretic peptide (NT-proBNP) or copeptin to the initial troponin assessment at presentation significantly increased the sensitivity and the negative predictive value for MI.[82,83] Measuring unbound free fatty acids in addition to conventional or highly sensitive troponin also improves sensitivity and specificity in the detection of ACS.[84] Higher levels of NT-proBNP or ST2 (a novel biomarker of cardiac stress) in patients with chest pain have been associated with increased mortality.[85,86] Investigating the interesting concept that larger platelets are more active, researchers have found a correlation between mean platelet volume and ACS in patients with acute chest pain.[87]

Advanced Imaging

Computed Tomography Angiography

Computed tomography angiography (CTA) has become the gold standard as the initial imaging test in the workup of patients suspected of having aortic dissection or PE. The sensitivity and specificity of CTA in detecting acute aortic dissection have been reported as 100% and 98% to 99%, respectively.[88] The data associated with PE have shown larger variations in accuracy. The largest study to date, PIOPED II, reported sensitivity of 83% and specificity of 96%, but most of the scans were performed with four-slice CT.[89] It is possible that with the arrival of 64-slice multidetector CT the diagnostic accuracy will increase significantly, thereby allowing a negative CTA alone to be used to effectively rule out PE as the cause of chest pain in all risk groups.[88]

As diagnostic accuracy increases with improved technology, an increasing number of isolated subsegmental PEs are being diagnosed with CTA.[90] No consensus has been reached regarding the proper management of patients with isolated subsegmental PE because 3-month outcomes are generally favorable and the risk of hemorrhage with anticoagulation might outweigh the benefits.[91]

Coronary Computed Tomography Angiography

Coronary CTA (CCTA) has received much attention in recent years, with a flurry of data about its use coming out in a short time. Although the role of CCTA has not been established or extensively validated in the workup of chest pain in the emergency department, its proposed use has been hotly debated. A recent metaanalysis involving only prospective studies estimated the sensitivity and specificity of CCTA for ACS to be 95%

TABLE 1-3.

PERC Rule[101]

Age under 50 years
Heart rate less than 100 beats/min
Oxygen saturation of more than 94% on room air
No history of DVT/PE
No recent trauma/surgery
No hemoptysis
No exogenous estrogen
No clinical signs of DVT

If all eight criteria are met, patient has less than a 2% chance of having PE.

and 87%, respectively.[92]

Heralded for its high negative predictive value and its potential to rule out ACS with a negative scan, CCTA has been shown to decrease time to diagnosis and disposition.[93,94] Critics of CCTA point out its low positive predictive value—all patients with significant underlying CAD, stable or not, will likely have a positive scan and thus require additional testing.[95] The radiation exposure must also be considered, as well as the fact that the study cannot be performed in patients with renal failure, those unable to tolerate beta-blockers, and those with ectopic rhythms.[96] While not yet standard of care, CCTA will likely find a role in rapidly triaging patients who are at low to intermediate risk for ACS and who have initially normal cardiac markers and an ECG that does not raise concern.[97,98]

Triple-Rule-Out Computed Tomography Angiography

A recently developed protocol combines CCTA with imaging of the pulmonary arteries and thoracic aorta. Triple-rule-out CTA enables patients to be simultaneously evaluated for ACS, PE, and aortic dissection in less than 20 minutes. The protocol has significant limitations: it is technically difficult to perform, it delivers a 50% larger dose of radiation than CCTA, and its image quality varies.[99] However, because more than 20% of patients evaluated for ACS are simultaneously assessed for PE or aortic dissection, performing only one imaging study would decrease their overall radiation exposure.[100] As with CCTA, the use of triple-rule-out CTA has not yet been validated in large prospective trials, but it may still find a role in ruling out disease in low- to intermediate-risk patients.[1]

Clinical Decision Rules

Considering the difficulty in accurately diagnosing the cause of chest pain while performing an efficient and cost-effective workup, multiple clinical decision rules have been devised to assist emergency physicians. Many of these rules have been well validated in large prospective trials. These rules should never replace the physician's best judgment, but they can be helpful when the differential diagnosis remains large. In this section, we describe a few of the more recognized clinical decision rules, along with their limitations.

Pulmonary Embolism Rule-out Criteria

The pulmonary embolism rule-out criteria (PERC) rule (Table 1-3) was devised to avoid additional testing in patients with a low pretest probability for PE. If a patient meets all eight criteria, his or her probability of having PE is less than 2%, which is an appropriate cutoff to discontinue further testing.[101] The rule's sensitivity for detecting PE is 97%; however, caution is advised, because the rule applies only to patients for whom the clinical suspicion for PE is low (<15%).[102] In patients for whom the probability is high, the PERC rule does not safely exclude the condition.[103]

TABLE 1-4.
PE Risk Stratification[104,105]

Wells	
Criteria	Score
Clinical signs and symptoms of DVT	+3
PE is most likely diagnosis	+3
Heart rate above 100 beats/min	+1.5
Immobilization in past 3 days or surgery in the past 4 weeks	+1.5
Previous DVT/PE	+1.5
Hemoptysis	+1
Malignancy with treatment in past 6 months or palliative care	+1
Low risk (15%)	<2 points
Intermediate risk (29%)	2-6 points
High risk (59%)	>6 points

Revised Geneva	
Criteria	Score
Lower extremity tenderness and unilateral edema	+4
Unilateral leg pain	+3
Heart rate between 75 and 94 beats/min	+3
Heart rate above 95 beats/min	+5
Surgery or fracture within 1 month	+2
Previous DVT/PE	+3
Hemoptysis	+2
Active malignancy	+2
Patient older than 65 years	+1
Low risk (8%)	<4 points
Intermediate risk (28%)	4-10 points
High risk (74%)	>10 points

> **KEY POINT**
>
> In a low-risk population, a negative PERC score can preclude the need for further workup for pulmonary embolus.

Wells and Revised Geneva Scores

The Wells and revised Geneva scores (Table 1-4) were developed by assessing the clinical probability of PE and have been validated in large clinical trials.[104,105] Both scores successfully stratify patients into low-, intermediate-, and high-risk groups for PE, but the Wells score is superior for the identification of patients in the high-risk group.[106] Critics of the Wells score point to the subjective nature of the score. It asks care providers to determine if PE is the most likely diagnosis. In contrast, the revised Geneva score is based solely on objective data.[107] In patients with an "unlikely" probability in the Wells or revised Geneva score (≤4 or <4, respectively), a negative highly sensitive D-dimer assay may be used to exclude PE without additional testing.[108]

Thrombolysis In Myocardial Infarction Risk Score

The Thrombolysis In Myocardial Infarction (TIMI) risk score (Table 1-5) has been well validated as a method to stratify patients diagnosed with unstable angina/NSTEMI according to their risk for adverse events. The score is used to guide therapeutic and prognostic decision making.[109] The TIMI risk score also correlates with outcomes when applied to emergency department patients[110]; however, its sensitivity alone has been shown repeatedly to be inadequate at ruling out ACS in the unique population of emergency department patients.[110,111] Although attempts have been made to create a "modified TIMI score" with improved performance in risk stratification, the new decision rule was still unable to screen patients safely for adverse events in the emergency department.[112]

HEART Score and North American Chest Pain Rule

The HEART score and the North American Chest Pain Rule (NACPR) were devised to identify patients who experienced chest pain but are suitable for early discharge without stress testing or cardiac imaging.[113,114] Both tools have yet to be validated in large multicenter prospective trials, but they have been shown initially to have an acceptable miss rate (<1%) for adverse events when combined with serial troponin measurements.[115] It is unlikely that these rules will change clinical practice, as they generally describe the current standard of care for ACS evaluation in the emergency department.

Conclusion

Chest pain is a common emergency department presentation and has multiple causes. Emergency providers should take a careful and systematic approach to evaluating patients with chest pain. As technology has improved and tests have become more sensitive, providers must navigate the increasingly complex workup and allocate resources appropriately. By using the strategies outlined in this chapter, emergency physicians should be able to diagnose the life-threatening causes of chest pain safely and successfully.

References

1. Halpern EJ. Triple-rule-out CT angiography for evaluation of acute chest pain and possible acute coronary syndrome. *Radiology*. 2009;252(2):332-345.
2. Feldman JA, Brinsfield K, Bernard S, et al. Real-time paramedic compared with blinded physician identification of ST-segment elevation myocardial infarction: results of an observational study. *Am J Emerg Med*. 2005;23(4):443-448.
3. O'Connor RE, Bossaert L, Arntz HR, et al. Part 9: Acute coronary syndromes: 2010 International Consensus on Cardiopulmonary Resuscitation and Emergency Cardiovascular Care Science with Treatment Recommendations. *Circulation*. 2010;122(16 Suppl 2):S422-S465.
4. Than M, Herbert M, Flaws D, et al. What is an acceptable risk of major adverse cardiac event in chest pain patients soon after discharge from the emergency department?: a clinical survey. *Int J Cardiol*. 2013;166(3):752-754.
5. Schull MJ, Vermeulen MJ, Stukel TA. The risk of missed diagnosis of acute myocardial infarction associated with emergency department volume. *Ann Emerg Med*. 2006;48(6):647-655.
6. Panju AA, Hemmelgarn BR, Guyatt GH, Simel DL. The rational clinical examination. Is this patient having a myocardial infarction? *JAMA*. 1998;280(14):1256-1263.
7. Goodacre SW, Angelini K, Arnold J, et al. Clinical predictors of acute coronary syndromes in patients with undifferentiated chest pain. *QJM*. 2003;96(12):893-898.
8. Body R, McDowell G, Carley S, Mackway-Jones K. Do risk factors for chronic coronary heart disease help diagnose acute myocardial infarction in the emergency department? *Resuscitation*. 2008;79(1):41-45.
9. Miller CD, Lindsell CJ, Khandelwal S, et al. Is the initial diagnostic impression of "noncardiac chest pain" adequate to exclude cardiac disease? *Ann Emerg Med*. 2004;44(6):565-574.
10. Canto JG, Shlipak MG, Rogers WJ, et al. Prevalence, clinical characteristics, and mortality among patients with myocardial infarction presenting without chest pain. *JAMA*. 2000;283(24):3223-3229.
11. Canto JG, Rogers WJ, Goldberg RJ, et al. Association of age and sex with myocardial infarction symptom presentation and in-hospital mortality. *JAMA*. 2012;307(8):813-822.
12. Woo KM, Schneider JI. High-risk chief complaints I: chest pain—the big three. *Emerg Med Clin North Am*. 2009;27(4):685-712.
13. Becattini C, Agnelli G. Acute pulmonary embolism: risk stratification in the emergency department. *Intern Emerg Med*. 2007;2(2):119-129.
14. Goldhaber SZ, Visani L, De Rosa M. Acute pulmonary embolism: clinical outcomes in the International Cooperative Pulmonary Embolism Registry (ICOPER). *Lancet*. 1999;353(9162):1386-1389.
15. Stein PD, Beemath A, Matta F, et al. Clinical characteristics of patients with acute pulmonary embolism: data from PIOPED II. *Am J Med*. 2007;120(10):871-879.
16. Ryom P, Ravn JB, Penninga L, et al. Aetiology, treatment and mortality after oesophageal perforation in Denmark. *Dan Med Bull*. 2011;58(5):A4267.
17. Bhatia P, Fortin D, Inculet RI, Malthaner RA. Current concepts in the management of esophageal perforations: a twenty-seven year Canadian experience. *Ann Thorac Surg*. 2011;92(1):209-215.
18. Vidarsdottir H, Blondal S, Alfredsson H, et al. Oesophageal perforations in Iceland: a whole population study on incidence, aetiology and surgical outcome. *Thorac Cardiovasc Surg*. 2010;58(8):476-480.

TABLE 1-5.

TIMI Risk Score[109]

Age 65 years or older	+1
Three or more CAD risk factors (hypertension, diabetes, smoking, HDL below 40, family history of premature CAD)	+1
Known CAD (stenosis of 50% or more)	+1
Aspirin use in past 7 days	+1
Two or more anginal events in past 24 hours	+1
ST changes of 0.5 mm or more	+1
Positive serum cardiac marker	+1

Risk of adverse event: 1=4.7%; 2=8.3%; 3=13.2%; 4=19.9%; 5=26.2%; 6, 7=at least 40.9%

19. Søreide JA, Viste A. Esophageal perforation: diagnostic work-up and clinical decision-making in the first 24 hours. *Scand J Trauma Resusc Emerg Med.* 2011;19:66.
20. Holloway VJ, Harris JK. Spontaneous pneumothorax: is it under tension? *J Accid Emerg Med.* 2000;17(3):222-223.
21. Leigh-Smith S, Harris T. Tension pneumothorax—time for a re-think? *Emerg Med J.* 2005;22(1):8-16.
22. Weldon E, Williams J. Pleural disease in the emergency department. *Emerg Med Clin North Am.* 2012;30(2):475-499.
23. Hassani B, Foote J, Borgundvaag B. Outpatient management of primary spontaneous pneumothorax in the emergency department of a community hospital using a small-bore catheter and a Heimlich valve. *Acad Emerg Med.* 2009;16(6):513-518.
24. Currie GP, Alluri R, Christie GL, Legge JS. Pneumothorax: an update. *Postgrad Med J.* 2007;83(981):461-465.
25. Aguinagalde B, Zabaleta J, Fuentes M, et al. Percutaneous aspiration versus tube drainage for spontaneous pneumothorax: systematic review and meta-analysis. *Eur J Cardiothorac Surg.* 2010;37(5):1129-1135.
26. McLean AR, Richards ME, Crandall CS, Marinaro JL. Ultrasound determination of chest wall thickness: implications for needle thoracostomy. *Am J Emerg Med.* 2011;29(9):1173-1177.
27. Asouhidou I, Asteri T. Acute aortic dissection: be aware of misdiagnosis. *BMC Res Notes.* 2009;2:25.
28. Rogers AM, Hermann LK, Booher AM, et al. Sensitivity of the aortic dissection detection risk score, a novel guideline-based tool for identification of acute aortic dissection at initial presentation: results from the international registry of acute aortic dissection. *Circulation.* 2011;123(20):2213-2218.
29. Zhan S, Hong S, Shan-Shan L, et al. Misdiagnosis of aortic dissection: experience of 361 patients. *J Clin Hypertens (Greenwich).* 2012;14(4):256-260.
30. Imamura H, Sekiguchi Y, Iwashita T, et al. Painless acute aortic dissection - diagnostic, prognostic and clinical implications. *Circ J.* 2011;75(1):59-66.
31. Braverman AC. Aortic dissection: prompt diagnosis and emergency treatment are critical. *Cleve Clin J Med.* 2011;78(10):685-696.
32. Hiratzka LF, Bakris GL, Beckman JA, et al. 2010 ACCF/AHA/AATS/ACR/ASA/SCA/SCAI/SIR/STS/SVM guidelines for the diagnosis and management of patients with thoracic aortic disease. *Circulation.* 2010;121(13):e266-e369.
33. Harris KM, Strauss CE, Eagle KA, et al. Correlates of delayed recognition and treatment of acute type A aortic dissection: the International Registry of Acute Aortic Dissection (IRAD). *Circulation.* 2011;124(18):1911-1918.
34. Kurabayashi M, Miwa N, Ueshima D, et al. Factors leading to failure to diagnose acute aortic dissection in the emergency room. *J Cardiol.* 2011;58(3):287-293.
35. Hoit BD. Pericardial disease and pericardial tamponade. *Criti Care Med.* 2007;35(8 Suppl):S355-S364.
36. Brown J, MacKinnon D, King A, Vanderbush E. Elevated arterial blood pressure in cardiac tamponade. *N Engl J Med.* 1992;327(7):463-466.
37. Roy CL, Minor MA, Brookhart MA, Choudhry NK. Does this patient with a pericardial effusion have a cardiac tamponade? *JAMA.* 2007;297(16):1810-1818.
38. Fesmire FM, Decker WW, Diercks DB, et al. Clinical policy: critical issues in the evaluation and management of adult patients with non–ST-segment elevation acute coronary syndromes. *Ann Emerg Med.* 2006;48(3):270-301.
39. Wagner GS, Macfarlane P, Wellens H, et al. AHA/ACCF/HRS recommendations for the standardization and interpretation of the electrocardiogram: part VI: acute ischemia/infarction: a scientific statement from the American Heart Association Electrocardiography and Arrhythmias Committee, Council on Clinical Cardiology; the American College of Cardiology Foundation; and the Heart Rhythm Society. Endorsed by the International Society for Computerized Electrocardiology. *J Am Coll Cardiol.* 2009;53(11):1003-1011.
40. Rowlandson I, Xue J, Farrell R. Computerized STEMI recognition: an example of the art and science of building ECG algorithms. *J Electrocardiol.* 2010;43(6):497-502.
41. Poh KK, Tan HC, Teo SG. ECG ST segment elevation in patients with chest pain. *Singapore Med J.* 2011;52(1):3-8.
42. Petrov DB. Sudden onset of chest pain associated with PR-segment depression in ECG. *Heart Lung.* 2009;38(5):440-443.
43. Lo E, Ren X, Hui PY. Electrical alternans and pulsus paradoxus. *J Hosp Med.* 2010;5(4):253-254.
44. Stein PD, Henry JW. Clinical characteristics of patients with acute pulmonary embolism stratified according to their presenting syndromes. *Chest.* 1997;112(4):974-979.
45. Hirata K, Wake M, Kyushima M, et al. Electrocardiographic changes in patients with type A acute aortic dissection. Incidence, patterns and underlying mechanisms in 159 cases. *J Cardiol.* 2010;56(2):147-153.
46. Ohtani N, Kiyokawa K, Asada H, Kawakami T. Stanford type A acute dissection developing acute myocardial infarction. *Jpn J Thorac Cardiovasc Surg.* 2000;48(1):69-72.
47. Gregorio MC, Baumgartner FJ, Omari BO. The presenting chest roentgenogram in acute type A aortic dissection: a multidisciplinary study. *Am Surg.* 2002;68(1):6-10.
48. Hegenbarth R, Birkenfeld P, Beyer R. Roentgen findings in spontaneous esophageal perforation (Boerhaave syndrome). *Aktuelle Radiol.* 1994;4(6):337-338.
49. Hingston CD, et al. Boerhaave's syndrome – rapidly evolving pleural effusion; a radiographic clue. *Minerva Anestesiol.* 2010;76(10):865-867.
50. Elliot CG, Goldhaber SZ, Visani L, DeRosa M. Chest radiographs in acute pulmonary embolism. *Chest.* 2000;118:33-38.
51. Daftary A, Gregory M, Daftary A, et al. Chest radiograph as a triage tool in the imaging-based diagnosis of pulmonary embolism. *AJR Am J Roentgenol.* 2005;185(1):132-134.
52. Torbicki A, Perrier A, Konstantinides S, et al. Guidelines on the diagnosis and management of acute pulmonary embolism: the Task Force for the Diagnosis and Management of Acute Pulmonary Embolism of the European Society of Cardiology (ESC). *Eur Heart J.* 2008;29(18):2276-2315.
53. Roy PM, Colombet I, Durieux P, et al. Systematic review and meta-analysis of strategies for the diagnosis of suspected pulmonary embolism. *BMJ.* 2005;331(7511):259-267.
54. Spodick DH. Risk prediction in pericarditis: who to keep in the hospital? *Heart.* 2008;94(4):398-399.
55. Kontos MC, Arrowood JA, Paulsen WH, Nixon JV. Early echocardiography can predict cardiac events in emergency department patients with chest pain. *Ann Emerg Med.* 1998;31(5):550-557.
56. Muscholl MW, Oswald M, Mayer C, van Scheidt W. Prognostic value of 2D echocardiography in patients presenting with acute chest pain and non-diagnostic ECG for ST-elevation myocardial infarction. *Int J Cardiol.* 2002;84(2-3):217-225.
57. Shah BN, Ahmadvazir S, Pabla JS, et al. The role of urgent transthoracic echocardiography in the evaluation of patients presenting with acute chest pain. *Eur J Emerg Med.* 2012;19(5):277-283.
58. Perkins AM, Liteplo A, Noble VE. Ultrasound diagnosis of type a aortic dissection. *J Emerg Med.* 2010;38(4):490-493.
59. Barrett C, Stone MB. Emergency ultrasound diagnosis of type a aortic dissection and apical pleural cap. *Acad Emerg Med.* 2010;17(4):e23-e24.
60. Blaivas M, Lyon M, Duggal S. A prospective comparison of supine chest radiography and bedside ultrasound for the diagnosis of traumatic pneumothorax. *Acad Emerg Med.* 2005;12(9):844-849.
61. Monti JD, Younggren B, Blankenship R. Ultrasound detection of pneumothorax with minimally trained sonographers: a preliminary study. *J Spec Oper Med.* 2009;9(1):43-46.
62. Kirkpatrick AW, Sirois M, Laupland KB, et al. Hand-held thoracic sonography for detecting post-traumatic pneumothoraces: the Extended Focused Assessment with Sonography for Trauma (EFAST). *J Trauma.* 2004;57(2):288-295.
63. Bassand JP, Hamm CW, Ardissino D, et al. Guidelines for the diagnosis and treatment of non–ST-segment elevation acute coronary syndromes. *Eur Heart J.* 2007;28(13):1598-1660.
64. Christ M, Bertsch T, Popp S, et al. High-sensitivity troponin assays in the evaluation of patients with acute chest pain in the emergency department. *Clin Chem Lab Med.* 2011;49(12):1955-1963.
65. Baker JO, Reinhold J, Redwood S, Marber MS. Troponins: redefining their limits. *Heart.* 2011;97(6):447-452.
66. Thygesen K, Mair J, Katus H, et al. Recommendations for the use of cardiac troponin measurement in acute cardiac care. *Eur Heart J.* 2010;31(18):2197-2204.
67. Michielsen EC, Wodzig WK, Van Dieijen-Visser MP. Cardiac troponin T release after prolonged strenuous exercise. *Sports Med.* 2008;38(5):425-435.
68. Kavsak PA, Wang X, Ko DT, et al. Short- and long-term risk stratification using a next generation, high-sensitivity research cardiac troponin I (hs-cTnI) assay in emergency department chest pain population. *Clin Chem.* 2009;55(10):1809-1815.
69. Thygesen K, Alpert JS, White HD. Universal definition of myocardial infarction. *Eur Heart J.* 2007;28(20):2525-2538.
70. NACB Writing Group, Wu AH, Jaffe AS, Apple FS, et al. National Academy of Clinical Biochemistry Laboratory medicine practive guidelines: use of cardiac troponins and B-type natriuretic peptide or N-terminal proB-type natriuretic peptide for etiologies other than acute coronary syndromes and heart failure. *Clin Chem.* 2007;53(12):2086-2096.
71. Vasile VC, Saenger AK, Kroning JM, Jaffe AS. Biological and analytical variability of a novel high-sensitivity cardiac troponin T assay. *Clin Chem.* 2010;56(7):1086-1090.
72. Scharnhorst V, Krasznai K, van't Veer M, Michels R. Rapid detection of myocardial infarction with a sensitive troponin test. *Am J Clin Pathol.* 2011;135(3):424-428.
73. Christ M, Popp S, Pohlman H, et al. Implementation of high sensitivity cardiac troponin T measurement in the emergency department. *Am J Med.* 2010;123(12):1134-1142.
74. Righini M, Perrier A, De Moerloose P, Bounameaux H. D-Dimer for venous thromboembolism diagnosis: 20 years later. *J Thromb Haemost.* 2008;6(7):1059-1071.
75. Schutgens RE, Ackermark P, Haas FJ, et al. Combination of a normal D-dimer concentration and a non-high pretest clinical probability score is a safe strategy to exclude deep venous thrombosis. *Circulation.* 2003;107(4):593-597.

76. Klok FA, Djurabi RK, Nijkeuter M, et al. High D-dimer level is associated with increased 15-d and 3 months mortality through a more central localization of pulmonary emboli and serious comorbidity. *Br J Haematol.* 2008;140(2):218-222.
77. Ghanima W, Abdelmoor M, Holmen LO, et al. D-dimer level is associated with the extent of pulmonary embolism. *Thromb Res.* 2007;120(2):281-288.
78. Jeebun V, Doe SJ, Singh L, et al. Are clinical parameters and biomarkers predictive of severity of acute pulmonary emboli on CTPA? *QJM.* 2010;103(2):91-97.
79. Marill KA. Serum D-dimer is a sensitive test for the detection of acute aortic dissection: a pooled meta-analysis. *J Emerg Med.* 2008;34(4):367-376.
80. Sutherland A, Escano J, Coon TP. D-dimer as the sole screening test for acute aortic dissection: a review of the literature. *Ann Emerg Med.* 2008;52(4):339-343.
81. Moysidis T, Lohmann M, Lutkewitz S, et al. Cost associated with D-dimer screening for acute aortic dissection. *Adv Ther.* 2011;28(11):1038-1044.
82. Reichlin T, Hochholzer W, Stelzig C, et al. Incremental value of copeptin for rapid rule out of acute myocardial infarction. *J Am Coll Cardiol.* 2009;54(1):60-68.
83. Truong QA, Bayley J, Hoffmann U, et al. Multi-marker strategy of natriuretic peptide with either conventional or high-sensitivity troponin-T for acute coronary syndrome diagnosis in emergency department patients with chest pain: from the "Rule Out Myocardial Infarction using Computer Assisted Tomography" (ROMICAT) trial. *Am Heart J.* 2012;163(6):972-979.
84. Bhardwaj A, Truong QA, Peacock WF, et al. A multicenter comparison of established and emerging cardiac biomarkers for the diagnostic evaluation of chest pain in the emergency department. *Am Heart J.* 2011;162(2):276-282.
85. Bassan R, Tura BR, Maisel AS. B-type natriuretic peptide: a strong predictor of early and late mortality in patients with acute chest pain without ST-segment elevation in the emergency department. *Coron Artery Dis.* 2009;20(2):143-149.
86. Aldous SJ, Richards AM, Troughton R, Than M. ST2 has diagnostic and prognostic utility for all-cause mortality and heart failure in patients presenting to the emergency department with chest pain. *J Card Fail.* 2012;18(4):304-310.
87. Chu H, Chen WL, Huang CC, et al. Diagnostic performance of mean platelet volume for patients with acute coronary syndrome visiting an emergency department with acute chest pain: the Chinese scenario. *Emerg Med J.* 2011;28(7):569-574.
88. Blanke P, Apfaltrer P, Ebersberger U, et al. CT detection of pulmonary embolism and aortic dissection. *Cardiol Clin.* 2012;30(1):103-116.
89. Stein PD, Fowler SE, Goodman LR, et al. Multidetector computed tomography for acute pulmonary embolism. *N Engl J Med.* 2006;354(22):2317-2327.
90. Auer RC, Schulman AR, Tuorto S, et al. Use of helical CT is associated with an increased incidence of postoperative pulmonary emboli in cancer patients with no change in the number of fatal pulmonary emboli. *J Am Coll Surg.* 2009;208(5):871-880.
91. Donato AA, Khoche S, Santora J, Wagner B. Clinical outcomes in patients with isolated subsegmental pulmonary emboli diagnosed by multidetector CT pulmonary angiography. *Thromb Res.* 2010;126(4):e266-e270.
92. Samad Z, Hakeem A, Mahmood SS, et al. A meta-analysis and systematic review of computed tomography angiography as a diagnostic triage tool for patients with chest pain presenting to the emergency department. *J Nucl Cardiol.* 2012;19(2):364-376.
93. Hoffmann U, Truong QA, Schoenfeld DA, et al. Coronary CT angiography versus standard evaluation in acute chest pain. *N Engl J Med.* 2012;367(4):299-308.
94. Goldstein JA, Chinnaiyan KM, Abidov A, et al. The CT-STAT (Coronary Computed Tomographic Angiography for Systematic Triage of Acute Chest Pain Patients to Treatment) trial. *J Am Coll Cardiol.* 2011;58(14):1414-1422.
95. Hendel RC. Is computed tomography coronary angiography the most accurate and effective noninvasive imaging tool to evaluate patients with acute chest pain in the emergency department? CT coronary angiography is the most accurate and effective noninvasive imaging tool for evaluating patients presenting with chest pain to the emergency department: antagonist viewpoint. *Circ Cardiovasc Imaging.* 2009;2(3):264-275.
96. Hendel R, Dahdah N. The potential role for the use of cardiac computed tomography angiography for the acute chest pain patient in the emergency department: a cautionary viewpoint. *J Nucl Cardiol.* 2011;18(1):163-167.
97. Nasis A, Meredith IT, Nerlekar N, et al. Acute chest pain investigation: utility of cardiac CT angiography in guiding troponin measurement. *Radiology.* 2011;260(2):381-389.
98. Hoffmann U, Bamberg F. Is computed tomography coronary angiography the most accurate and effective noninvasive imaging tool to evaluate patients with acute chest pain in the emergency department?: CT coronary angiography is the most accurate and effective noninvasive imaging tool for evaluating patients presenting with chest pain to the emergency department. *Circ Cardiovasc Imaging.* 2009;2(3):251-263.
99. Lee HY, Yoo SM, White CS. Coronary CT angiography in emergency department patients with acute chest pain: triple rule-out protocol versus dedicated coronary CT angiography. *Int J Cardiovasc Imaging.* 2009;25(3):319-326.
100. Rogg JG, De Neve JW, Huang C, et al. The triple work-up for emergency department patients with acute chest pain: how often does it occur? *J Emerg Med.* 2011;40(2):128-134.
101. Kline JA, Courtney DM, Kabrhel C, et al. Prospective multicenter evaluation of the pulmonary embolism rule-out criteria. *J Thromb Haemost.* 2008;6(5):772-780.
102. Singh B, Parsaik AK, Agarwal D, et al. Diagnostic accuracy of pulmonary embolism rule-out criteria: a systematic review and meta-analysis. *Ann Emerg Med.* 2012;59(6):517-520.
103. Hugli O, Righini M, Le Gal G, et al. The pulmonary embolism rule-out criteria (PERC) rule does not safely exclude pulmonary embolism. *J Thromb Haemostasis.* 2011;9(2):300-304.
104. Wells PS, Anderson DR, Rodger M, et al. Derivation of a simple clinical model to categorize patients probability of pulmonary embolism: increasing the models utility with the SimpliRED D-dimer. *Thromb Haemost.* 2000;83(3):416-420.
105. Le Gal G, Righini M, Roy PM, et al. Prediction of pulmonary embolism in the emergency department: the revised Geneva score. *Ann Intern Med.* 2006;144(3):165-171.
106. Penaloza A, Melot C, Motte S. Comparison of the Wells score with the simplified revised Geneva score for assessing pretest probability of pulmonary embolism. *Thromb Res.* 2011;127(2):81-84.
107. Klok FA, Kruisman E, Spaan J, et al. Comparison of the revised Geneva score with the Wells rule for assessing clinical probability of pulmonary embolism. *J Thromb Haemost.* 2008;6(1):40-44.
108. Lucassen W, Geersing GJ, Erkens PM, et al. Clinical decision rules for excluding pulmonary embolism: a meta-analysis. *Ann Intern Med.* 2011;155(7):448-460.
109. Antman EM, Cohen M, Bernink PJ, et al. The TIMI risk score for unstable angina/non-ST elevation MI: a method for prognostication and therapeutic decision making. *JAMA.* 2000;284(7):835-842.
110. Chase M, Robey JL, Zogby KE, et al. Prospective validation of the Thrombolysis in Myocardial Infarction Risk Score in the emergency department chest pain population. *Ann Emerg Med.* 2006;48(3):252-259.
111. Lyon R, Morris AC, Caesar D, et al. Chest pain presenting to the Emergency Department—to stratify risk with GRACE or TIMI? *Resuscitation.* 2007;74(1):90-93.
112. Body R, Carley S, McDowell G, et al. Can a modified thrombolysis in myocardial infarction risk score outperform the original for risk stratifying emergency department patients with chest pain? *Emerg Med J.* 2009;26(2):95-99.
113. Backus BE, Six AJ, Kelder JC, et al. Chest pain in the emergency room: a multi-center validation of the HEART Score. *Crit Pathw Cardiol.* 2010;9(3):164-169.
114. Hess EP, Brison RJ, Perry JJ, Calder LA, et al. Development of a clinical prediction rule for 30-day cardiac events in emergency department patients with chest pain and possible acute coronary syndrome. *Ann Emerg Med.* 2012;59(2):115-125.e1.
115. Mahler SA, Miller CD, Hollander JE, et al. Identifying patients for early discharge: performance of decision rules among patients with acute chest pain. *Int J Cardiol.* 2013;168(2):795-802.

CHAPTER 2

The Electrocardiogram in the Evaluation and Management of Acute Coronary Syndrome

Korin Hudson, Norine McGrath, and William J. Brady

IN THIS CHAPTER

Clinical uses of the 12-lead ECG

Specific ECG findings of acute coronary syndrome

Regional patterns

ECG abnormalities predictive of acute coronary syndrome

The use of additional leads in the evaluation of acute coronary syndrome

Serial ECG monitoring

Confounding patterns

STEMI mimic patterns

Clinical Uses of the 12-Lead ECG

The electrocardiogram (ECG) is a very useful tool in the evaluation of many medical conditions. It is inexpensive, portable, and noninvasive and can be applied in a number of medical settings, ranging from ambulances and emergency departments to acute care wards and intensive care units. The ECG can be used for single-channel or multichannel evaluation of cardiac rhythms. In addition, monitoring with 12 leads (or more) can be used to establish diagnoses, rule out certain conditions, and guide the treatment of a wide range of medical conditions.

One of the more important applications of the ECG is the rapid evaluation, assessment, and diagnosis of patients presenting with symptoms and signs consistent with acute coronary syndrome (ACS). ACS can manifest with a multitude of ECG abnormalities, ranging from an entirely normal 12-lead ECG to the obvious ST-elevation myocardial infarction (STEMI) pattern, with many different presentations between those two extreme interpretations. In patients with ACS, factors that affect the ECG presentation are listed in Table 2-1.

An ECG is an electrical graph, a "snapshot," that provides a description of the heart's electrical activity for a very brief time. The 12-lead ECG demonstrates a time-based evolution of STEMI, from the early "hyperacute" T wave to obvious ST-segment elevation, culminating in either normalization, T-wave inversion, or Q wave (Figure 2-1). At times, the ECG diagnosis of ACS is straightforward, as in a STEMI with a predictable regional pattern of ST-segment elevation. In other presentations, the ECG findings are subtle and thus challenge the emergency physician's ability to diagnose ACS because of either the early nature of the event or the subtle manifestations of an acute infarction. It is important to remember that a "normal" or "nondiagnostic" ECG does not rule out ACS. Yet, this very important statement must be qualified: a normal or nondiagnostic ECG does not rule out ACS *in a patient with a clinical presentation that otherwise strongly suggests ACS*. If ACS is not suspected based on other features of the presentation, then a normal or minimally (nonspecifically) abnormal ECG can be

TABLE 2-1.

Clinical Variables that Affect the ECG in Patients with ACS

Coronary anatomy involved (the culprit artery) and the cardiac segment(s) that are affected

Degree of coronary artery occlusion (incomplete versus complete)

Time course in the evolution of the event (early versus late)

Individual characteristics of the patient

11

considered a strong indicator in the "rule out ACS" evaluation.

> **KEY POINT**
>
> A normal ECG does not rule out ACS in a patient with a clinical presentation that otherwise strongly suggests the syndrome.

Specific ECG Findings of ACS

The Hyperacute T Wave

An early finding of STEMI is the hyperacute (ie, prominent, large) T wave.[1] It is theorized that a reduction in perfusion to the soon-to-infarct area results in cell injury and the release of potassium, leading to a change in the electrical potential and grossly enlarged T waves in the affected area. Hyperacute T waves can be seen as early as 1 to 2 minutes after vessel occlusion and are often found in the first 30 minutes of acute infarction. The hyperacute T waves of early STEMI (Figure 2-2) are large and prominent. The base is broad, and the two "limbs" of the wave are often asymmetric, with a gradual upslope and an abrupt downslope. These T waves are frequently associated with elevation of the J point (ie, the juncture at which the QRS complex terminates and the ST segment initiates). ST-segment depression, called *reciprocal ST-segment depression or reciprocal change*, is sometimes seen in other ECG leads and is strongly suggestive of STEMI (reciprocal change is discussed later in this chapter). The hyperacute T wave is a transient finding on the ECG of a STEMI patient. It is usually short-lived, with progression to frank STEMI-related ST-segment elevation within minutes. If it is encountered in a patient with appropriate clinical correlation, the appearance of the hyperacute T wave should be considered an early STEMI presentation; thus, the patient should be considered for emergency reperfusion therapy.

> **KEY POINT**
>
> In patients with an appropriate clinical presentation, hyperacute T waves should be considered indicative of an early presentation of STEMI.

FIGURE 2-1.
The ECG progression of STEMI. A, Hyperacute T wave. B, ST-segment elevation of established STEMI. C, T-wave inversion of completed infarction with minimal myocardial injury. The lower magnitude of injury indicates a favorable response to reperfusion therapy (ie, administration of a fibrinolytic agent or percutaneous coronary intervention). D, Q wave of completed infarction with significant myocardial injury, which either was not treated with reperfusion therapy or did not respond to it.

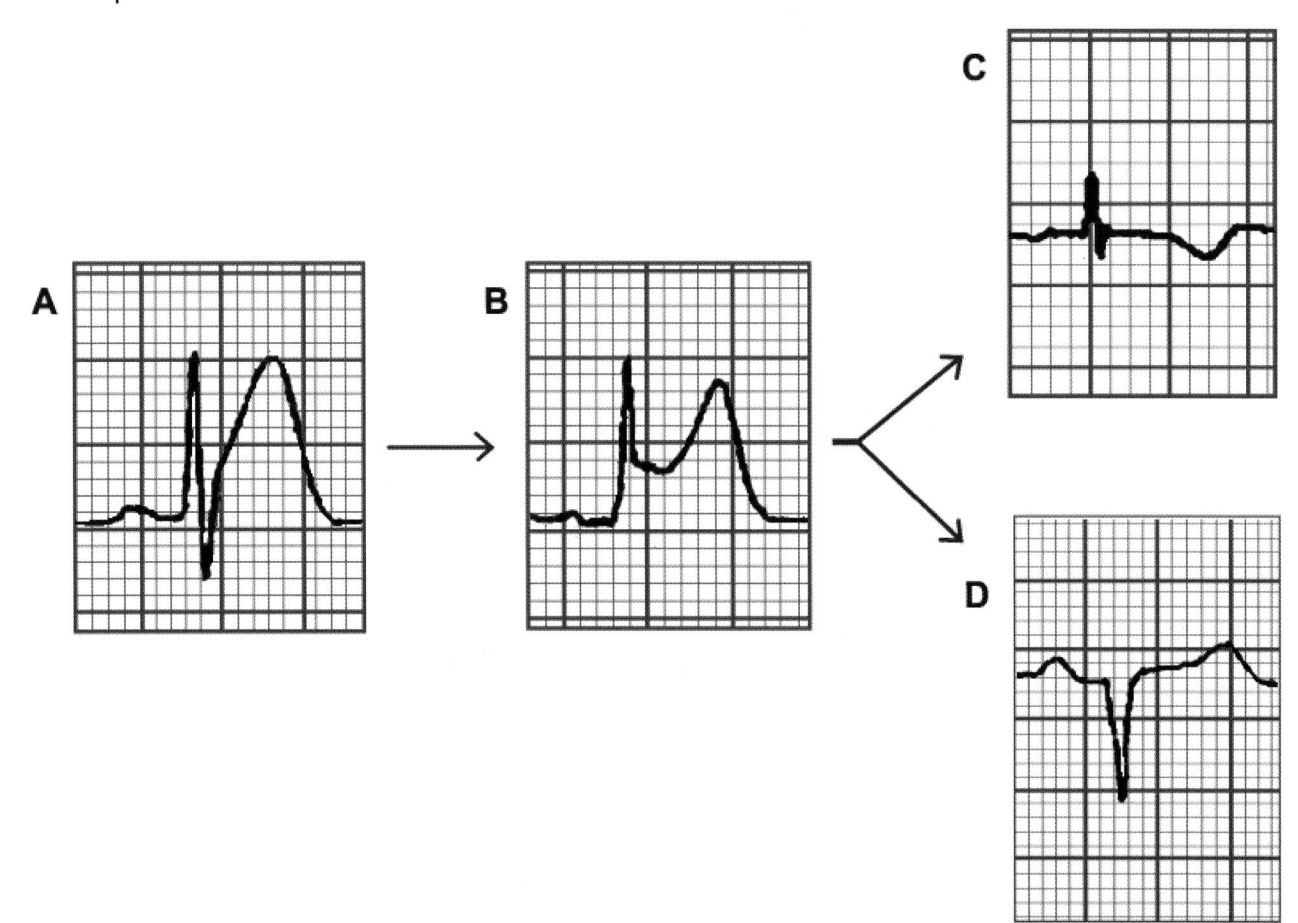

ST-Segment Elevation

As noted above, over a relatively short time the hyperacute T wave of early STEMI will evolve into elevation of the entire ST segment as the infarction progresses (Figure 2-1, A and B).[1] ST-segment elevation of at least 1 mm in two contiguous leads is required for the diagnosis of STEMI. In leads V_2 and V_3, the ST-segment elevation is often even greater. In patients with STEMI, ST-segment elevation is often seen in a single anatomic region in at least two contiguous leads.[2-4]

At baseline, the ST segment is flat because of the isoelectric nature of the myocardium during repolarization. Ischemia can reduce the membrane potential and shorten the action potential of the affected area, causing a voltage gradient. Within minutes to hours after the onset of symptomatic infarction, alterations in the electrical potential of the myocytes are reflected on the ECG as ST-segment elevation. The presence of ST-segment elevation on the ECG, if related to STEMI, is indicative of active infarction.

The ST segment, when elevated, can assume one of three morphologies (Figure 2-3): concave, obliquely straight, or convex.[5-7] Although any ST-segment elevation morphology can be associated with STEMI, typically the obliquely straight (Figure 2-3B) or convex form (Figure 2-3C) is seen; the concave shape (Figure 2-3A) is less common. The shape of the ST-segment elevation can be determined by considering the morphology of its initial upsloping portion (Figure 2-4), beginning at the J point and ending at the apex of the T wave. With ST-segment elevation, a concave elevated segment is more often associated with a non-AMI cause of the ECG abnormality, while a non-concave shape is seen in STEMI patients. Caution is advised in this approach, because a concave shape can also be seen in STEMI presentations, particularly early in the course of the infarction.[5-7]

The amount of ST-segment elevation is greater in the STEMI patient than in the noninfarction ST-segment elevation patient. The magnitude of ST-segment elevation is defined as the millivolt summation of elevation in all involved ECG leads. The anatomic distribution of the ST-segment abnormality can be considered in this evaluation, although this information is less helpful in distinguishing ACS from non-ACS syndromes. Widespread ST-segment changes are associated with non–acute myocardial infarction (AMI) causes, while localized changes occur in ACS presentations, but this difference is not significant in most situations. The magnitude of the ST-segment elevation can be minimal (Figures 2-5A and 2-5B) or pronounced (Figure 2-5C).[5]

The differentiation between ST-segment elevation resulting from STEMI and elevation induced by noninfarction causes

FIGURE 2-2.

Prominent, or hyperacute, T waves of early STEMI. Note the tall, vaulted appearance with a broad base. The T wave is asymmetric—the upsloping portion is more gradual, with an abrupt return to the baseline in the downsloping limb. At times, the J point is elevated as well, with early ST-segment elevation, as seen in B, C, and E.

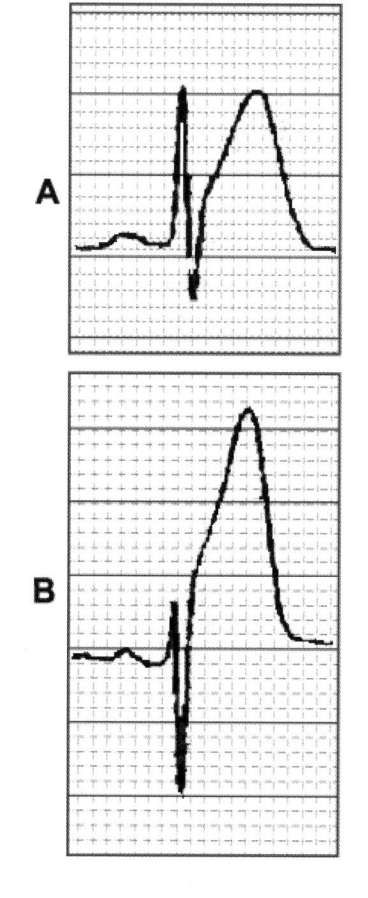

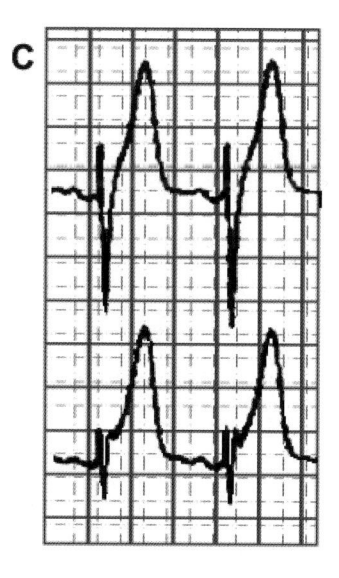

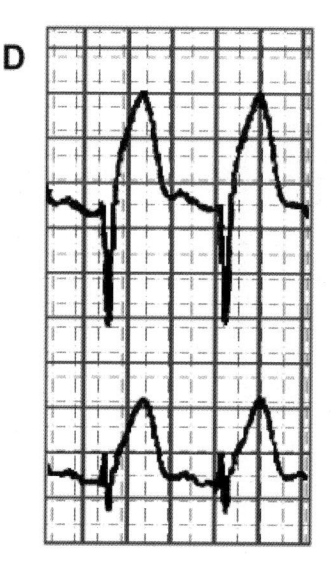

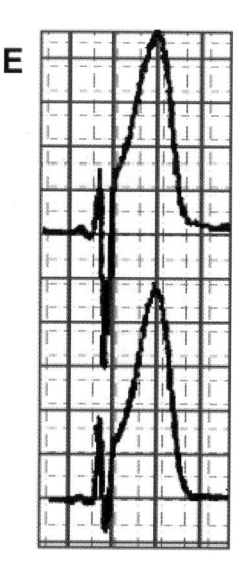

is a vital component of early AMI diagnosis and management. But this distinction is often quite challenging, if not impossible, to make. For instance, in a prehospital study, Otto and Aufderheide noted that 51% of chest pain patients demonstrated ST-segment elevation resulting from causes other than STEMI. The most common causes of the elevation in the prehospital setting were left ventricular hypertrophy (LVH) by voltage and left bundle-branch block (LBBB) patterns.[8] In the emergency department, only 15% of chest pain patients with ST-segment elevation were diagnosed with STEMI. The remaining 85% had other causes of ST-segment elevation, the most common causes being LVH (25%), LBBB (15%), benign early repolarization (12%), and right bundle-branch block (5%).[7] Thus, the mere presence of ST-segment elevation in the adult chest pain patient does not equal STEMI. In fact, STEMI is an uncommon cause of ST-segment deviations in this population.

KEY POINT

The presence of ST-segment elevation in the adult patient with chest pain does not necessarily indicate STEMI.

ST-Segment Depression

ST-segment depression (Figure 2-6) is generally considered to represent subendocardial, noninfarctional ischemia (ie, unstable angina), but it might be the presenting ECG finding in the patient with non-STEMI (NSTEMI) or any early finding in a patient ultimately found to have STEMI. The shape of subendocardial ischemic ST-segment depression is classically horizontal or downsloping; upsloping depression can also be seen but is less often associated with an acute ischemic event. With subendocardial ischemia, the ST-segment depression is often diffuse and can be seen in both the anterior and inferior leads. Coexistent ST-segment depression, called *reciprocal ST-segment depression*, also occurs with STEMI. ST-segment depression in

FIGURE 2-3.

ST-segment elevation of established STEMI. A, Concave. B, Obliquely straight. C, Convex.

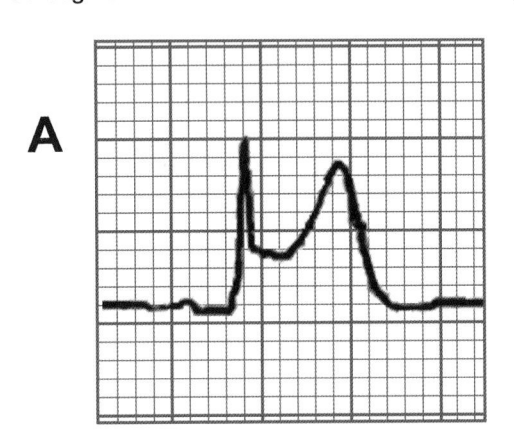

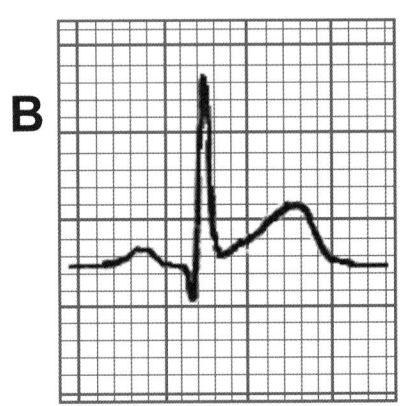

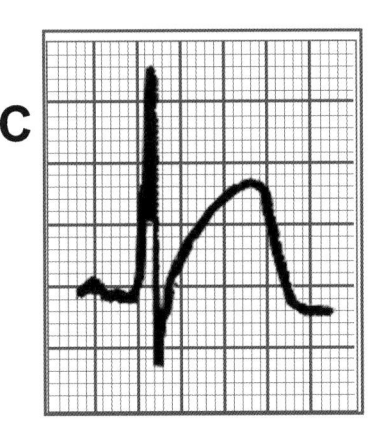

FIGURE 2-4.

ST-segment elevation of established STEMI. A, Concave appearance, with dotted line connecting J point and apex of the T wave. The ECG waveform is below the dotted line. B, Obliquely straight appearance, with dotted line connecting J point and apex of the T wave. The ECG waveform is superimposed on the dotted line. C, Convex appearance, with dotted line connecting J point and apex of the T wave. The ECG waveform is above the dotted line.

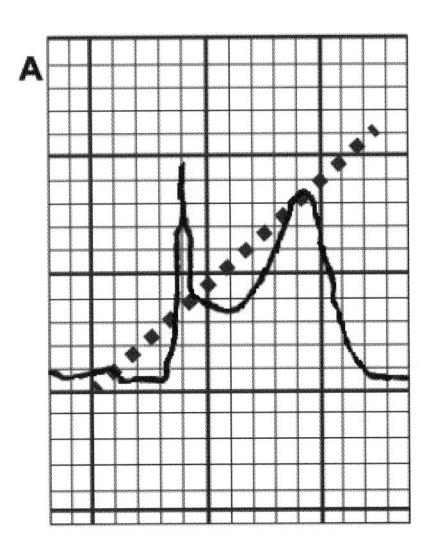

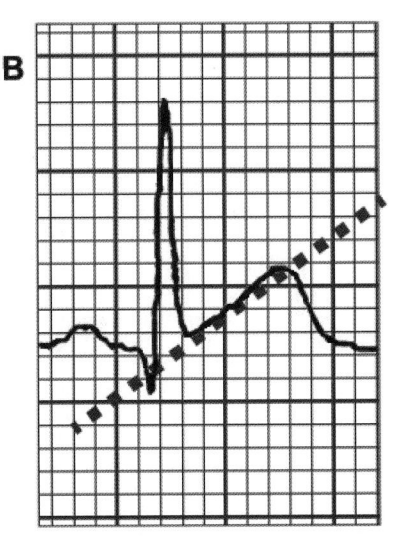

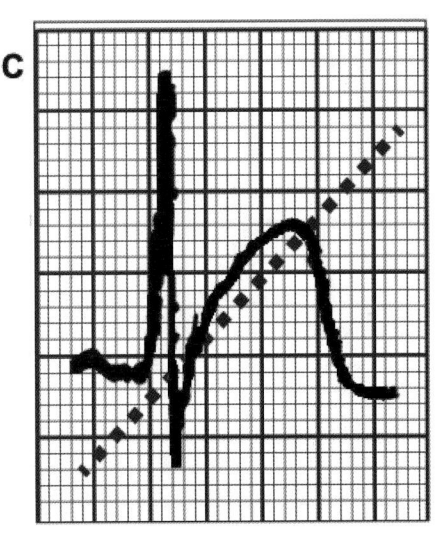

the right precordial leads might represent posterior wall AMI. ACS-related causes of ST-segment depression are listed in Table 2-2.

Nonischemic causes of ST-segment depression include bundle-branch block, LVH with strain, digitalis effect, hyperventilation, and hypokalemia. In patients who use digitalis or who have hypokalemia, the ST-segment depression generally occurs globally as opposed to the more localized presentation of AMI. Digitalis can cause a specific scooping appearance of the ST segment, known as the digitalis effect. As always, these findings must be used in conjunction with other clinical information, since a patient taking digitalis probably has cardiac disease and is not excluded from having a myocardial infarction.

T-Wave Inversion

In a normal ECG, the orientation of the T wave should correspond to the matched QRS wave. T-wave inversion can indicate a range of clinical events, from benign, normal variant situations to life-threatening presentations (Table 2-3).[9,10] As is true in all ECG applications, clinical correlation of T-wave inversion with the patient's presentation will guide the clinician toward the most appropriate interpretation of the 12-lead ECG.

T-wave inversion is another potential finding of myocardial ischemia (ie, unstable angina) or the manifestation of NSTEMI. T-wave inversion can occur early in the ECG presentation of STEMI, with ultimate evolution to ST-segment elevation in the same anatomic distribution as the initial T-wave abnormalities. T-wave inversion is also seen as a sign of injury induced by coronary artery disease. Since these inverted waves can persist after resolution of a previous ischemic event, it can be very helpful to compare the current findings with previous ECGs to identify new inversions. It is also possible for chronically inverted T waves to normalize during a recurrent ischemic event, although the predictive value of this change is poor; these persistent T-wave inversions can normalize (ie, revert to normal configurations), indicating ACS, in a process called

FIGURE 2-5.

ST-segment elevation of established STEMI. A, Subtle, with minimal magnitude and obliquely straight appearance. B, Subtle, with minimal magnitude and concave appearance. C, Marked.

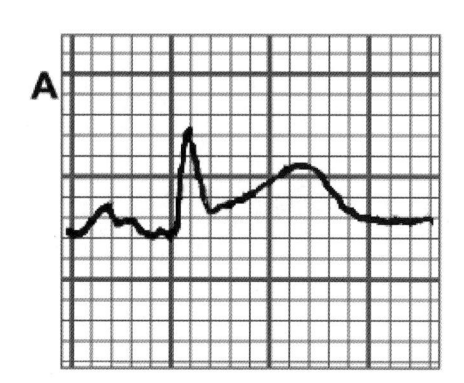

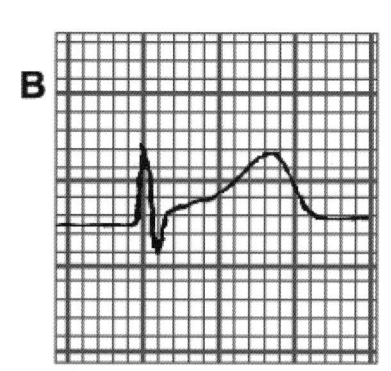

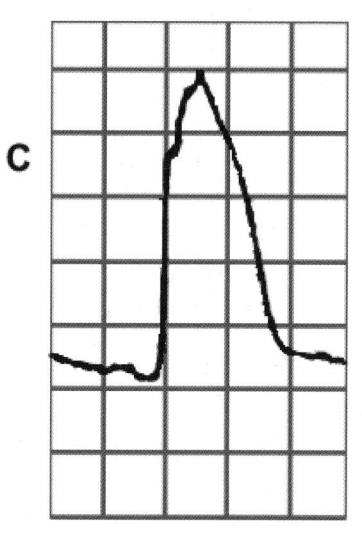

FIGURE 2-6.

ST-segment depression. A, Horizontal or flat. B, Downsloping. C, Upsloping.

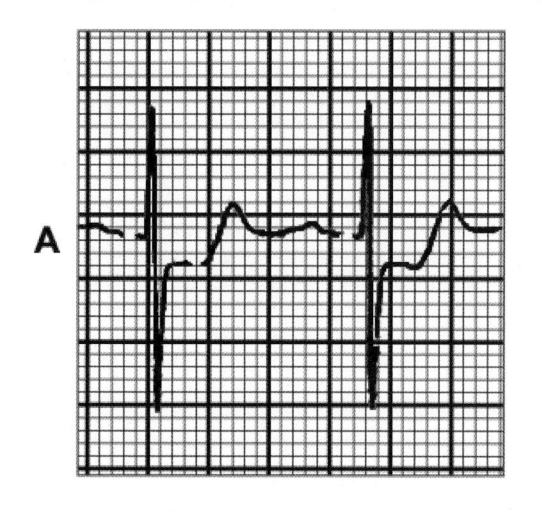

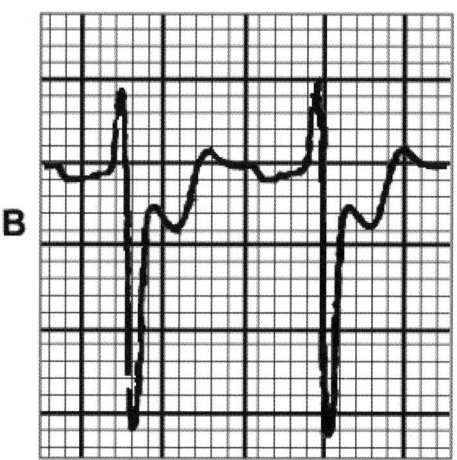

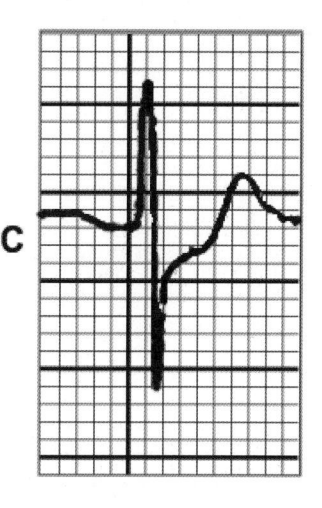

pseudo-normalization of T-wave inversions. Morphologically, the T-wave inversions of ACS are symmetric (Figure 2-7), meaning that the downsloping and upsloping limbs are mirror images. In contrast, the T-wave inversions seen in non-ACS presentations are asymmetric, with a more gradual downsloping limb and an abrupt return to baseline as the upsloping limb.

KEY POINT

In ACS, the downsloping and upsloping limbs of the T wave are symmetric; in contrast, T-wave inversions in non-ACS presentations are asymmetric, with a gradual downsloping limb and an abrupt upsloping return to baseline.

Wellens syndrome, characterized by proximal left anterior descending occlusion and ultimate anterior wall myocardial infarction, manifests as a pattern of specific T-wave abnormalities in the anterior region.[11] These abnormalities (Figure 2-8) include deeply inverted T waves in leads V_1 to V_4 or biphasic T waves (both positive [upright] and negative [inverted] components in a single wave) in leads V_2 and V_3. Additional diagnostic criteria include the absence of other ECG evidence of evolving or established myocardial infarction, such as pathologic ST-segment elevation, Q waves, and/or significant loss of R waves. Furthermore, serum markers are negative because Wellens syndrome is a preinfarction event. T-wave abnormalities are encountered when pain is either present or absent, meaning that

TABLE 2-2.
ACS-related Presentations of ST-segment Depression

Unstable angina (ie, coronary ischemia)
NSTEMI
Posterior wall myocardial infarction (acute)
Reciprocal ST-segment depression in the STEMI patient

TABLE 2-3.
Causes of T-wave Inversion

Acute coronary ischemia
Myocardial infarction (acute or past)
Pulmonary embolism
Acute myopericarditis
Digitalis effect
Hypothermia
Ventricular paced pattern
Left bundle-branch block
Right bundle-branch block
Left ventricular hypertrophy pattern with strain
Normal variant

FIGURE 2-7.

T-wave inversion in ACS. ACS-related T-wave inversions are symmetric, with upsloping and downsloping limbs similar in appearance. A and B, Typical inverted T waves of ACS. C and D, T-wave inversions seen in Wellens syndrome (C, deeply inverted T-wave morphology; D, biphasic T-wave inversion morphology [a T wave with both upright and inverted portions]). E, Non-ACS T-wave inversion (indicative of LVH).

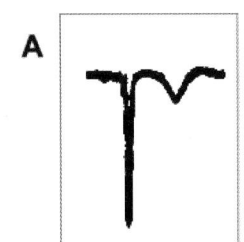

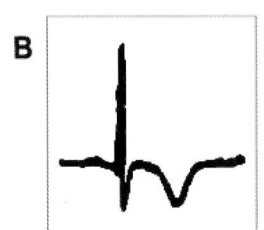

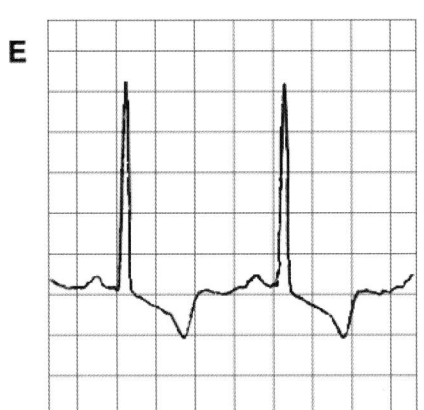

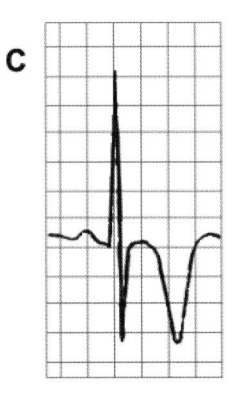

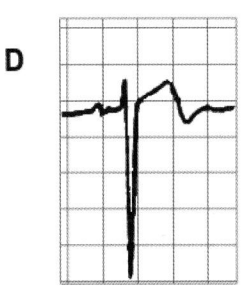

these changes persist into the asymptomatic state. The natural history of Wellens syndrome is anterior wall STEMI within 30 to 90 days.

Q Waves

A Q wave (Figure 2-9) most often indicates past myocardial infarction; it rarely is the sole manifestation of an ACS event. In most instances, a Q wave develops within 9 to 12 hours after the onset of AMI. As a STEMI evolves and culminates in infarcted myocardium, Q waves develop in the cardiac region of the ECG that had previously demonstrated ST-segment elevation. In the rare case, a Q wave appears within 2 to 3 hours after STEMI (Figure 2-9D); in such instances, significant ST-segment elevation will also be present. The clinician should identify this "early Q wave" appearance and still consider the patient as a potential candidate for urgent reperfusion therapy. The combination of Q wave with significant ST-segment elevation in a patient who has experienced a relatively short period of chest discomfort should alert the clinician to these early Q waves. Q waves, if indicative of a completed myocardial infarction, most often remain on the ECG indefinitely as an ECG myocardial scar.

KEY POINT

A Q wave is rarely the sole manifestation of an ACS event.

From the ECG perspective, Q waves represent an initial negative deflection of the QRS complex (Figure 2-9). Q waves are considered "pathologic" (medically significant) if either amplitude or width criteria are met. The amplitude and width requirements for pathologic Q waves are as follows: amplitude, 25% to 33% of the accompanying R wave of the QRS complex, and width, at least one small box (at least 40 msec). Nonpathologic Q waves, of smaller amplitude and/or less pronounced width, are normally seen in leads aVR, V_4, V_5, and V_6 because of the depolarization of the septum.

Regional Patterns

Blood is supplied to the myocardium via the coronary arteries. These arteries arise from the base of the aorta and course along the epicardial surface of the heart, dividing into smaller branches, ultimately branching further and diving into the myocardium. Each of the major coronary arteries follows a typical course around the heart and usually supplies a specific area of heart muscle (Figure 2-10 and Table 2-4). The two coronary arteries that branch directly off of the aorta are the right coronary artery (RCA) and the left main coronary artery (LMCA). The RCA wraps around the right ventricle, supplying it with blood, and ultimately supplying blood flow to the inferior wall of the left ventricle. In some individuals, the RCA continues as the posterior descending branch to the posterior wall of the left ventricle. The LMCA is a very short but important segment of the coronary circulation, as it supplies nearly all of the blood flow for the left ventricle. The LMCA branches into two arteries. The first is the left anterior descending artery (LAD), which supplies the ventricular septum (the wall between the

FIGURE 2-8.

Wellens syndrome. A, 12-lead ECG with biphasic T waves. B, Deeply inverted T-wave inversions. C, Progression of the 12-lead ECG in A, with development of anterolateral STEMI, the natural history of Wellens syndrome.

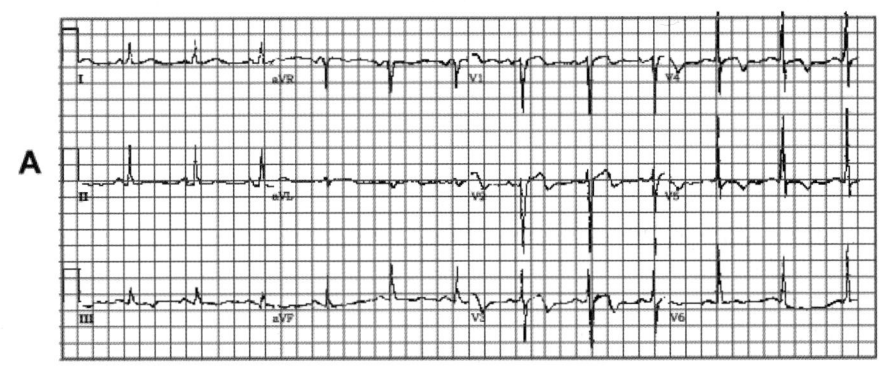

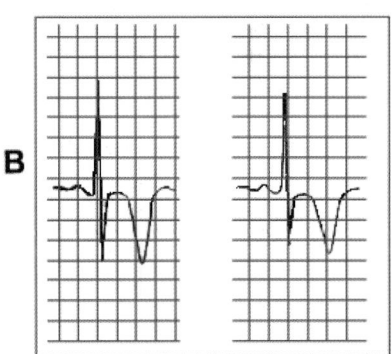

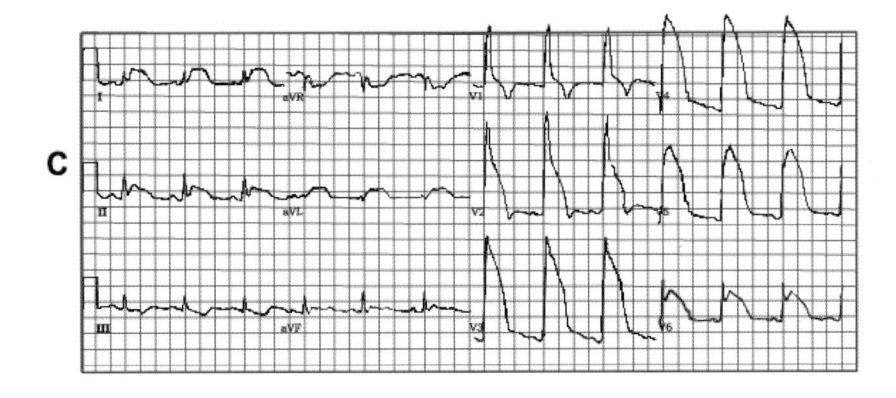

CARDIOVASCULAR EMERGENCIES

FIGURE 2-9.

Q waves indicating established AMI. A-C, Q waves appear as early as 9 to 12 hours after completed myocardial infarction. The Q wave will persist for the remainder of the patient's life, as a scar from the AMI. D, Q wave with ST-segment elevation. In certain situations, the Q wave develops early in the evolution of STEMI, long before the typical 9- to 12-hour period. If the Q wave appears early in the reported course of the patient's chest discomfort and if hyperacute ST-segment elevation is also present, the patient still might benefit from urgent reperfusion therapy.

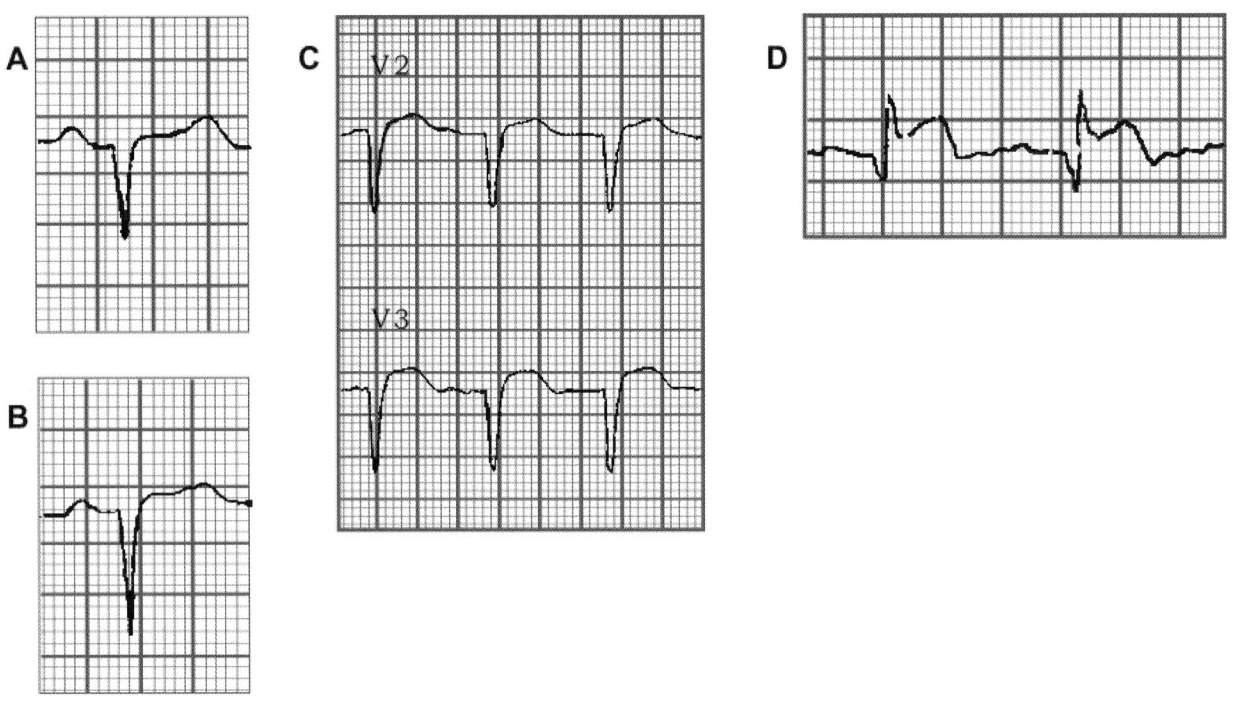

FIGURE 2-10.

Regional segments, coronary anatomy, and corresponding ECG leads in the ECG evaluation of ACS. A, Anterior perspective. B, Posterior perspective.

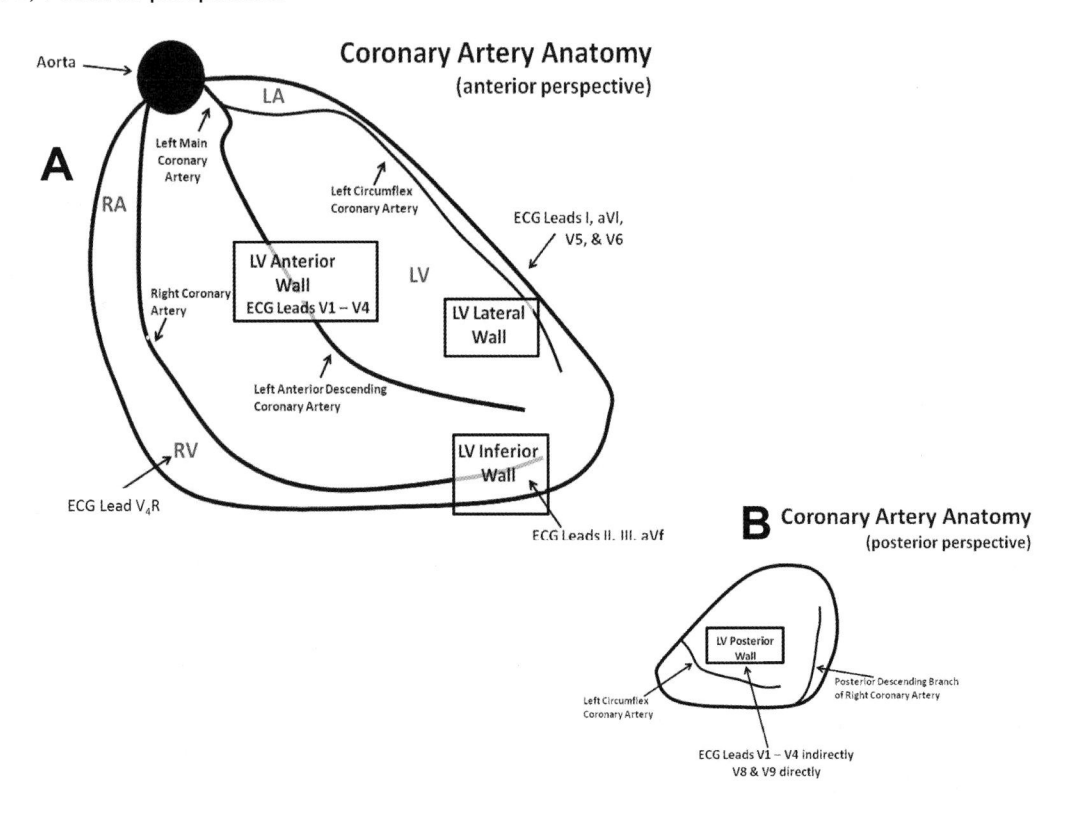

ventricles) and the anterior wall of the left ventricle. The second is the left circumflex coronary artery (LCX), which supplies the lateral wall of the left ventricle. The LCX also provides perfusion to the posterior wall of the left ventricle in some patients. Branches from the LAD are called *diagonals*, and branches off the left circumflex are called *obtuse marginals* or *marginals*. The branches are named numerically from proximal to distal (eg, the first diagonal branch of the LAD is D1 [the first diagonal branch] and the second branch of the LCX is OM2 [the second obtuse marginal branch]).

There is important variation in the blood supply to the back of the heart. Most people have *right dominant* anatomy, meaning that the RCA continues around the right ventricle to supply the inferior portion of the ventricular septum as well as the posterior left ventricle. When it does so, it is called the *posterior descending artery*. However, in others, the back of the heart is supplied by the left side of the coronary circulation, where the posterior descending artery arises as a continuation of the left circumflex coronary artery. A minority of people have *co-dominant* coronary anatomy, in which two smaller vessels contributed by the right and left circulations supply the posterior heart, rather than a specific single vessel.

An anterior wall STEMI is caused by occlusion of the LAD or proximal diagonal branches of the LAD. The 12-lead ECG will demonstrate ST-segment elevation in the lead V_1 to V_4 distribution (Figure 2-11). An infarction in this region is called an *anterior* or *anteroseptal STEMI*. An anterolateral STEMI, a significantly larger infarction, can result from any number of coronary artery obstructions, including the LAD, the proximal diagonal branches of the LAD, the LCX, and the proximal marginal branches of the LCX. The 12-lead ECG will reveal ST-segment elevation in leads V_1 to V_4 (anterior) and V_5 and V_6 (lateral); lateral leads I and aVL will also demonstrate elevation of the ST segment (Figure 2-12). A lateral wall STEMI results most commonly from occlusion of the LCX; less commonly, lateral wall myocardial infarction results from either LAD or RCA obstruction. ECG changes of lateral wall STEMI are seen in leads I, aVL, V_5, and/or V_6 (Figure 2-13). At times, all four leads demonstrate abnormality; in other instances, only I and aVL or V_5 and V_6 are involved.

An inferior wall STEMI is caused by occlusion of the RCA. Abnormalities of the inferior wall are seen in leads II, III, and aVF (Figure 2-14); in the case of STEMI, ST-segment elevation will be seen in these leads. Right ventricular myocardial infarction (RVMI) can be seen in conjunction with inferior wall STEMI; in fact, approximately one third of inferior wall STEMI cases also involve acute RVMI. RVMI is suggested in the following inferior wall STEMI presentations (Figure 2-15):

TABLE 2-4.
Regional ECG Correlation

Chamber	Coronary Artery	Anatomic Segment	ECG Leads
Left ventricle	Left anterior descending coronary artery	Anterior	V_1 through V_4
Left ventricle	Right coronary artery	Inferior	II, III, and aVF
Left ventricle	Left circumflex artery	Lateral	I, II, V_5, and V_6
Left ventricle	Left circumflex artery *or* posterior descending branch of right coronary artery	Posterior	V_1 through V_3: indirect V_7 through V_9: direct
Right ventricle	Right ventricular branch of right coronary artery	Right ventricle	V_4R or V_1R through V_4R

FIGURE 2-11.
Anterior STEMI. ST-segment elevation in leads V_1 to V_4.

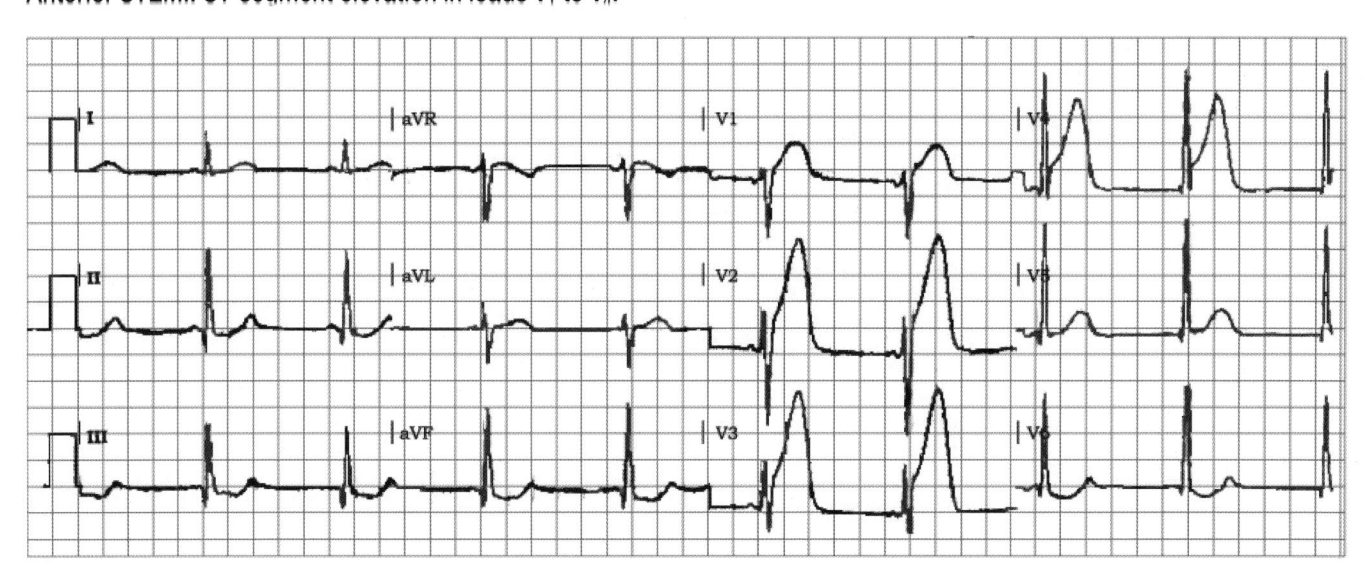

CARDIOVASCULAR EMERGENCIES

FIGURE 2-12.

Anterolateral STEMI: ST-segment elevation in leads V$_1$ to V$_4$ (anterior) and leads I, aVL, V$_5$, and V$_6$ (lateral).

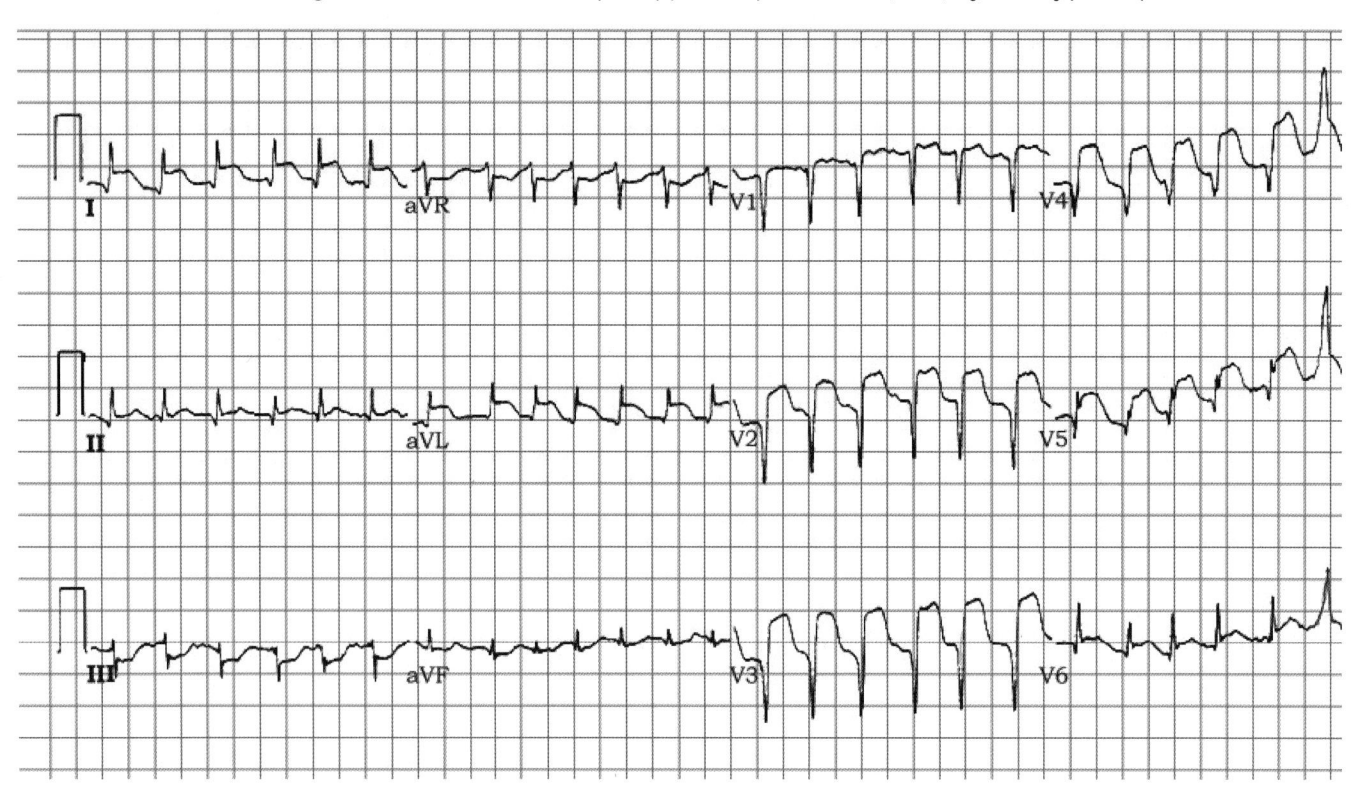

FIGURE 2-13.

Lateral STEMI. ST-segment elevation in leads V$_5$ and V$_6$.

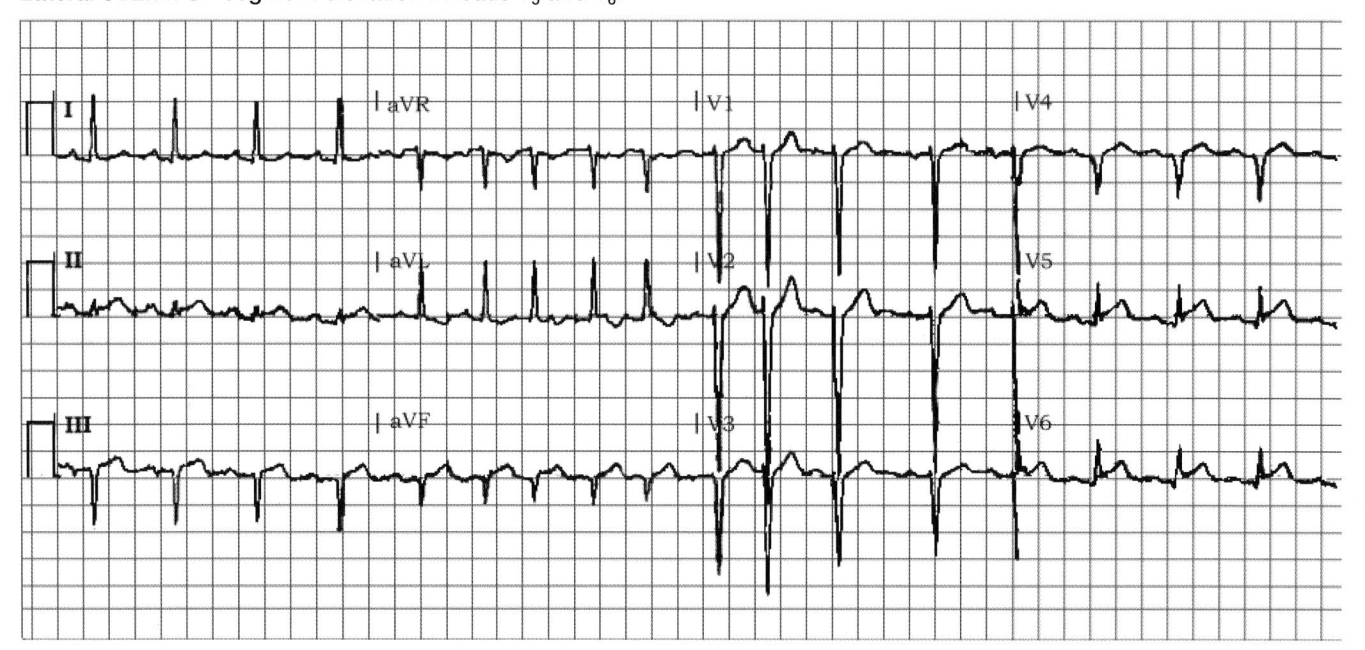

1) hypotension either spontaneously or after vasodilator therapy (eg, with nitroglycerin or morphine sulfate); 2) ST-segment elevation in lead V_1; and 3) more pronounced ST-segment elevation in lead III compared with leads II or aVF. If clinical concern exists for RVMI, tracings from additional right-sided ECG leads (either lead V_4R [Figure 2-15B] or leads V_1R to V_6R) may be obtained. The use of additional ECG leads is discussed later in this chapter.

From the perspective of the 12-lead ECG, an acute posterior myocardial infarction presents with ST-segment depression in leads V_1 to V_4 (Figure 2-16). In this distribution, the posterior wall of the left ventricle is viewed indirectly from the perspective of the anterior wall. In patients suspected of having ACS, ST-segment depression in leads V_1 to V_4 results from either anterior wall ischemia or acute posterior wall myocardial infarction. Three additional features increase the likelihood of acute posterior myocardial infarction, as follows: horizontal morphology of the depressed ST segment, an upright T wave, and a prominent R wave. Additional leads V_8 and V_9 (Figure 2-16D) directly image the posterior wall and will demonstrate ST-segment elevation (see below).

KEY POINT

A posterior wall acute infarction is detected using either anterior leads V_1 to V_4, demonstrating ST-segment depression with prominent R waves and upright T waves, or posterior leads V_7 to V_9, revealing ST-segment elevation.

ECG Abnormalities Predictive of ACS

Reciprocal ST Segment Depression

Reciprocal ST-segment depression, also known as reciprocal change, is defined as ST-segment depression in leads separate and distinct from leads reflecting ST-segment elevation (Figure 2-17). The depression is either horizontal or downsloping in morphology; further, it need only be present in a single lead, but it frequently is present in numerous leads. Reciprocal change is an important ECG concept to consider and note on the 12-lead ECG. It identifies patients with a high-risk ACS presentation and provides supportive evidence that STEMI is, in fact, present. Reciprocal change in the setting of STEMI identifies a patient with an increased likelihood of cardiovascular complication (heart block, malignant ventricular arrhythmia, cardiogenic shock) and poor outcome (significant left ventricular dysfunction, death). Such patients may benefit from a more aggressive therapeutic approach. Furthermore, its presence on the ECG supports the diagnosis of AMI with very high sensitivity and a positive predictive value greater than 90%.[7,8] Reciprocal change is seen in approximately 75% of patients with inferior wall AMIs and in 30% of patients with anterior wall myocardial infarctions.

KEY POINT

Reciprocal change is a very valuable ECG finding, not only supporting the diagnosis of STEMI but also indicating a high-risk patient.

Lead aVR ST-Segment Elevation

ST-segment elevation in lead aVR (Figure 2-18) in the patient with clinically suspected ACS suggests a strong possibility of LMCA obstruction. This observation includes patients with non-AMI ACS presentations as well as NSTEMI and STEMI.[12] ST-segment elevation of 1 to 1.5 mm in lead aVR is strongly suggestive of LMCA obstruction. This finding is important in that such obstruction is associated with a markedly higher mortality rate. Urgent reperfusion is best performed with percutaneous coronary intervention rather than fibrinolysis. This ECG finding is associated with significant risk of an adverse event such as heart block, malignant ventricular arrhythmia, cardiogenic shock, or death.

FIGURE 2-14.

Inferior STEMI. ST-segment elevation in leads II, III, and aVF.

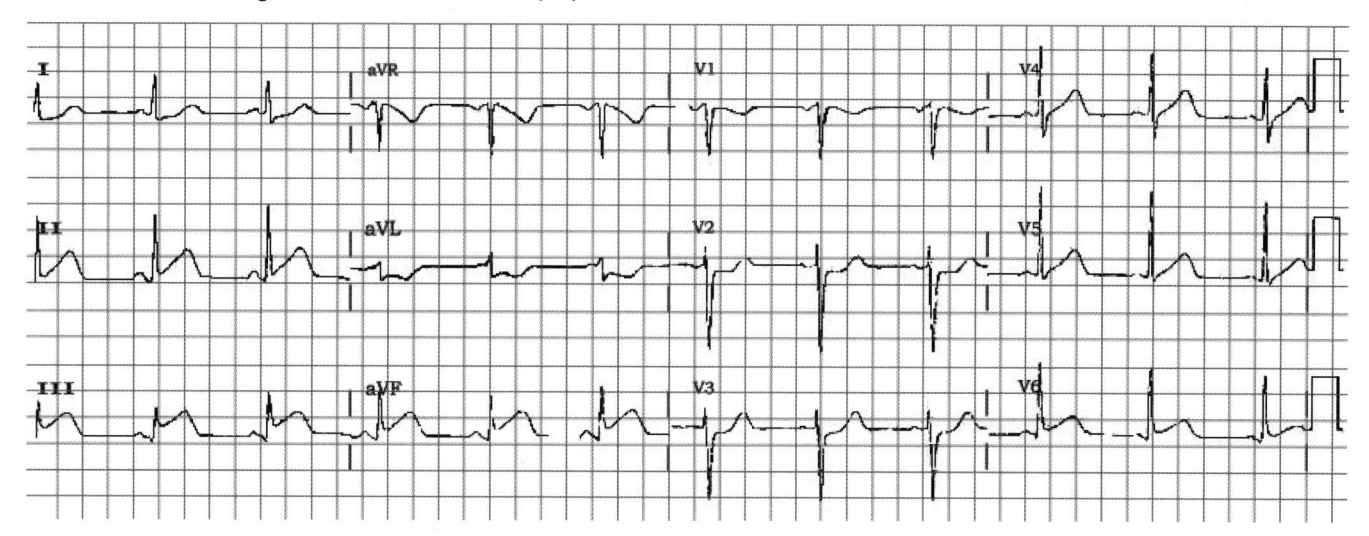

CARDIOVASCULAR EMERGENCIES

> **KEY POINT**
>
> ST-segment elevation in lead aVR can indicate a very high-risk presentation with the LMCA as the culprit artery.

Additional Predictive ECG Features

ST-segment depression in lead aVL (Figure 2-19), in the appropriate patient, can indicate impending inferior wall STEMI. In the normal patient, lead aVL should have an isoelectric ST segment, that is, the absence of ST-segment deviation. The T wave can be inverted in this lead as a normal variant. Lead aVL ST-segment depression ranges from minimal (subtle, <1 mm) to maximal (profound, many millimeters of depression).

In the normal patient, lead V_1 demonstrates an inverted T wave. In the patient with highly suspect ACS and a simultaneously nondiagnostic ECG, an upright T wave in lead V_1 can indicate an impending anterior wall process, such as anterior wall STEMI (Figure 2-20).

In the patient with highly suspected ACS who has a nondiagnostic ECG (with the exception of ST-segment depression in lead aVL or an upright T wave in lead V_1), the 12-lead ECG should be scrutinized for subtle ST-segment deviation, including the inferior leads and the anterior leads. If warranted, serial ECGs should be obtained, and particular attention should be given to these areas (Figures 2-19 and 2-20).

The Use of Additional Leads in the Evaluation of ACS

The 12-lead ECG is a less-than-perfect indicator of STEMI because of a number of limitations. The sensitivity of a single 12-lead ECG for the diagnosis of STEMI, ranging from 45% to 60%, is not impressive. One of the shortcomings of the 12-lead ECG involves anatomic limitations. The entire right ventricle and the posterior wall of the left ventricle are incompletely imaged by the standard 12-lead ECG. This less-than-impressive sensitivity of the 12-lead ECG might be improved with the use of additional body surface leads in selected individuals.

The most commonly employed additional-lead ECG is the 15-lead ECG, which comprises the standard 12-lead ECG plus the right ventricular lead, V_4R, and two posterior leads, V_8 and V_9. These leads are placed as follows (Figure 2-21): lead V_4R is placed on the right anterior thorax in the same position as

FIGURE 2-15.

Inferior STEMI with RV infarction. A, 12-lead ECG with ST-segment elevation in leads II, III, and aVF, indicative of inferior STEMI. RV infarction is found in 25% to 33% of patients with inferior STEMI presentations. Additional features that suggest RV infarction include ST-segment elevation in lead V_1 and disproportionate ST-segment elevation in lead III compared with leads II and aVF. In the setting of inferior STEMI with ST-segment elevation in leads II, III, and aVF, if the degree of elevation is greatest in lead III compared with the other inferior leads, then the presence of RV infarction should be considered. B, Additional, right-sided lead V_4R shows subtle ST-segment elevation, consistent with acute RV infarction.

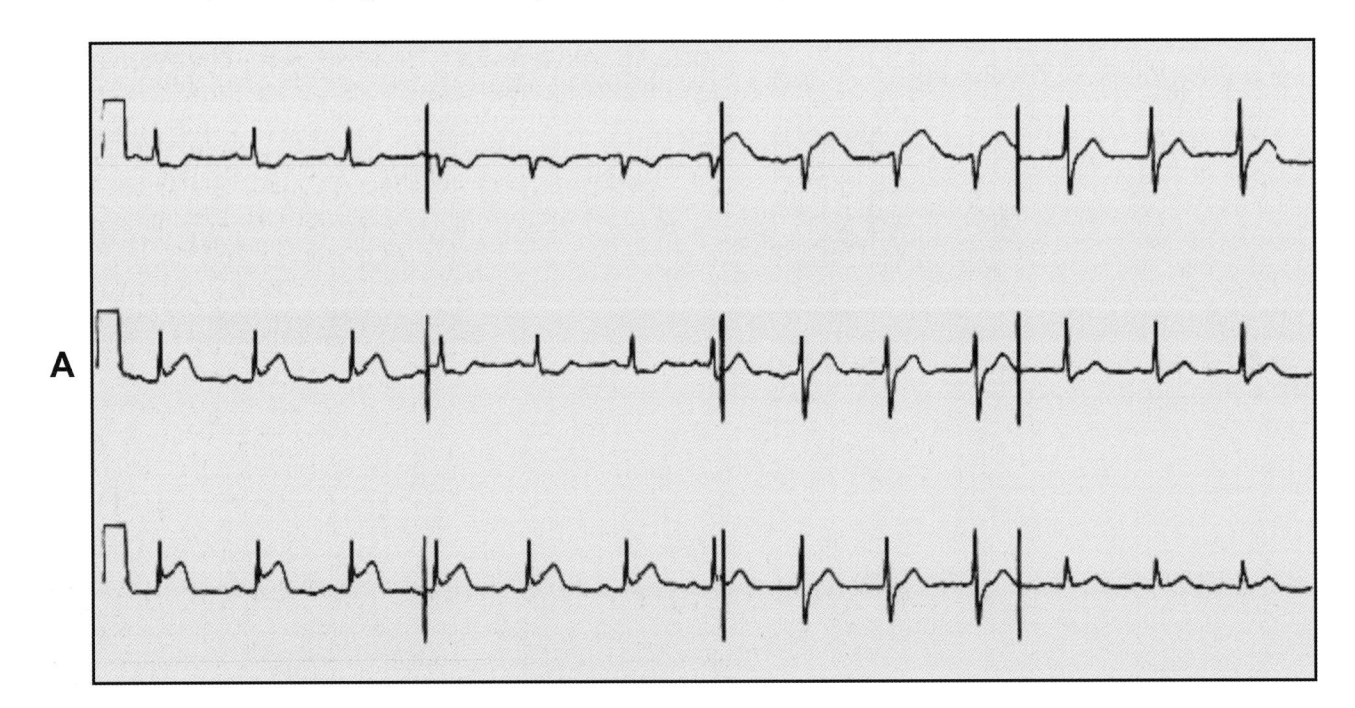

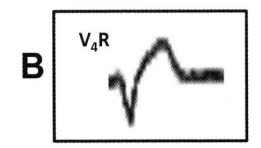

standard lead V_4, except that it is located on the right chest; lead V_8 is placed on the posterior thorax at the tip of the left scapula, and lead V_9 is located halfway between lead V_8 and the posterior midline of the back. Eighteen- and 24-lead ECGs have also been developed. A 15-lead ECG is appropriate for the patient with a high clinical likelihood of ACS but a nondiagnostic ECG. Right ventricular and posterior wall myocardial infarctions are likely to be underdiagnosed from the standard ECG perspective. Indications for the 15-lead ECG are listed in Table 2-5.

Acute RVMI occurs most frequently in conjunction with inferior wall STEMI; in fact, one third of inferior STEMIs occur along with an RVMI. Two issues make the ECG diagnosis of RVMI difficult: 1) the relatively small muscle mass of the right ventricle produces minimal ST-segment elevation; and 2) the standard 12-lead ECG does not directly image the right ventricle. Three 12-lead ECG findings suggest RVMI (Figure 2-15): the presence of STEMI of inferior wall, ST-segment elevation in lead V_1, and disproportionately greater ST-segment elevation in lead III than in leads II and aVF. As with posterior-wall myocardial infarction, the placement of additional leads can further explore the possibility of RVMI. The additional leads in this case are called *right-sided leads* and directly image the right ventricle. ST-segment elevation resulting from RVMI in the right-sided leads is usually minimal because of the relatively small muscle mass of the right ventricle; the smaller muscle mass produces less voltage when RVMI occurs. The additional leads can be V_1R to V_6R, or V_4R can be applied as a single right ventricular lead (Figure 2-15). ECG findings suggestive of RVMI are listed in Table 2-6.

Posterior-wall AMI represents 15% to 20% of all AMI presentations. Posterior-wall AMI is often associated with STEMI

FIGURE 2-16.

Inferior STEMI with posterior AMI. A, ST-segment elevation in leads II, III, and aVF, indicative of inferior STEMI. ST-segment depression in leads V_1 to V_3 with prominent R waves, indicative of posterior wall myocardial infarction. B and C, ST-segment depression in the right precordial leads (V_1 through V_3), prominent R waves, and upright T waves in in leads V_1 to V_3, indicative of posterior wall myocardial infarction. D, Additional, posterior leads V_8 and V_9, demonstrating ST-segment elevation, consistent with acute posterior wall AMI.

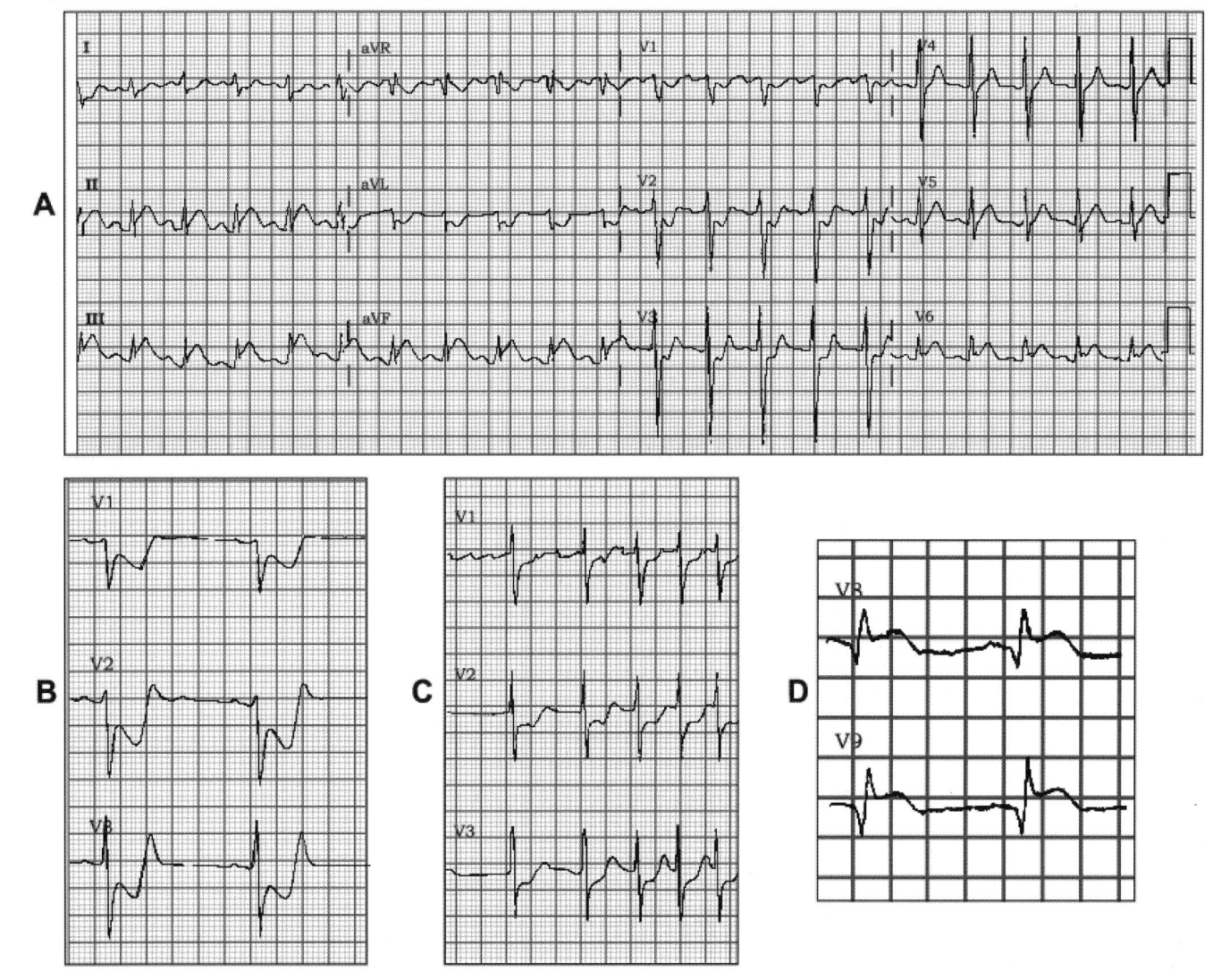

of either the inferior or lateral walls of the left ventricle; however, isolated posterior-wall AMI does occur and represents a not-insignificant minority (approximately 7%) of all AMIs. On a standard 12-lead ECG (Figure 2-16), posterior-wall AMI often presents with horizontal, or flat, ST-segment depression in the anterior leads (V_1 through V_4), prominent R waves in leads V_1 and/or V_2, an R/S ratio larger than 1 in leads V_1 and/or V_2, and an upright T wave in leads V_1 and/or V_2. Confirmatory evidence of an acute posterior-wall myocardial infarction is found in posterior leads V_8 and V_9 (Figure 2-16). These additional leads (V_8 and V_9), placed on the posterior thorax, directly image the posterior wall of the left ventricle. ST-segment elevation in V_8 and V_9 indicates AMI. The magnitude of the ST-segment elevation in these leads is frequently minimal. The leads are placed distant from the myocardium and thus the detected voltage is rather low, with a resultant lower magnitude of ST-segment elevation. ECG findings suggestive of acute posterior wall AMI are presented in Table 2-7.

Another application of additional-lead electrocardiography is termed *ECG body mapping*, a "mega" additional-lead ECG. Body mapping employs significantly more lead applications to the torso, including traditionally imaged segments of the left ventricle as well as less often observed regions such as the right ventricle and posterior wall of the left ventricle. In general, body mapping increases the diagnostic yield of ACS in patients with a high clinical likelihood for AMI and a nondiagnostic 12-lead ECG. An example of body mapping is the 80-lead ECG, which has 64 anterior thorax leads and 16 posterior thorax leads.[13]

KEY POINT

Additional ECG leads in the high-risk patient with a nondiagnostic 12-lead ECG can reveal significant ACS changes, including STEMI in certain patients.

Serial ECG Monitoring

Approximately half of AMI patients present with an initially nondiagnostic ECG, and a significant portion of them progress to AMI within hours after presentation. The dual recognition of the dynamic state of ACS and the static nature of a single ECG provides justification for serial ECG monitoring. Serial ECGs demonstrate the evolution of ST-segment elevation and thus identify a candidate for reperfusion treatment (Figures 2-19 and 2-20). Serial electrocardiography can also help emergency physicians assess a patient with both confounding and mimicking patterns, through the demonstration of dynamic

TABLE 2-6.

ECG Findings Suggestive of RVMI

Inferior STEMI

Disproportionate ST-segment elevation in lead III relative to leads II and aVF

ST-segment elevation in lead V_1 in the setting of inferior STEMI

ST-segment elevation in right-sided (right ventricular) leads V_4R or V_1R through V_6R

TABLE 2-5.

Indications for the 15-lead ECG in the Patient Suspected of Having AMI

Anterior (V_1, V_2, V_3, and/or V_4) ST-segment depression Prominent R wave in leads V_1 and/or V_2	Indicative of acute posterior wall AMI
Inferior STEMI Hypotension, either spontaneously or after vasodilator therapy, with interior STEMI	Indicative of acute right ventricular AMI
Inferior STEMI Lateral STEMI	Indicative of acute posterior wall AMI or acute right ventricular AMI

FIGURE 2-17.

Inferior STEMI with reciprocal ST-segment depression, or reciprocal change, in lead aVL.

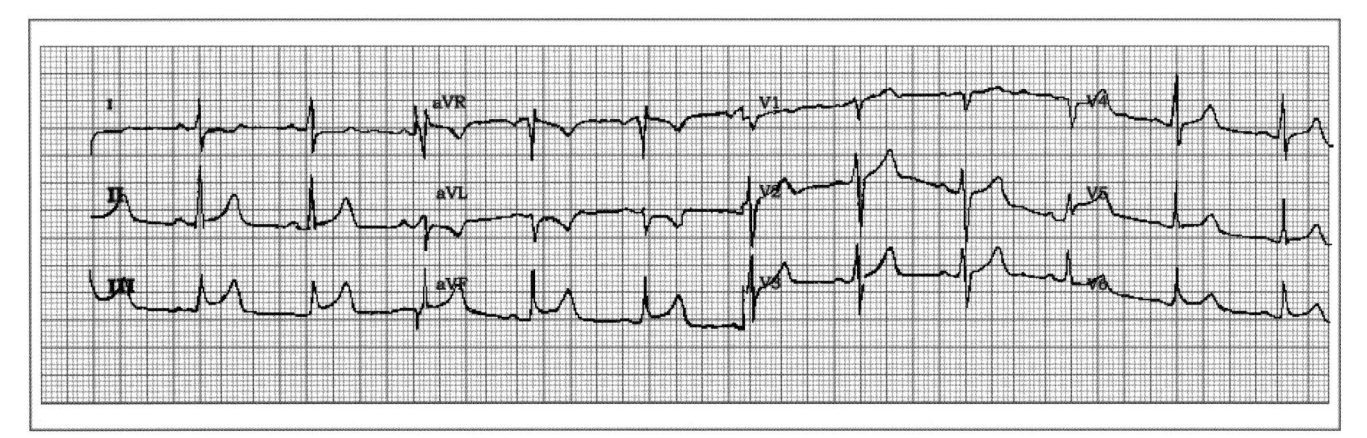

changes in the ST segments and T-wave configurations. It is important to note that not all patients benefit from serial ECG monitoring; rather, higher-suspicion patients with nondiagnostic 12-lead ECGs can be considered candidates for "sequential ECG" evaluation.

Serial electrocardiography is performed with either repeat applications of the standard 12-lead ECG or computer-assisted ST-segment trend monitoring. The most frequently used approach is repeat applications of the 12-lead. In this technique, the clinician obtains repeat 12-lead ECGs in serial fashion, looking for changes in the ST-segment and T-wave morphologies as well as the development of diagnostic ST-segment elevation consistent with STEMI. ST-segment trend monitoring, using diagnostic-capable cardiac monitors and computer software, provides another form of serial ECG monitoring. In this technique, the computer obtains a 12-lead ECG at frequent intervals and compares the ST segments. If the segments demonstrate an absolute or relative increase in height, the clinician is alerted, allowing direct provider-based interpretation of the ECG.

TABLE 2-7.
ECG Findings Suggestive of Acute Posterior Wall AMI

ST-segment depression in leads V_1, V_2, V_3, and/or V_4
Prominent R wave in leads V_1 and/or V_2
Upright T wave in leads V_1, V_2, and/or V_3, with ST-segment depression
Coexistent inferior or lateral STEMI

KEY POINT

As with the additional ECG leads, serial electrocardiography can rule in significant ACS in high-risk patients with nondiagnostic ECGs.

FIGURE 2-18.
Lead aVR ST-segment elevation as a predictor of left main coronary artery occlusion: Both examples demonstrate significant ST-segment elevation in the anterior region of the 12-lead ECG, indicating anterior STEMI. Additionally, lead aVR demonstrates ST-segment elevation, which is a warning that the culprit lesion will be found in the left main coronary artery.

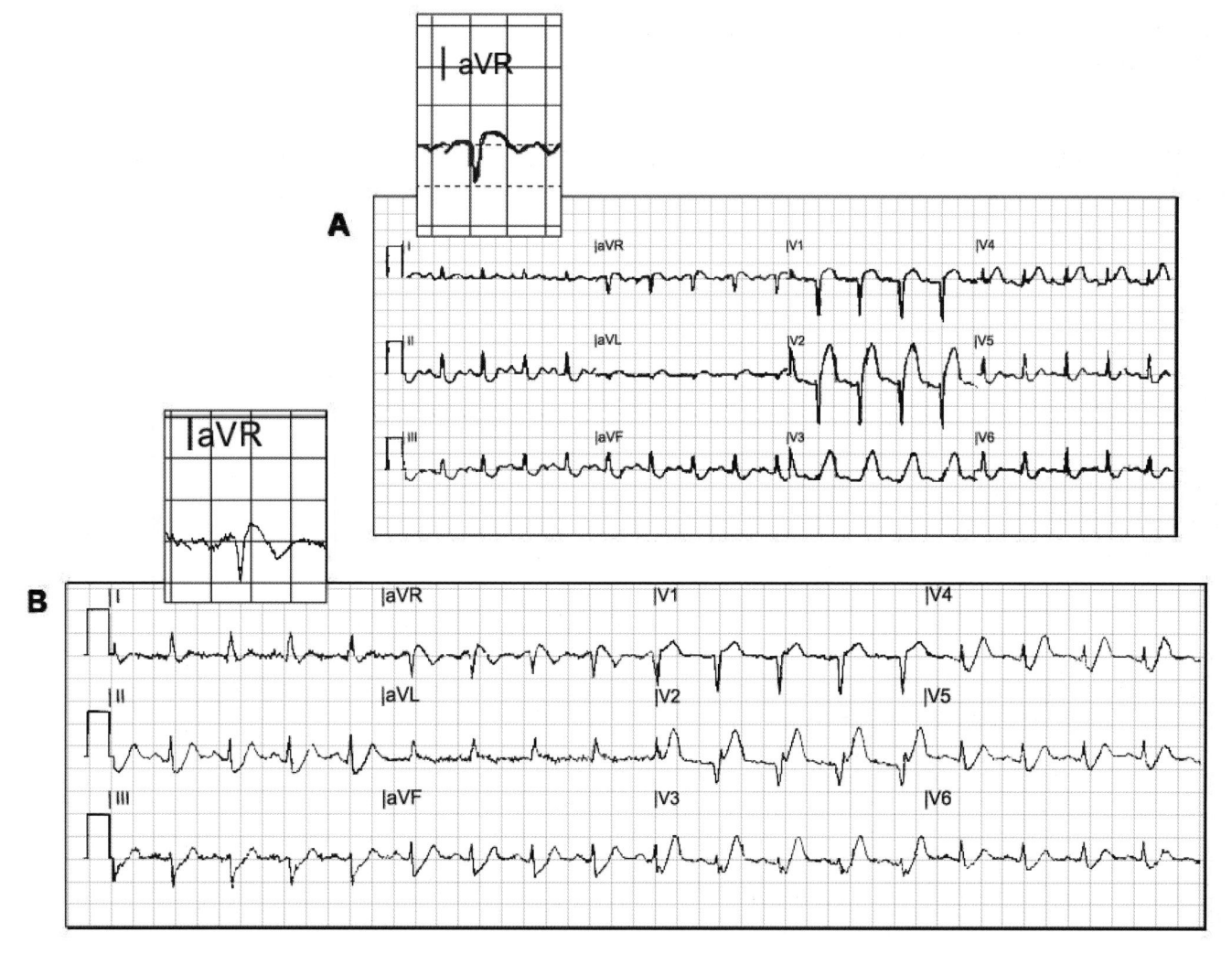

Confounding Patterns

Three ECG patterns confound the ability of a 12-lead ECG to detect ACS and reduce its diagnostic potential, as follows: LBBB, right ventricular paced rhythms (RVPR) from an implanted pacemaker, and LVH by voltage.

Left Bundle-Branch Block

The discussion of LBBB and the diagnosis of AMI must include a review of the significance of this pattern's appearance in the patient suspected of myocardial infarction as well as the ability to diagnose acute infarction in its presence. The finding of a new LBBB pattern in a patient suspected of AMI used to be considered a STEMI equivalent, but no longer. Patients with LBBB should be considered to have STEMI if they are hemodynamically unstable or in acute heart failure. LBBB identifies a high-risk ACS presentation and a concomitant risk of complete heart block, malignant ventricular arrhythmias, cardiogenic shock, and death.

LBBB not only reduces the diagnostic potential of the ECG but also produces ST-segment and T-wave abnormalities that mimic changes seen in ACS. In the patient with LBBB, the anticipated or expected ST-segment/T-wave configurations are discordant, directed opposite from the major, terminal portion of the QRS complex (Figures 2-22 and 2-23). Thus, leads with a predominantly positive QRS complex (eg, I, aVL, V_5, and V_6) will demonstrate ST-segment depression with an inverted T wave. The leads with primarily negatively oriented QRS complexes (ie, V_1 through V_3) will have ST-segment elevation

FIGURE 2-19.

Lead aVL ST depression/T-wave inversion as an early warning of inferior STEMI. A, The inferior leads along with lead aVL demonstrate only a T-wave inversion in lead aVL. B, Serial ECG performed 24 minutes later in a patient with worsened chest pain demonstrates subtle ST-segment changes in the inferior leads. More pronounced ST-segment depression with inverted T wave is seen in lead aVL. C, Inferior STEMI is noted 17 minutes later.

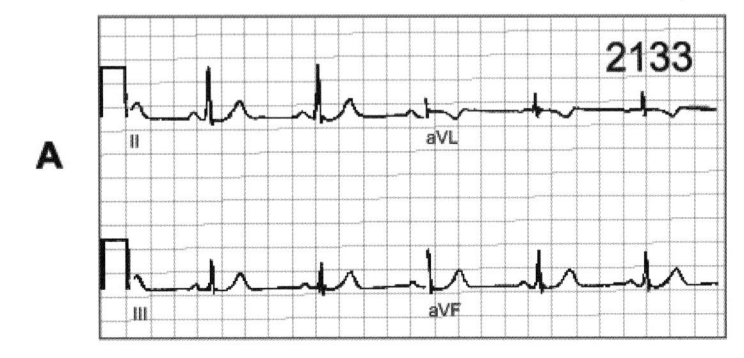

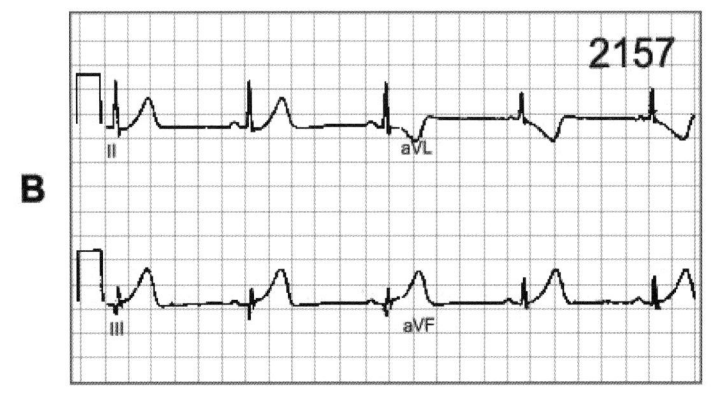

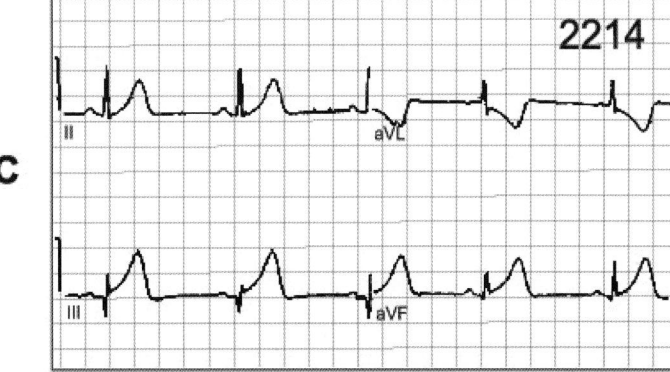

with upright T waves. These ST-segment changes are called discordant ST-segment depression and discordant ST-segment elevation, respectively. These are normal findings in the patient with LBBB. Loss of this normal QRS-complex/ST-segment discordance in patients with LBBB might imply an acute process such as AMI.

Sgarbossa et al[14] developed a clinical prediction rule to assist in the diagnosis of AMI in the setting of LBBB using specific ECG findings. The criteria suggesting a diagnosis of AMI, ranked with a scoring system based on the probability of such a diagnosis (Figures 2-24 and 2-25; Table 2-8), are 1) ST-segment elevation larger than 1 mm, concordant with the QRS complex (score of 5) (Figures 2-24A and 2-25A); 2) ST-segment depression larger than 1 mm, limited to leads V_1, V_2, and V_3 (score of 3) (Figures 2-24B and 2-25B); and 3) ST-segment elevation larger than 5 mm and discordant with the QRS complex (score of 2) (Figures 2-24C and 2-25C). A total score of 3 or more suggests that the patient is likely experiencing an AMI based on

FIGURE 2-20.

"Too tall T wave in lead V_1," a predictor of anterior STEMI. A, The normal T wave is inverted in lead V_1. In the appropriate setting (ie, ACS is highly suspected), an upright T wave in lead V_1 can indicate an ACS event of the anterior wall, with potential anterior-wall STEMI as a consequence. B, From the same patient as in A. Development of anterior STEMI as predicted by the "too tall T wave in lead V_1."

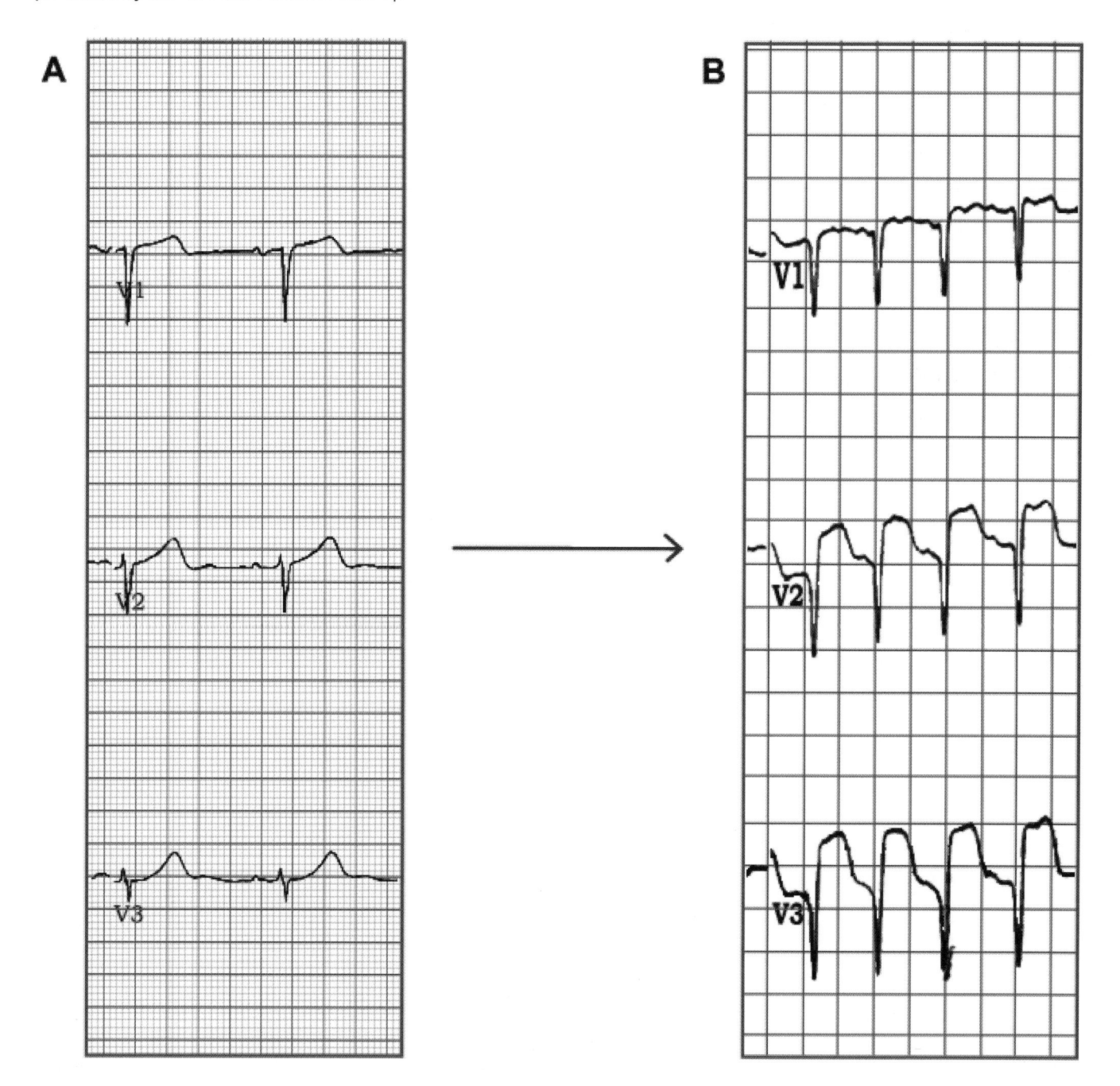

CARDIOVASCULAR EMERGENCIES

FIGURE 2-21.
Placement of the additional leads used in the 15-lead ECG. A, Lead V₄R provides direct imaging of the right ventricle. B, Leads V₈ and V₉ provide direct imaging of the posterior wall of the left ventricle.

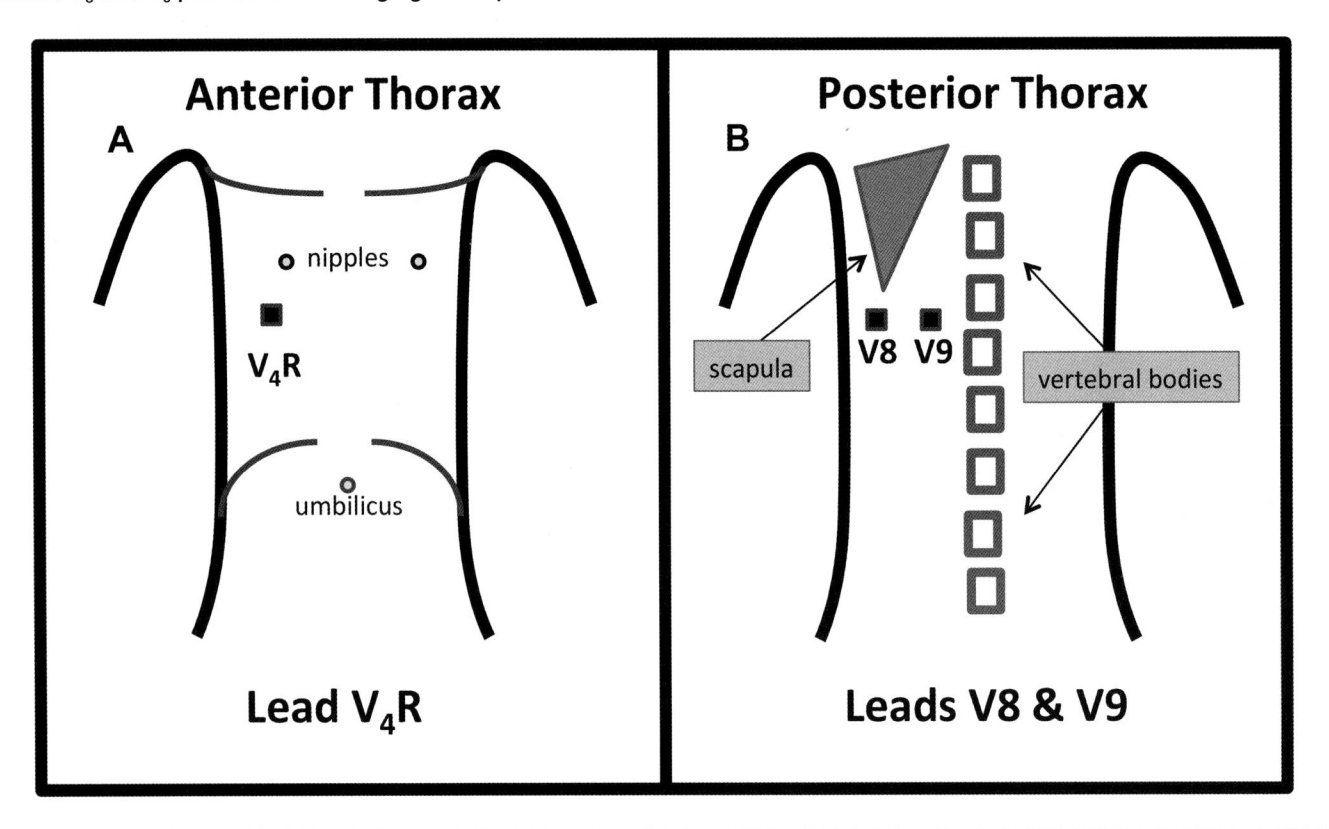

FIGURE 2-22.
A, Left bundle-branch block with ST-segment abnormalities. B, Comparison of ST-segment elevation associated with LBBB (left) and non-LBBB STEMI (right).

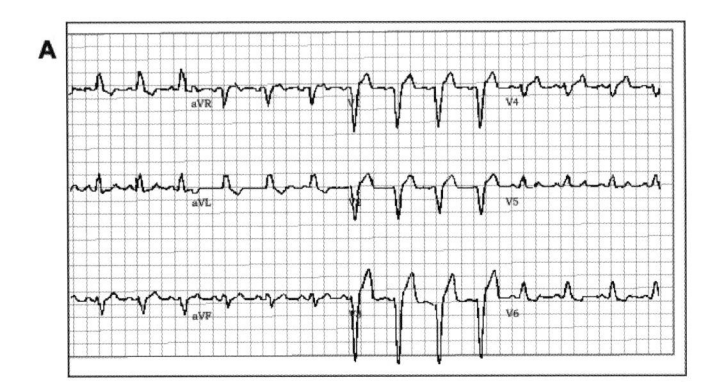

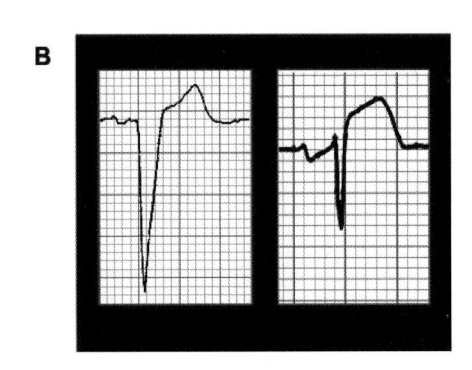

the ECG criteria. A score less than 3 makes the ECG diagnosis less assured, requiring additional evaluation.

> **KEY POINT**
>
> In the patient with LBBB, the Sgarbossa criteria are based largely on an understanding of the normal relationship of the QRS complex and the ST segment. The major, terminal portion of QRS complex and ST segment should be located on opposite sides of the ECG baseline. Alterations of this normal relationship in the appropriate patient can indicate an acute process, such as ACS.

TABLE 2-8.

Sgarbossa Clinical Prediction Rule to Assist in the Diagnosis of AMI in the Setting of LBBB[14]

ST-segment elevation larger than 1 mm, concordant with the QRS complex	Score = 5
ST-segment depression larger than 1 mm, limited to leads V_1, V_2, and V_3	Score = 3
ST-segment elevation larger than 5 mm and discordant with the QRS complex	Score = 2

This scoring system is based on the probability of AMI. A score of 3 or more suggests AMI based on the ECG criteria. A score of less than 3 makes the ECG diagnosis less certain, requiring additional evaluation.

Right Ventricular Paced Rhythm from Implanted Right Ventricular Pacemaker

As with the LBBB pattern, the right ventricular paced rhythm pattern can both mimic and mask the manifestations of AMI. In RVPR, the ventricular depolarization pattern is abnormal, with activation of the ventricles occurring from right to left, resembling an LBBB pattern in part. The expected ST-segment/T-wave configurations are discordant (Figure 2-26), directed opposite from the terminal portion of the QRS complex. As such, leads with QS complexes such as leads V_1 to V_6, will demonstrate ST-segment elevation, mimicking AMI. Leads with large monophasic R waves demonstrate ST-segment depression. The T wave, particularly in the right to mid precordial and inferior leads, has a convex upward shape or a tall, vaulting appearance, similar to the hyperacute T wave of early myocardial infarction. The T waves in leads with the monophasic R wave are frequently inverted. As with the LBBB pattern, the loss of a discordant relationship between the major, terminal portion of the QRS complex and the ST segment can suggest AMI, assuming the clinical presentation is applicable.

Sgarbossa et al[15] investigated the ECG changes encountered in patients with RVPR experiencing AMI. Three ECG criteria were found to be useful in the early diagnosis of AMI, as follows: 1) discordant ST-segment elevation larger than 5 mm, 2) concordant ST-segment elevation larger than 1 mm, and 3) ST-segment depression larger than 1 mm in lead V_1, V_2, or V_3. These findings can be used to guide the clinician in the evaluation of suspected ACS in patients with this confounding pat-

FIGURE 2-23.

Appropriate discordance in patients with bundle-branch block and ventricular paced rhythms. The major terminal portion of the QRS complex and the ST segment/T wave are located on opposites sides of the isoelectric baseline. These findings are the normal, or expected, ST-segment/T-wave configurations in patients with bundle-branch block and ventricular paced rhythms. A, Discordant ST-segment elevation. B, Discordant ST-segment depression.

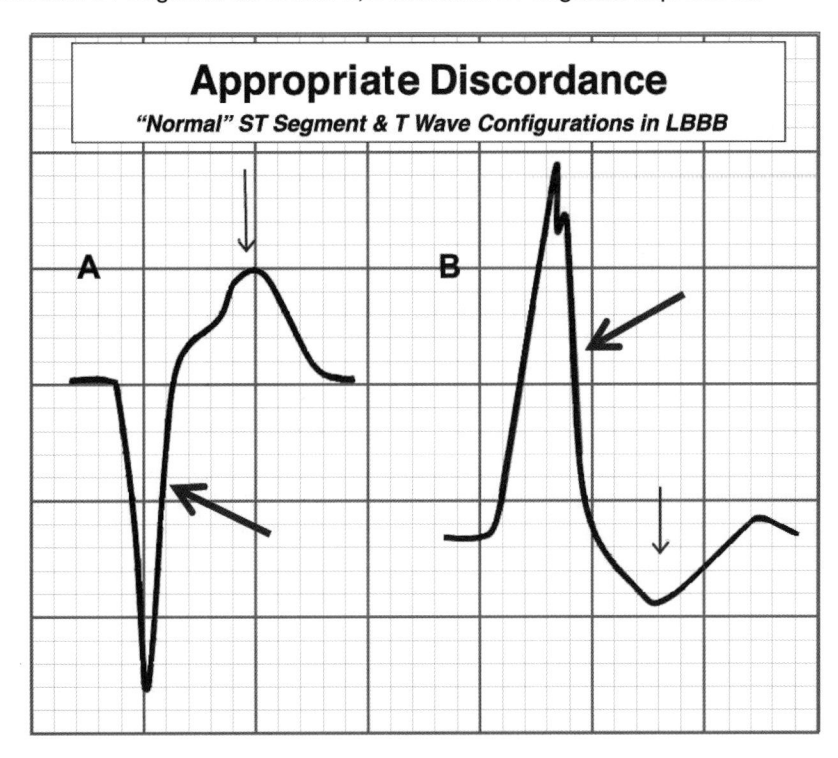

CARDIOVASCULAR EMERGENCIES

FIGURE 2-24.

Abnormal findings in patients with bundle-branch block and ventricular paced rhythms, suggestive of an acute coronary event according to the Sgarbossa criteria.[14] A, Concordant ST-segment elevation: the ST segment is elevated on the same side of the isoelectric baseline as the major terminal portion of the QRS complex. B, Concordant ST-segment depression: the ST segment is depressed on the same side of the isoelectric baseline as the major terminal portion of the QRS complex. C, Excessive, discordant ST-segment elevation larger than 5 mm: the ST segment is directed opposite the major terminal portion of the QRS complex, which is considered a normal finding. The degree of elevation, however, is more than 5 mm and thus suggests ACS.

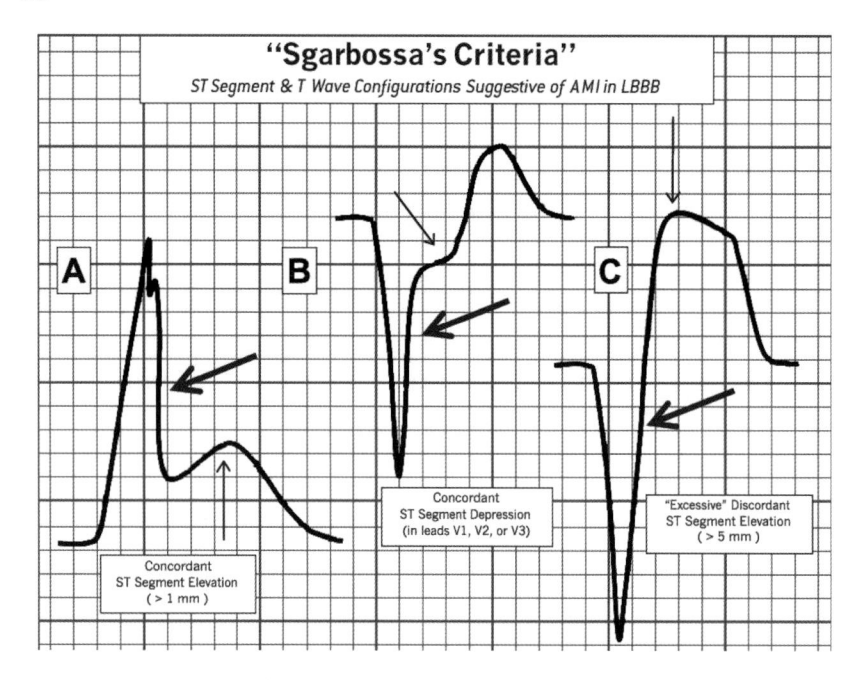

FIGURE 2-25.

Examples of ST-segment abnormality in LBBB AMI presentations. A, Concordant elevation. B, Concordant depression. C, Excessive (>5 mm) discordant elevation.

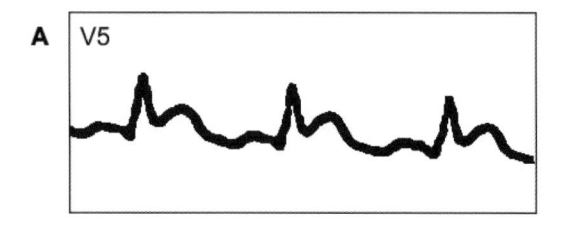

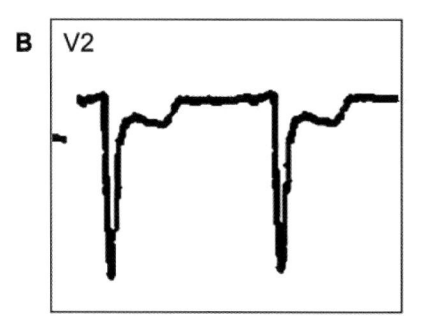

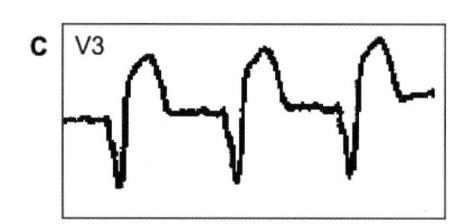

tern. The presence of these findings, while suggestive, does not rule in AMI; the clinical presentation must also be appropriate. Furthermore, the absence of these findings does not rule out AMI. These findings are similar to the abnormalities seen in LBBB AMI (Figures 2-24 and 2-25).[14]

> **KEY POINT**
>
> As in the patient with LBBB, the basic principles of the Sgarbossa criteria can be applied to the patient with an implanted, right ventricular paced ECG pattern in whom ACS is suspected.

Left Ventricular Hypertrophy

ECG LVH and its related repolarization changes are seen frequently in patients with chest pain. As with LBBB and RVPR presentations, the ECG LVH pattern and related ST-segment/T-wave abnormalities both confound the ECG diagnosis of AMI and mimic findings typical of ACS. The ECG LVH pattern is present when significantly large QRS complexes are observed on the ECG; in 70% of these patients, marked ST-segment and T-wave abnormalities are noted, representing the strain pattern. Recognition of the ECG LVH pattern is extremely important. Without it, LVH-associated ST-segment and T-wave abnormalities can be interpreted incorrectly as primarily resulting from ACS. The recognition of this pattern involves application of the scoring systems that consider the various QRS-complex voltages. The Sokolow-Lyon criteria[16] constitute the most accurate and most straightforward method. In this model, LVH by voltage criteria is detected if the sum of the amplitude of the largest S wave in lead V_1 or V_2 and the largest R wave in lead V_5 or V_6 is more than 35 mm in a patient older than 35 years.

In patients with ECG LVH (Figure 2-27), ST-segment/T-wave changes are encountered in approximately 70% of cases. These changes result from altered repolarization of the ventricular myocardium and represent the new normal for the patient with ECG LVH. LVH is associated with poor R-wave progression and loss of the septal R wave in the right to mid precordial leads, most commonly producing a QS pattern. In general, these QS complexes are located in leads V_1 and V_2, rarely extending beyond lead V_3; in these leads, ST-segment elevation is encountered in this distribution along with prominent T waves. The ST-segment elevation seen in these leads can exceed 5 mm in height. The initial upsloping portion of the ST segment is frequently concave. Leads V_5 and V_6 as well as leads I and aVL demonstrate large positive QRS complexes, described as monophasic R waves. These leads demonstrate ST-segment depression with inverted T waves. The morphology of the ST-segment/T-wave complex is highly characteristic of LVH—the initial downsloping portion is gradual, with an abrupt return to baseline.

At this time, a clinical decision rule for the LVH pattern that supports the ECG diagnosis of AMI does not exist. An understanding of the abnormalities seen in the LVH pattern allows the clinician to evaluate the 12-lead ECG appropriately in this presentation.

FIGURE 2-26.

A, Ventricular paced pattern from implanted right ventricular pacemaker. B, Comparison of ST-segment elevation associated with the ventricular paced pattern (left) and STEMI (right).

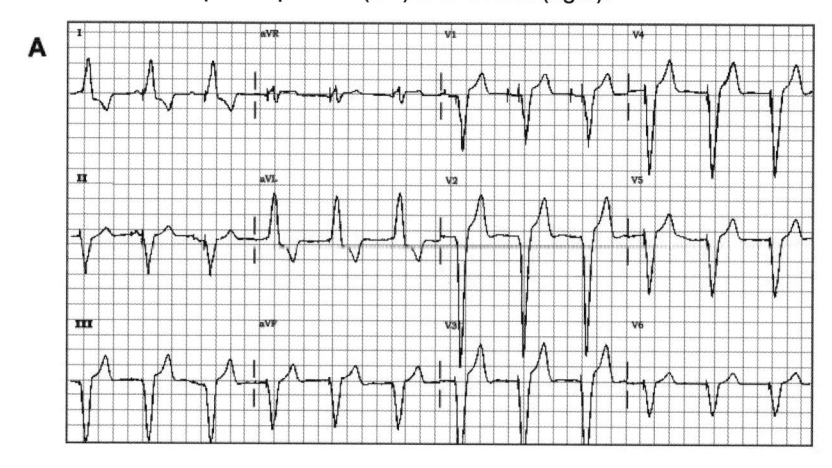

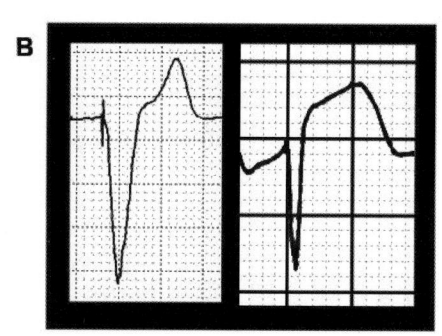

CARDIOVASCULAR EMERGENCIES

FIGURE 2-27.

A, Left ventricular hypertrophy with ST-segment abnormalities, also known as "strain." B, Comparison of ST-segment elevation associated with LVH (left) and STEMI (right).

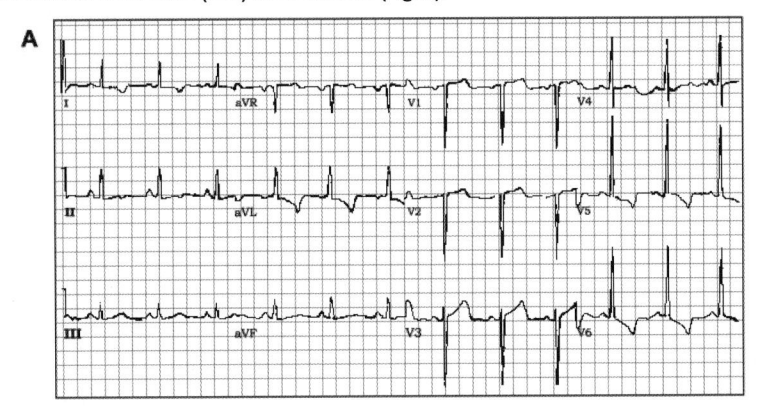

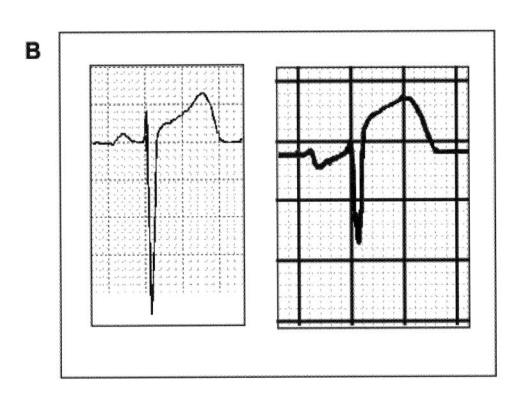

FIGURE 2-28.

A, Benign early repolarization with ST-segment and T-wave abnormalities. B, Comparison of ST-segment elevation associated with benign early repolarization (left) and STEMI (right).

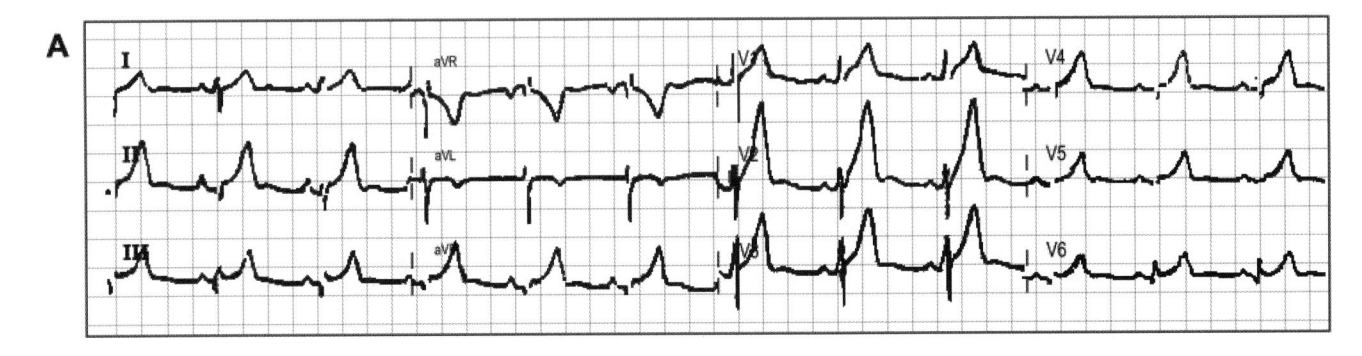

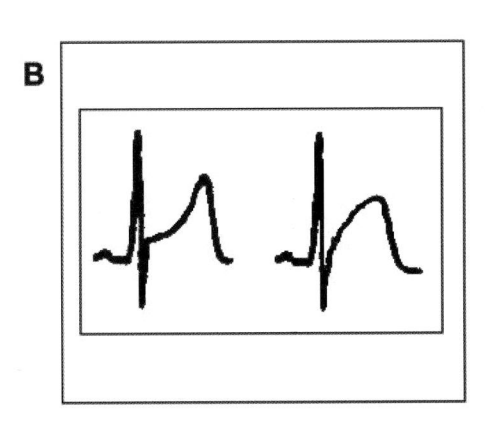

The Electrocardiogram in the Evaluation and Management of Acute Coronary Syndrome

STEMI Mimic Patterns

STEMI mimic patterns present as ST-segment or T-wave abnormalities that resemble ACS-related changes when, in fact, no acute coronary event is occurring. These include the confounding patterns discussed above (Figures 2-22, 2-26, and 2-27; Table 2-9) as well as a range of mimicking presentations, such as benign early repolarization, acute myopericarditis, and left ventricular aneurysm (LVA).

TABLE 2-9.
STEMI-Mimicking Patterns

Left bundle-branch block[a]
Right bundle-branch block
Right ventricular paced pattern[a]
Left ventricular hypertrophy (voltage) pattern with strain[a]
Benign early repolarization
Pulmonary embolism
Left ventricular aneurysm
Myocarditis, myopericarditis
Hyperkalemia
Cardiomyopathies

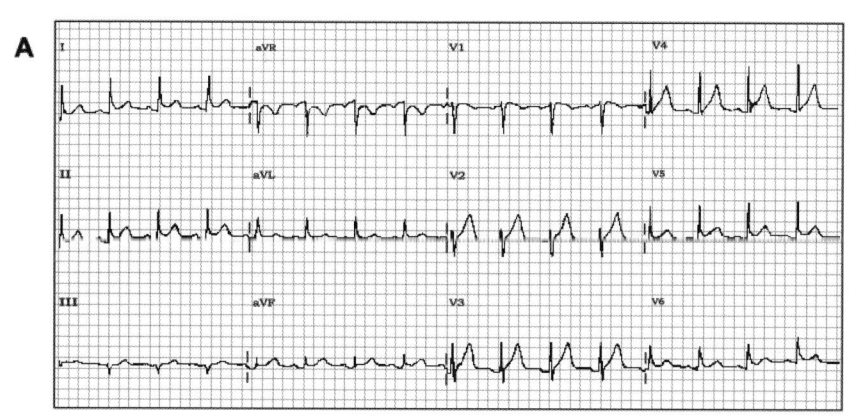

[a]Also considered a confounding ECG pattern

KEY POINT

A significant number of adults with chest pain present with ST-segment elevation. An understanding of the differential diagnosis of ST-segment elevation in the adult chest pain patient will assist the clinician in the appropriate evaluation of the 12-lead ECG.

Benign Early Repolarization

Benign early repolarization is considered a normal variant, not indicative of underlying cardiac disease or associated with poor prognosis. It is a chronic pattern found in people (mostly African-American males) between 20 and 40 years of age. It diminishes over time and disappears by the age of 50.

The ECG definition of benign early repolarization includes the following characteristics: 1) ST-segment elevation, 2) upward concavity of the initial portion of the ST segment, 3) notching or slurring of the J point, 4) symmetric, concordant T waves of large amplitude, 5) widespread or diffuse distribution of ST-segment elevation, and 6) relative temporal stability (Figure 2-28).

The ST-segment elevation begins at the J point and is usually 0.5 to 3.5 mm in magnitude. In rare cases, the elevation can approach 5 mm. The elevation is greater in the precordial leads (2 mm) than in the limb leads (0.5 mm). The morphology of the elevated ST segment is characteristic of benign early repolarization: it appears as if it has been evenly lifted upward from the isoelectric baseline at the J point, with preservation of the

FIGURE 2-29.
A, Pericarditis with ST-segment abnormalities. B, Comparison of ST-segment elevation associated with pericarditis (left) and STEMI (right).

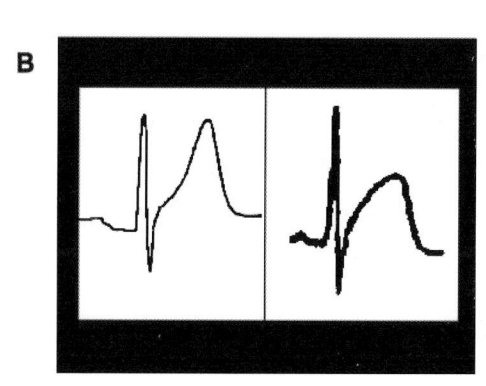

normal concavity of the initial upsloping portion of the ST-segment/T-wave complex. The T waves are large and quite prominent; they are concordant with the QRS complex and most often seen in the right to mid precordial leads. The changes are distributed as follows: right to mid precordial leads in most instances; precordial leads and the limb (eg, inferior) leads in certain cases; and "isolated" in the limb leads very rarely. The ST-segment/T-wave changes are fixed and do not demonstrate change over hours, days, or weeks.

Acute Myopericarditis

Acute pericarditis, appropriately called *acute myopericarditis*, produces diffuse inflammation of the pericardium and superficial epicardium. This inflammation can produce a range of ECG abnormalities (Figure 2-29), including ST-segment elevation, T-wave inversion, and PR-segment changes (elevation and depression, depending on the lead). The ST-segment elevation is most often 1 to 3 mm in height, rarely exceeding 5 mm. It is usually observed in numerous leads, although "isolated" changes can be seen in single anatomic regions (eg, the inferior wall with leads II, III, and aVF). The initial upsloping portion of the ST segment is most frequently concave in morphology. PR-segment deviation is also seen in certain individuals. PR-segment depression is seen usually in leads II, III, aVF, and V_6. PR-segment elevation is seen in lead aVR and is usually very apparent when present.

Left Ventricular Aneurysm

LVA is defined as a localized area of infarcted myocardium that bulges outward during both systole and diastole. LVAs most often are noted after large anterior wall infarctions that either do not come to medical attention or do not respond to treatment. In most cases, the LVA is manifested electrocardiographically by varying degrees of ST-segment elevation, ranging from minimal to maximal (Figure 2-30). The morphology of the elevated ST segment is varied, including concave, obliquely straight, and convex. Accompanying the ST-segment elevation are Q waves, indicative of the completed myocardial infarction. A comparison of the T wave with the QRS complex can aid in distinguishing LVA from STEMI. In LVA, the QRS complex is usually a large Q wave while the T wave is inverted and small in amplitude; the ratio of the T wave to QRS complex is rather small. In the STEMI patient, the T wave is often larger relative to the QRS complex, producing a larger ratio of T wave to QRS complex.

Summary

The ECG is a valuable and useful tool in the evaluation of patients suspected of ACS. Its uses include establishing the diagnosis, evaluating other syndromes that can present with chest pain, providing criteria for various interventions and therapies, considering the impact of treatment, predicting the risk of an adverse event, and suggesting disposition location. In addition to providing the key diagnostic information, it can reveal

FIGURE 2-30.

A, ST-segment elevation in LVA. B, Comparison of ST-segment elevation associated with LVA (left) and STEMI (right).

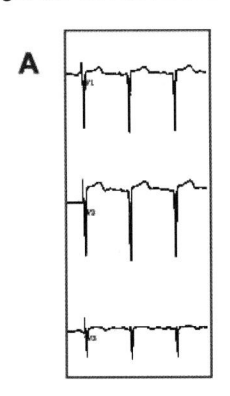

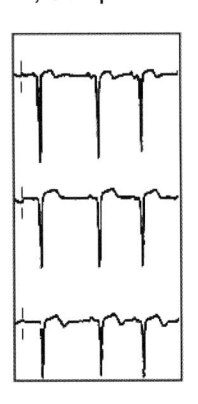

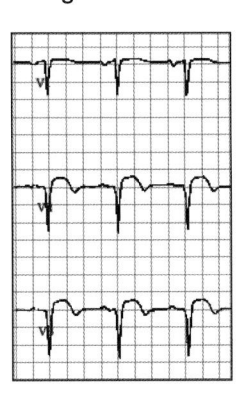

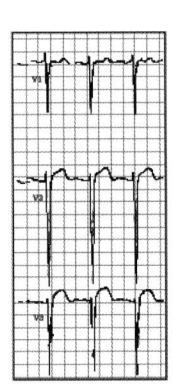

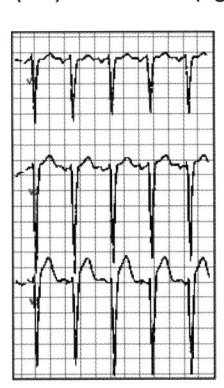

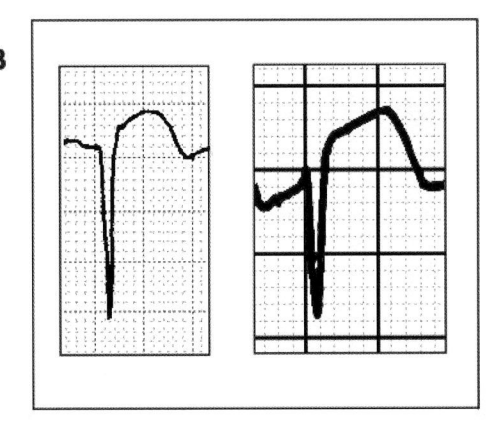

life-threatening arrhythmias that can complicate ACS. It is inexpensive, portable, and noninvasive and can be applied in a number of medical settings, ranging from a patient's living room to the emergency department and beyond to the ICU. While it is quite useful, the ECG does have limitations, including imperfect test characteristics for the diagnosis of STEMI. A knowledge of these limitations will allow the clinician to use the ECG appropriately in the management of the patients in whom ACS is suspected.

References

1. Nable JV, Brady WJ. The evolution of ECG changes in ST-segment elevation myocardial infarction. *Am J Emerg Med*. 2009;27:734-746.
2. Fesmire FM, Hahn S, Jagoda AS, et al. Clinical policy: critical issues in the evaluation and management of adult patients with non–ST-segment elevation acute coronary syndromes. *Ann Emerg Med*. 2006;48:270-301.
3. Fesmire FM, Brady WJ, Hahn S, et al. Clinical policy: indications for reperfusion therapy in emergency department patients with suspected acute myocardial infarction. *Ann Emerg Med*. 2006;48:358-371.
4. O'Connor RE, Brady W, Brooks SC, et al. Acute coronary syndromes: 2010 American Heart Association Guidelines for Cardiopulmonary Resuscitation and Emergency Cardiovascular Care. *Circulation*. 2010;122:s787-s817.
5. Brady WJ, Perron AD, Ullman EA. Electrocardiographic ST segment elevation: a comparison of AMI and non-AMI ECG syndromes. *Am J Emerg Med*. 2002;20:609-612.
6. Brady WJ, Syverud SA, Beagle C, et al. Electrocardiographic ST-segment elevation: the diagnosis of acute myocardial infarction by morphologic analysis of the ST segment. *Acad Emerg Med*. 2001;8:961-967.
7. Brady WJ, Perron AD, Martin ML, et al. Cause of ST segment abnormality in ED chest pain patients. *Am J Emerg Med*. 2001;19:25-28.
8. Otto LA, Aufderheide TP. Evaluation of ST segment elevation criteria for the prehospital electrocardiographic diagnosis of acute myocardial infarction. *Ann Emerg Med*. 1994;23:17-24.
9. Aro AL, Anttonen O, Tikkanen JT, et al. Prevalence and prognostic significance of T-wave inversions in right precordial leads of a 12-lead electrocardiogram in the middle-aged subjects. *Circulation*. 2012;125:2572-2577.
10. Nikus KC, Sclarovsky S, Huhtala H, et al. Electrocardiographic presentation of global ischemia in acute coronary syndrome predicts poor outcome. *Ann Med*. 2012;44:494-502.
11. Rhinehardt J, Brady WJ, Perron AD, Mattu A. Electrocardiographic manifestations of Wellens' syndrome. *Am J Emerg Med*. 2002;20:638-643.
12. Williamson K, Mattu A, Binder A, et al. Electrocardiographic applications of lead aVR. *Am J Emerg Med*. 2006;24:864-874.
13. Self WH, Mattu A, Martin M, et al. Body surface mapping in the emergency department evaluation of the chest pain patient: use of the 80-lead electrocardiogram system. *Am J Emerg Med*. 2006;24:87-112.
14. Sgarbossa EB, Pinski SL, Barbagelata A, et al. Electrocardiographic diagnosis of evolving acute myocardial infarction in the presence of left bundle-branch block. GUSTO-1 (Global Utilization of Streptokinase and Tissue Plasminogen Activator for Occluded Coronary Arteries) Investigators. *N Engl J Med*. 1996;334:481-487.
15. Sgarbossa EB, Pinski SL, Gates KB, et al. Early electrocardiographic diagnosis of acute myocardial infarction in the presence of ventricular paced rhythm. GUSTO-I investigators. *Am J Cardiol*. 1996;77:423-424.
16. Sokolow M, Lyon TP. The ventricular complex in left ventricular hypertrophy as obtained by unipolar precordial and limb leads. *Am Heart J*. 1949;37:161-186.

CARDIOVASCULAR EMERGENCIES

CHAPTER 3

Acute Coronary Syndrome: Biomarkers and Imaging

Maame Yaa Yiadom and Chadwick D. Miller

IN THIS CHAPTER

Use of biomarkers for myocardial infarction

Risk stratification tools for the diagnosis of acute coronary syndrome

Cardiac and coronary imaging modalities for the evaluation of myocardial ischemia

In this chapter, we review the cardiac biomarkers and cardiovascular imaging modalities that are available to evaluate emergency department patients for acute coronary syndrome (ACS). We also discuss some of the tools available to assist in stratifying patients according to risk for myocardial ischemia and infarction from ACS. Given that ST-elevation myocardial infarction (STEMI) is an electrocardiographic (ECG) diagnosis for the emergency physician, this diagnostic discussion focuses on non–ST-elevation myocardial infarction (NSTEMI) and unstable angina.

Myocardial Ischemia and Acute Coronary Syndrome

The identification of ACS in the emergency department patient uses symptoms, signs, demographic medical risk, and diagnostic testing to determine whether ACS physiology is occurring at the level of the coronary artery. Specifically, the emergency physician is looking to see if flow is obstructed within a coronary artery. The most common cause of this obstruction is rupture or erosion of a coronary artery wall plaque, resulting in thrombus formation.[1] The thrombus narrows the vessel lumen, decreasing blood flow. This process is referred to as *primary ACS*. Limited blood flow creates a mismatch between the myocardial tissue's supply and demand for oxygen and nutrients, which results in myocardial cell and tissue ischemia. The discomfort and symptoms of this process are what lead patients to seek care.

Coronary artery disease (CAD) is the predisposing condition for ACS physiology. CAD develops when cholesterol plaques that form within the coronary artery wall gradually narrow the lumen over time. This is also known as coronary atherosclerosis. The presence and degree of CAD correlate with increasing age and the presence of diabetes, hypertension, and hyperlipidemia. Smoking accelerates the processes associated with plaque formation. As atherosclerotic plaques grow, they can narrow the arterial lumen. Also, within these plaques is active inflammation that contributes to plaque instability.[2] These dynamic changes create opportunities for 1) inadequate oxygen and nutrient delivery as a result of obstructed inflow and 2) injury of the vessel wall from the sheer force of blood flow (ie, plaque rupture). Thus, the presence of CAD increases the chances that ACS physiology can occur. Known CAD in a patient, or the presence of risk factors for CAD, should heighten the emergency physician's suspicion for ACS.[3]

Obstructive CAD is more likely than nonobstructive CAD to cause ACS. However, data from serial angiographic evaluations demonstrate that plaque rupture commonly occurs in vessels previously determined to have nonobstructive CAD.[4,5]

This highlights the fact that the presence of CAD, rather than the determination of obstructive versus nonobstructive disease, is more pertinent to immediate risk stratification. In addition, secondary ACS can occur in the absence of significant CAD (often referred to as *demand ischemia*). It can occur in the setting of severe hypertension, valvular disease, and anemia.

It is worth noting additional differences between primary and secondary ACS. In the former, the primary event is an acute anatomic change, typically involving plaque rupture and thrombosis, within a coronary artery. Secondary ischemia occurs when an alternative primary process exacerbates coronary flow limitations, as with the increased metabolic demand of sepsis, the sheer forces of an arrhythmia, or arterial dissection from trauma. All can cause distal tissue ischemia. First-line treatment for secondary ischemia is addressing the primary process.

KEY POINTS

CAD is a predisposing condition for most patients with ACS.

The evaluation of patients for ACS involves using symptoms, signs, demographic medical risk, and diagnostic testing to determine whether ACS physiology is occurring at the level of the coronary artery.

Evaluating Patients for Myocardial Ischemia: The ROMI Workup

The term *risk stratification* is used broadly in discussing the evaluation of ACS patients. This process is often called the rule out myocardial ischemia (ROMI) workup. Its diagnostic decision steps are listed in Table 3-1. In this section, we discuss the use of cardiac biomarkers and cardiac imaging in the context of these steps.

We will take two patients with us through this chapter.

CASE ONE

This patient is a 35-year-old male smoker with a history of untreated hypertension but no known CAD. He is brought in complaining of stabbing left-sided chest pain. His pain was nonpleuritic and nonradiating, lasted 20 minutes, and resolved before arrival. He had called an ambulance and the paramedics reported normal vital signs en route and an unremarkable electrocardiogram (ECG).

CASE TWO

This patient is an 84-year-old woman with a history of diabetes, hypertension, chronic obstructive pulmonary disease (COPD), stroke, myocardial infarction (MI) with stent placement, and mild systolic heart failure. She arrives looking uncomfortable and complaining of shortness of breath that had started earlier that day. For the past 2 days, she has experienced chest pressure that radiates to her left shoulder. On her review of systems, she mentions nausea and dizziness. She called 911, and the paramedics, on arrival, noted that her ECG showed T-wave inversion in leads V_1, V_2, and V_3 (Figure 3-1).

Identifying Myocardial Infarction: STEMI and NSTEMI

The first step in the assessment of patients with chest pain involves the identification of MI as STEMI or NSTEMI. STEMI is diagnosed via an early screening ECG (obtained <10 minutes after arrival). This early diagnosis identifies patients best served with emergent thrombolysis or percutaneous coronary intervention (PCI). The ECG may also be helpful in the early identification of NSTEMI and unstable angina when diagnostic ST-segment depressions and/or T-wave inversions in a coronary artery distribution are present. These findings suggest a culprit lesion causing ischemia in coronary artery territory. However, NSTEMI can occur even when the ECG is normal; therefore, a screening ECG is followed by measurement of cardiac biomarkers to identify biochemical evidence of MI.

Identifying Myocardial Ischemia

In a stable patient for whom there is reasonable concern for ACS, whose screening ECG is nondiagnostic, and whose initial serum troponin level is normal, it is imperative to continue to monitor for evolving signs of myocardial ischemia and obtain serial assessments of biochemical markers. This phase of care can be done through a prolonged emergency department stay, in a dedicated chest pain or observation unit, during an inhospital stay, or with out-of-hospital followup. The decision regarding the location for the monitoring depends on the risk for future MI, institutional resources, and the patient's access to followup care. The goal is to find signs of a flow-limiting lesion. This involves coronary imaging that directly looks at the coronary vasculature for evidence of significant CAD or cardiac tissue findings suggestive of epicardial coronary artery

TABLE 3-1.

Phases of Evaluating the Patient with Symptoms Suggesting ACS

Early identification of STEMI for reperfusion therapy (fibrinolytics versus percutaneous coronary intervention)
Early identification of NSTEMI with cardiac biomarkers
ACS risk stratification to determine the most appropriate location for continued care
Identification of NSTEMI versus UNSTABLE ANGINA versus alternative diagnosis with repeat cardiac biomarkers, provocative testing, and/or coronary imaging
Risk stratification for future ACS events, given the presence of CAD or CAD risk factors or the potential for recurrence of the symptoms that prompted an ACS workup (which might need to be repeated in the future)
Outpatient referral for screening and management of CAD risk factors

flow limitations such as wall motion abnormalities, myocardial tissue perfusion deficiencies, and myocardial edema.

Patients who complete the diagnostic evaluation without evidence of MI or ischemia should be referred to an outpatient care provider for risk factor screening and/or management. The decision pathway for testing patients with potential ACS is summarized in Figure 3-2.[6]

KEY POINTS

The ROMI workup involves screening for MI and myocardial ischemia and then referring patients for ACS risk-factor management.

Diagnostic tools used for this workup include ECG, cardiac biomarkers, and cardiac/coronary imaging.

Cardiac biomarkers are used to detect MI.

Imaging is used to identify the location of a flow-limiting lesion where ACS physiology may be taking place. Imaging evaluates for the presence of 1) wall motion abnormalities, 2) inducible myocardial tissue perfusion deficiencies, or 3) culprit CAD lesions.

CASE ONE CONTINUED

This patient's risk factors for CAD are hypertension and smoking. He has never been identified as having CAD, and his symptoms are atypical. The first steps in his evaluation are to obtain an ECG within 10 minutes of his arrival and to establish intravenous access. The ECG showed no signs of STEMI, is identical to the ECG obtained by the paramedics, and shows no ST or T-wave changes. As his nurse secures the intravenous line, she explains that she is drawing a blood sample to test for cardiac biomarkers.

CASE TWO CONTINUED

This elderly woman has many risk factors for CAD. But, more importantly, she has established CAD, as evidenced by her previous MI and stent placement. She falls into a demographic group at high risk for CAD. Her symptoms are more typical than those of the patient in Case One, but she has many competing diagnoses to consider, such as a COPD flare, exacerbation of heart failure, occult pneumonia, and pulmonary embolism. An ECG from a previous visit is obtained and compared with the ECG obtained during today's assessment. They show the same T-wave inversion, more prominent on the current tracing than on the older one. An intravenous line is inserted, and a blood sample is sent for cardiac biomarker testing.

Cardiac Biomarkers for Myocardial Infarction

Troponin is the definitive biomarker for MI, but it is not the only one in clinical use.[7,8] All currently available cardiac biomarkers are screening assays for MI by way of their ability to detect signs of myocardial injury. Their specificity for myocardial ischemia depends on the clinical context of the patient being tested. These laboratory assays detect proteins expressed into the blood serum as a result of myocardial cell death or necrosis. The proteins are components of intracellular contents released when the myocyte wall ruptures. These components leak into the myocardial tissue interstitium and then travel through the lymphatic system and eventually into the blood, where they can

FIGURE 3-1.

ECG of patient in Case Two. Image courtesy of Chadwick Miller, MD, Wake Forest University.

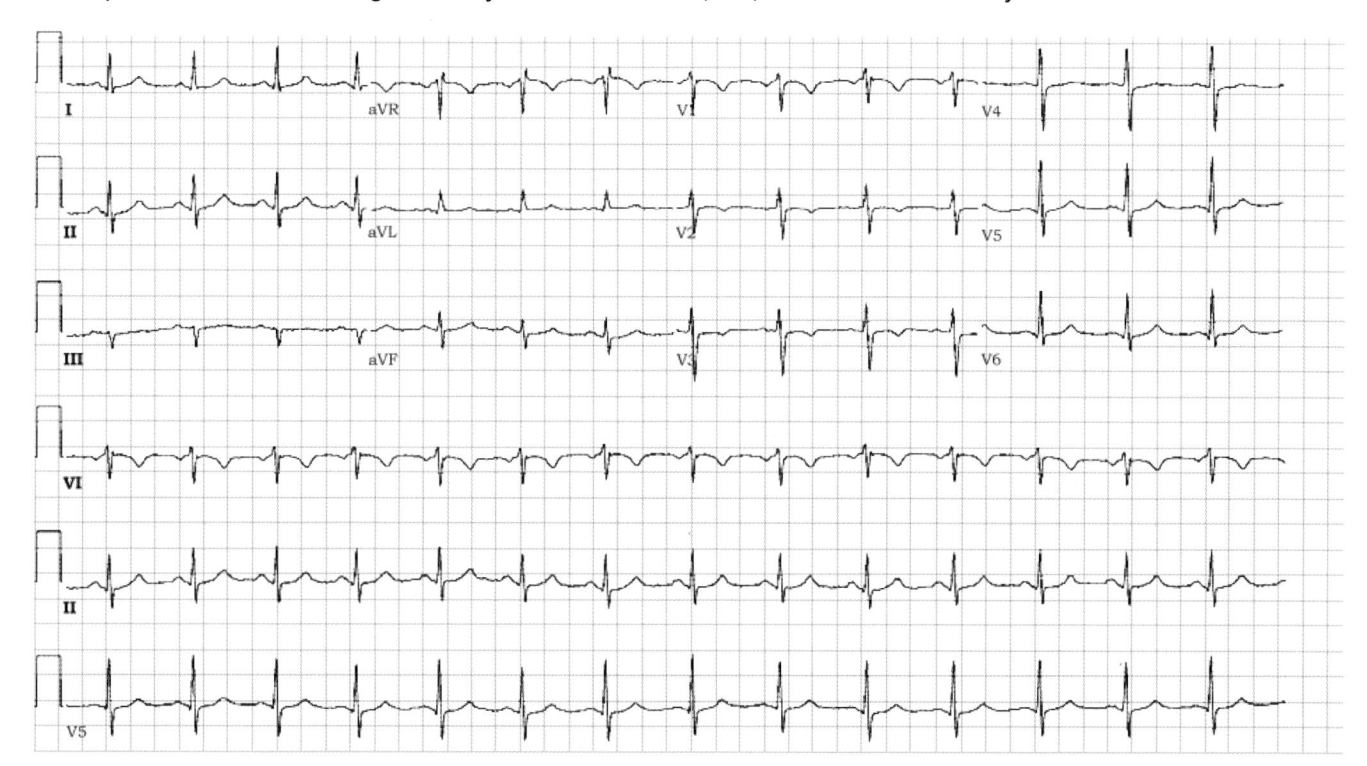

be detected with serologic testing. In the setting of suspected ACS, myocardial injury can be attributed to ischemia.[9,10]

The European Society of Cardiology and the American College of Cardiology developed a universal definition of MI, which is the international standard for diagnosing MI. For acute presentations, it requires a rise or fall of cardiac biomarkers, with at least one value being above the 99% upper reference limit, along with one of the following observations: 1) symptoms of ischemia, 2) ECG findings of new ST-segment or T-wave abnormalities or a new left bundle-branch block, 3) the development of pathologic Q waves, 4) imaging evidence of acute loss of previously viable myocardium or new regional wall motion abnormalities, and 5) the identification of coronary thrombus with angiography or at autopsy.[10-13]

KEY POINTS

Troponin is the definitive biomarker for MI.

All currently available cardiac biomarkers are screening assays for MI by way of their ability to detect the signs of myocardial injury.

The proteins detected by biomarker assays are components of intracellular contents released when the myocyte wall ruptures.

The assays' specificity for myocardial ischemia resulting from ACS depends on the clinical context of the patient being tested.

FIGURE 3-2.

Decision algorithm for initial diagnostic testing for ACS

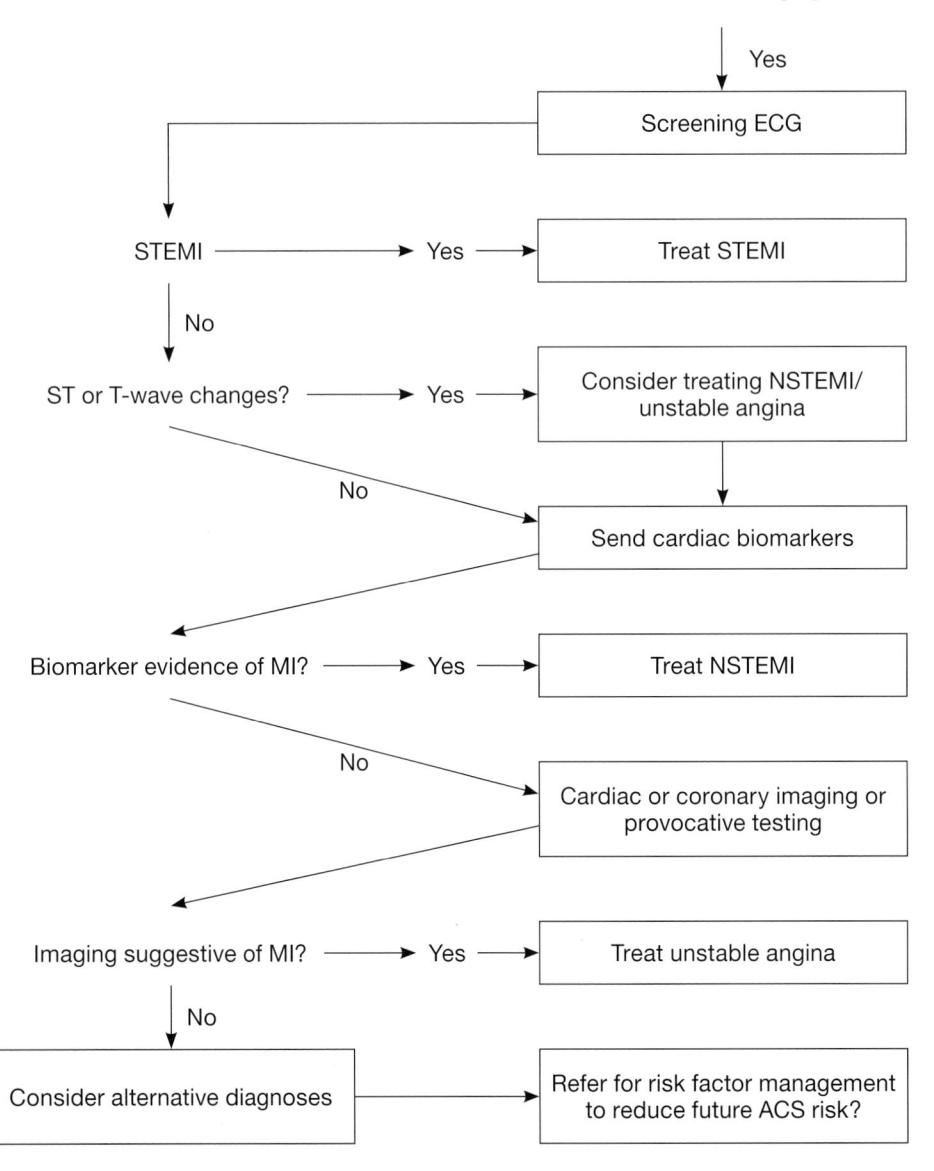

The Evolution of Cardiac Biomarkers

Creatine Phosphokinase

In the 1960s, creatine phosphokinase (CPK or CK) was found to be a myocyte-specific enzyme released during muscle necrosis. CK, a heme protein in red blood cells and muscle cell, is involved in the storage and transportation of oxygen. It is located in the cytosol of myocardial cells and therefore is released into the circulation relatively early compared with the previously used biomarkers—lactate dehydrogenase, aspartate transaminase, and myoglobin. It can be detected in serum as early as 3 to 8 hours after cardiac injury. Its concentration peaks in 10 to 24 hours and then normalizes within 3 days.[14-17] By the end of the decade, measures of total CK were used as a rapid test to help with the diagnosis of MI. However, elevations are also associated with exercise, intramuscular injection, major surgeries, hypothyroidism, rhabdomyolysis, and hypermetabolic states.[18]

By the 1970s, organ-predominant isoenzymes were identified. CK-MB was found to be not only myocyte specific but also cardiac predominant. Its serum detectability and duration were similar to those of total CK, except levels normalize closer to 4 days rather than 3. It was found that a ratio of CK-MB to total CK of more than 5% was highly suggestive of MI. Also helpful was CK-MB's higher serum peak level and rapid clearance, which made it possible to repeat measurements within 3 to 6 hours after an initially elevated level is detected (a delta CK-MB:CK ratio) to assist with the detection of an acute event.

In 1976, the World Health Organization compiled criteria for the identification of MI, which required the presence of two of the following three features: symptoms of myocardial ischemia (continuous chest pain for 20 minutes), ECG changes with ST-segment elevation or Q-wave development, and elevation of sensitive and specific cardiac biomarkers. The combination of clinical presentation, ECG findings, and cardiac biomarkers for the diagnosis of MI is still used today.[10]

Until the late 1980s, CK was the gold standard biomarker for MI. Then a highly sensitive monoclonal antibody assay was developed that dramatically improved the sensitivity and ease of testing, increasing its utility for the acutely symptomatic patient. Along with our ability to detect myocardial ischemia, major advances occurred in our ability to treat myocardial ischemia and the associated coronary lesions. These improvements heightened the need to make the diagnosis early and accurately. The new CK-MB and CK assays increased the sensitivity of our detection but they demonstrated markedly reduced specificity, increasing the number of false-positive tests. With a need to balance the risks and benefits of emerging antiplatelet, antithrombotic therapies along with PCI, limited sensitivity challenged the use of the CK-MB:CK ratio as a diagnostic test for MI.

Cardiac Troponins

The search was on for a similarly sensitive but more specific marker. Cardiac-specific troponin assays stepped into this void,

FIGURE 3-3.

The kinetics of biomarker elevation. From: French JK, White HD. Clinical implications of the new definition of myocardial infarction. *Heart.* 2004;90(1):99-106. Used with permission.

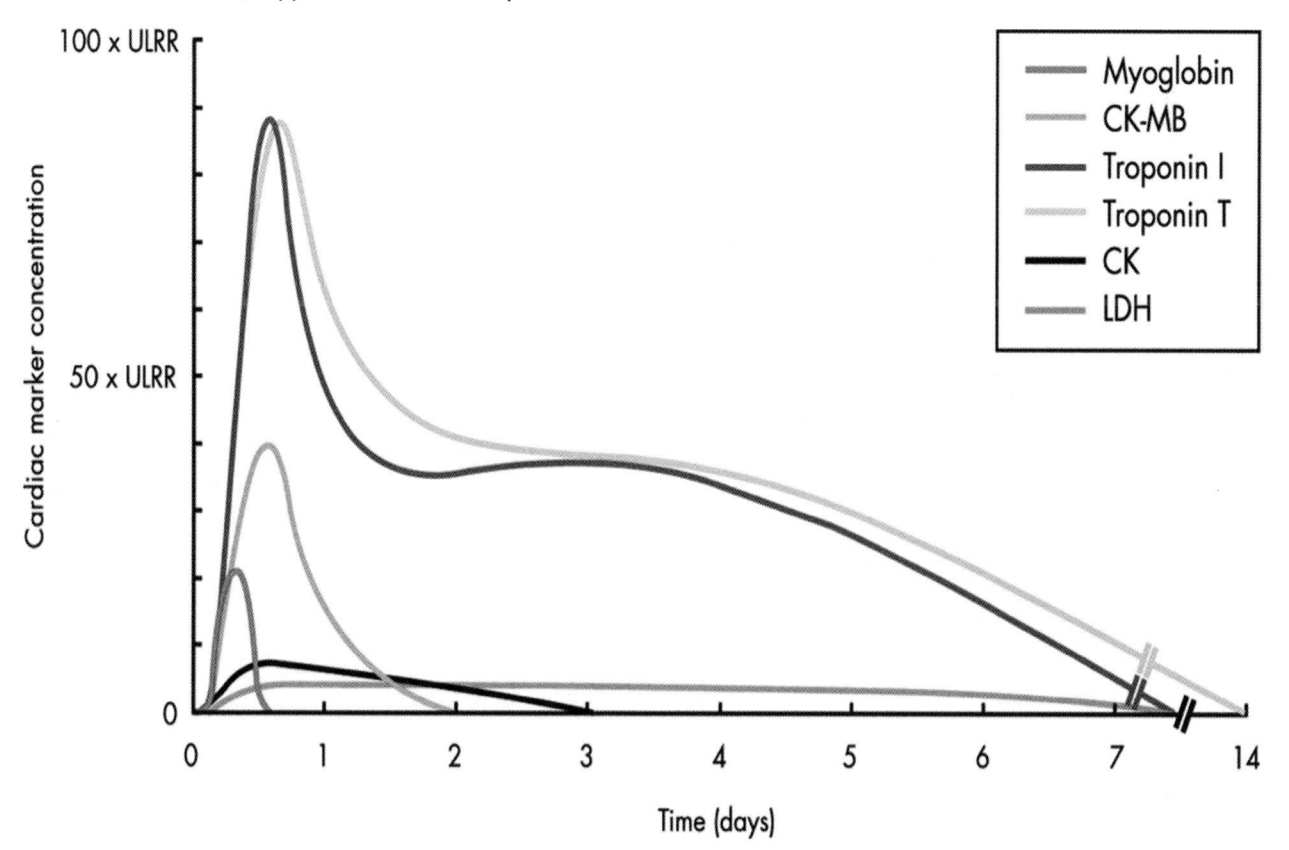

providing a more sensitive and specific test for myocardial injury. The first commercial assays became available in 1997. In 2000, the European Society of Cardiology updated the World Health Organization definition by making the diagnosis of most cases dependent on an elevated serum troponin level. Serum assays are monoclonal antibodies that have little cross reactivity with troponins from skeletal muscle.[9] Cardiac troponins demonstrate a biphasic elevation in the setting of myocardial ischemia, with the detection of small quantities in the cytosol released soon after cell wall rupture.[19,20,]

Initial assays allowed detection of troponin as early as 3 to 6 hours from the onset of coronary artery myocyte death or myocardial tissue necrosis, with levels normalizing in 4 to 14 days. Serum levels demonstrate a double peak over time, the first occurring at 10 to 24 hours. The second peak occurs at 72 to 96 hours after the start of infarction and is due to the delayed release of muscle protein, which continues to break down after myocyte death. Serial samples are highly sensitive for the early detection of myocardial injury. There is nearly a linear correlation between the troponin level and the risk for cardiac events and death. Elevations can reflect the time since infarction; however, they do not necessarily reflect infarct size.[21] The relative onset, peaks, and serum clearance of these biomarkers are illustrated in Figure 3-3.

Troponin is a protein component of the actin and myosin mechanism that produces muscle contraction. It consists of three subunits: troponin I (TnI), troponin T (TnT), and troponin C (TnC). Troponin I and T are detected with current assays. They are expressed by a cardiac-specific gene, yielding high sensitivity and specificity for these "cardiac troponins" (cTn). Cardiac troponins are not typically detected in the serum of healthy individuals, making it easier to establish specific cutoffs. However, the variety of cTnI assays can lead to different levels for a "positive test" in order to maintain comparable sensitivities. This should be kept in mind when comparing positive TnI results across institutions.[21-23]

Troponin assays have progressed through several generations to impressive levels of analytic and clinical sensitivity.[24] The ability to detect smaller levels of serum troponin allows clinicians to now classify more patients traditionally diagnosed with unstable angina as having MI. Several studies have shown contemporary and future-generation TnI and TnT assays to have sensitivities of approximately 95%, with the initial troponin drawn on arrival alone, regardless of the prehospital time of symptom onset. With future-generation assays, this clinical sensitivity could be even higher. This enhanced ability to detect serum troponin comes at the expense of clinical specificity, so that more patients are classified as having an elevated serum troponin but do not have physiologic changes of ACS at the level of the coronary artery. As more sensitive troponin assays become available, the most effective method of integrating these assays will need to be informed by further studies.[25-28]

The sensitivities and specificities of the cardiac biomarkers discussed in this section are compared in Table 3-2. Given the performance of troponin in comparison with the other markers, it is clear why it is now the gold standard for the detection of myocardial injury as evidence of MI.[16,23,27,28]

Most troponin testing in emergency medicine is done to rule out the presence of myocardial injury caused by ACS. When patients have a positive troponin result or have signs highly suspicious for MI, it is easy to commit to additional testing and time. However, fewer than 15% of patients evaluated for ACS in emergency departments ultimately have a positive test result.[29,30] The traditional interval—the time from symptom onset or emergency department arrival—for ruling out MI from ACS has been 6 hours.[31] However, since the 1990s, troponin assays have become far more sensitive and specific. More recent studies on the biochemical availability of troponin subunits in blood serum suggest that 3 hours between the initial troponin measurement and the second draw to assess a delta troponin is an appropriate time frame in which to identify myocardial injury. This practice is supported by clinical studies following cohorts to diagnosis and guidelines endorsed by the European Science Council and American College of Cardiology for NSTEMI and unstable angina.[32-35]

In the setting of an ACS evaluation, an elevation in the troponin level is presumed to be from ischemia until proved otherwise. However, myocyte loss can have many causes, including heart failure, sheer forces, and reduced renal clearance. Studies with highly sensitive troponin T assays have found that the positive predictive value of a positive test has ranged from 38% to 98%.[36-39] Therefore, a positive test must be interpreted within the appropriate context. The likelihood of ACS as the cause of the elevation is highly driven by the pretest probability. Of significant value to the emergency care provider is the negative predictive value, a measure of the test's infarction "rule out" capability, which has been demonstrated to be 96% to 99%.[36-42] It is important to remember that the troponin test does not rule out unstable angina or account for unstable angina that evolves into infarction. Patients who are at risk for ischemia and have suggestive symptoms should undergo provocative testing or coronary imaging.

TABLE 3-2.

Sensitivities and Specificities of Cardiac Biomarkers for Acute MI as a Cause of Myocardial Injury

Biomarker	Time to Detection	Sensitivity	Specificity
CK	6 to 8 hr	94%	57%
CK-MB:CK ratio	6 to 8 hr	90.7%	99.6%
Troponin	2 to 6 hr	94% to 96%	97% to 99%

The Multi-Marker Approach

Multi-marker approaches have been marginally successful in the diagnosis of ACS. The potential for a synergistic combination of markers is appealing; however, these approaches are hampered by low accuracy. As troponin assays have become more sensitive, the utility of multi-marker approaches has diminished.[20,27,28]

Emerging Cardiac Biomarkers

The clinical utility of several emerging biomarkers is still under investigation.[17,27,28] Cardiac albumin, also referred to as ischemia-modified albumin, is detectable in serum soon after transient coronary occlusion. This modified form results from a change in the amino terminus of the molecule, which reduces the capacity of albumin to bind cobalt during ischemia. The level rises well before that of CK-MB, cTn, and even myoglobin. The discovery of this biomarker introduced a test that has the potential to detect early *ischemia* in addition to infarction. Early studies have shown promise but have been too small to demonstrate generalizable results.[43-45]

B-type natriuretic peptide (BNP) is a neurohormone released from cardiac myocyte stretch as proBNP. ProBNP is cleaved to the N-terminal proBNP (NT-proBNP), then to BNP. Measurements of proBNP and NT-proBNP are widely used markers in the diagnosis of decompensated heart failure. They also have good predictive power for recurrent ACS events, cardiac-related death, and coexisting acute decompensated heart failure. When measured at first contact, BNP can be a strong predictor of short- and long-term mortality in patients who receive a final diagnosis ACS.[46,47]

C-reactive protein (CRP) and highly sensitive CRP are acute-phase inflammatory reactants. They have been shown to be useful for the long-term prognosis for cardiac events in healthy patients. Studies are underway to investigate their potential short-term prognostic value in patients being evaluated for ACS.[48-50]

Biomarker Summary

Troponin is the biomarker of choice for determining whether patients have myocardial injury and necrosis. Current guidelines recommend that serial troponin measurements should be obtained at a time interval that places the last measurement 6 to 8 hours from symptom onset. Practically, the time lapse between symptom onset and measurement of the first troponin is generally more than 2 hours. Therefore, the practice of obtaining serial measurements of troponin at arrival, 3 hours after arrival, and 6 hours after arrival has been widely adopted.[34] Present data suggest that a 3-hour sampling time interval for the newer-generation troponin assays (ultrasensitive cTnI or highly sensitive TnT) is reasonable clinical practice. Medical care providers should consider the time of symptom onset when implementing shorter time intervals for biomarker testing. A negative troponin result measured with a newer generation assay 3 hours after presentation, and without a significant change from the first measurement, makes MI unlikely as the cause of the patient's symptoms. A negative troponin result obtained 6 hours after arrival has a high negative predictive value for MI as the cause of the symptoms. However, these time intervals are unreliable in patients with worsening or stuttering symptoms, as patients initially presenting with unstable angina could convert to MI at any time. Guidelines do not support the routine use of markers such as CK or CK-MB in addition to troponin.[20,27,28]

KEY POINTS

CK-MB is a cardiac-specific biomarker when measured with a total CK to calculate the CK-MB:CK ratio. A ratio of more than 5% suggests MI but is not as sensitive or specific as a troponin assay.

Cardiac troponins, including troponin T and I assays, are the gold standard for detection of MI.

The negative predictive value of ultrasensitive troponin I and highly sensitive troponin T assays is 38% to 96%.

The use of 6-hour "delta troponin" intervals is common practice. With the use of current ultrasensitive troponin I and the highly sensitive troponin T assays, a 3-hour sampling interval for low-risk patients is reasonable practice.

Clinical Decision Aids

Pertinent to the practice of emergency medicine is the identification of patients who require an evaluation for ACS. Recent approaches to assist with this decision-making process are discussed in this section. They are in various stages of validation; results to date are promising. It is important to note that the studies conducted so far have been retrospective or prospective observational. These clinical decision aids have not been investigated prospectively as interventions. In the absence of prospective data and validation, these decision aids should be implemented only after careful consideration in the context of local practice norms, and they should be used with quality assurance monitoring.

The emerging decision aids use abbreviated workups to distinguish patients who can be discharged safely without stress testing or coronary/cardiac imaging from those in need of further evaluation. The goal is to make this assessment within a 2- to 4-hour timeframe. The themes of the clinical decision aids are the need to incorporate one or two troponin measurements, ECG findings, and some component of clinical features. The troponin assessments are used to detect patients with MI. The clinical features and ECG findings are used to identify patients with a higher likelihood of having unstable angina, who might benefit from stress testing. For these approaches to be accepted in the United States, the diagnostic process must miss less than 1% of ACS events while maximizing the proportion of patients identified for early discharge from the emergency department.[28]

Accelerated Diagnostic Protocol

The accelerated diagnostic protocol (ADP) was developed and has been validated in an observational setting. It is the most studied of the decision aid options. Originally, it used two multimarker point-of-care biomarker measurements obtained at 0 and 120 minutes from arrival in the emergency department, ECG findings of ischemia, and the TIMI risk score to identify patients for early discharge.[50] This protocol was able to identify only 10% of enrolled patients as eligible for early discharge. A revision of the ADP, published in 2012, replaced the multimarker measurements with troponin testing.[51] This change increased the proportion of enrolled patients who were identified for early discharge. Of 1,975 patients, 302 (15.3%) had an adverse cardiac event. The ADP classified 392 patients (20%) as low risk, one of whom (0.25%) had an adverse event. The ADP showed a sensitivity of 99.7% and a negative predictive value of 99.7%. According to the revised ADP, patients with a normal ECG, non-elevated contemporary troponin measurements (at 0 and 120 minutes), and a TIMI risk score of 0 have less than a 1% risk of ACS.[52] Further study is needed to determine the safety and efficiency of the ADP when used in real-time clinical practice.

The HEART Pathway

The HEART pathway is a tool for predicting and managing the risk of MI. It combines elements of the patient's history, ECG, age, and risk factors to create an integer-based scoring system. It was originally called The HEART Score and demonstrated an event rate (MI, death, need for percutaneous transluminal coronary angioplasty) of 1% to 1.7% in patients with a low-risk HEART score.[53,54] It was subsequently modified with the addition of troponin measurements at 0 and 3 hours to the calculation of the HEART score and renamed the HEART Pathway.[55] The HEART Pathway has achieved better than 99% sensitivity and identified 20% of patients for early discharge.[56] These findings are promising but are yet to be published from a prospective clinical trial.

The North American Chest Pain Rule

The North American Chest Pain Rule is a risk-stratification tool used to identify patients at low risk of ACS, who are safe for discharge home. It includes five outcome predictors: age, history of CAD, quality of ACS symptoms, ECG, and a 6-hour troponin measurement. It has been found to be more than 99% sensitive and 21% specific, identifying 11% of patients evaluated as safe for discharge from the emergency department. One retrospective validation suggested that this rule has lower specificity than the HEART Pathway.[56] These findings have yet to be tested in a prospective clinical trial.

Vancouver Chest Pain Rule

The Vancouver Chest Pain Rule is a decision aid that comprises historical features, ECG results, and biomarker measurements. It is also designed to identify low-risk patients safe for early discharge. The Vancouver rule is different from the other decision-making tools in that it considers all patients younger than 40 years old with a normal ECG and no history of ischemic heart disease to be low risk and incorporates CK-MB results. The derivation of the rule demonstrated 98.8% sensitivity; however, recent validation attempts did not yield similar results. One validation in Iran resulted in 95% sensitivity.[57] Another study removed CK-MB results and used troponin as the sole biomarker, revealing 91% sensitivity.[58] Without additional data or adaptations, the use of the Vancouver Chest Pain Rule cannot be recommended.

KEY POINT

The ADP and the HEART Pathway are useful emergency medicine decision aids that help identify patients requiring a cardiac evaluation. These decision aids generally are able to make this assessment in a 2- to 3-hour timeframe. Common elements of these clinical decision aids include the need for one or two troponin measurements, clinical features, and ECG findings.

TABLE 3-3.

Cardiac and Coronary Imaging Modalities to Identify CAD in Patients Being Evaluated for ACS

	Findings	Sensitivity	Specificity	Limitations
Exercise treadmill testing	Ischemic ECG changes with increasing myocardial work	66% to 71%	80%	Unable to walk Abnormal ECG
Resting echocardiography	Wall motion abnormalities in a patient with active symptoms	87% to 92%	85% to 94%	Chest wall deformity Obesity Emphysema
Stress echocardiography	Wall motion abnormalities induced by increasing myocardial work	61% to 97%	51% to 94%	Chest wall deformity Obesity Emphysema Pharmacologic stress agent risk
Calcium scoring CT	Calcified obstructive CAD or other CAD lesions	79% to 95%	66% to 75%	Radiation exposure, 3 mSv Beta-blocker use needed
CCTA (64-slice CT scanner)	Obstructive (and nonobstructive) CAD lesions of varied composition Coronary artery perfusion	94%	97% to 100%	Radiation exposure, 12 mSv Intravenous contrast dye exposure Beta-blocker use needed
Methoxyisobutyl isonitrile-SPECT (rNPI)	Myocardial tissue perfusion deficits	87% to 93%	70% to 90%	Exposure to a radionuclear isotope Pharmacologic stress agent risk Claustrophobia

CASE ONE CONTINUED

According to these decision rules, this man is a good candidate for early discharge. He is young, his symptoms are atypical for ACS, he has no established CAD, his ECG was normal, and his initial troponin test result was negative. His doctor requests a second troponin measurement at 120 minutes, and it was also negative. The patient remains pain free in the emergency department. He has a primary care physician who could coordinate testing for obstructive CAD risk stratification via a stress test or coronary computed tomography angiography (CCTA). In addition, the patient and his physician need to discuss how to better control his hypertension. The emergency department has a means of following up on discharged patients' outcomes, so his physician considers discharging him home.

CASE TWO CONTINUED

According to these protocols, this patient is not a good candidate for discharge. She has many symptoms and features in her history that put her at high risk for mortality and morbidity, regardless of the cause of her symptoms. Within the differential diagnosis for her presentation, she is at high risk for ACS. She needs inpatient testing, treatment, and monitoring. Her initial troponin was negative, a repeat ECG was unchanged, and her shortness of breath resolved with two 0.4-mcg sublingual nitroglycerin tablets. She was eventually admitted to the hospital.

Acute Coronary Syndrome Risk Stratification

Current guidelines from the American College of Cardiology and the American Heart Association recommend stress testing or cardiac imaging as a key component of the evaluation of patients with possible ACS. The ACS diagnosis includes patients with unstable angina who have presentations that place them at risk for ACS but whose screening troponin levels are normal. A comprehensive evaluation for these patients requires investigation beyond biomarkers. One objective of ACS risk-stratification protocols just discussed is to identify very low-risk patients who do not require further imaging; these tools are still in the derivation/validation process. Stress testing is commonly performed during the index visit; however, outpatient stress testing within 72 hours is acceptable in low-risk patients with normal serial troponin results, with no ECG changes diagnostic of ACS, and with no pain.[33]

Myocardial ischemia is suspected when aberrations in myocardial hemodynamics and tissue perfusion are observed on cardiac imaging studies. Several cardiac and coronary imaging modalities can help with the evaluation of ischemia when troponin assays are not elevated. These tools answer three questions, as follows:

1. Are any structural or functional abnormalities present in the heart? (echocardiography, stress echocardiography)
2. Is CAD present? (CCTA, invasive coronary angiography)
3. Are there signs of limited myocardial perfusion? (stress radionuclide myocardial perfusion imaging [rMPI], cardiac magnetic resonance [CMR] imaging)

Selection of a particular stress test or imaging modality depends on institutional resources and patient attributes. Within an institution, expertise is generally focused on a limited number of cardiac testing modalities, commonly exercise treadmill testing, stress echocardiography, and stress rMPI. In choosing a test for a patient, remember that no one test is best for everyone. It is important to consider the patient's pretest probability for ACS, potential exposures inherent in the tests (eg, exercise, radiation, applying pressure to the chest), conduction abnormalities, and previous cardiac injury (Table 3-3).

Imaging Tests of Structure and Function

These tests include rMPI and echocardiography and might be of value in the evaluation of patients who have persistent or very recent symptoms suggestive of ACS, a nondiagnostic ECG, and initially negative cardiac enzyme measurements. They are performed at rest and provide information about the anatomic and dynamic function of the heart. Patients whose chest pain has resolved are more likely to require stress testing.

Resting Echocardiogram

An echocardiogram uses ultrasound waves to create structural images of a patient's heart anatomy, including chamber size, wall thickness, and shape. Transthoracic echocardiography is a dynamic imaging modality that records still images and video to provide details on the heart's pump capacity and function, as measured by cardiac output or ejection fraction (Figure 3-4). It is often used to screen for segmental areas of hypokinetic wall motion as a sign of ischemic myocardial tissue when evidence of NSTEMI is not seen on the ECG or if cardiac markers are not elevated. Severe ischemia produces regional wall motion abnormalities that can be visualized within 12 to 20 seconds after coronary artery occlusion. This occurs prior to the onset of ECG changes and the development of symptoms and can persist for hours following resolution of active ischemia. Ultrasound waves convey no radiation exposure. Image quality is operator dependent and limited by poor acoustic windows, as occurs in

FIGURE 3-4.

Echo apical four-chambered view. Image courtesy of Deepak Gupta, MD, Vanderbilt University Medical Center.

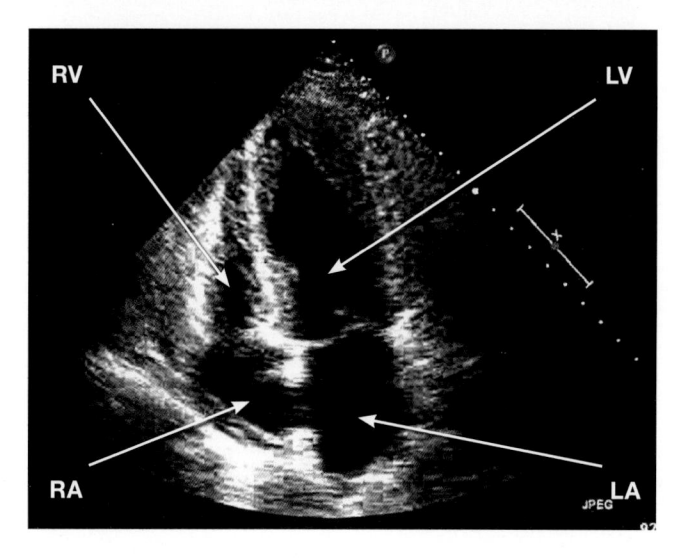

patients who have COPD or are obese. Studies examining the sensitivity and specificity of resting cardiac echocardiography for ACS have been small and limited; however, both are markedly increased (to >90%) in the setting of active symptoms. The role of resting echocardiography in the evaluation of patients for ACS is limited to acquiring information about alternative diagnoses, such as cardiomyopathy and valvular disease and, importantly, the identification of segmental wall motion abnormalities in patients with ongoing symptoms. Without a physiologic stress component, resting echocardiography is limited in its ability to identify clinically significant CAD in patients who are not actively symptomatic.[59-62]

Resting Radionuclide Perfusion Imaging

rMPI involves the use of an injectable radioisotope to image myocardial perfusion at the time of injection. Patients with ongoing symptoms of ischemia are injected at rest with a radioisotope, commonly technetium-99, and images are obtained to characterize resting myocardial perfusion. A patient who is found to have normal perfusion and normal cardiac biomarkers is at low risk for adverse cardiac events (Figure 3-5). Determining whether perfusion defects are new or old can require additional imaging and data such as resting imaging after symptoms abate, and consideration of serum troponin results. Stress rMPI, discussed later in this chapter, is needed in patients who come to the emergency department after their symptoms have resolved.[63,64]

Is There Coronary Artery Disease?

Calcium Scoring Coronary Computed Tomography

Calcium scoring coronary computed tomography (CT) noninvasively visualizes the wall composition of the coronary arteries. Most patients must be beta-blocked to a heart rate of less than 65 beats/min to get appropriately gated images. The scan assesses a patient's overall plaque burden to categorize cardiovascular risk based on age and gender. This scan is often done as the first phase of CCTA. A calcium score of 0 indicates that there is little or no calcified CAD. The absence of calcium deposition lowers the likelihood of ACS. Calcium scoring CTs are most helpful for ROMI patients when the calcium score is low, because the likelihood of ACS is low in the absence of significant CAD. However, it is well acknowledged that soft plaque can cause ACS and might not be associated with an elevated calcium score. Recent studies suggest that less-calcified plaques, which have a proportionately larger lipid core, are more vulnerable to rupture and more likely to lead to the development of occlusive thrombi.[66] The precise role for coronary CT

FIGURE 3-5.

Radionuclide perfusion imaging of a normal heart (top) and ischemic heart (bottom). Image courtesy of Deepak Gupta, MD, Vanderbilt University Medical Center.

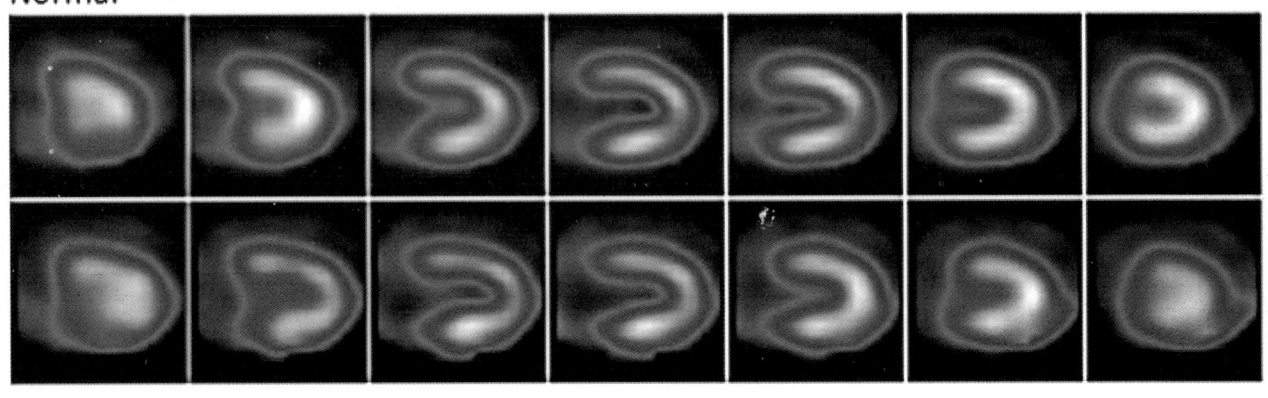

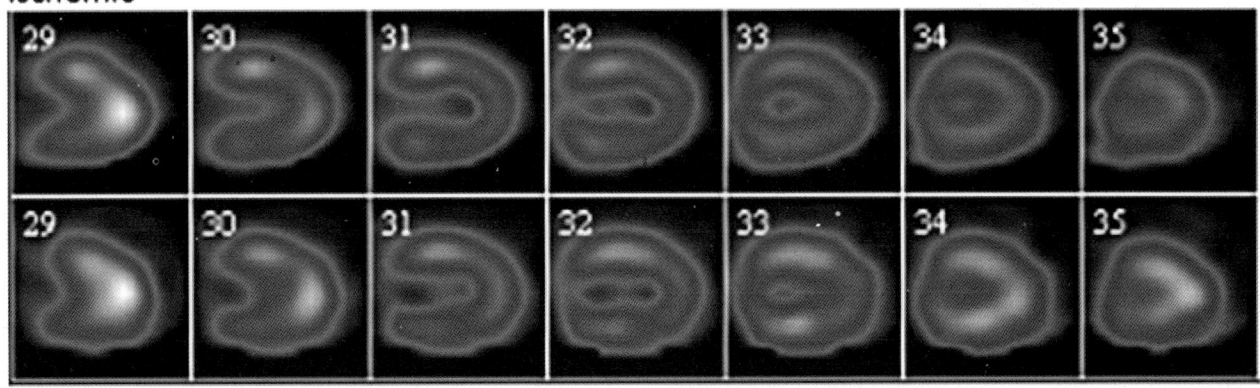

Acute Coronary Syndrome: Biomarkers and Imaging

in ruling out ACS remains under investigation, but it is a useful adjunct in screening low-risk patients. The radiation exposure from CCTA is approximately 3 mSv, the amount of natural background radiation to which the average person is exposed in 1 year.[67-69]

Coronary Computed Tomography Angiography

High-resolution CCTA is the best noninvasive means of performing coronary angiography. It adds information to the calcium score because CAD plaques within the inner lining of the arteries are made of fat and cholesterol in addition to calcium. These materials can produce luminal narrowing or positive remodeling (outward growth) that is not visualized on calcium scoring CT. An injection of intravenous contrast dye is timed to perfuse the coronary vessels. This allows visualization of any narrowing, obstruction, or luminal irregularity that could produce ischemia (Figure 3-6). CCTA is challenging in patients with a high calcium score and those who cannot tolerate beta-blockade to achieve a heart rate less than 65 beats/min. CCTA can identify the presence and extent of CAD in 83% to 94% of patients.[69-72] Two randomized clinical trials supported the adoption of a CCTA-based testing strategy. Litt and colleagues demonstrated that emergency department patients with less than 50% coronary stenosis revealed by CCTA have less than a 1% rate of death or MI at 30 days.[67] Hoffman and colleagues also demonstrated a CCTA strategy to be safe and reduce length of stay. However, patients randomized to CCTA had higher radiation exposure and more downstream testing.[68] The results are most helpful for ROMI patients when they reveal an absence of lumen narrowing or evidence of CAD lesions. These patients are typically younger, a population in which radiation exposure is of reasonable concern. Because CCTA is often obtained in conjunction with a preceding calcium scoring CT, the patient receives two phases of radiation exposure, and this practice is being questioned. Conventional CCTA delivers 10 to 15 mSv.[70-76] Low-dose radiation protocols are being widely adopted for imaging in carefully selected patients, using radiation doses ranging from 3 to 8 mSv, with some as low as 1 mSv.

Although standard CCTA does not provide information about tissue perfusion, inference can be made by correlating ECG findings with significant lesions. The presence of CAD can also identify a higher risk patient who might benefit from further testing. The mere presence of CAD does not imply that the patient's chest pain was cardiac in origin unless the location of the lesion correlates with findings on the ECG. This can drive the need for stress testing after CCTA, as shown in the Hoffman study discussed above. In summary, the primary role for CCTA is to exclude CAD in low-risk patients. Factors limiting the adoption of CCTA include concerns about patient risk from radiation exposure and the availability of expertise for obtaining and interpreting CCTA images.

Diagnostic Cardiac Catheterization

Cardiac catheterization with coronary angiography is most frequently considered by emergency physicians as an intervention, when it is used as a means to perform PCI in patients with identified MI. However, diagnostic angiography via cardiac catheterization can be performed as a form of coronary imaging in a patient with a high-risk presentation. It is more invasive than CCTA, as it involves central arterial access through an iliac or radial artery, the use of antithrombotic and antiplatelet agents, and mechanical manipulation of major arteries with a catheter. Altogether, this introduces the risk of vessel perforation and bleeding (intracranial, gastrointestinal, or access site hemorrhage). Angiography of this kind is the gold standard for the diagnosis of CAD. In the emergency department, it is reserved for patients with suspected high-grade obstructive disease or active ACS physiology.

FIGURE 3-6.

Post-contrast CT images of the left anterior descending artery (left) and right cononary artery (right). Both are without obstruction or CAD. Images courtesy of Deepak Gupta, MD, Vanderbilt University Medical Center.

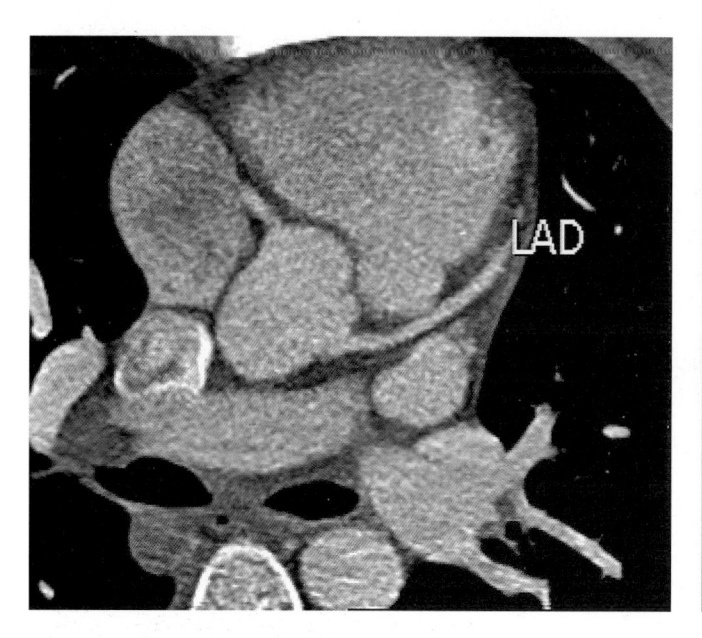

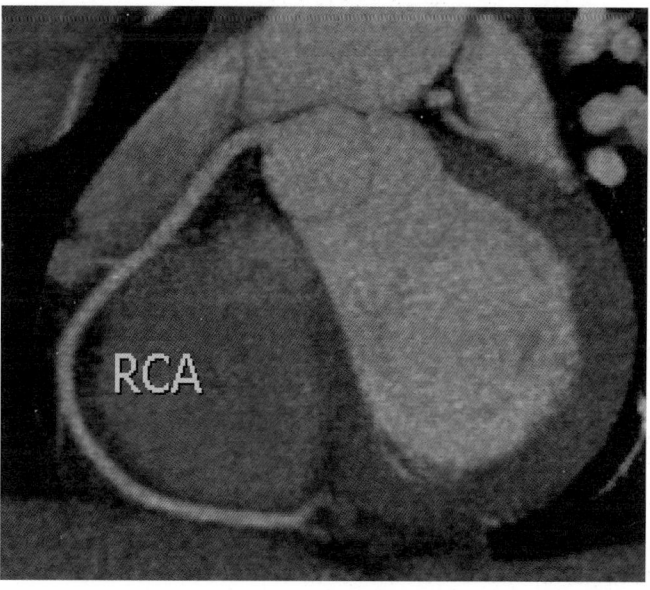

Tissue Perfusion (Provocative Testing)

Tissue perfusion or provocative testing attempts to increase the heart rate and myocardial demand for blood flow to exacerbate flow/perfusion deficits. The goal is to reproduce and image tissue ischemia. The heart rate can be increased by physically challenging the patient on a treadmill or stationary bike or by administering a vasodilator agent such as adenosine or a pharmacologic stress agent such as dobutamine. Each imaging modality has its own means of identifying ischemic tissue changes.

Exercise Treadmill Testing

For exercise treadmill testing, ECG leads are placed on the patient's chest. A running 12-lead tracing is started as the patient begins to walk and eventually run on a treadmill to increase the heart rate and the heart muscle's demand for blood flow. The objective is to identify changes in the ECG with increasing or prolonged myocardial work. Patients undergoing this test must be able to walk and have an ECG without ventricular conduction blocks and with normal ST and T-wave segments.

Exercise treadmill testing is fast and relatively easy to perform, and it exposes the patient to little risk; however, its sensitivity (68%) and specificity (77%) for obstructive CAD are limited. The test's accuracy is lower for women than for men. An alternative should be considered for patients who have a high risk for ACS, whose ECG shows baseline abnormalities, or who are not able to walk. Many medical centers have replaced routine exercise treadmill testing with imaging-based modalities.[29,77-79]

Stress Echocardiography

Using the same cardiac imaging technique as resting echocardiography, stress echocardiography images are obtained before and after the patient exercises or is given a pharmacologic stress agent. Stress echocardiography takes less time than treadmill testing and includes an assessment of valvular function; however, its performance is similarly limited, with a sensitivity of 61% to 97% and a specificity of 51% to 94%.[59-63] Accuracy is reduced in obese patients and in those with tachycardia, emphysema, or chest wall deformities. Inducible ischemia, indicated by a wall motion abnormality with stress, identifies patients who need further evaluation with diagnostic cardiac catheterization and who should be considered for PCI. A normal study reliably identifies patients at low risk for subsequent cardiac events. The risks of this study are generally associated with the pharmacologic stress agents (Table 3-4).[29,60]

Stress Radionuclide Perfusion Imaging

In patients without recent (within 3 to 6 hours) or ongoing ischemic symptoms, stress imaging is used to complement rMPI. After acquisition of resting images, the patient exercises or is given a chemical myocardial challenge agent. Stress images are obtained after injection, and the rest and stress images are compared to identify areas with flow limitations (Figure 3-5). rMPI is more time consuming than other imaging modalities, and it exposes the patient to 15 to 30 mSv of radiation (the effective dose is highly dependent on renal clearance and weight). The results are far less operator dependent than CCTA or echocardiography. When combined with single-photon emission CT (SPECT), the sensitivity of this imaging for significant coronary stenosis is 87% to 93%.[80]

Cardiac Magnetic Resonance Imaging

CMR imaging is an evolving modality that appears well suited for provocative testing of patients at intermediate to high risk for ACS. In one recent large trial, the sensitivity of CMR for significant CAD was shown to be superior to that of SPECT, with similar accuracy.[81] CMR uses conventional principles of magnetic resonance imaging to obtain still images during the stages of the cardiac cycle. These images are then placed in cine loop to create a dynamic clip of myocardial function. The strengths of CMR imaging relate to its ability to get a robust assessment of cardiac structure and function during a single examination.[81,82]

CMR imaging examinations are typically tailored to the ex-

TABLE 3-4.

Pharmacologic Stress Agents—Mechanisms, Risks, and Cautions

	Cardiac Stress Mechanism	Risks	Seek Alternative if History of...
Adenosine	Stimulates coronary artery vasodilation Increases myocardial contractility and oxygen consumption	Bronchospasm	Bronchospasm
Dobutamine	Increases cardiac contractility and cardiac output	Ventricular tachycardia/ventricular fibrillation Increased cardiac rhythm ectopy	Arrhythmia
Dipyridamole (Persantine)	Stimulates coronary artery vasodilation Increases left ventricular contractility	Bronchospasm Bleeding	Bronchospasm
Regadenoson (Lexiscan/RapiScan)	Stimulates coronary artery vasodilation Increases myocardial contractility and oxygen consumption	Bronchospasm	Bronchospasm

pertise available at each center. Components of a CMR examination can include T2-weighted images that assess for myocardial edema, resting wall motion, resting perfusion, stress wall motion, stress perfusion, and delayed enhancement. Substantial advantages of CMR imaging result from the integration of T2 imaging with delayed enhancement. The combination of these components allows the reader to distinguish between new and old infarcts. T2 has also been shown to detect edema, an early sign of ischemia, even before troponin elevation.[82] CMR imaging is also useful in detecting other causes of myocardial pathology, such as myocarditis or toxicity from chemotherapy agents. The additional information provided by CMR is most likely to benefit more complex patients such as those at intermediate to high risk for ACS or those with prior cardiac events. Studies have demonstrated that CMR protocols can be adapted to be an integral component of observation unit care. A recent randomized trial of 752 participants by Greenwood and colleagues demonstrated CMR imaging to have higher sensitivity (67% versus 87%) and similar specificity (both 83%) when compared with SPECT for the ability to detect significant epicardial coronary stenosis.[81,83]

It is tempting to consider using magnetic resonance angiography to visualize coronary anatomy as well as other CMR components. Downsides include increased exposure to gadolinium-containing contrast agents, prolonged scanner time, and lower accuracy compared with other angiography methods.[80,84] Further, studies have not consistently shown the magnetic resonance angiography component to add significant diagnostic value. As a result, most centers do not routinely use magnetic resonance angiography when testing patients for ACS.

KEY POINTS

Resting echocardiography provides information about the structure of the heart.

Calcium scoring CT, CCTA, and diagnostic cardiac catheterization help to identify CAD lesions that could be the source of active or future ACS.

Exercise treadmill testing, stress echocardiography, and rMPI are used to detect signs of ischemic or infarcted myocardium evidenced by diminished tissue perfusion.

CMR imaging is a highly accurate modality best adapted to testing intermediate- to high-risk patients.

CASE ONE RESOLUTION

The emergency physician explains that no evidence of a heart attack or MI was found (his troponin tests were negative). However, given his CAD risk factors and his chest pain, she recommends that he have a stress test to see if he has any signs of coronary flow-limiting CAD. He is considered for CCTA to test for this purpose and to see if he has any calcified coronary plaques; however, he could have an exercise treadmill test or stress echocardiography as an outpatient in 2 or 3 days. His primary care physician is unable to coordinate a stress test this quickly, so CCTA is performed. He had no flow-limiting lesions but a single calcified plaque causing less than 30% stenosis was detected. He is referred to his primary care physician for CAD risk factor screening and management.

CASE TWO RESOLUTION

The emergency physician in this case informs the patient her that her initial troponin test was negative, as were her other laboratory tests. But, given her high risk for ACS and the other diagnoses being considered, she will be admitted for further testing. The patient waits for her second troponin test while her physician considers the most appropriate form of provocative testing. She is unable to walk fast because of arthritis, so she is not a candidate for an exercise treadmill test. Because of her history of COPD, she is at risk for bronchospasm if exposed to adenosine, dipyridamole, or regadenoson, so dobutamine is selected. Stress echocardiography or rMPI will be done after she is admitted to the hospital.

Conclusion

The evaluation of emergency department patients with symptoms suggesting myocardial ischemia involves the medical history, measurement of cardiac biomarkers, and, typically, cardiac imaging to determine if the physiology of ACS is present. Several decision tools can help with the identification of patients whose presentation warrants a workup for ACS, including the HEART Pathway and the ADP. Once the decision is made to investigate the possibility of ACS, the first step is to use the ECG and biomarkers to identify signs of MI. Cardiac biomarkers traditionally detect myonecrosis by assaying for intracellular myocyte components. Of these, a troponin is the most sensitive and specific and is widely recognized as the gold standard for detection of myocardial necrosis. Imaging can be used to detect CAD or myocardial ischemia and thus reduce the likelihood of unstable angina as the cause of the patient's symptoms after MI has been excluded. No one test is best for all patients. Choosing the best imaging modality should take into consideration a patient's pretest probability for ACS, institutional resources, the patient's known cardiac pathology and comorbidities, and the risks the test poses for the patient.

References

1. Virmani R, Kolodgie FE, Burke AP, et al. Pathology of the vulnerable plaque. *J Am Coll Cardiol*. 2006;47:C13-C18.
2. Libby P. Mechanisms of acute coronary syndromes and their implications for therapy. *N Engl J Med*. 2013;368:2004-2013.
3. Libby P. Current concepts of the pathogenesis of the acute coronary syndromes. *Circulation*. 2001;104:365-372.
4. Rossini R, Musumeci G, Lettieri C. Acute coronary syndrome in patients with non-obstructive coronary artery disease: long-term prognosis. *EuroIntervention*. 2013:7:suppl M. Available at: www.pcronline.com/eurointervention/M_issue/3/. Accessed on October 31, 2013.
5. Newman J, Danqas G, Brener S, et al. Outcomes in patients with non-obstructive coronary artery disease with and without cardiac biomarker elevations: The ACUITY trial. *J Am Coll Cardiol*. 2012;60(17_S). doi:10.1016/j.jacc.2012.08.512.
6. Cassar A, Holmes DR, Rihal CS, et al. Chronic coronary artery disease: diagnosis and management. *Mayo Clin Proc*. 2009: 84(12):1130-1146.
7. Third Universal Definition of Myocardial Infarction. *Eur Heart J*. 2012;33:2551-2567.
8. Morrow DA, Rifai N, Tanasijevic M, et al. Clinical efficacy of three assays for cardiac troponin I for risk stratification acute coronary syndromes: a thrombolysis in myocardial infarction (TIMI) IIB substudy. *Clin Chem*. 2000;46:453-460.
9. Wu AH, Apple FS, Gibler WB, et al. National Academy of Clinical Biochemistry Standards of Laboratory Practice: recommendations for the use of cardiac markers in coronary artery diseases. *Clin Chem*. 1999;45:1104-1121.

10. Joint International Society and Federation of Cardiology/World Health Organization. Nomenclature and criteria for diagnosis of ischemic heart disease. *Circulation.* 1979;59:607-609.

11. Mendis S, Thygesen K, Kuulasmaa K. Writing group on behalf of the participating experts of the WHO consultation for revision of WHO definition of myocardial infarction. The World Health Organization definition of myocardial infarction: 2008–09 revision. *Int J Epidemiol.* 2011;40: 147-149.

12. Thygesen K, Alpert JS, White HD, et al. Universal definition of myocardial infarction redefined. *Circulation.* 2007;116:2634-2653.

13. A consensus document of The Joint European Society of Cardiology/American College of Cardiology Committee for the Redefinition of Myocardial Infarction. *Eur Heart J.* 2000;21:1502-1513.

14. Alpert JS, Thygesen K, Antman E, et al. Myocardial infarction redefined--a consensus document of The Joint European Society of Cardiology/American College of Cardiology Committee for the redefinition of myocardial infarction *J Am Coll Cardiol.* 2000;36(3):959-969.

15. Christenson RH, Vaidya H, Landt Y, et al. Standardization of creatine kinase-MB (CK-MB) mass assays: the use of recombinant CK-MB as a reference material. *Clin Chem.* 1999;45:1414-1423.

16. Pant S, Deshmukh A, Neupane P, et al. Chapter 2: Cardiac biomarkers. Novel strategies in ischemic Heart Disease. 2012: InTech.com. Available at: www.intechopen.com/books/novel-strategies-in-ischemic-heartdisease/biomarkers-in-ischemic-heart-disease. Accessed on August 14, 2013.

17. Mair J, Morandell D, Genser N, et al. Equivalent early sensitivities of myoglobin, creatine kinase MB mass, creatine kinase isoform ratios, and cardiac troponins I and T for acute myocardial infarction. *Clin Chem.* 1995;41:1266-1272.

18. Jaffe AS, Babuin L, Apple FS. Biomarkers in acute cardiac disease: the present and the future. *J Am Coll Cardiol.* 2006;48:1-11.

19. Tsung SH. Several conditions causing elevation of serum CK-MB and CK-BB. *Am J Clin Pathol.* 1981;75:711-715.

20. Roger VL, Killian JM, Weston SA, et al. Redefinition of myocardial infarction: prospective evaluation in the community. *Circulation.* 2006;114:790-797.

21. Reichlin T, Hochholzer W, Bassetti S. The early diagnosis of myocardial infarction with highly sensitive cardiac troponins. *N Engl J Med.* 2009;361: 858-867.

22. Hamm CW, Goldmann BU, Heeschen C, et al. Emergency room triage of patients with acute chest pain by means of rapid testing for cardiac troponin T or troponin I. *N Engl J Med.* 1997;337:1648-1653.

23. Galvani M, Ottani F, Ferrini D, et al. Prognostic influence of elevated values of cardiac troponin I in patients with unstable angina. *Circulation.* 1997;95:2053-2059.

24. Lindahl B, Andren B, Ohlsson J, et al. Risk stratification in unstable coronary artery disease: Additive value of troponin T determinations and pre-discharge exercise tests. FRISK Study Group. *Eur Heart J.* 1997;18:762-770.

25. Apple FS, Pearce LA, Chung A, et al. Multiple biomarker use for detection of adverse events in patients presenting with symptoms suggestive of acute coronary syndrome. *Clin Chem.* 2007;53:874-881.

26. Morrow DA, Cannon CP, Rifai N, et al. Ability of minor elevations of troponins I and T to predict benefit from an early invasive strategy in patients with unstable angina and non-ST elevation myocardial infarction: results from a randomized trial. *JAMA.* 2001;286:2405-2412.

27. Macrae AR, Kavsak PA, Lustig V, et al. Assessing the requirement for the 6-hour interval between specimens in the American Heart Association Classification of Myocardial Infarction in Epidemiology and Clinical Research Studies. *Clin Chem.* 2006;52:812-818.

28. Eggers KM, Oldgren J, Nordenskjold A, Lindahl B. Diagnostic value of serial measurement of cardiac markers in patients with chest pain: limited value of adding myoglobin to troponin I for exclusion of myocardial infarction. *Am Heart J.* 2004;148:574-581.

29. Anderson JL, Adams CD, Antman EM, et al. ACC/AHA 2007 guidelines for the management of patients with unstable angina/non ST-elevation myocardial infarction: a report of the American College of Cardiology/American Heart Association Task Force on Practice Guidelines (Writing Committee to Revise the 2002 Guidelines for the Management of Patients With Unstable Angina/Non ST-Elevation Myocardial Infarction): developed in collaboration with the American College of Emergency Physicians, the Society for Cardiovascular Angiography and Interventions, and the Society of Thoracic Surgeons: endorsed by the American Association of Cardiovascular and Pulmonary Rehabilitation and the Society for Academic Emergency Medicine. *Circulation.* 2007;116:e148-e304.

30. Bhuiya FA, Pitts SR, McCaig LF, et al. Emergency department visits for chest pain and abdominal pain: United States, 1999–2008. *National Hospital Ambulatory Medical Care Survey: 1999–2008.* U.S. Department of Health and Human Services: Centers for Disease Control and Prevention, National Center for Health Statistics. 2010, No. 40, p 8.

31. Hamm CW, Goldmann BU, Heeschen C, et al. Emergency room triage of patients with acute chest pain by means of rapid testing for cardiac troponin T or troponin I. *N Engl J Med.* 1997;337:1648-1653.

32. Thygesen K, Johannes M, Evangelos G, et al. How to use high-sensitive cardiac troponins in acute cardiac care. *Eur Heart J.* 2012;33:2252-2257.

33. Keller T, Zeller T, Ojeda F, et al. Serial changes in highly sensitive troponin I assay and early diagnosis of myocardial infarction. *JAMA.* 2011;306:2684-2693.

34. Hamm CW, Bassand JP, Agewall S, et al. ESC Guidelines for the management of acute coronary syndromes in patients presenting without persistent ST-segment elevation: The Task Force for the Management of Acute Coronary Syndromes (ACS) in Patients Presenting Without Persistent ST-Segment Elevation of the European Society of Cardiology (ESC). *Eur Heart J.* 2011;32:2999-3054.

35. Reiter M, Twerenbold R, Reichlin T, et al. Early diagnosis of acute myocardial infarction in the elderly using more sensitive cardiac troponin assays. *Eur Heart J.* 2011;32:1379-1389.

36. Guo X, Jianzhang F, Hengshan G. The predictive value of the bedside troponin T test for patients with acute chest pain. *Exp Clin Cardiol.* 2006;4:298-301.

37. Lippi G, Guidi GC. The power of negative thinking. *Am J Emerg Med.* 2008;26:373-374.

38. Mueller M, Biener M, Vafaie M, et al. Absolute and relative kinetic changes of high-sensitive cardiac troponin T in acute coronary syndrome and in patients with increased troponin the in absence of acute coronary syndrome. *Clin Chem.* 2012;58:209-218.

39. Januzzi JL Jr, Bamberg F, Lee H, et al. Highly sensitivity troponin T concentration in acute chest pain patients evaluated with cardiac computed tomography. *Circulation.* 2010;121:1227-1234.

40. Freund Y, Chenevier-Gobeauz C, Bonnet P, et al. High-sensitivity vs conventional troponin in the emergency department for the diagnosis of acute myocardial infarction. *Crit Care.* 2011;15(3):R147.

41. Yiadom MY, Kosowsky JM, Melanson SL, et al. Diagnostic performance of a highly sensitive cardiac troponin I assay in an emergency department setting. *Clin Chem.* 2010;56(suppl 6):A131.

42. Collinson PO, Gaze DC, Bainbridge K, et al. Utility of admission cardiac troponin and ischemia modified albumin for rapid evaluation and rule out myocardial infarction in the emergency department. *Emerg Med J.* 2006;23:256-261.

43. Sinha M, Roy D, Gaze DC, et al. Role of ischemia modified albumin, a new biochemical marker of myocardial ischemia, in the early diagnosis of acute myocardial ischemia syndromes. *Emerg Med J.* 2004;21:29-34.

44. Keating L, Benger JR, Beetham R, et al. The PRIMA Study: pre-ischaemia-modified albumin in the emergency department. *Emerg Med J.* 2006;23:764-768.

45. Goetze JP, Christoffersen C, Perko M, et al. Increased cardiac BNP expression associated with myocardial ischemia. *FASEB J.* 2003;17:1105-1107.

46. Omland T, Persson A, Ng L, et al. N-terminal pro-B-type natriuretic peptide and long-term mortality in acute coronary syndromes. *Circulation.* 2002;106:2913-2918.

47. Kennon S, Timmis AD, Whitbourn R, et al. C reactive protein for risk stratification in acute coronary syndromes? Verdict: unproven. *Heart.* 2003;89:1288-1290.

48. Emerging Risk Factor Collaboration, Kaptoge S, DiAngelantonio E, Lowe G, et al. C-reactive protein concentrations and risk of coronary heart disease, stroke and mortality: an individual participant metanalysis. *Lancet.* 2010;375:132-140.

49. Kavsak PA, MacRae AR, Newman AM. Elevated C-reactive protein in acute coronary syndrome presentation is an independent predictor of long-term mortality and heart failure. *Clin Biochem.* 2007;40:326-329.

50. McCann CJ, Glover BM, Menown IB, et al. Novel biomarkers in early diagnosis of acute myocardial infarction compared with cardiac troponin T. *Eur Heart J.* 2008;29:2843-2850.

51. Than M, Cullen L, Reid CM, et al. A 2-h diagnostic protocol to assess patients with chest pain symptoms in the Asia-Pacific region (ASPECT): a prospective observational study. *Lancet.* 2011;377:1077-1084.

52. Than M, Cullen L, Aldous S, et al. 2-hour accelerated diagnostic protocol to assess patients with chest pain symptoms using contemporary troponins as the only biomarker. *J Am Coll Cardiol.* 2012;59:2091-2098.

53. Six AJ, Backus BE, Kelder JC. Chest pain in the emergency room: value of the HEART score. *Neth Heart J.* 2008;16:191-196.

54. Backus BE, Six AJ, Kelder JC, et al. A prospective validation of the HEART score for chest pain patients at the emergency department. *Int J Cardiol.* 2013;168:2153-2158.

55. Backus BE, Six AJ, Kelder JC, et al. Chest pain in the emergency room: a multicenter validation of the HEART Score. *Critical Path Card.* 2010;9:164-169.

56. Mahler SA, Miller CD, Hollader JE, et al. Identifying patients for early discharge: performance of decision rules among patients with acute chest pain. *Int J Cardiol.* 2013;168:795-802.

57. Jalili M, Hejripour Z, Honarmand AR, et al. Validation of the Vancouver Chest Pain Rule: a prospective cohort study. *Acad Emerg Med.* 2012;19:837-842.

58. Greenslade JH, Cullen L, Than M, et al. Validation of the Vancouver Chest Pain Rule using troponin as the only biomarker: a prospective cohort study. *Am J Emerg Med.* 2013;31:1103-1107.

59. Wohlgelertner D, Cleman M, Highman HA, et al. Regional myocardial dysfunction during coronary angioplasty: evaluation by two-dimensional echocardiography and 12 lead electrocardiography. *J Am Coll Cardiol.* 1986;7:1245-1254.

60. Sabia P, Afrookteh A, Touchstone DA, et al. Value of regional wall motion abnormality in the emergency room diagnosis of acute myocardial infarction: a prospective study using two-dimensional echocardiography. *Circulation.* 1991;84(3 suppl):I85-I92.

61. Kimura BJ, Bocchicchio M, Willis CL, et al. Screening cardiac ultrasonographic examination in patients with suspected cardiac disease in the emergency department. *Am Heart J.* 2001;142:324-330.
62. Cheitlin MD, Armstrong WF, Aurigemma GP, et al. ACC/AHA/ASE 2003 guideline update for the clinical application of echocardiography. *Circulation.* 2003;108:1146-1162.
63. Marwick TH. Stress echocardiography. *Heart.* 2003;89:113-118.
64. Hilton TC, Thompson RC, Williams HJ, et al. Technetium-99m sestamibi myocardial perfusion imaging in the emergency room evaluation of chest pain. *J Am Coll Cardiol.* 1994;23:1016-1022.
65. Varetto T, Cantalupi D, Altieri A, et al. Emergency room technetium-99m sestamibi imaging to rule out acute myocardial ischemic events in patients with nondiagnostic electrocardiograms. *J Am Coll Cardiol.* 1993;22:1804-1808.
66. Stone, GW, Maehara A, Lansky AJ, et al. PROSPECT Investigators. A prospective natural history study of coronary atherosclerosis. *N Engl J Med.* 2011;364:226-235.
67. Litt HI, Gatsonis C, Snyder B, et al. CT Angiography for safe discharge of patients with possible acute coronary syndromes. *N Engl J Med.* 2012;366:1393-1403.
68. Hoffman U, Truong QA, Schoenfeld DA, et al. Coronary CTA angiography verses standard evaluation in acute chest pain. *N Engl J Med.* 2012;367:299-308.
69. Greenland P, Bonow RO, Brundage BH, et al. ACCF/AHA 2007 clinical expert consensus document on coronary artery calcium scoring by computed tomography in global cardiovascular risk assessment and in evaluation of patients with chest pain: a report of the American College of Cardiology Foundation Clinical Expert Consensus Task Force (ACCF/AHA Writing Committee to Update the 2000 Expert Consensus Document on Electron Beam Computed Tomography) Developed in Collaboration With the Society of Atherosclerosis Imaging and Prevention and the Society of Cardiovascular Computed Tomography. *J Am Coll Cardiol.* 2007;49:378-402.
70. Hoffman U, Ferencik M, Cury R, et al. Coronary CT angiography. *J Nucl Med.* 2006;47:797-806.
71. Ropers D, Rixe J, Anders K, et al. Usefulness of multidetector row spiral computed tomography with 64- x 0.6-mm collimation and 330-ms rotation for the noninvasive detection of significant coronary artery stenosis. *Am J Cardiol.* 2006;97:343-348.
72. Fine JJ, Hopkins CB, Ruff N, Newton FC. Comparison of accuracy of 64-slice cardiovascular computed tomography with coronary angiography in patients with suspected coronary artery disease. *Am J Cardiol.* 2006;97:173-174.
73. Ong TK, Chin SP, Liew CK, et al. Accuracy of 64-row multidetector computed tomography in detecting coronary artery disease in 134 symptomatic patients: influence of calcification. *Am Heart J.* 2006;151:1323.e1-e6.
74. Raff GL, Gallagher MJ, O'Neill WW, Goldstein JA. Diagnostic accuracy of noninvasive coronary angiography using 64-slice spiral computed tomography. *J Am Coll Cardiol.* 2005;46:552-557.
75. Achenbach S, Moselewski F, Ropers D, et al. Detection of calcified and non-calcified coronary atherosclerotic plaque by contrast-enhanced, submillimeter multi-detector spiral computed tomography: a segment-based comparison with intravascular ultrasound. *Circulation.* 2004;109:14-17.
76. Fazel R, Krumholz HM, Wang Y, et al. Exposure to low-dose ionizing radiation from medical imaging procedures. *N Engl J Med.* 2009;361:849-857.
77. Amsterdam EA, Kirk JD, Diercks DB, et al. Exercise testing in chest pain units: rational, implementation, and results. *Cardiol Clin.* 2005;23:503-516.
78. Gianrossi R, Detrano R, Mulvhill D, et al. Exercise-induced ST depression in the diagnosis of coronary artery disease: a meta-analysis. *Circulation.* 1989;80:87-98.
79. Fleischmann KE, Hunink MG, Kuntz KM, et al. Exercise echocardiography or exercise SPECT imaging? A meta-analysis of diagnostic test performance. *JAMA.* 1998;280:913-920.
80. Beller GA. Myocardial perfusion imaging for detection of silent myocardial ischemia. *Am J Cardiol.* 1988;61:22F-28F.
81. Miller CD, Hwang W, Hoekstra JW, et al. Stress cardiac magnetic resonance imaging with observation unit care reduces cost for patients with emergency chest pain: a randomized trial. *Ann Emerg Med.* 2010;56:209-219.e2.
82. Cury RC, Shash K, Nagurney JT, et al. Cardiac magnetic resonance with T2-weighted images improves detection of patients with acute coronary syndrome in the emergency department. *Circulation.* 2008;118:837-844.
83. Greenwood JP, Maredia N, Younger JF, et al. Cardiovascular MRI and single photo emission CT for diagnosis of coronary heart disease (CE_MARC): a prospective trial. *Lancet.* 2012;379:453-460.
84. The American College of Radiology and Radiological Society of North America. Reducing Radiation from Medical X-rays. Radiologyinfo.com. Available at: www.fda.gov/ForConsumers/ConsumerUpdates/ucm095505.htm, updated August 23, 2013. Accessed on October 31, 2013.

Cerqueira MD, Allman KC, Ficaro EP, et al. Recommendations for Reducing Radiation Exposure in Myocardial Perfusion Imaging. *J Nucl Cardiol.* 2010;17:709-718.

Chang SM, Nabi F, Xu J, Raza U, Mahmarian JJ. Normal stress-only versus standard stress/rest myocardial perfusion imaging: similar patient mortality with reduced radiation exposure. *J Am Coll Cardiol.* 2010;55:221-230.

Hauser AM, Gangadharan V, Ramos RG, et al. Sequence of mechanical, electrocardiographic and clinical effects of repeated coronary artery occlusion in human beings: echocardiographic observations during coronary angioplasty. *J Am Coll Cardiol.* 1985;5:193-197.

Hausleiter J, Meyer T, Hadamitzky M, et al. Prevalence of noncalcified coronary plaques by 64-slice computed tomography in patients with an intermediate risk for significant coronary artery disease. *J Am Coll Cardiol.* 2006;48:312-318.

Hoffmann U, Moselewski F, Nieman K, et al. Noninvasive assessment of plaque morphology and composition in culprit and stable lesions in acute coronary syndrome and stable lesions in stable angina by multidetector computed tomography. *J Am Coll Cardiol.* 2006;47:1655-1662.

Leber AW, Knez A, von Ziegler F, et al. Quantification of obstructive and nonobstructive coronary lesions by 64-slice computed tomography: a comparative study with quantitative coronary angiography and intravascular ultrasound. *J Am Coll Cardiol.* 2005;46:147-154.

Min JK, Devereux RB, Koch R, et al. Identification of plaque types and distribution patterns by multi-detector computed tomography enhances prediction of clinically significant coronary artery disease (abstract). *J Am Coll Cardiol.* 2006;47(suppl 1):128A.

Schuijf JD, Pundziute G, Jukema JW, et al. Diagnostic accuracy of 64-slice multislice computed tomography in the noninvasive evaluation of significant coronary artery disease. *Am J Cardiol.* 2006;98:145-148.

Stein PD, Beemath A, Kayali F, et al. Multidetector computed tomography for the diagnosis of coronary artery disease: a systematic review. *Am J Med.* 2006;119:203-216.

Van der Zaag-Loonen HJ, Dikkers R, de Bock GH, Oudkerk M. The clinical value of a negative multi-detector computed tomographic angiography in patients suspected of coronary artery disease: a meta-analysis. *Eur Radiol.* 2006;16:2748-2756.

Additional Reading

Arbab-Zadeh A, Nakano M, Virmani R, et al. Acute coronary events. *Circulation.* 2012;125:1147-1156.

CARDIOVASCULAR EMERGENCIES

CHAPTER 4

Bedside Ultrasound for Emergency Cardiovascular Disorders

Phillips Perera, Sarah R. Williams, and Laleh Gharahbaghian

IN THIS CHAPTER

Basic concepts of the echocardiography examination
Sonographic windows
Evaluation of the inferior vena cava
Evaluation of the internal jugular veins
Diagnosis of pericardial effusions and tamponade
Assessment of cardiac contractility
Echocardiography for pulmonary embolus
Ultrasound guidance for transvenous pacemaker placement
Resuscitation ultrasound
Focused echocardiography in cardiac arrest

Echocardiography (echo) has evolved to become one of the key clinical skills for emergency physicians. Enhanced ultrasound technology, improved image quality, and the availability of affordable and portable units have dramatically facilitated the performance of focused echo in the relative safety of monitored clinical areas.[1] Emergent treatment of the patient can therefore be rendered concurrently with bedside echo, making it an essential tool for the diagnosis, resuscitation, and ongoing monitoring of the cardiac patient.

The use of focused ultrasound is supported by the major emergency medicine organizations, including the American College of Emergency Physicians (ACEP), the Society for Academic Emergency Medicine, and the Council of Residency Directors. These organizations all currently endorse both residency and post-residency training in this modality as well as its use in routine clinical practice.[2-5] In 2010, an important collaborative paper published jointly by ACEP and the American Society of Echocardiography (ASE) endorsed focused echo for a defined set of emergent conditions.[6] While it is recognized that a large proportion of practicing emergency physicians have yet to be trained in echo, it is hoped that this chapter will demonstrate the usefulness of this technology to the practice of emergency medicine and stimulate further education in this area.

Tables 4-1 through 4-4 categorize the functional uses, clinical indications, and goals for bedside echo, as defined by ACEP and ASE.

KEY POINTS

The technology currently available for bedside echo has evolved greatly, allowing examinations to be performed directly in the monitored resuscitation areas of the emergency department as part of the immediate evaluation of the patient.

The use of focused echo is supported by all of the major emergency medicine societies.

The Echocardiography Examination: Basic Concepts

Probe Selection

A phased-array probe is typically used for cardiac echo, as it has the benefit of a small footprint that can easily fit between the ribs. When deeper imaging is needed, a probe operating at a lower frequency (usually between 2.5 and 3 MHz) is best.

Machine Settings and Modalities

Cardiac Preset

The heart moves rapidly in reference to other body structures. For this reason, selection of a high frame rate (above 24 frames/sec) on the ultrasound machine settings will allow optimal imaging. This cardiac preset is preloaded on most ultrasound machines.

B-Mode Ultrasound

Ultrasonography of the heart typically employs modalities that can capture both anatomy and physiology.[7] Two-dimensional B-mode imaging is used first to visualize the heart as it moves through the cardiac cycle. B-mode imaging projects the heart as a continuum of color in the grey spectrum, termed *echogenicity*. Echogenicity results from the fact that the ultrasound probe acts as a transducer that sends sound waves into the body. The sound waves then penetrate the body, traveling a distance until they are bounced back to the probe. Different tissues have varying resistance to the movement of sound. Higher density (hyperechoic) structures reflect an increasing amount of the sound back to the probe, resulting in a brighter appearance (eg, a calcified valve). Fluid-filled structures (hypoechoic or anechoic) allow increased propagation of sound through the body, leading to a darker appearance of the image (eg, blood in the cardiac chambers, fluid around the heart) (Figure 4-1).

M-Mode Ultrasound

M-mode, or "motion" mode, ultrasound creates an "ice pick" image of movement across a defined anatomic axis in relation to time. This approach generates a grey scale illustration of movement over time that can be used to document motion on a static image (Figures 4-2, 4-3, and 4-4).

Doppler Ultrasound

Doppler ultrasound allows the advanced evaluation of motion in direct reference to the relative position of the ultrasound probe (the Doppler shift). The Doppler shift can be interpreted in a number of imaging modalities, discussed below.

Color-flow Doppler demonstrates the directionality of flow both toward and away from the probe and is often used in advanced echo. Movement toward the probe results in a shorter frequency of sound, typically represented as red. Movement away from the probe results in a longer frequency of sound, represented as blue. The scale that displays the color-flow Doppler setting should be set high (>60 cm/sec) to best capture the fast flow of the blood traveling through the heart (Figure 4-5).

Pulsed-wave Doppler allows assessment of flow velocity in a waveform that identifies the specific speed of blood flow over time. This modality is often used in advanced echo to define the velocity of blood flow through cardiac valves (Figure 4-6).

Probe Orientation in Relation to the Ultrasound Machine

Historically, practices varied with regard to the orientation of the indicator dot on the ultrasound machine screen and the marker on the ultrasound probe. The reason is that the first widespread applications of ultrasound in emergency medicine such as the Focused Assessment with Sonography for Trauma

TABLE 4-1.

ACEP Functional Categories for Ultrasound Examination

Diagnostic
Procedure guidance
Resuscitative
Symptom-based or sign-based
Therapeutic and monitoring

TABLE 4-2.

ACEP/ASE Consensus Guidelines for Ultrasound Examination: Clinical Indications

Cardiac trauma: focused assessment with sonography for trauma (FAST examination)
Cardiac arrest
Chest pain
Dyspnea/shortness of breath
Hypotension/shock

TABLE 4-3.

ACEP/ASE Consensus Guidelines for Core Ultrasound Examination: Clinical Goals

Assessment for pericardial effusions and pericardial tamponade
Assessment of global cardiac systolic function
Assessment of intravascular volume
Confirmation of transvenous pacemaker wire placement
Guidance of pericardiocentesis
Identification of marked right ventricular and left ventricular enlargement

TABLE 4-4.

ACEP/ASE Consensus Guidelines for Advanced Ultrasound Examination: Examination Goals

The following conditions can be suspected on focused echocardiography (additional imaging should be obtained if possible):
Aortic dissection
Cardiac chamber thrombus
Endocarditis
Intracardiac masses
Regional wall motion abnormalities

(FAST) and obstetric/gynecologic examinations were based on traditional radiology ultrasound practice, which places the ultrasound screen indicator to the left. In contrast, in traditional cardiology practice, the indicator dot is oriented to the right of the ultrasound screen.

Despite this difference, standard practice has been to orient the ultrasound probe (at a 180° variance, depending on screen orientation) so that the cardiac images obtained with either convention display the heart in the same configuration. In this chapter, the probe orientation for each cardiac view is described with the indicator dot positioned to the left on the screen (Figure 4-5). This avoids having to reposition the dot on the ultrasound screen between the ultrasound applications commonly performed in emergency medicine practice. The probe marker will then be specifically oriented on the chest wall to view the heart in a standard configuration that will not differ between cardiology and emergency medicine echocardiography.

KEY POINTS

Setting up the ultrasound machine with the optimal echo settings prior to an examination can maximize the quality and usefulness of the images obtained.

Select a phased-array 3-MHz probe for echo.

Use the cardiac presets on the ultrasound machine.

Various modalities (including M-mode and Doppler) are available to maximize echo imaging.

The Echocardiography Examination: Sonographic Windows

Three windows are used traditionally for cardiac echo (Figure 4-7), as follows: the parasternal (long- and short-axis views), subxiphoid, and apical windows.

The Parasternal Long-Axis View

Patient Position

This view can be obtained with the patient in a supine position. However, turning the patient into a left lateral decubitus position will often improve imaging by moving the heart away from the sternum and closer to the chest wall, displacing the lung from the path of the sound waves.

Probe Position

The probe should be positioned initially just lateral to the sternum at about the third intercostal space. The position can then be adjusted for optimal imaging by moving the probe up or down one additional intercostal space. The probe indicator should be oriented toward the patient's left elbow (Figure 4-8).

Anatomic and Sonographic Correlation

The parasternal long-axis view allows visualization of three cardiac chambers (all but the right atrium) and the aorta (Figures 4-9 and 4-10). The best parasternal long-axis images have the aortic and mitral valves in the same view.

The clinician can begin by examining the chambers. Hy-

FIGURE 4-1.
Pericardial fluid

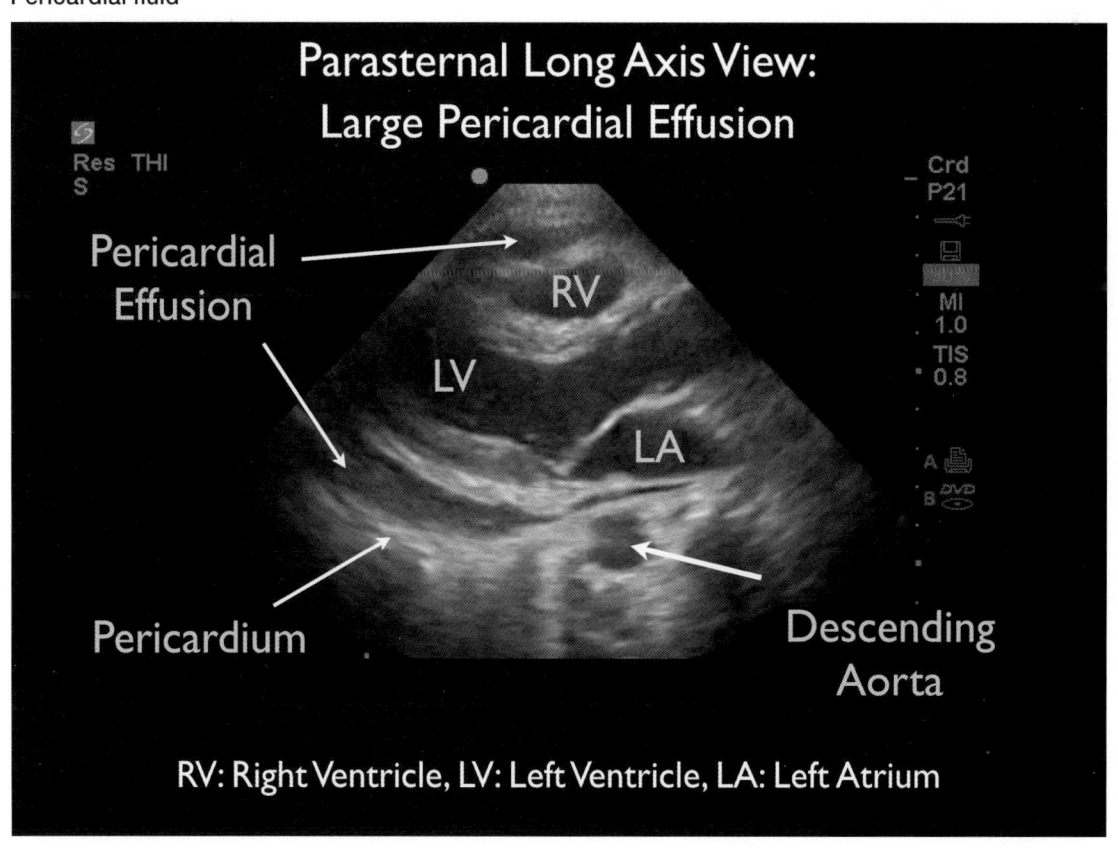

CARDIOVASCULAR EMERGENCIES

FIGURE 4-2.

M-mode, good contractility

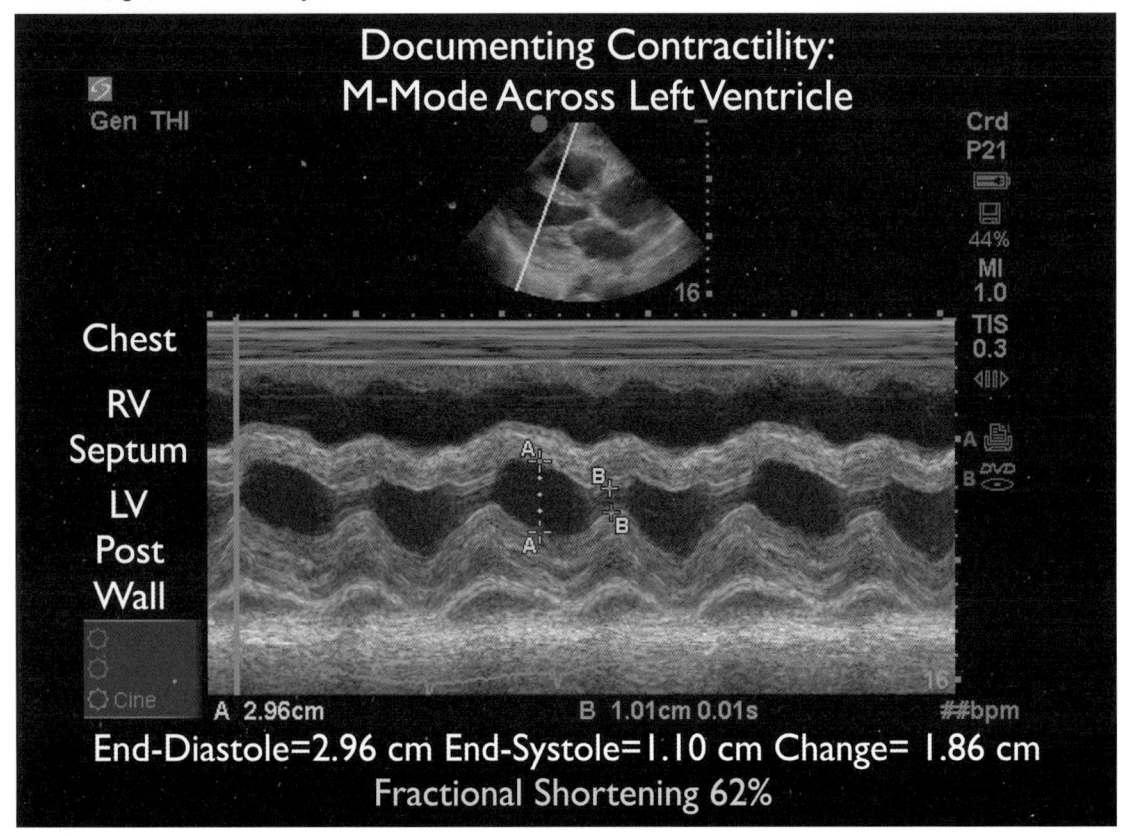

End-Diastole=2.96 cm End-Systole=1.10 cm Change= 1.86 cm
Fractional Shortening 62%

FIGURE 4-3.

M-mode, poor contractility

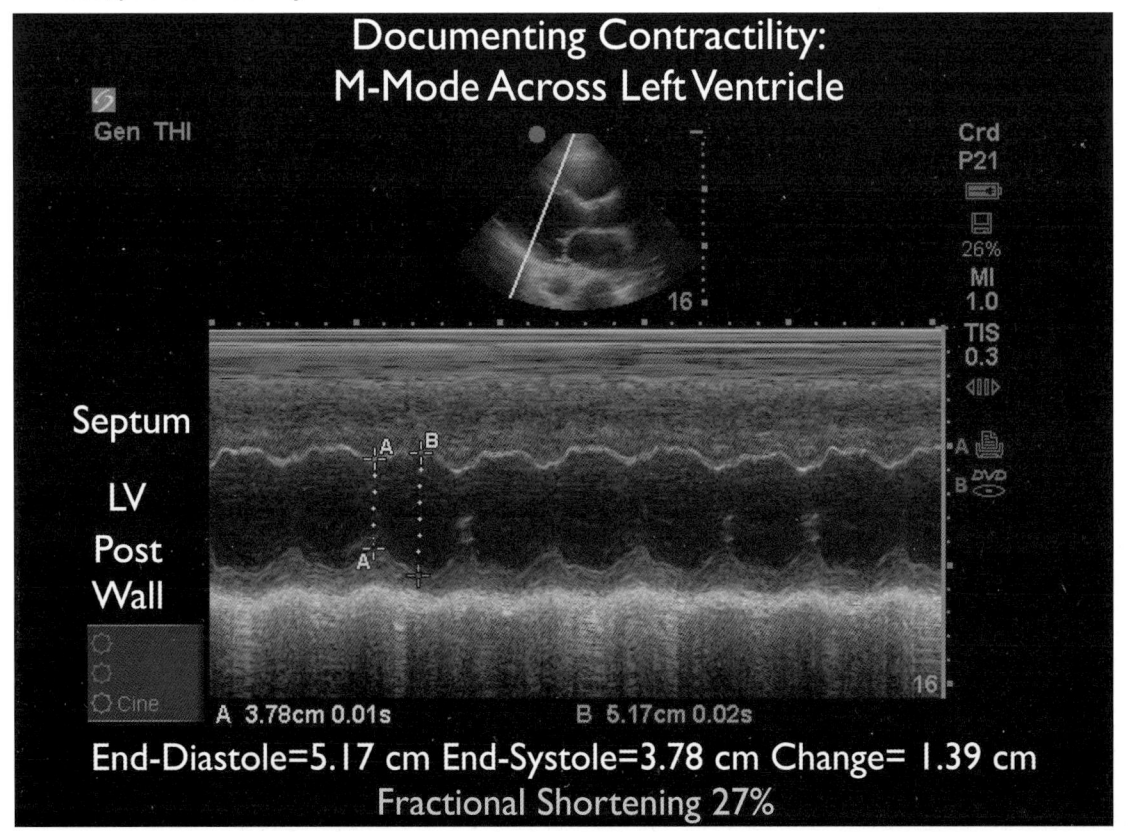

End-Diastole=5.17 cm End-Systole=3.78 cm Change= 1.39 cm
Fractional Shortening 27%

pertrophy of the left ventricular walls can be diagnosed by a wall thickness greater than 10 mm. In contrast, hypertrophy of the right ventricular walls is defined as a wall thickness greater than 5 mm.[8,9]

The aortic valve and aortic root can be visualized in the left ventricular outflow tract. This area can be examined for pathology of the aortic valve, often indicated by calcifications. The proximal aorta is seen just distal to or to the right of the aortic valve. A widened aortic root, defined as a diameter larger than 3.8 cm measured just distal to the aortic valve, can be seen in cases of aneurysm or dissection (Figure 4-11).[10] An intimal flap indicating a proximal, or Stanford type A, aortic dissection, might be visualized in this area.[11,12] However, because bedside ultrasound cannot image the proximal aorta in all patients adequately, transesophageal echo or computed tomography imaging should be pursued if pathology of the aorta is highly suspected.

KEY POINTS

The parasternal long-axis view offers a great deal of information about the patient's heart and should generally be obtained first on bedside echo.

Place the probe left of the sternum at about the third intercostal space. The patient can be positioned either supine or, more optimally, in the left lateral decubitus position.

Align the probe indicator down, toward the patient's left elbow.

Move the probe up or down, medially or laterally, until the optimal cardiac view comes into view.

Parasternal Short-Axis View

Probe Position

This view is obtained by first identifying the heart in the parasternal long-axis view and then rotating the probe 90° clockwise. The probe indicator dot is aligned toward the patient's right hip (Figure 4-12).

Anatomic and Sonographic Correlation

The short-axis view, known as the ring or doughnut view of the heart (Figure 4-13), visualizes the left and right ventricles in cross section. The traditional view is of the left ventricle at the level of the mitral valve, which appears as a "fish-mouth," opening and closing during the cardiac cycle. Visualizing the heart as a cylinder with the ultrasound beam cutting tangentially through different levels, the sonographer can look as far inferiorly as the apex of the left ventricle and superiorly to the level of the aortic valve.

To best evaluate left ventricular contractility, the probe is moved inferiorly to the level of the papillary muscles, allowing confirmation of the assessment taken from the parasternal long-axis view. In addition, cardiologists routinely evaluate for segmental wall motion abnormalities on this view. This examination for segmental wall motion abnormalities is considered an advanced application of echo and is currently not recom-

FIGURE 4-4.

Mitral valve, E-point septal separation

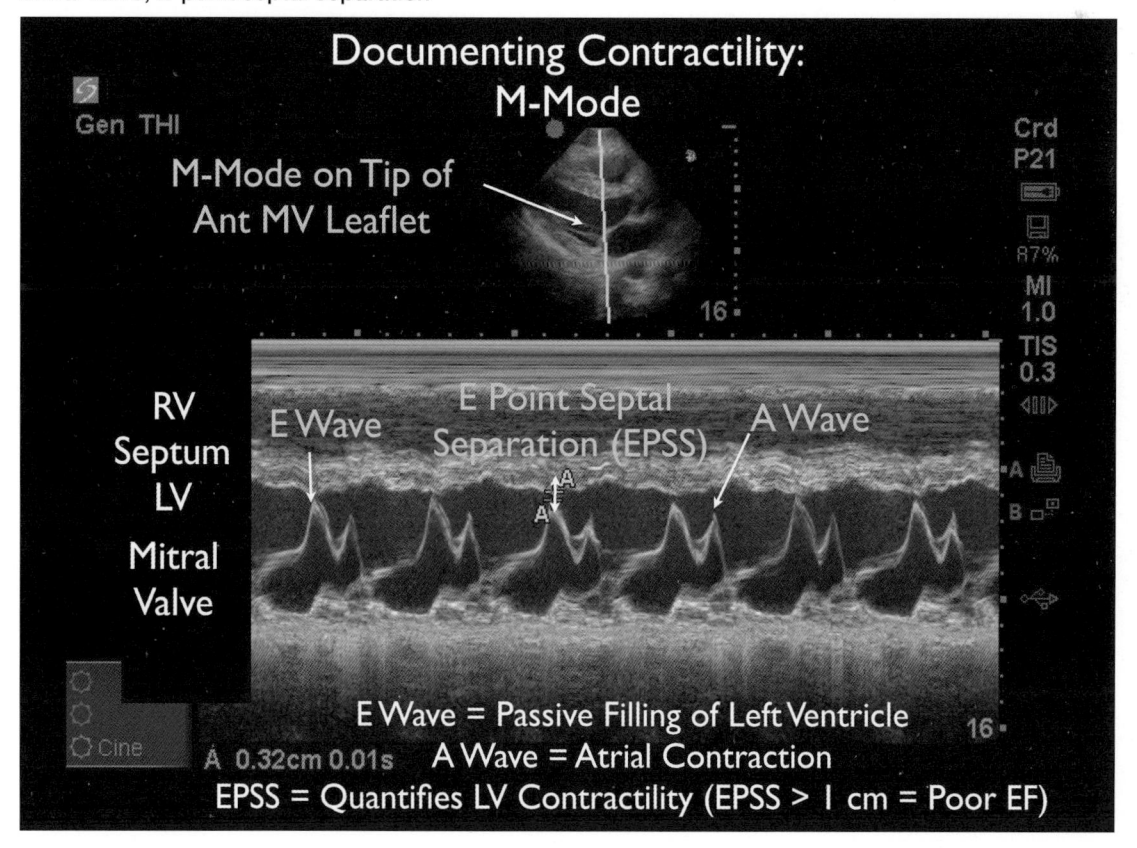

CARDIOVASCULAR EMERGENCIES

FIGURE 4-5.

Color-flow Doppler, with high setting (>60 cm/sec) for echo

Parasternal Long Axis View:

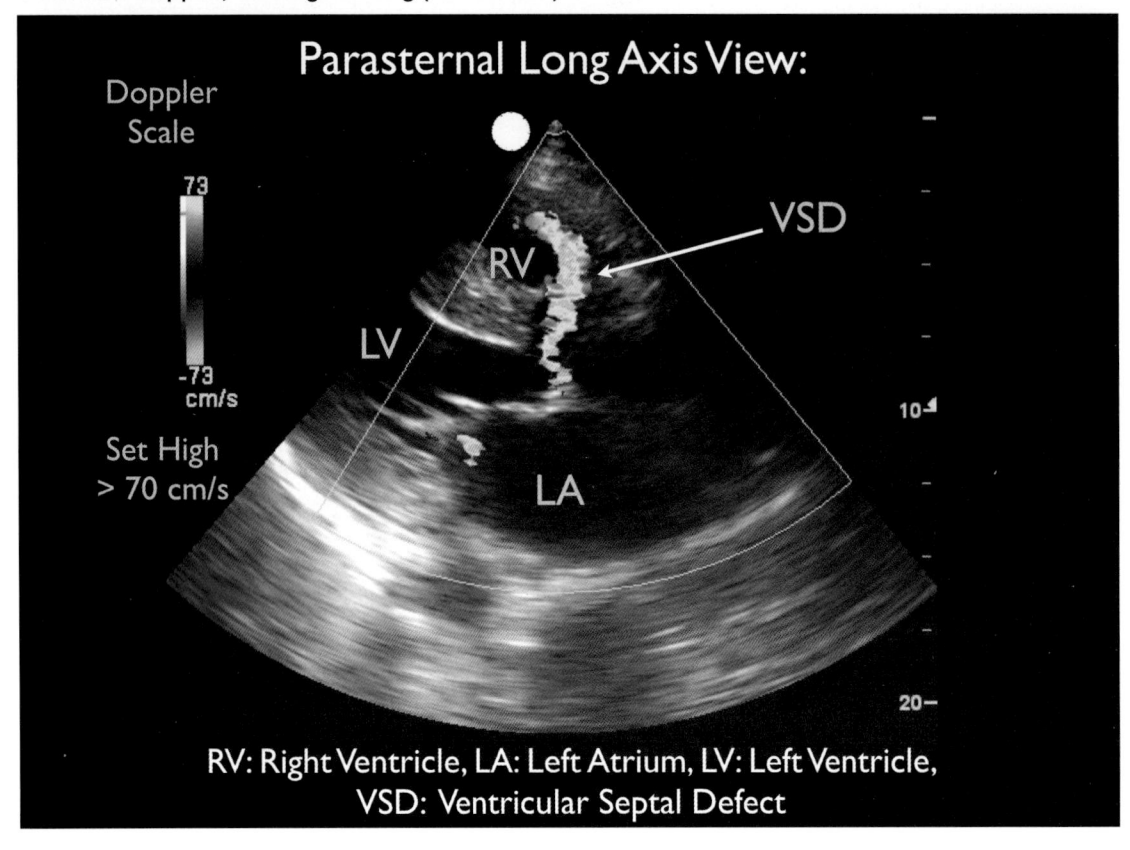

RV: Right Ventricle, LA: Left Atrium, LV: Left Ventricle, VSD: Ventricular Septal Defect

FIGURE 4-6.

Tricuspid flow, augmented respiratory variation in tamponade

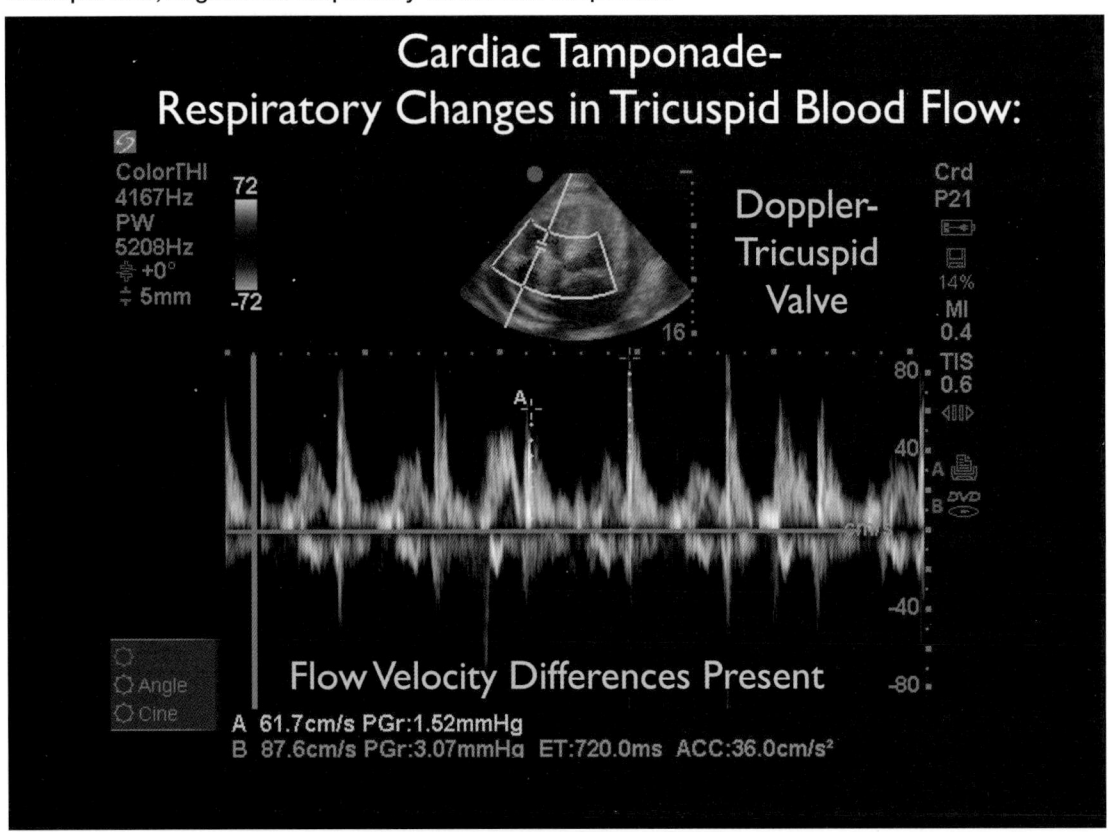

Cardiac Tamponade- Respiratory Changes in Tricuspid Blood Flow:

Doppler- Tricuspid Valve

Flow Velocity Differences Present

A 61.7cm/s PGr:1.52mmHg
B 87.6cm/s PGr:3.07mmHg ET:720.0ms ACC:36.0cm/s²

mended during routine bedside ultrasound by emergency physicians.

If the probe is angled superiorly and medially from the above location, the aortic valve and right ventricular outflow tract will come into view. The aortic valve should appear as the Mercedes-Benz sign, with a normal tricuspid configuration (Figure 4-14). A calcified bicuspid valve that is prone to stenosis and pathology can be identified here.[13]

KEY POINTS

The parasternal short-axis view provides information that is complementary to the long-axis view and can visualize the heart in cross section from the apex inferiorly to the aortic valve superiorly.

Place the probe left of the sternum at about the third intercostal space, with the patient either supine, or more optimally, in the left lateral decubitus position.

Align the probe indicator down, toward the patient's right hip.

The probe can then be moved and angled up or down to visualize multiple levels of the heart.

Subxiphoid Window

Patient Position

This view is obtained with the patient supine. Bending the patient's knees will relax the abdominal muscles and can improve imaging.

Probe Position

Place the probe just inferior to the xiphoid tip of the sternum, with the indicator oriented toward the patient's right side (Figure 4-15). Flattening and pushing down on the probe will aim the ultrasound beam superiorly and under the sternum to best image the heart. If a gas-filled stomach or intestinal loop impedes imaging, the probe can be moved toward the patient's right while simultaneously aiming it toward the patient's left shoulder to use more of the liver as an acoustic window to the heart.

Anatomic and Sonographic Correlation

All four cardiac chambers can be seen from this view. Because of the superior ability to visualize the right side of the heart, the subxiphoid view is often employed when close assessment of these chambers is needed (Figure 4-16).

KEY POINTS

The subxiphoid view allows imaging of all four chambers of the heart and is very useful for visualizing the right heart chambers, which will be closest to the probe.

Place the probe just inferior to the xiphoid tip of the sternum and aim superiorly and toward the patient's left shoulder. The probe marker should be oriented toward the patient's right side.

Placing the hand on top of the probe, while flattening the

FIGURE 4-7.

Cardiac echo: standard windows

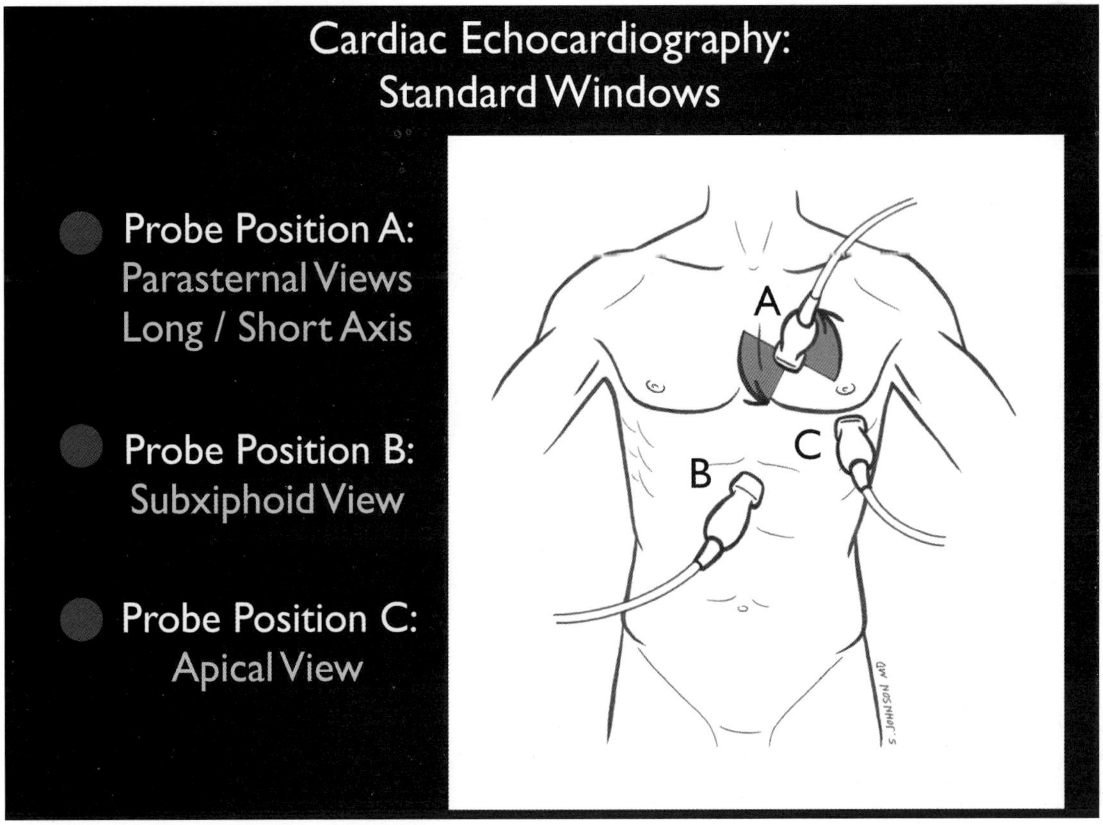

CARDIOVASCULAR EMERGENCIES

FIGURE 4-8.

Parasternal long-axis view: probe position

Parasternal Long Axis View of Heart

- Probe Placed Left of Sternum
- Intercostal Space 3 or 4
- Marker to Left Elbow
- Ultrasound Screen Indicator to Left
- Left Lateral Decubitus May Help Imaging

Marker L. Elbow

FIGURE 4-9.

Parasternal long-axis view: anatomy

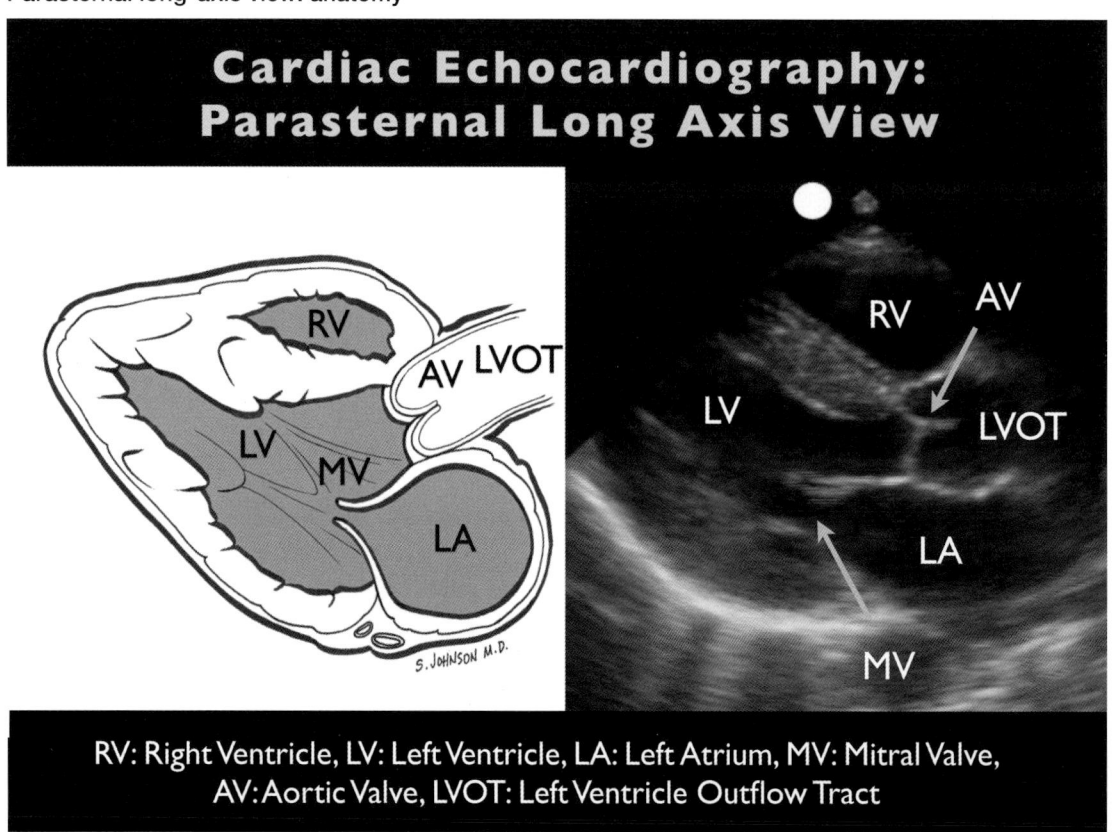

Cardiac Echocardiography: Parasternal Long Axis View

RV: Right Ventricle, LV: Left Ventricle, LA: Left Atrium, MV: Mitral Valve, AV: Aortic Valve, LVOT: Left Ventricle Outflow Tract

Bedside Ultrasound for Emergency Cardiovascular Disorders

probe on the abdomen to best angle it down and under the xiphoid tip, can aid imaging.

Stomach gas can get in the way from this view. To compensate, move the probe toward the patient's right to use more of the liver as an acoustic window, while simultaneously aiming toward the patient's left shoulder.

Apical Window

Patient Position

Roll the patient into the left lateral decubitus position to bring the heart closer to the lateral chest wall. Optimal imaging can then be obtained from this position.

Probe Position

Palpate the point of maximal impulse on the lateral chest wall and place the transducer at this point. This is generally just below the nipple line in men and under the breast in women. For the apical view, orient the probe marker toward the patient's right elbow (Figure 4-17).

Anatomic and Sonographic Correlation

The apical window allows detailed assessment of the sizes and movements of all four cardiac chambers in relation to one another (Figure 4-18). Traditionally, the first view from this window is the apical four-chamber view. The optimal views from this position capture both the mitral and tricuspid valves in the image. From this position, the probe can then be angled more superiorly to obtain the apical five-chamber view (Figure 4-19). The "fifth chamber" is the aortic outflow tract in the middle of the image.

KEY POINTS

The apical four-chamber view allows imaging of the right and left chambers of the heart in relation to each other. The apical five-chamber view allows additional visualization of the aortic root and outflow tract.

Position the patient in the left lateral decubitus position and place the probe under the left nipple in men or under the left breast in women, with the probe marker oriented toward the patient's right side.

Angle the probe slightly medially to obtain the apical four-chamber view.

Angle the probe both medially and superiorly to obtain the apical five-chamber view.

Evaluation of the Inferior Vena Cava

Performing the Examination

From the subxiphoid window, several views are used in imaging the inferior vena cava (IVC). First, identify the right atrium in the four-chamber subxiphoid view and then angle the probe inferiorly toward the spine to visualize the IVC as it joins this chamber. The IVC can be followed further inferiorly as it runs from the right atrium through the liver to the confluence

FIGURE 4-10.

Parasternal long-axis view: detailed anatomy

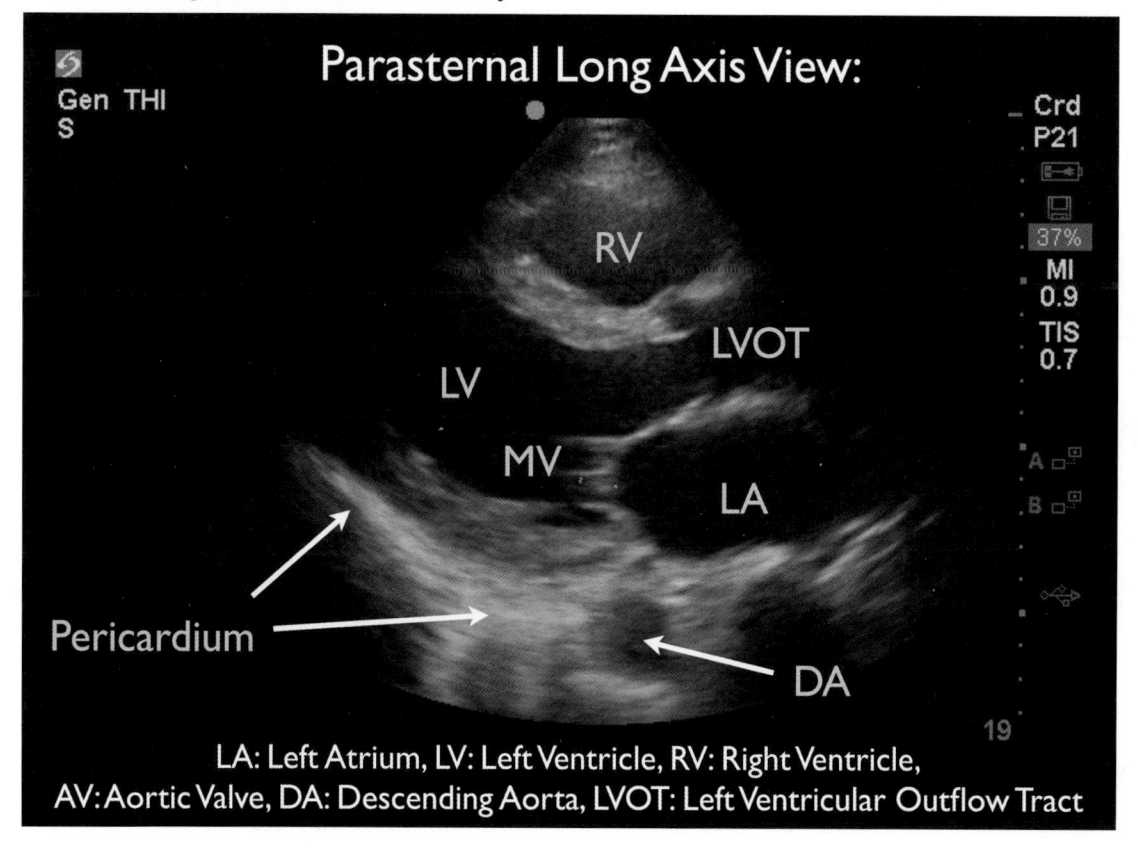

LA: Left Atrium, LV: Left Ventricle, RV: Right Ventricle, AV: Aortic Valve, DA: Descending Aorta, LVOT: Left Ventricular Outflow Tract

61

CARDIOVASCULAR EMERGENCIES

FIGURE 4-11.
Parasternal long-axis view: proximal aortic aneurysm

Parasternal Long Axis View: Proximal Aortic Aneurysm

Widened Aortic Root 4.74 cm

RV: Right Ventricle, LV: Left Ventricle, LA: Left Atrium, AV: Aortic Valve

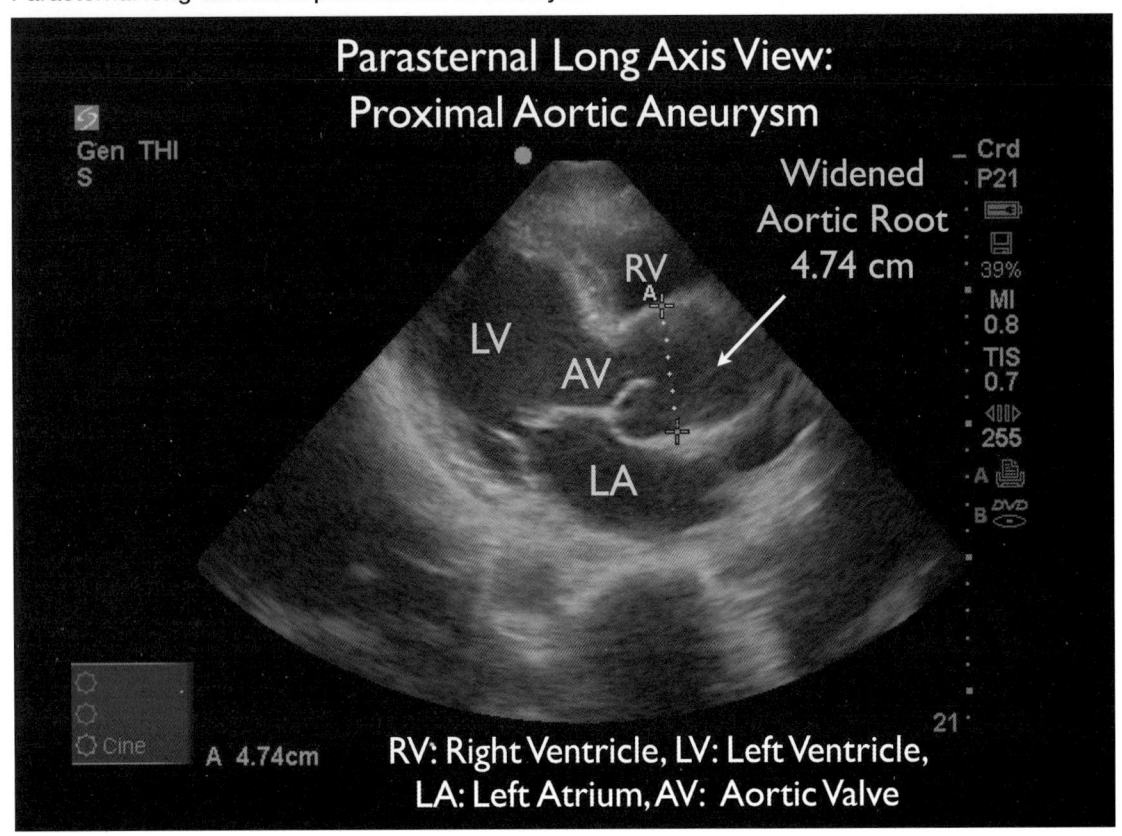

FIGURE 4-12.
Parasternal short-axis view: probe position

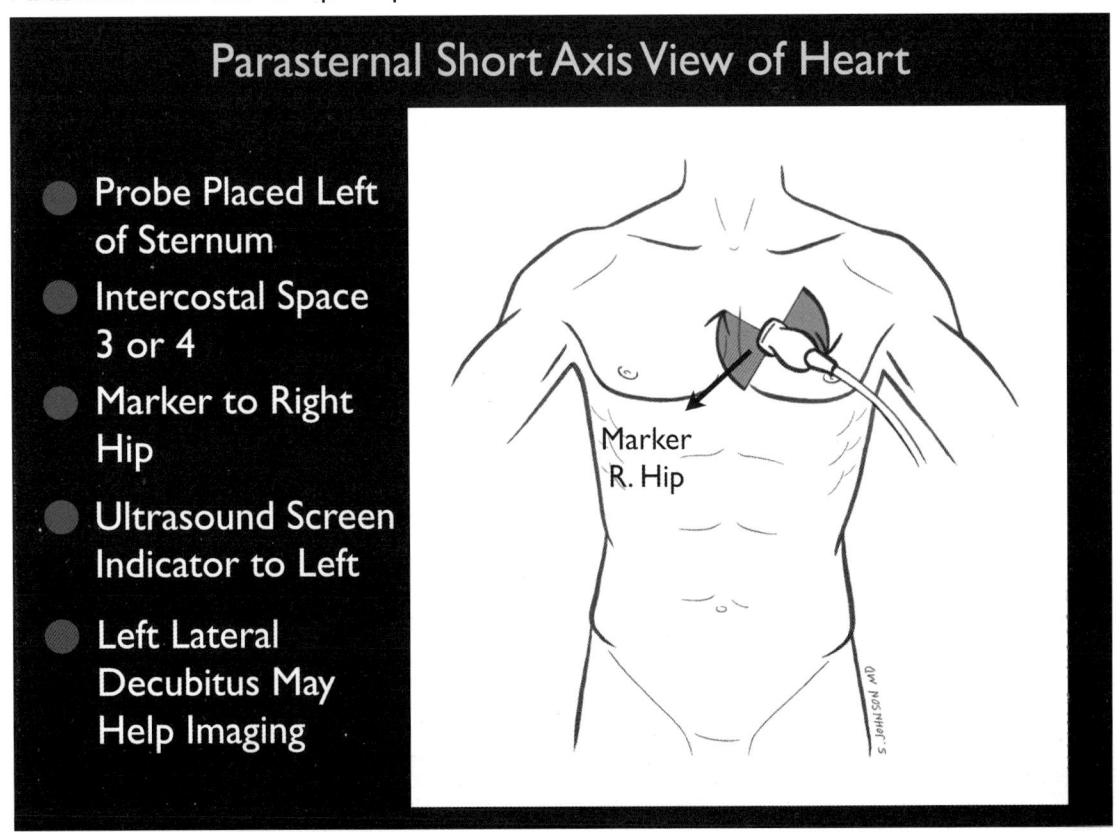

Parasternal Short Axis View of Heart

- Probe Placed Left of Sternum
- Intercostal Space 3 or 4
- Marker to Right Hip
- Ultrasound Screen Indicator to Left
- Left Lateral Decubitus May Help Imaging

with the three hepatic veins.

Next, rotate the probe from the subxiphoid four-chamber view to the subxiphoid two-chamber view, by orienting the probe with the indicator oriented superiorly toward the ceiling. This allows imaging of the right ventricle above the left ventricle, with the aorta typically seen in a long-axis orientation inferior to the heart (Figure 4-20). Moving the probe toward the patient's right side will bring the IVC into view (Figure 4-21).

Anatomic and Sonographic Correlation

The current recommendation for measurement of the IVC is at the point just inferior to the confluence with the hepatic veins, approximately 2 cm from the junction of the right atrium and the IVC.[14] Examining the IVC first as a circular structure in a short-axis plane is helpful. This can avoid slicing the ultrasound beam to the side of the IVC, which results in a falsely low measurement, a pitfall known as the cylinder tangent effect. The probe can then be rotated to view the IVC in a longitudinal plane, allowing confirmation of the accuracy of vessel measurements.

Differentiation of IVC from Aorta

The aorta and the IVC can be confused with one another. The aorta can be identified as a thicker walled and pulsatile structure, with more prominent branch vessels; it is located toward the patient's left side. In contrast, the IVC has thinner walls, is often compressible with the probe, can be seen to move through the liver, and is located toward the patient's right side. Although the IVC may have pulsations because of its proximity to the aorta, Doppler ultrasound allows differentiation of arterial pulsations from the phasic movement of IVC blood with respirations (Figure 4-22).

Ultrasound Evaluation of the IVC for Volume Status

A patient's relative intravascular volume can be estimated noninvasively by examining both the relative size and the respiratory dynamics of the IVC. The assessment of the IVC should follow determination of cardiac contractility, allowing the clinician to evaluate both parameters together to more accurately gauge the volume status.

As the patient breathes, the IVC has a normal pattern of inspiratory collapse. This respiratory variation can be accentuated by having the patient sniff or inspire forcefully. M-mode ultrasound, positioned in both the short- and long-axis planes of the IVC, can graphically document these dynamic respiratory changes in vessel size. Previous studies have demonstrated a positive correlation between the size and respiratory change of the IVC taken simultaneously with the patient's measured central venous pressure (CVP). This examination is called sonospirometry (Figures 4-23, 4-24, 4-25, and 4-26).[15-23] ASE guidelines support this approach to evaluation of IVC size and respiratory change in the assessment of CVP and suggest specific ranges for estimated pressure measurements (Table 4-5).[24]

In intubated patients, the respiratory dynamics of the IVC are reversed. In these patients, the IVC becomes less compliant and more distended in both respiratory phases. However, im-

FIGURE 4-13.

Parasternal short-axis view: anatomy

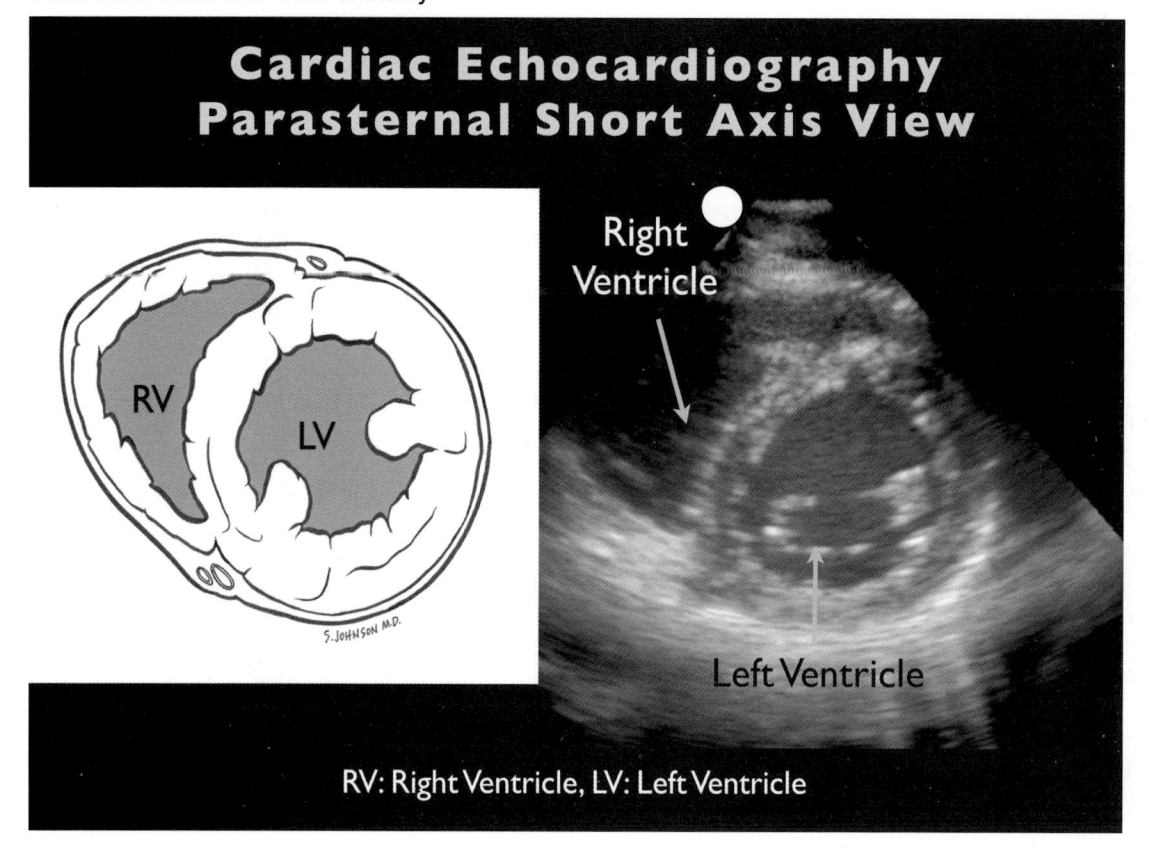

Cardiac Echocardiography
Parasternal Short Axis View

RV: Right Ventricle, LV: Left Ventricle

CARDIOVASCULAR EMERGENCIES

FIGURE 4-14.

Parasternal short-axis view: aortic valve

Parasternal Short Axis View - Level of Aortic Valve:

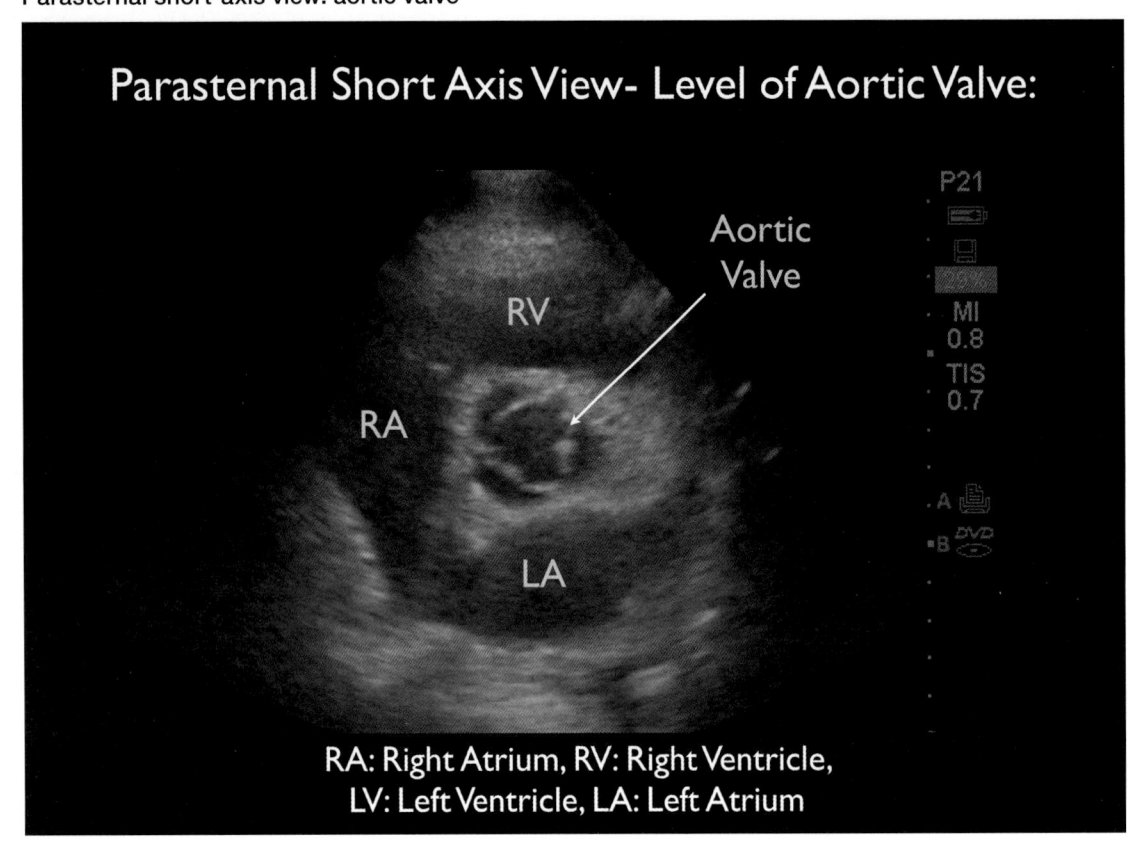

RV, RA, LA, Aortic Valve

RA: Right Atrium, RV: Right Ventricle,
LV: Left Ventricle, LA: Left Atrium

FIGURE 4-15.

Subxiphoid view: probe position

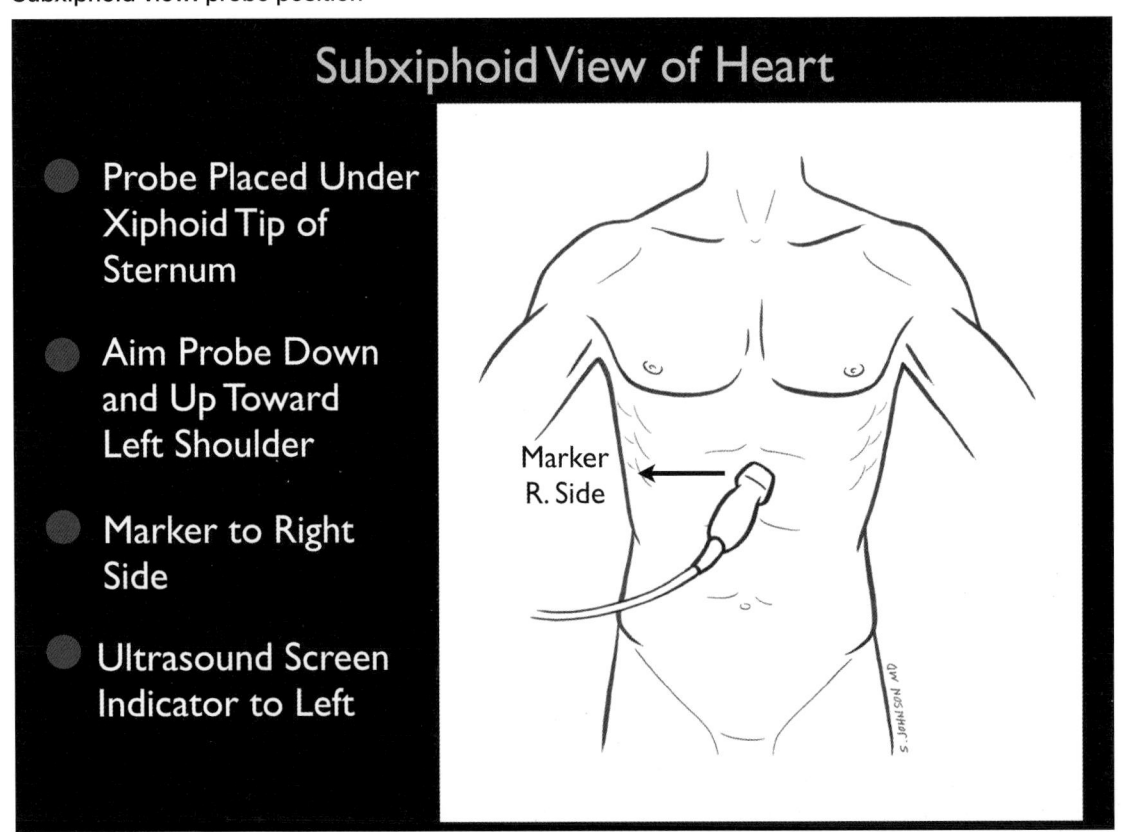

Subxiphoid View of Heart

- Probe Placed Under Xiphoid Tip of Sternum
- Aim Probe Down and Up Toward Left Shoulder
- Marker to Right Side
- Ultrasound Screen Indicator to Left

Marker R. Side

portant physiologic data can still be obtained, as fluid responsiveness correlates with an increase in IVC diameter over time.[25]

KEY POINTS

Evaluation of the IVC allows noninvasive assessment of intravascular volume status, which can be integral in managing the cardiac patient and the patient in shock.

Place the probe in the position described above for the subxiphoid view. Angling the probe relatively inferiorly toward the spine will image the IVC in cross section as it enters the right atrium. Further angling of the probe inferiorly will image the IVC at the confluence to the hepatic veins.

The IVC should also be visualized in long axis by swiveling the probe so that the marker is oriented superiorly and toward the ceiling.

A noninvasive determination of CVP can be made by evaluation of both the absolute size and the percentage inspiratory collapse of the IVC. This determination is made from analysis of the IVC just inferior to the confluence of the hepatic veins (Table 4-5).

Evaluation of the Internal Jugular Veins

The internal jugular veins can be evaluated as an alternative means of volume assessment. This is helpful in the patient in whom a gas-filled stomach or intestine inhibits imaging of the IVC. The patient should be positioned with the head of the bed elevated to 30°. A high-frequency linear-array probe is recommended for this examination. For volume assessment, both the relative fullness and the height of the vessel column in the neck should be examined. Both short- and long-axis views can be used (Figures 4-27 and 4-28). The percentage change in these parameters with respiratory dynamics can also be evaluated, similar to assessment of the IVC.[26-28]

KEY POINTS

Evaluation of the internal jugular veins is another noninvasive means of intravascular volume assessment. This approach is most important in the patient in whom the IVC cannot be adequately visualized.

Use a high-frequency linear-array ultrasound probe for evaluation of the internal jugular veins.

Position the patient with the head of bed upright at 30°. Place the probe in both short- and long-axis orientations over the internal jugular vein to observe for the relative level of the closing column of blood.

CVP can be determined by observing both the relative height and the respiratory dynamics of the closing column of blood in the internal jugular veins. In patients with low CVP, the closing column is low in the neck and moves further inferiorly with inspiration. In patients with a high CVP, the closing column is high in the neck, and this position changes little with inspiration.

FIGURE 4-16.

Subxiphoid view: anatomy

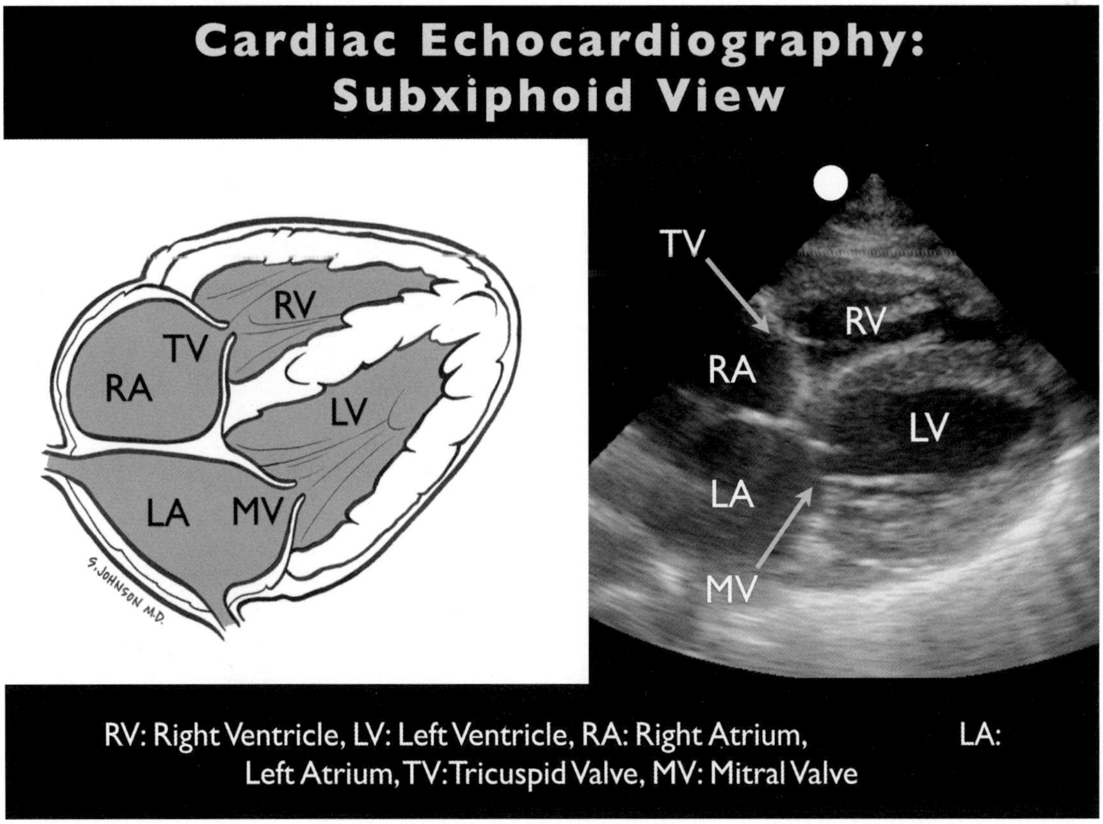

RV: Right Ventricle, LV: Left Ventricle, RA: Right Atrium, LA: Left Atrium, TV: Tricuspid Valve, MV: Mitral Valve

CARDIOVASCULAR EMERGENCIES

FIGURE 4-17.

Apical view: probe position

Apical View of Heart

- Probe Placed Under Left Nipple
- Point Maximal Impulse of Heart
- Marker to Right Side
- Ultrasound Screen Indicator to Left
- Left Lateral Decubitus Position Improves Image

Marker R. Side

FIGURE 4-18.

Apical view: anatomy

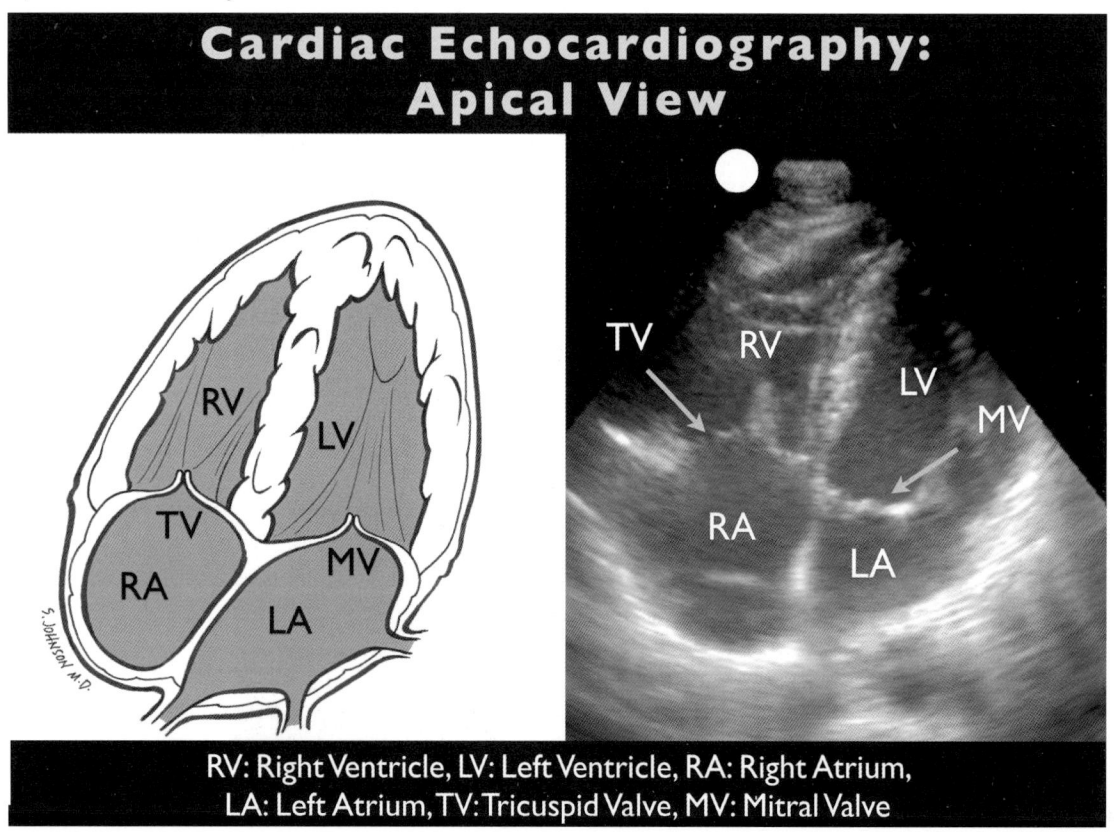

Cardiac Echocardiography: Apical View

RV: Right Ventricle, LV: Left Ventricle, RA: Right Atrium, LA: Left Atrium, TV: Tricuspid Valve, MV: Mitral Valve

Diagnosis of Pericardial Effusions and Cardiac Tamponade

Pathophysiology

Pericardial effusions are found relatively commonly in critically ill patients presenting with acute shortness of breath, respiratory failure, shock, and cardiac arrest.[29,30] Fortunately, the literature indicates that emergency physicians with focused echo training can identify effusions accurately.[31]

Pericardial effusions can result in hemodynamic instability as the pressure in the pericardial sac acutely increases, resulting in reduced cardiac filling.[32] Acute pericardial effusions (as small as 50 mL) can result in tamponade. This pathology can quickly compromise the trauma patient. Conversely, in chronic conditions, the pericardium can slowly stretch to accommodate large effusions over time, without the development of tamponade.[33]

Sonographic Appearance

Pericardial effusions are generally recognized by a dark, or anechoic, appearance; however, effusions associated with inflammatory or infectious conditions can have a brighter, or more echogenic, appearance. Traumatic pericardial effusions take on a brighter echogenic appearance over time as blood clots (Figure 4-29). A scale for describing the size of the effusion is shown in Table 4-6.[8]

Specific Echocardiographic Windows for Evaluating Pericardial Effusions

Parasternal Long-Axis View

Size and Location of Effusions. Smaller effusions first layer posteriorly behind the heart. As effusions grow in size, they surround the heart circumferentially, moving into the anterior pericardial space.[33] Most effusions are free flowing in the pericardial sac. Occasionally, loculated effusions occur, typically in postoperative cardiac surgery patients and in association with inflammatory conditions.[34]

Differentiation of Pleural from Pericardial Fluid. The critical landmarks for detection of a pericardial effusion are the descending aorta and the posterior pericardial reflection. The descending aorta appears as a circle directly behind the left atrium, posterior to the mitral valve (Figure 4-10). The posterior pericardial reflection can be identified as a hyperechoic structure, immediately anterior to the descending aorta. First, select the appropriate depth for the ultrasound image, so that the descending aorta and pericardial reflection are adequately identified posteriorly on the screen.

Pericardial effusions are located anterior to the descending aorta and above the posterior pericardial reflection (Figure 4-1). In contrast, pleural effusions are located posterior to the descending aorta and below the posterior pericardial reflection (Figure 4-30). To further confirm the presence of a left pleural effusion, the probe can be moved to a lateral position on the chest wall, as for the FAST views, and aimed above the dia-

FIGURE 4-19.

Apical five-chamber view

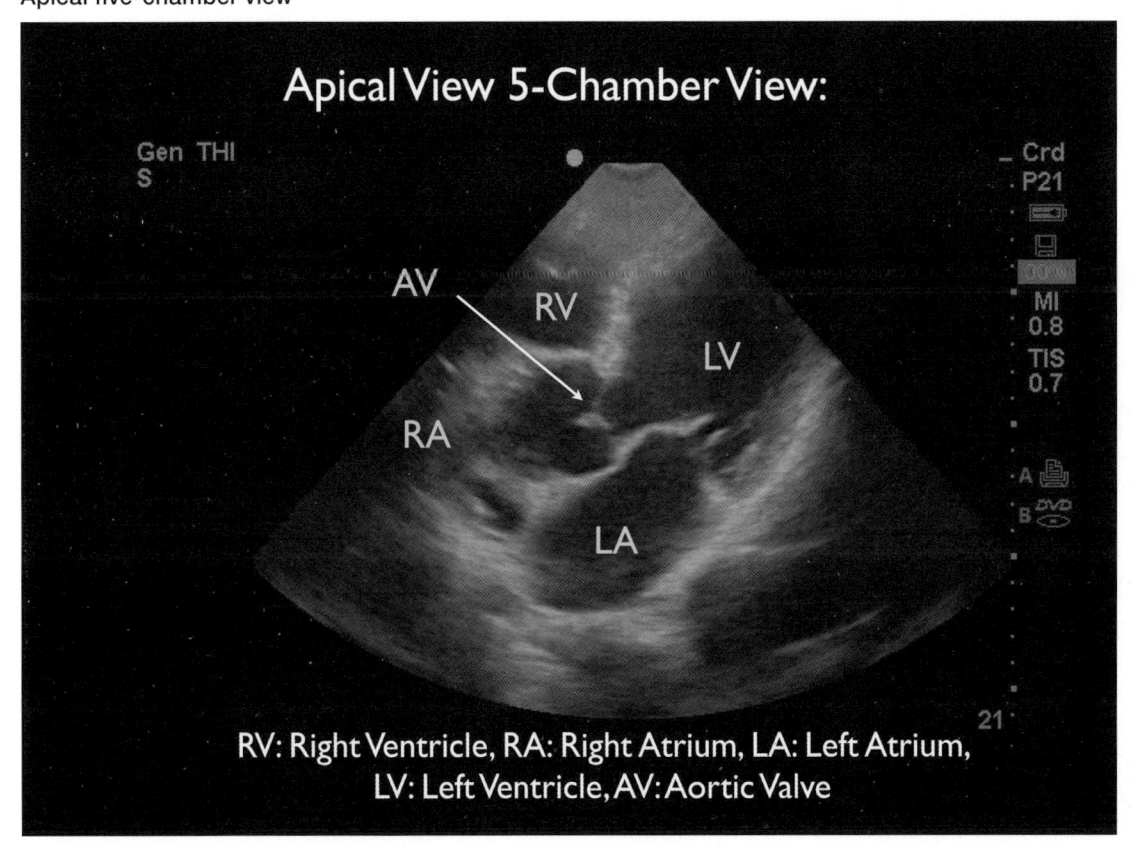

RV: Right Ventricle, RA: Right Atrium, LA: Left Atrium, LV: Left Ventricle, AV: Aortic Valve

CARDIOVASCULAR EMERGENCIES

FIGURE 4-20.

Subxiphoid two-chamber view: aorta long axis

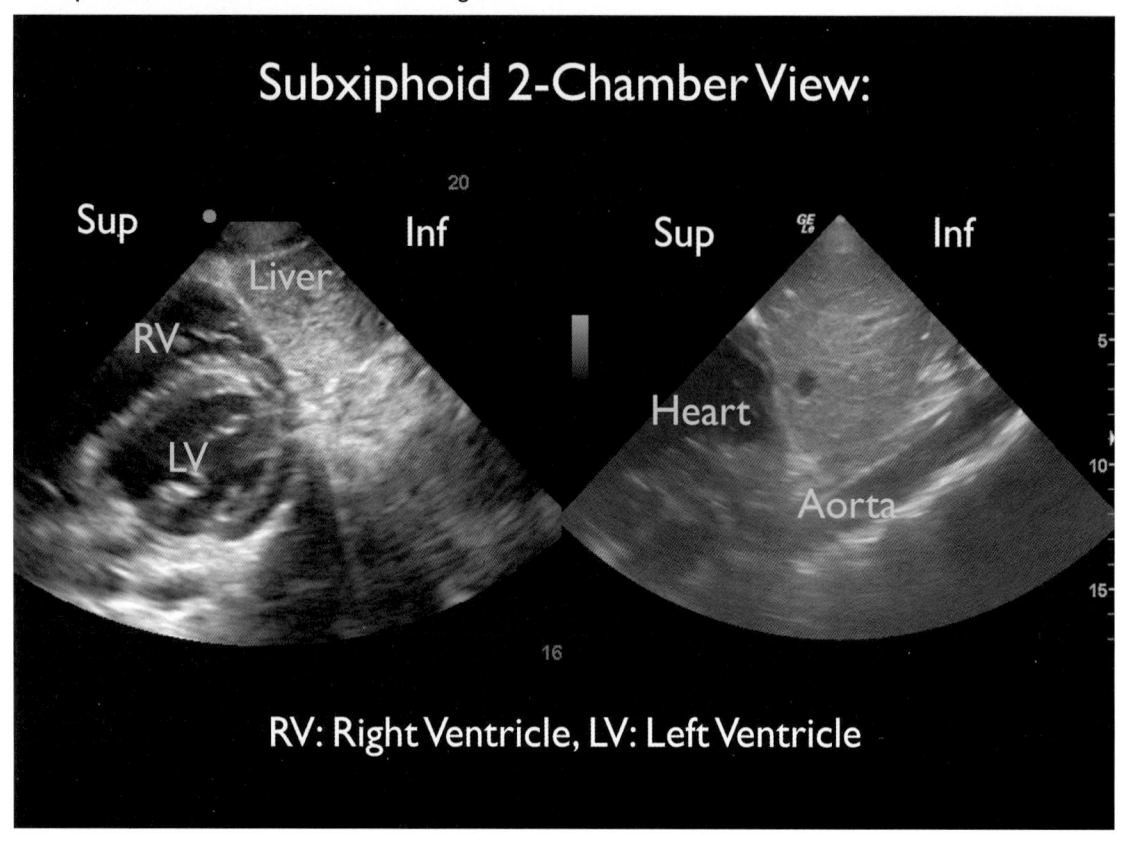

FIGURE 4-21.

Subxiphoid view for IVC

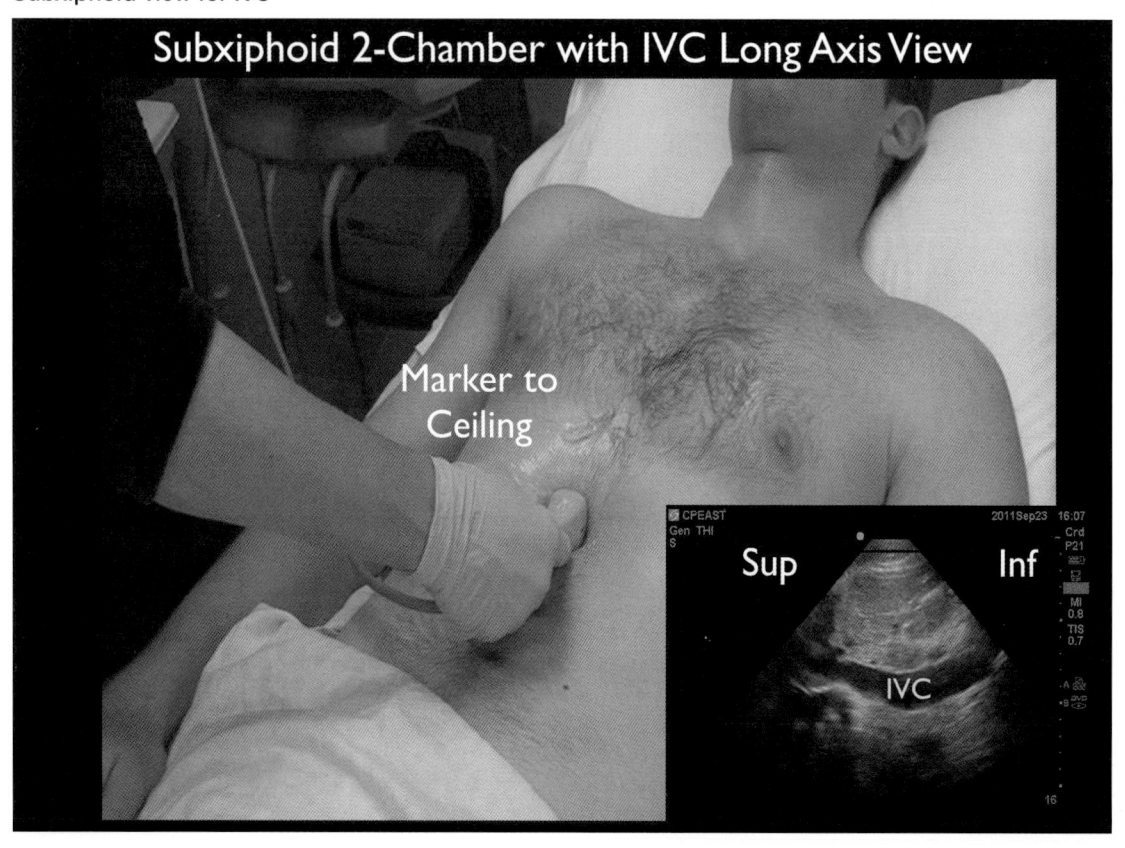

phragm to visualize the lower thoracic cavity (Figure 4-31).

Pericardial/Epicardial Fat Pad. A pericardial, or epicardial, fat pad might be confused with a pericardial effusion. The typical location for this structure is in the area just deep to the near-field pericardial reflection and anterior to the heart. The fat pad often has a classic appearance, with an interspersed speckling of bright, or hyperechoic, regions.

From the parasternal views, an isolated echo-dense structure in an anterior location is more suggestive of a fat pad, not an effusion. For an effusion to be visualized anteriorly on the parasternal views, a circumferential effusion usually needs to be present (with the exception of the more uncommon loculated anterior pericardial effusion). From the other cardiac views (like the subxiphoid), the fat pad would again be seen closer to the probe, just posterior to the near-field pericardial reflection and anterior to the heart (Figure 4-32).

Subxiphoid View

Size and Location of Effusions. Because the subxiphoid view is performed from a position inferior to the heart, small effusions typically first accumulate along the near-field pericardial reflection. This is especially noted in patients who have been in an upright position. Larger effusions spread to surround the heart circumferentially.

Differentiation of Pericardial Effusion from Ascites. Ascites can be confused with a pericardial effusion. Ascites is seen nearer to the probe, anterior to the near-field pericardial reflection, outside the pericardial sac, and surrounding the liver within the abdominal cavity. In contrast, a pericardial effusion is located posterior to the near-field pericardium, adjacent to the heart, and within the pericardial sac (Figure 4-33).

Echocardiographic Diagnosis of Cardiac Tamponade

Ultrasound Findings

As pericardial effusions accumulate, the pressure in the pericardial sac increases and affects the lower pressure circuit of the right heart first. This is best recognized sonographically as an inability of these chambers to fully expand during the relaxation phase of the cardiac cycle. Cardiac tamponade is thus classically defined on ultrasound as diastolic collapse of either the right atrium or the right ventricle (Figure 4-34).

Although both right heart chambers should be evaluated, diastolic collapse of the right ventricle is a more specific finding. As tamponade progresses, the right atrium can take on the appearance of a "furiously contracting chamber," with hyperdynamic contractions. At times, this makes differentiation of systolic contraction from diastolic collapse more difficult.

Diastolic collapse of the right ventricle in tamponade is best understood as a spectrum of ultrasound findings, from a subtle serpentine deflection of the wall to complete chamber compression (Figure 4-35).[35] One important pitfall to this general diagnostic strategy is seen in the patient with pulmonary hypertension, where diastolic collapse of the right heart can occur late in the disease process.

FIGURE 4-22.

IVC and aorta, color-flow Doppler

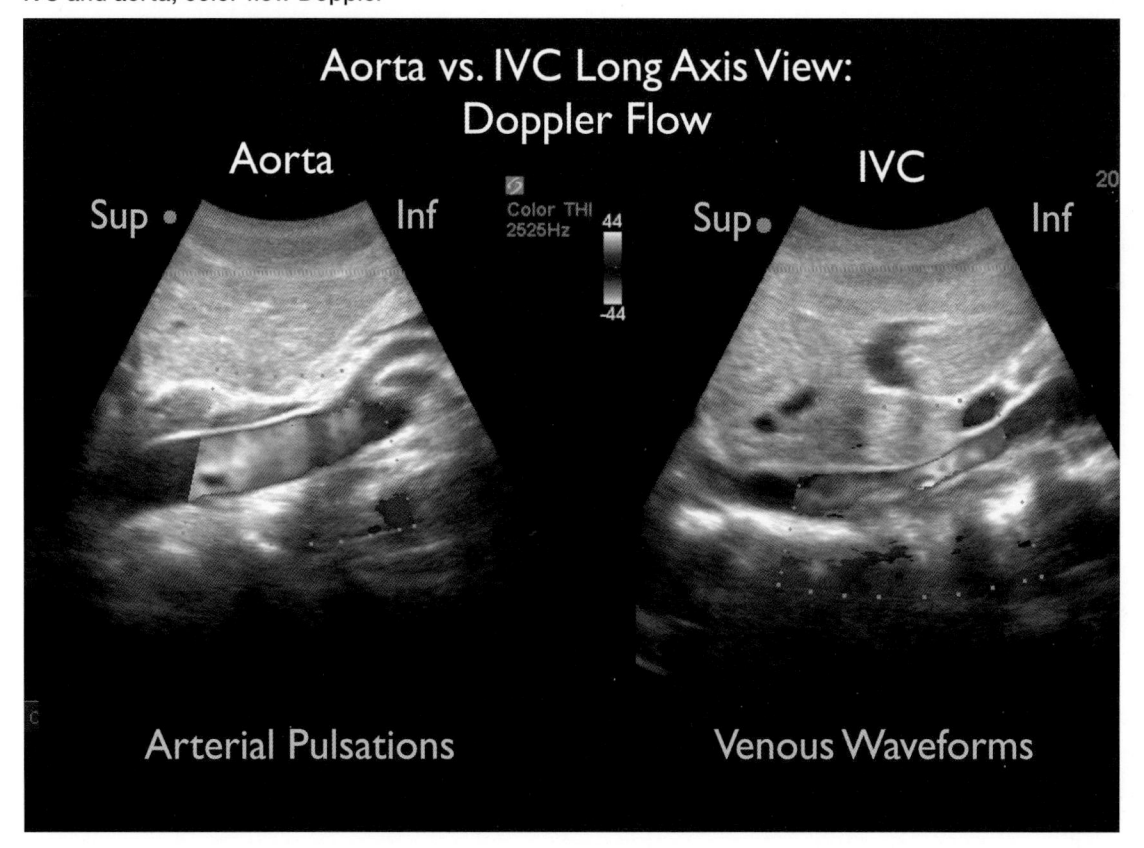

CARDIOVASCULAR EMERGENCIES

FIGURE 4-23.
IVC evaluation, low CVP

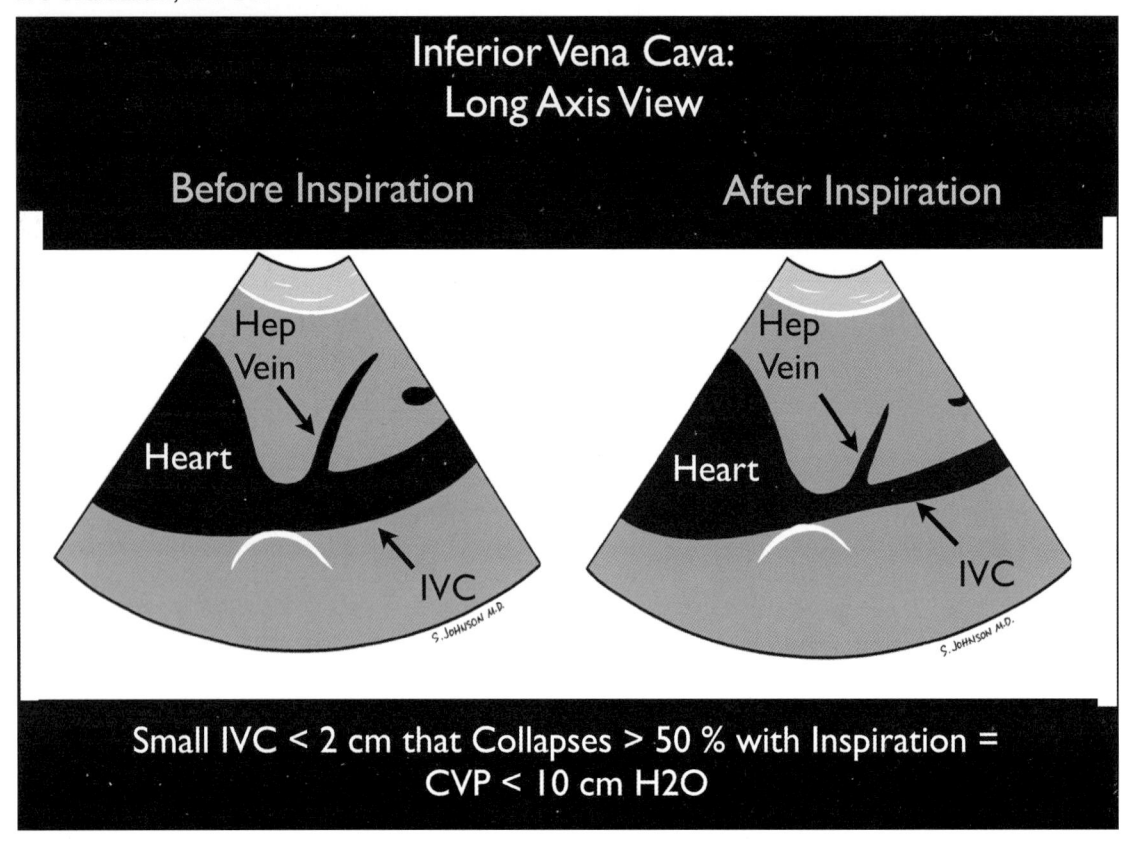

Inferior Vena Cava:
Long Axis View

Before Inspiration — After Inspiration

Small IVC < 2 cm that Collapses > 50 % with Inspiration = CVP < 10 cm H2O

FIGURE 4-24.
IVC evaluation, high CVP

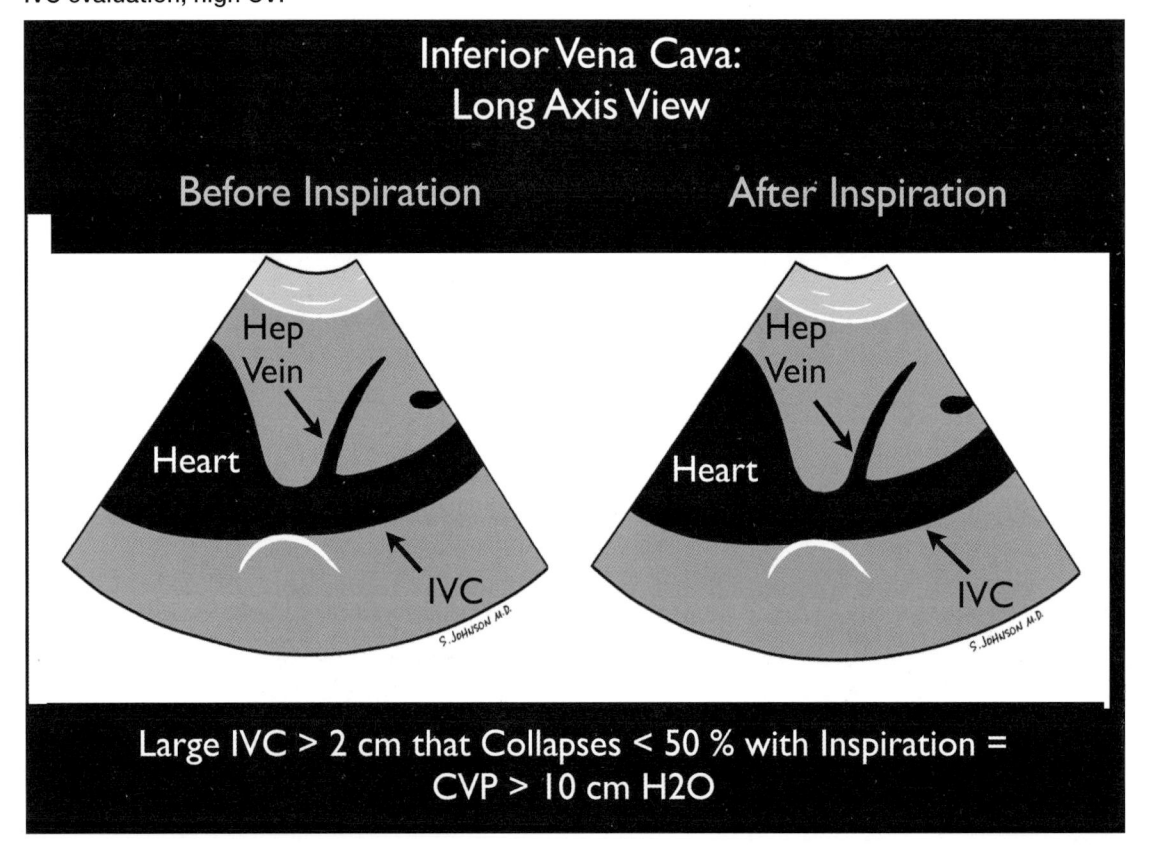

Inferior Vena Cava:
Long Axis View

Before Inspiration — After Inspiration

Large IVC > 2 cm that Collapses < 50 % with Inspiration = CVP > 10 cm H2O

Advanced Strategies in the Identification of Tamponade

Several more advanced strategies can be used to document diastolic compression of the right heart in tamponade.[36] The first is to attach an ECG monitoring lead to the ultrasound machine to allow simultaneous display of both the electrical and echo phases. The IVC can also be evaluated to confirm tamponade physiology. A dilated IVC without significant respiratory collapse implies tamponade physiology.[37]

A more advanced examination using Doppler ultrasound is one of the most sensitive tests for the evaluation of tamponade. From the apical four-chamber view, color-flow Doppler can be used first to identify the flow of blood through the tricuspid and mitral valves. Pulsed-wave Doppler can then be directed onto the jet of blood through either valve. This allows identification of augmented differences in the velocity of flow during the respiratory cycle that occurs in tamponade. During inspiration, blood flow through the tricuspid valve increases and flow through the mitral valve decreases as tamponade progresses (Figure 4-6).[38]

Ultrasound-Guided Pericardiocentesis

Emergency physicians have classically been taught the subxiphoid approach for pericardiocentesis. However, a large review from the Mayo Clinic, which included 1,127 pericardiocentesis procedures, found that the optimal position for placement of the needle was the apical position in 80% of patients.[39] The subxiphoid approach was chosen in only 20% of these procedures because of concern regarding the interposition of the liver. Ultrasound allows accurate guidance of the pericardiocentesis needle and guidewire into the pericardial sac (Figure 4-36). In addition, agitated saline can be used as a form of ultrasound contrast to confirm proper needle placement in the pericardial space.[40,41]

KEY POINTS

Pericardial effusions and cardiac tamponade can be diagnosed in a significant percentage of critical patients. Bedside ultrasound allows a quick, noninvasive, and sensitive means for diagnosing pericardial effusions and further assessment of tamponade physiology.

Pericardial effusions can be seen on all the major echo windows and typically have a dark, or anechoic, appearance on ultrasound.

Small effusions are generally first seen in the most dependent areas of the pericardial sac. Larger effusions will grow to circumferentially surround the heart. Because the pericardium is a tough and fibrous tissue, small effusions can cause tamponade early, while large effusions can gradually stretch the pericardium, causing tamponade relatively later.

Cardiac tamponade can be diagnosed on echo by looking for diastolic collapse of the right atrium and/or right ventricle. Other advanced means for the identification of tamponade include using simultaneous ECG monitoring to better identify the diastolic cardiac phase, Doppler

FIGURE 4-25.

IVC B-mode, long-axis view

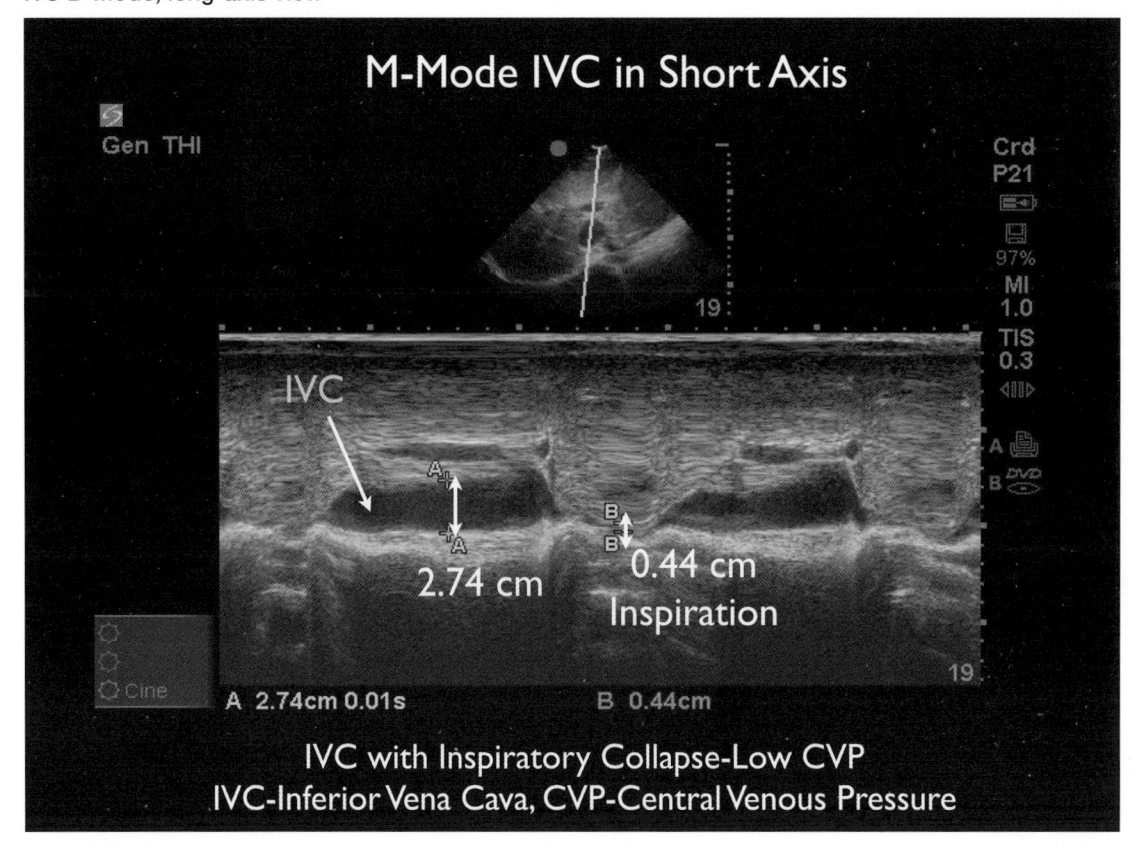

CARDIOVASCULAR EMERGENCIES

FIGURE 4-26.

IVC M-mode, low CVP

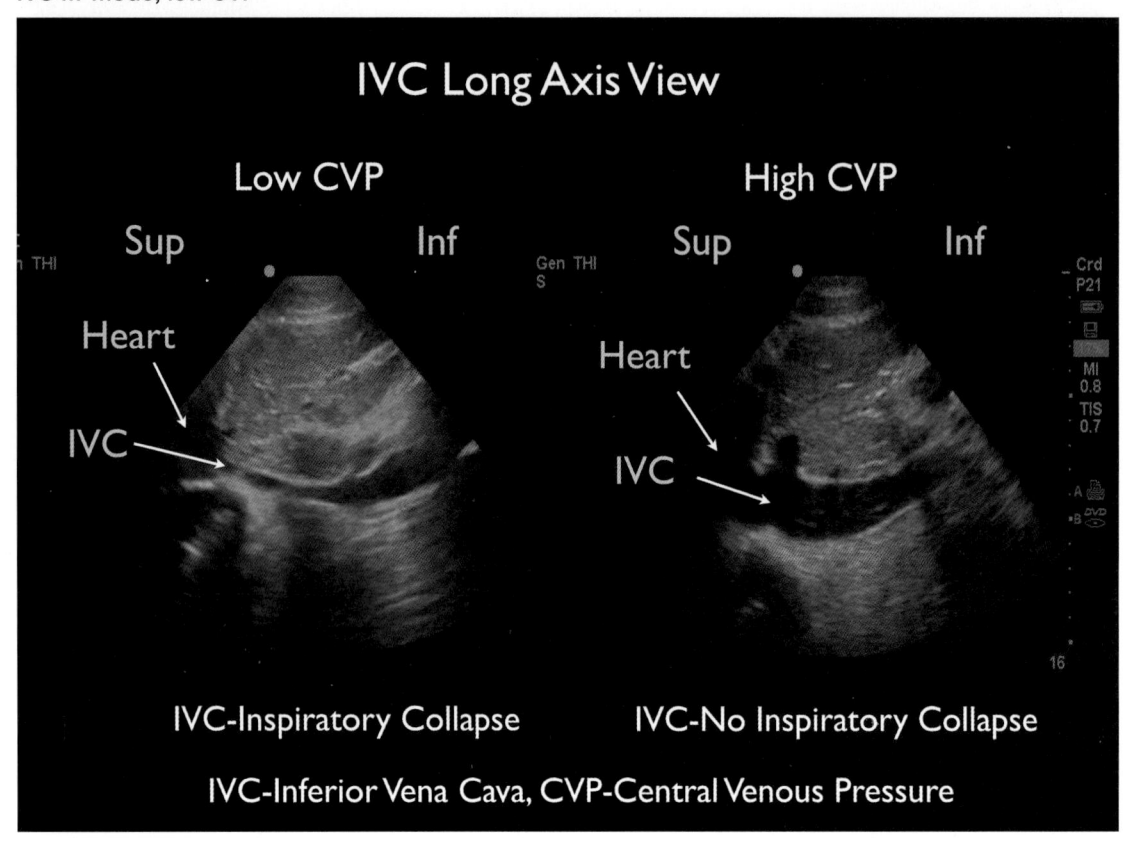

IVC Long Axis View

Low CVP — IVC-Inspiratory Collapse

High CVP — IVC-No Inspiratory Collapse

IVC-Inferior Vena Cava, CVP-Central Venous Pressure

FIGURE 4-27.

Internal jugular vein, low CVP

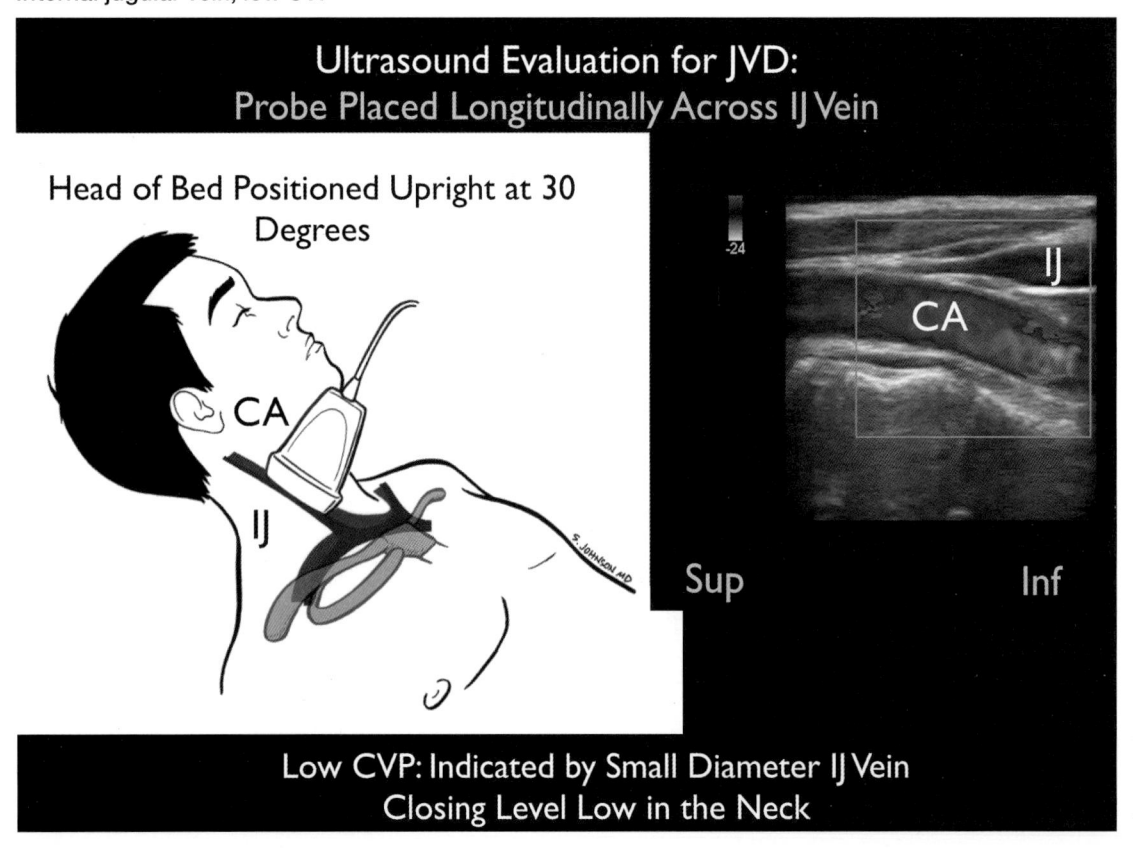

Ultrasound Evaluation for JVD: Probe Placed Longitudinally Across IJ Vein

Head of Bed Positioned Upright at 30 Degrees

Low CVP: Indicated by Small Diameter IJ Vein Closing Level Low in the Neck

assessment of augmented respiratory-induced variation in blood flow across the tricuspid and mitral valves, and, finally, assessment of the IVC for signs of elevated CVP.

Assessment of Cardiac Contractility

Many critically ill patients have compromised cardiac function contributing to their shock state, and that dysfunction can be diagnosed with bedside echo.[42] Studies have documented that emergency physicians with focused training can accurately evaluate left ventricular contractility.[43]

TABLE 4-5.

IVC Size and Collapsibility: Correlation With CVP (ASE Guidelines)

IVC diameter <2.1 cm, collapses >50% with sniff
Correlates with a normal CVP pressure of 3 mm Hg (range, 0-5 mm Hg)
Considered normal in the healthy patient but low in the critically ill hypotensive patient
IVC diameter >2.1 cm, collapses <50% with sniff:
Correlates with a high CVP of 15 mm Hg (range, 10-20 mm Hg)
When IVC diameter and collapsibility do not fit with the above indices, an intermediate value of 8 mm Hg (range, 5-10 mm Hg) can be used

Qualitative Evaluation of Left Ventricular Systolic Contractility

Evaluating motion of the left ventricular walls by a visual estimation of the volume change from diastole to systole provides a qualitative assessment of contractility.[42-44] A ventricle that has good contractility has a large volume change between the two cycles, while a poorly contracting heart has a small percentage change (Figures 4-37 and 4-38). The poorly contracting heart can also be dilated. Based on these assessments, cardiac contractility can be broadly categorized as normal, mild to moderately decreased, or severely decreased. A fourth, hyperdynamic, category can be seen in patients with advanced hypovolemia or in distributive shock states. In this scenario, the heart has small chambers and vigorous, hyperkinetic contractions with the endocardial walls almost touching together during systole.

Evaluation for Diastolic Heart Failure

The above measurements apply to the category of decreased left ventricular contractility, as seen in systolic dysfunction. Today, increasing numbers of patients are being diagnosed with diastolic heart failure, which is common in patients with chronic hypertension. The resulting left ventricular hypertrophy can be visualized with ultrasound. Episodic diastolic dysfunction can also occur in conditions such as acute pulmonary edema and sepsis.[45,46] The echo means of detecting this condition involves a complex assessment, specifically requiring Doppler evaluation of changes in blood flow across the mitral valve, seen during distinct stages of the disease.[47]

FIGURE 4-28.

Internal jugular vein, high CVP

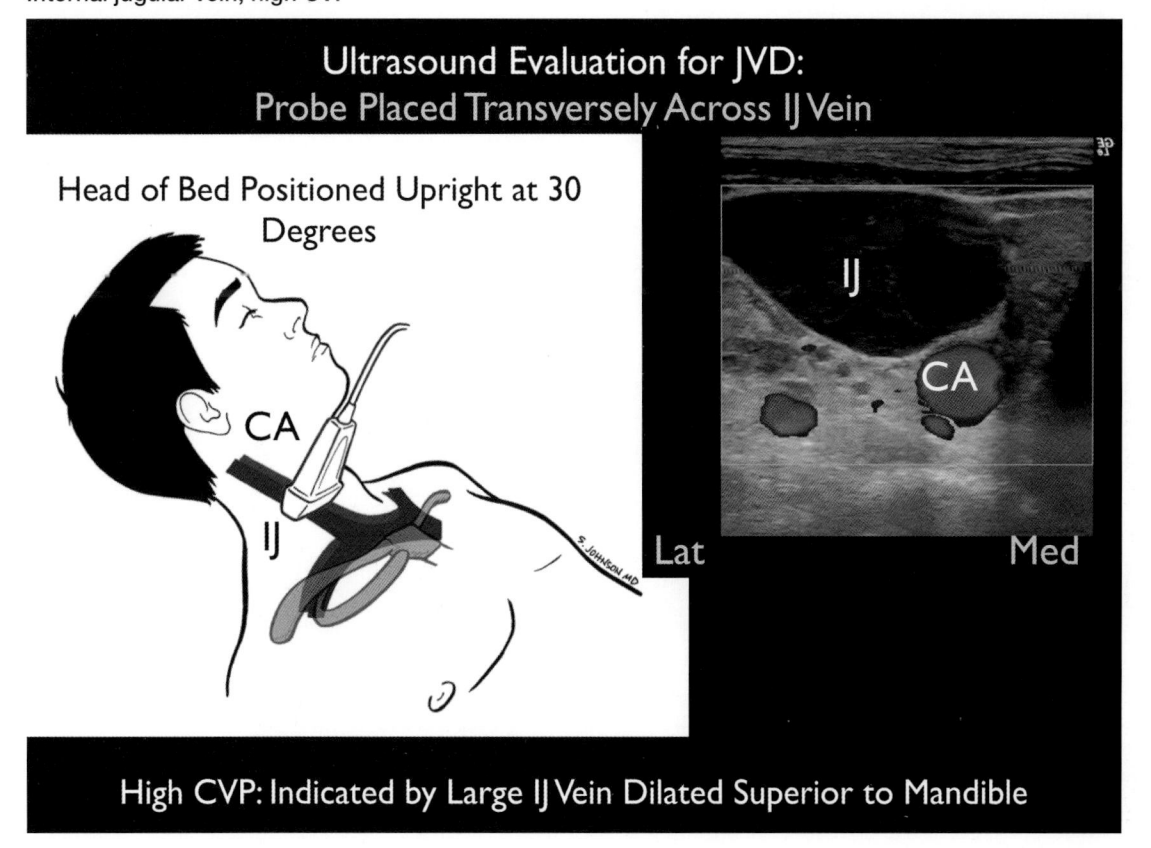

Ultrasound Evaluation for JVD: Probe Placed Transversely Across IJ Vein

Head of Bed Positioned Upright at 30 Degrees

High CVP: Indicated by Large IJ Vein Dilated Superior to Mandible

CARDIOVASCULAR EMERGENCIES

FIGURE 4-29.
Types of pericardial effusions

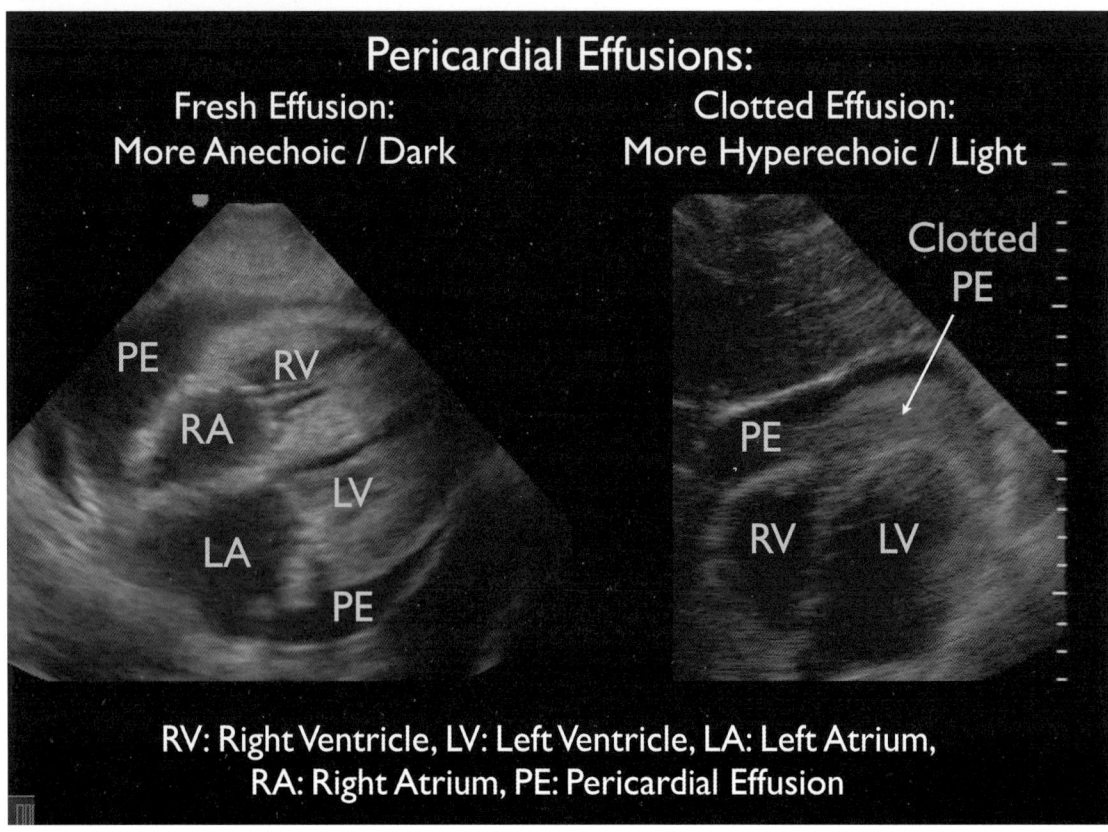

Pericardial Effusions:
Fresh Effusion: More Anechoic / Dark
Clotted Effusion: More Hyperechoic / Light

RV: Right Ventricle, LV: Left Ventricle, LA: Left Atrium, RA: Right Atrium, PE: Pericardial Effusion

FIGURE 4-30.
Pleural fluid

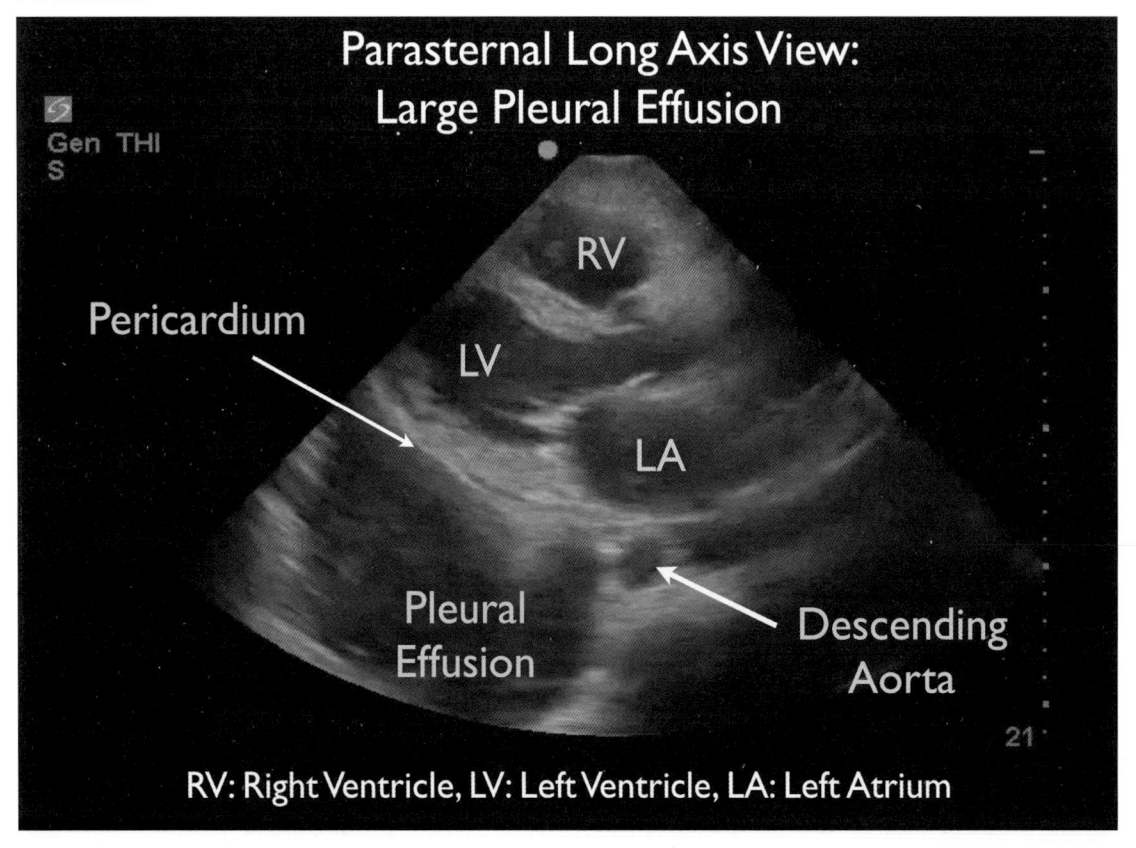

Parasternal Long Axis View: Large Pleural Effusion

RV: Right Ventricle, LV: Left Ventricle, LA: Left Atrium

Semiquantitative Assessment of Contractility

Fractional Shortening

M-mode ultrasound can be used to graphically depict the movements of the left ventricular walls through the cardiac cycle. To perform this evaluation, the M-mode cursor is placed across the mid-portion of the left ventricle just beyond the tips of the mitral valve leaflets. The resulting tracing allows a two-dimensional, length-based measurement of the chamber diameters over time.

Fractional shortening is calculated according to the following formula:

$$(EDD - ESD) / EDD \times 100$$

in which ESD is end-systolic diameter, measured at the smallest dimension between the ventricular walls, and EDD is the end-diastolic diameter where the distance is greatest (Figures 4-2 and 4-3).

In general, fractional shortening above 35% to 40% correlates to a normal ejection fraction.[48] Compared with the comprehensive volumetric assessment required for measuring ejection fraction, fractional shortening is a semiquantitative method for determining systolic function that is relatively fast and easy to perform.[49]

E-Point Septal Separation

Motion of the anterior leaflet of the mitral valve in the parasternal long-axis view can also be used to assess left ventricular contractility, with the caveat that mitral valve abnormalities (stenosis, regurgitation), aortic regurgitation, and extreme left ventricular hypertrophy are not present.

In a normal contractile state, the anterior mitral leaflet can be observed to flip open and almost touch the septal wall during diastole. Early opening of the mitral valve is represented on M-mode ultrasound as the E-point. The distance measured between the E-point, representing the position of early opening of the mitral valve, and the septum is known as the E-point septal separation (EPSS).[50] To measure the EPSS, the M-mode cursor is placed over the tip of the anterior mitral valve leaflet. In a normal contractile state, the mitral valve will open fully to a position close to the septum, resulting in an EPSS less than 7 mm (Figure 4-4).[50-52] As left ventricular contractility decreases, the EPSS correspondingly increases, because of more limited opening of the mitral valve. Research is ongoing to determine the accuracy of correlation between EPSS and fractional shortening.[53]

TABLE 4-6.

Grading Scale for Pericardial Effusions

Small: Less than 1 cm in depth, noncircumferential around heart
Moderate: Less than 1 cm in depth, circumferential around heart
Large: More than 1 cm in depth, circumferential around the heart

FIGURE 4-31.

Pleural effusion

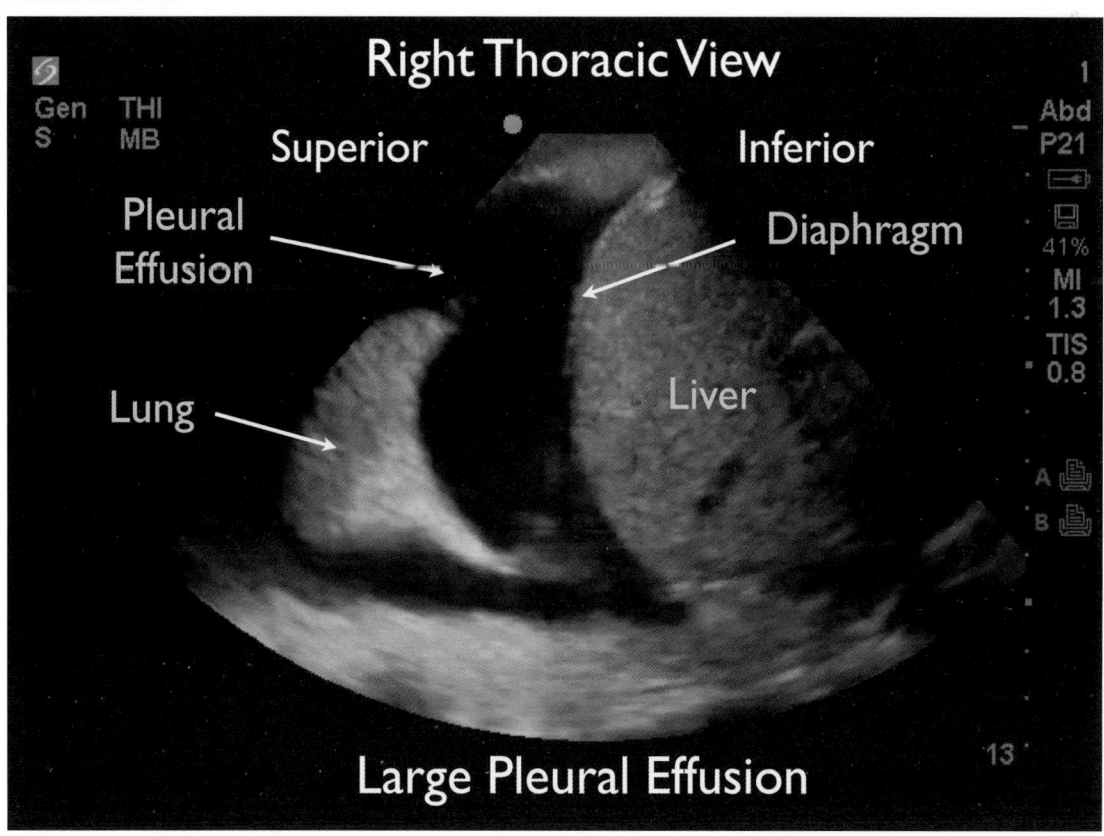

CARDIOVASCULAR EMERGENCIES

FIGURE 4-32.

Pericardial fat pad

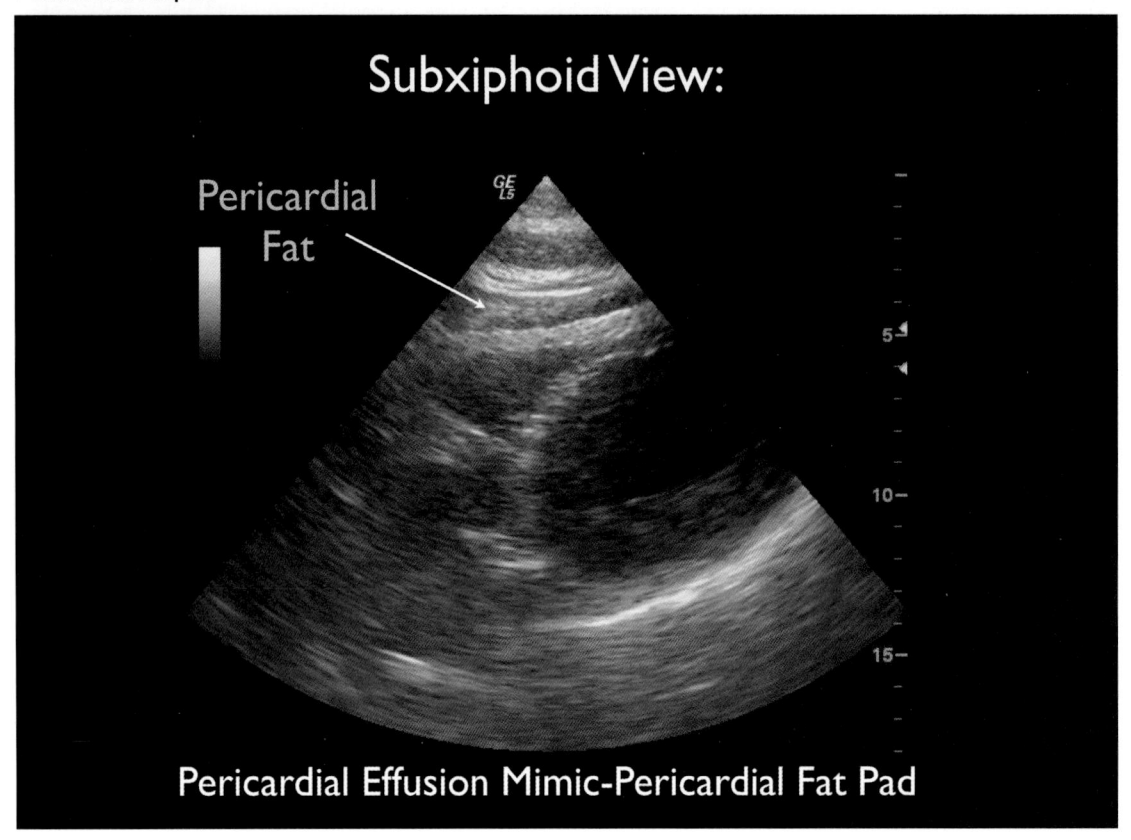

FIGURE 4-33.

Subxiphoid view, pericardial effusion vs. ascites

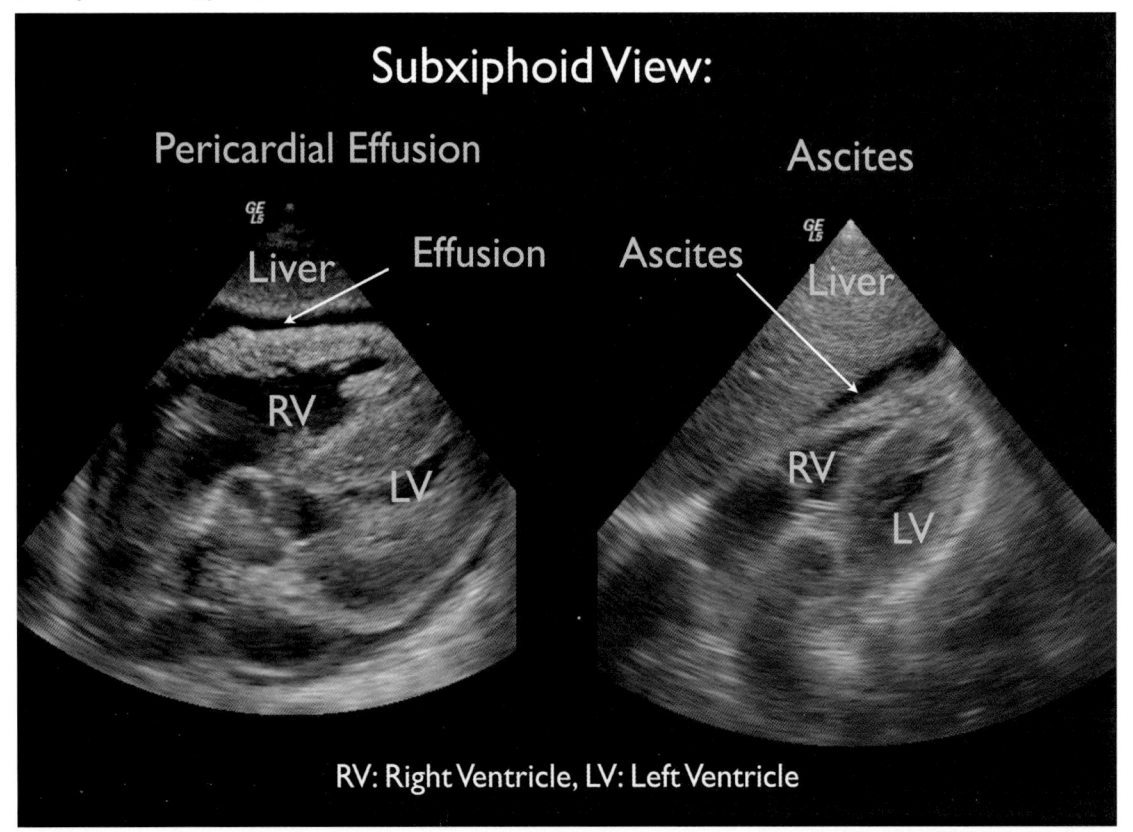

Quantitative Volumetric Measurements of Left Ventricular Contractility–Ejection Fraction

This three-dimensional volumetric assessment of cardiac function is employed in the echo lab.

Ejection fraction (EF) is defined by the following equation:

$$EF = \text{Stroke volume} \div \text{End-diastolic volume}$$

This value represents the volume change of the left ventricle during systole. It is best measured by the biplane method of discs, known as Simpson's modified rule, which employs the concept that the left ventricle represents a bullet-shaped structure.[54] Using this method, the endocardial borders of the left ventricle are traced in two orthogonal views during end-diastole and end-systole, generally from the apical four- and two-chamber views (Figure 4-39). Calculation software can then generate the multiple discs representing the left ventricle and will sum the calculated volumes to provide an accurate ventricular volume. First, the stroke volume is calculated as the difference between the diastolic and systolic volumetric measurements. Next, ejection fraction is calculated using the equation presented above.[55] Because this measurement is relatively complex and time intensive, it is not currently a routine part of the goal-directed echo evaluation performed by emergency physicians.

KEY POINTS

Focused echo can allow an accurate determination of left ventricular contractility, which can be crucial to management of the cardiac patient and the patient in shock.

Left ventricular contractility can be evaluated from all the major echo windows.

Rapid qualitative assessment of left ventricular contractility can be determined by looking at the relative movements of the ventricular walls from diastole to systole.

More advanced means for evaluation of left ventricular contractility include M-mode ultrasound. The fractional shortening of the left ventricular cavity through the cardiac cycle can be quantified. Next, the mitral valve E-point septal separation can be assessed by evaluation of the early diastolic movement of the valve, allowing another quantitative assessment of contractility.

Echocardiography for Pulmonary Embolus

Although computed tomography angiography is typically thought of as the current diagnostic standard for pulmonary embolism, focused echo can identify one of the more serious complications of this disease—right ventricular strain. This finding correlates with a poorer patient prognosis and the need for more immediate treatment.[56,57] Right ventricular enlargement on focused echo can also suggest this pathology in the undifferentiated patient presenting in shock, potentially leading to more timely diagnosis and treatment (see RUSH section below).

Current Literature Assessing Echocardiography for Pulmonary Embolus

Multiple studies have evaluated the use of echo for the diagnosis of pulmonary embolus. The current literature finds the

FIGURE 4-34.

Cardiac tamponade, right atrial collapse

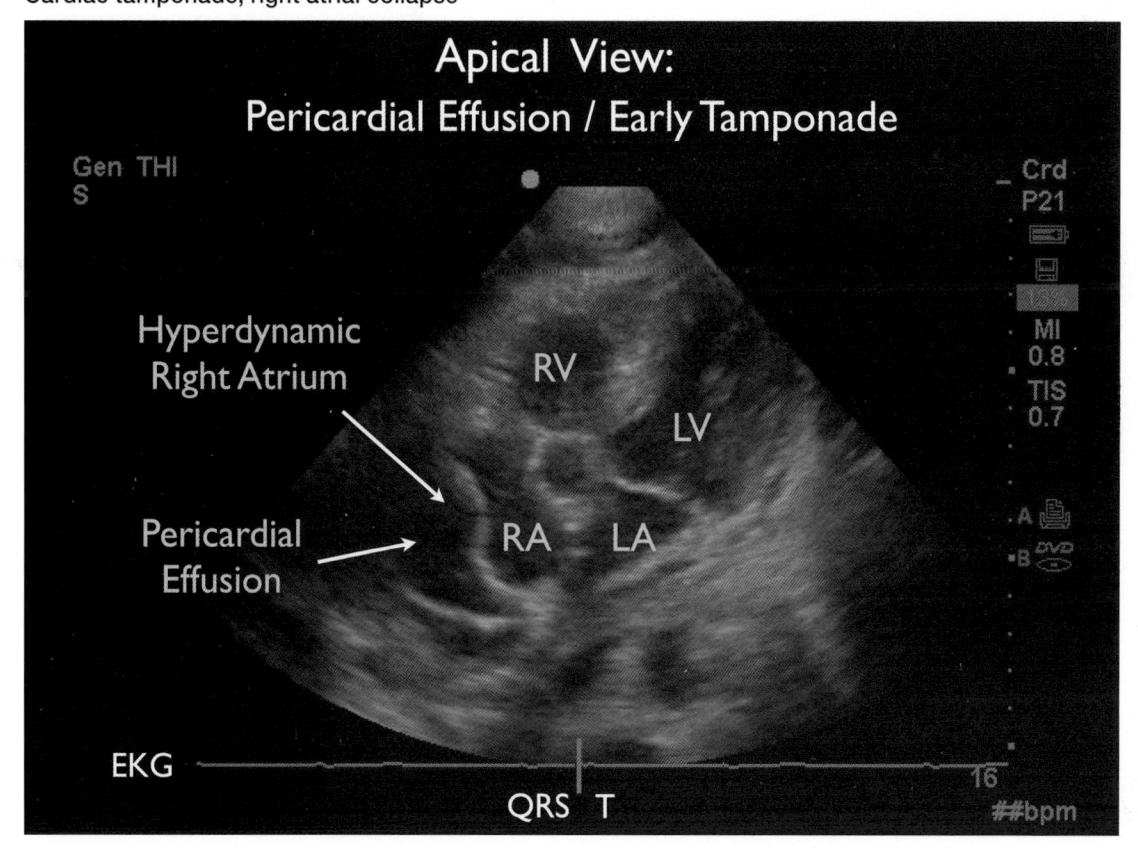

CARDIOVASCULAR EMERGENCIES

FIGURE 4-35.

Cardiac tamponade, right ventricular collapse

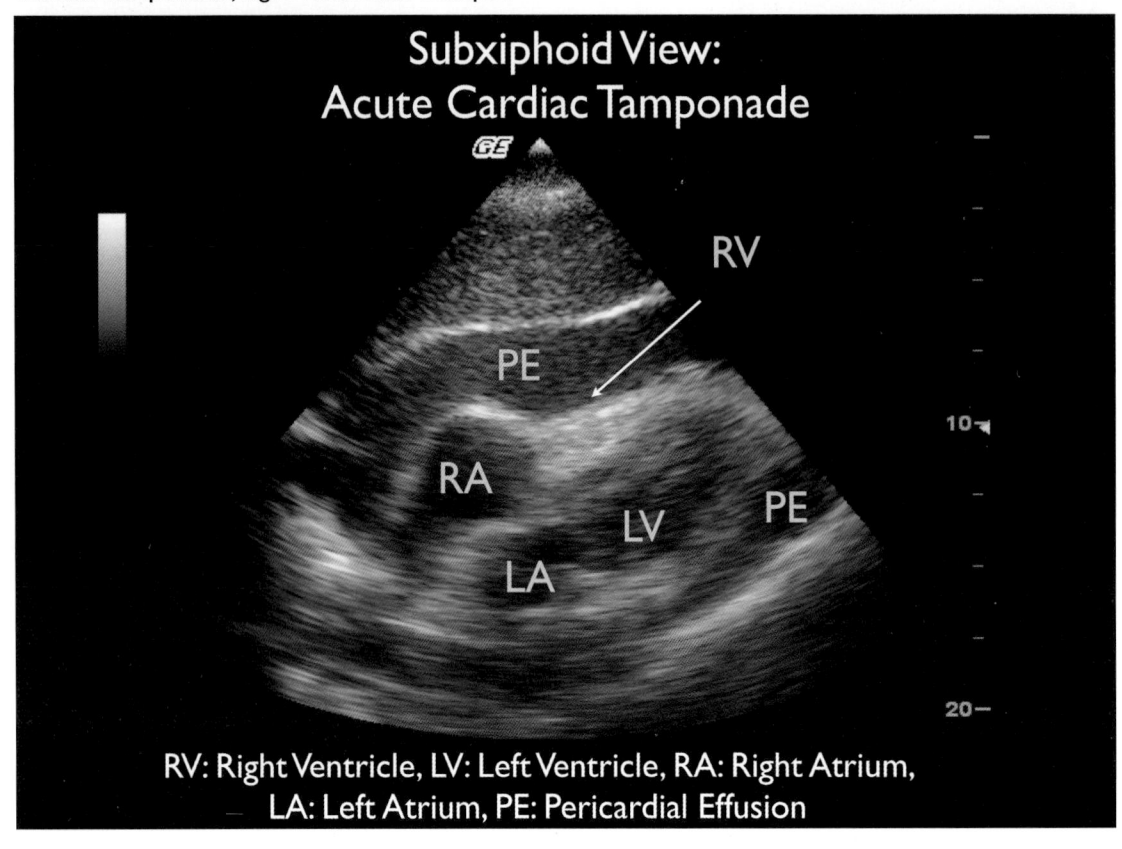

Subxiphoid View: Acute Cardiac Tamponade

RV: Right Ventricle, LV: Left Ventricle, RA: Right Atrium, LA: Left Atrium, PE: Pericardial Effusion

FIGURE 4-36.

Ultrasound guidance for pericardiocentesis

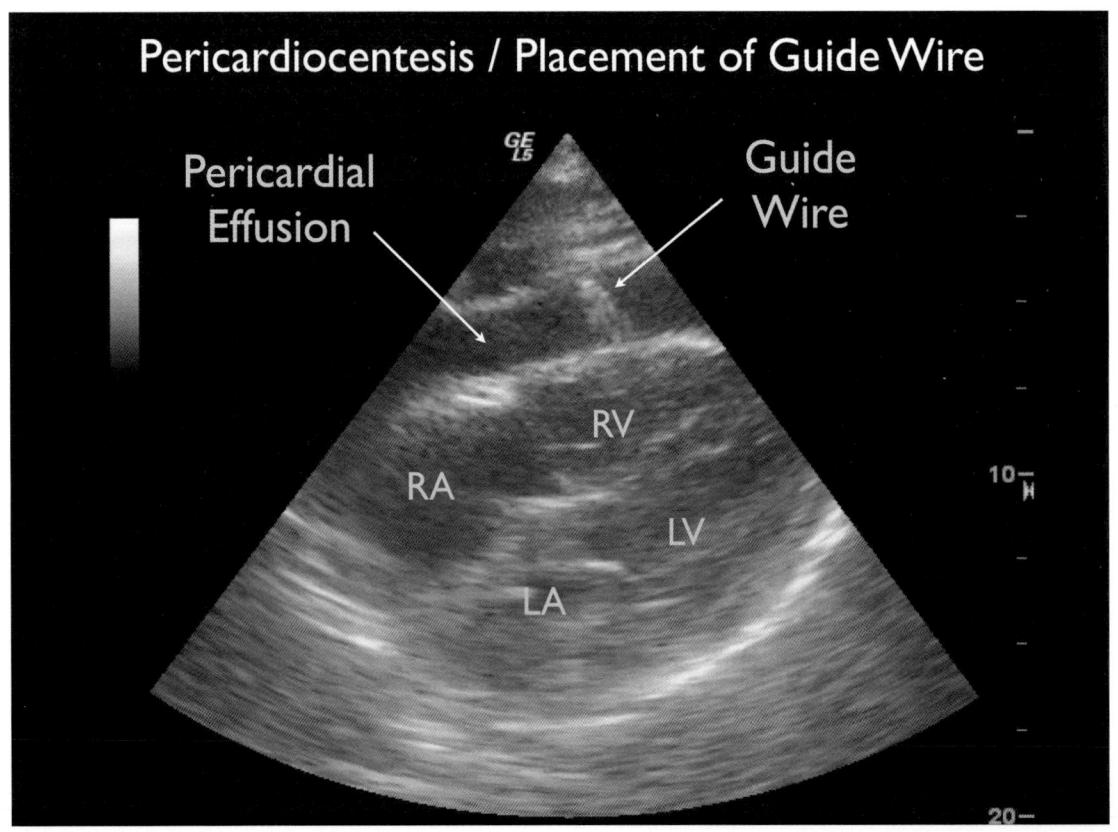

Pericardiocentesis / Placement of Guide Wire

documented sensitivity of this test in all patients with pulmonary embolus to be moderate. Therefore, echo cannot be used to rule out a pulmonary embolus, especially in patients who are hemodynamically stable. However, studies do support the finding of right ventricular enlargement as being highly suggestive of acute cardiac strain caused by pulmonary embolus in the correct clinical context. This finding can be of increased diagnostic utility in cases of hypotension with suspected thromboembolic disease, where it has a higher specificity and positive predictive value.[58-63]

The traditional treatment of patients with a pulmonary embolus has been anticoagulation. More recent guidelines, including those published by the American Heart Association in 2011, recommend the combined use of anticoagulants and fibrinolytics in patients with severe pulmonary embolism,[64-67] which is defined as the presence of acute right heart strain and clinical signs and symptoms of hypotension, severe shortness of breath, or altered mental status. Patients with submassive pulmonary embolism (defined as the presence of right ventricular strain without hypotension) can have echocardiographic evidence of pulmonary artery hypertension for some time following the event. This evidence is being considered as a possible indication for fibrinolytic treatment in a broader range of patients to prevent this complication.[68]

Echocardiographic Findings of a Hemodynamically Significant Pulmonary Embolism

Parasternal Views

The relative sizes of the left and right ventricles can be evaluated from this window. A normal ratio of the right to the left ventricle is 0.6:1, with a ratio larger than 1:1 indicating right ventricular dilation.[69,70] A higher relative ratio, combined with deflection of the interventricular septum from right to left, indicates the right ventricular strain that can be seen in a severe pulmonary embolus.

In acute right ventricular strain, the chamber wall is typically thin because compensatory hypertrophy has not had time to develop. Conversely, in cases of chronic pulmonary strain seen in conditions of long-standing pulmonary artery hypertension, the right ventricle compensates by hypertrophy. This results in a thicker wall, measuring more than 5 mm. These findings allow the clinician to differentiate acute and chronic right heart enlargement based on the ultrasound findings.

On the parasternal short-axis view, the interventricular septum can be seen to bow from right to left as a result of higher right-sided pressure as the septum is pushed down and away from the right ventricle. This finding is known as the left ventricular "D-shaped cup" (Figure 4-40).[71]

Subxiphoid and Apical Views

The subxiphoid view can also be used in the assessment of right ventricular strain. However, one must take care to aim the

FIGURE 4-37.

Left ventricle, good contractility

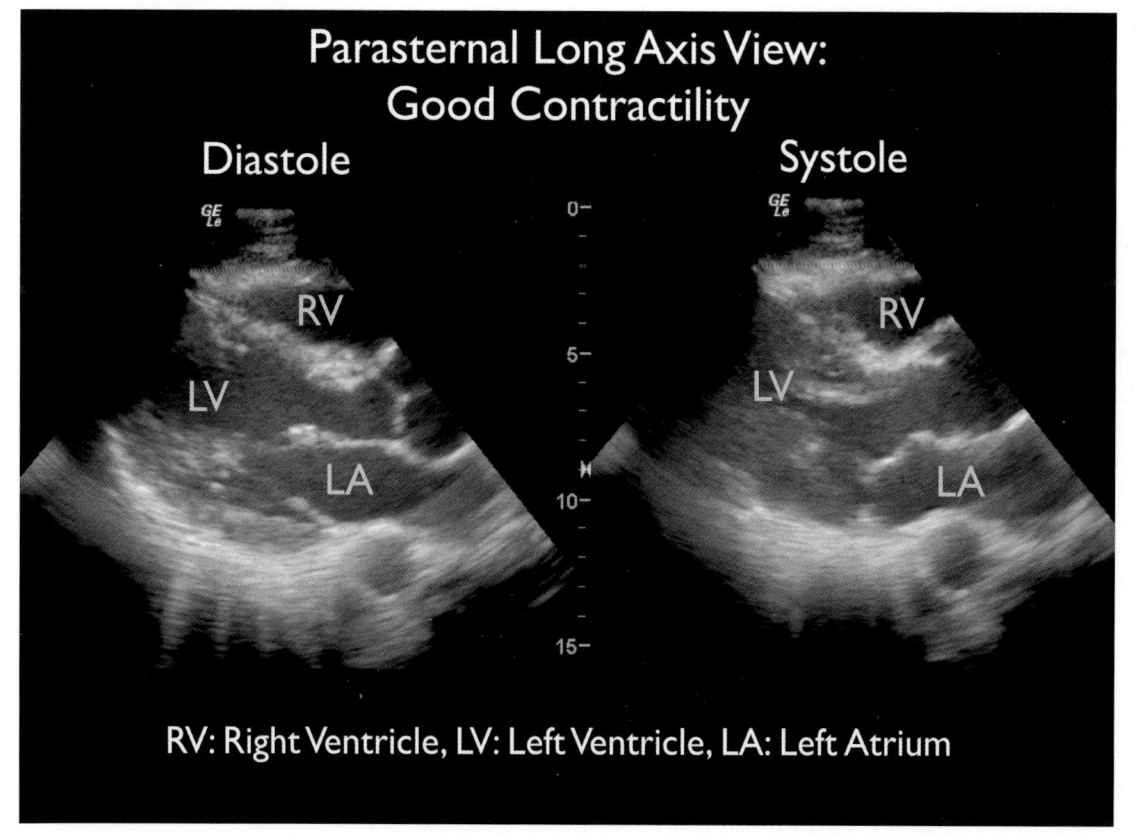

CARDIOVASCULAR EMERGENCIES

FIGURE 4-38.

Left ventricle, poor contractility

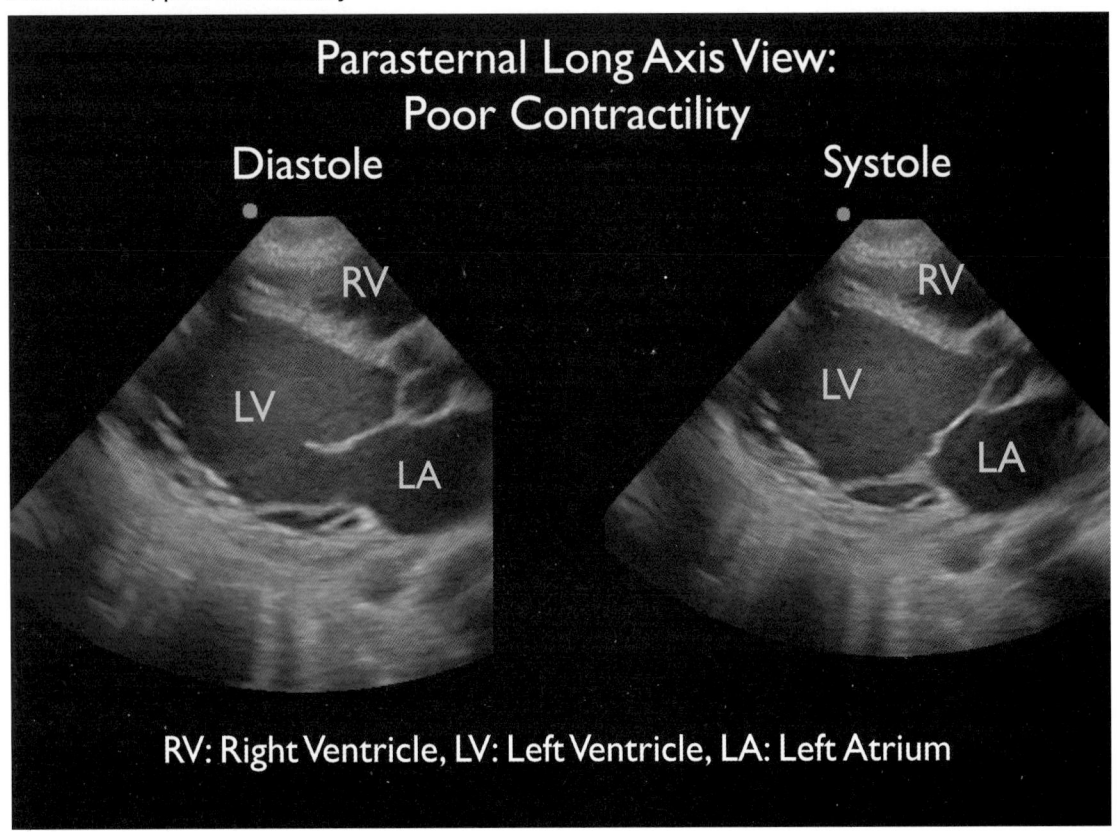

FIGURE 4-39.

Simpson's method, ejection fraction

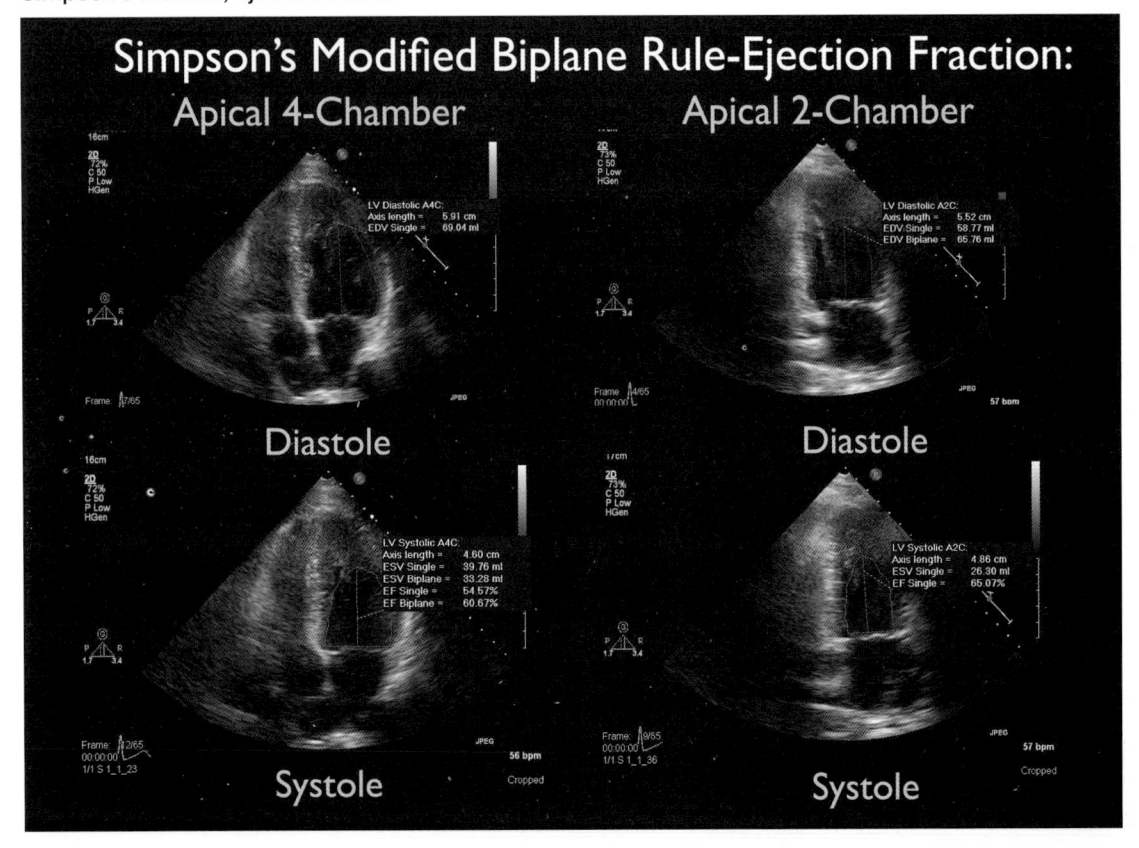

probe to capture the widest chamber size, avoiding underestimation of dimensions by imaging the right ventricle off-axis. The apical window is another excellent view for visualization of both right ventricular enlargement and septal bowing. In addition to findings of right ventricular strain, clot is occasionally visualized within the heart (Figure 4-41).[72]

KEY POINTS

Focused echo can be used to diagnose acute right ventricular enlargement, which, in the correct clinical context, can indicate a hemodynamically significant pulmonary embolism.

Right ventricular enlargement is diagnosed on echo by a relative right ventricular dimension that is as large as, or greater than, the adjacent left ventricle.

Deflection of the interventricular septum from right to left can also be seen in patients with relatively high right-side heart pressures.

In cases of acute right heart strain (as seen with acute pulmonary embolus), the right ventricular wall is thin, measuring less than 5 mm. In chronic pulmonary hypertension, the right ventricle generally hypertrophies to thicker than 5 mm. This allows differentiation between acute and chronic right heart strain.

Ultrasound Guidance for Transvenous Pacemaker Placement

Guidance for transvenous pacemaker placement can be obtained from either the subxiphoid or apical window, the views that best image the right side of the heart. The pacing wire should be observed to pass from the right atrium through the tricuspid valve and into the right ventricle. Optimally, the wire can be observed to float to a position against the electrically active right ventricular septum. Mechanical capture can then be confirmed with ultrasound (Figure 4-42).

Resuscitation Ultrasound

Current Resuscitation Ultrasound Protocols

As bedside ultrasound is increasingly incorporated into clinical practice, a number of protocols have been developed for the evaluation of patients in shock and respiratory distress. Major resuscitation ultrasound protocols for use in critically ill medical and trauma patients include the following: ACES,[73] BEAT,[74] BLEEP,[75] Boyd ECHO,[76] EGLS,[77] Elmer/Noble Protocol,[78] FALLS,[79] FATE,[80] FAST,[81] Extended-FAST,[82] FEEL-Resuscitation,[83] FEER,[84] FREE,[85] POCUS-Fast and reliable,[86] RUSH-HIMAP,[87] RUSH Pump/Tank/Pipes,[88-90] Trinity,[91] and UHP.[92] The major medical shock ultrasound protocols are compared in Table 4-7. Current major resuscitation protocols for dyspnea include the BLUE protocol[93] and RADIUS.[94] The BLUE protocol focuses solely on lung ultrasound for the diagnosis of pneumothorax, pulmonary edema, and pulmonary

FIGURE 4-40.

Parasternal views, right ventricular strain

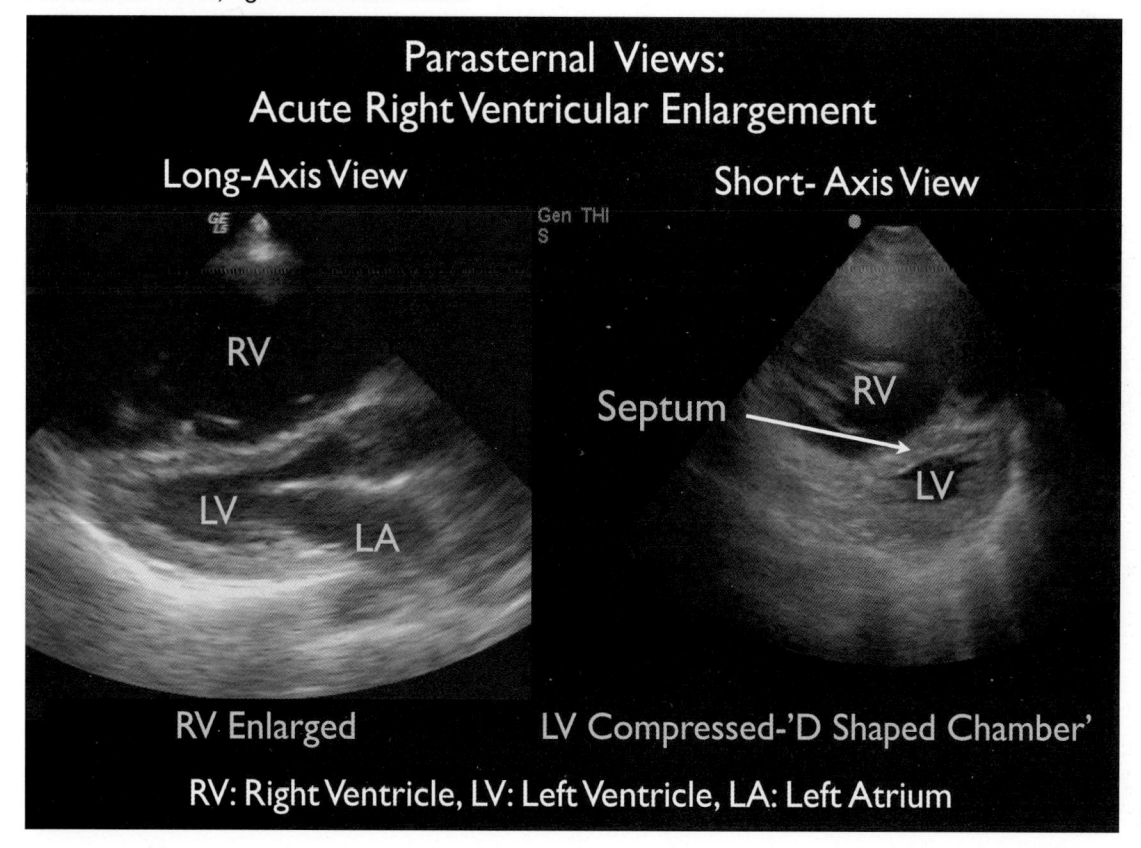

CARDIOVASCULAR EMERGENCIES

FIGURE 4-41.
Thrombus in right atrium entering right ventricle

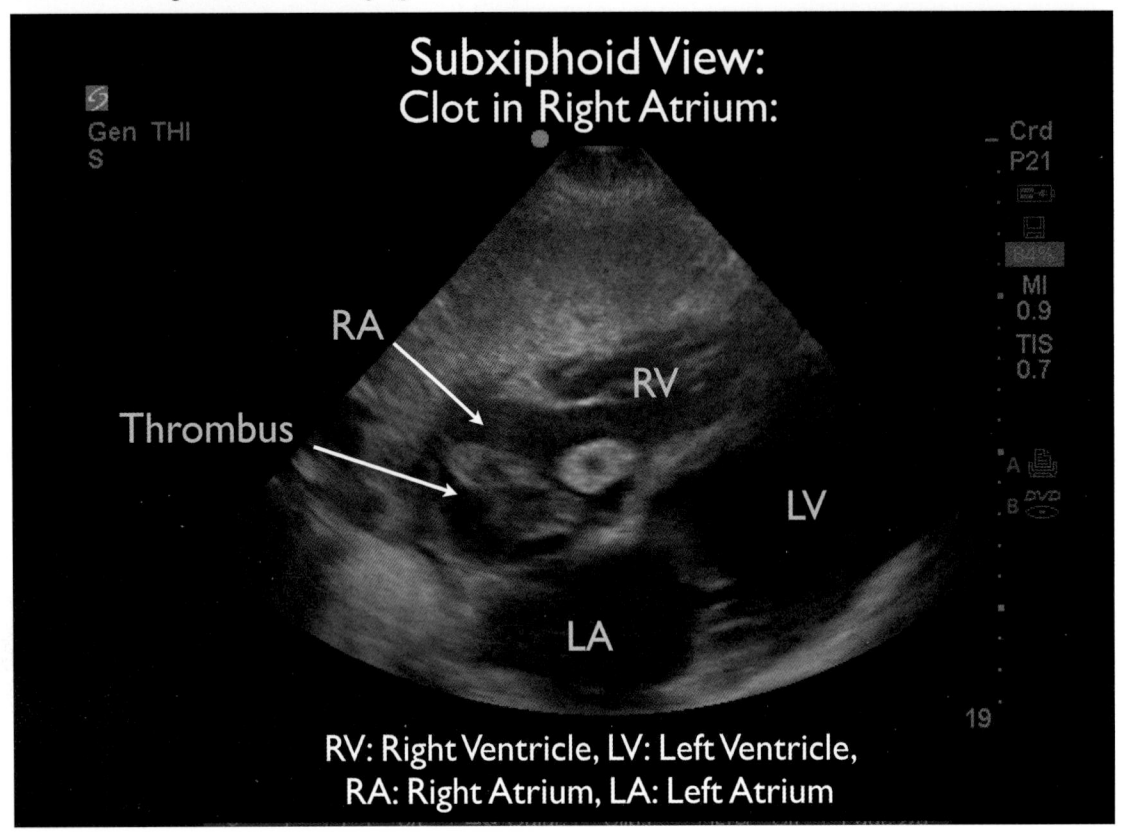

FIGURE 4-42.
Subxiphoid view, pacer wire present

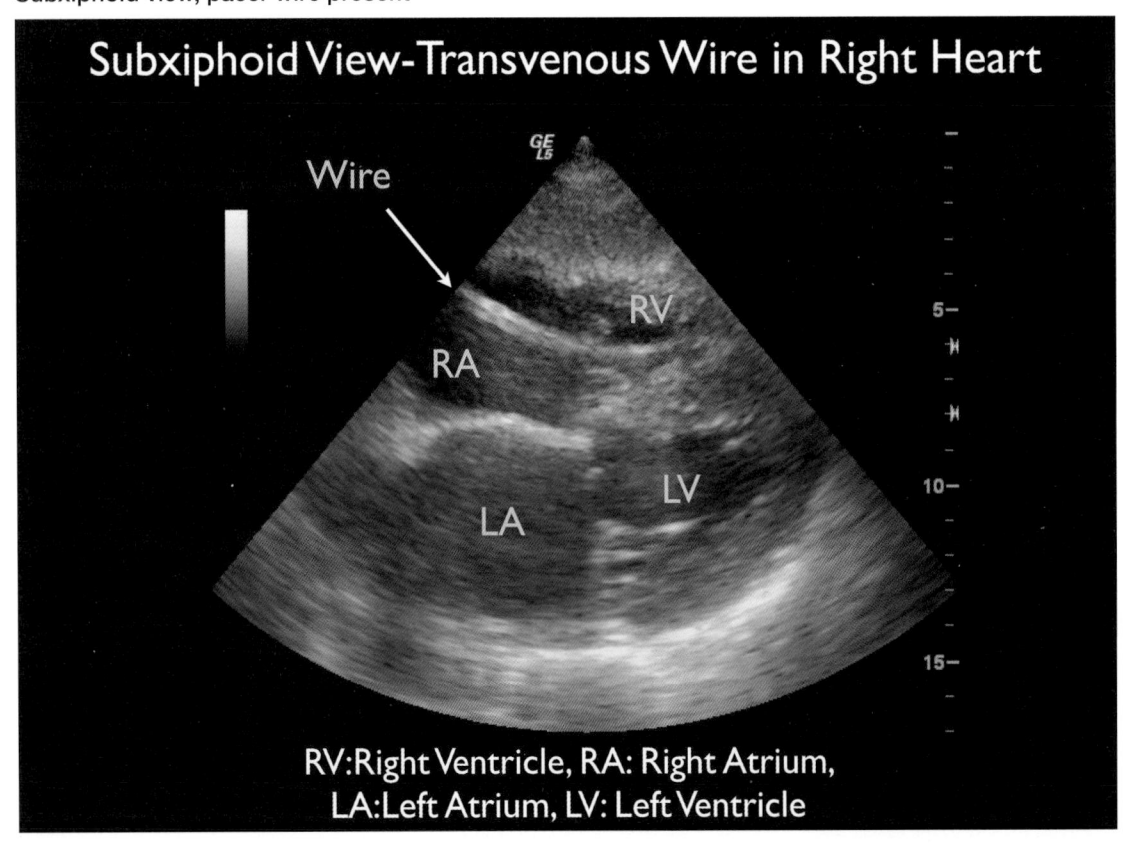

consolidation and effusions. The RADIUS protocol begins with cardiac and IVC evaluation, followed by a focused pulmonary examination.

While it seems that there are many competing shock protocols, what unifies them is inclusion of many of the same ultrasound components. Cardiac and IVC views are integral to most of them. More recent protocols have also included lung ultrasound as an important component for hemodynamic assessment. These protocols prioritize the sequence of the examination differently, but most of the contents are the same.

Rapid Ultrasound in SHock in the Critically Ill Patient

The Rapid Ultrasound for SHock (RUSH) examination was created by one of the authors (PP) as a protocol that can delineate the cause of shock in the undifferentiated patient presenting with hypotension.[88-90] The examination involves a three-part bedside physiologic assessment simplified as the pump, the tank, and the pipes.

Step 1—The Pump. Clinicians caring for the patient in shock should begin with goal-directed echo for rapid assessment of the function of the pump (Figure 4-7). This involves looking for three specific findings: pericardial effusion/cardiac tamponade, the degree of left ventricular contractility, and the presence of right ventricular enlargement. The details of this examination are discussed above. The information gained by this examination allows assessment of the need for an emergent cardiac procedure. Then ultrasound can be used to guide the pericardiocentesis procedure and the placement of a transvenous pacemaker wire.

Step 2—The Tank. The second part of the RUSH protocol focuses on determination of the effective intravascular volume status—the tank (Figure 4-43). This information, in conjunction with evaluation of cardiac status, provides a guide to fluid management in the critically ill patient. The tank is evaluated based on its fullness, leakiness, and compromise.

The fullness of the tank, or the CVP, is assessed after the heart has been evaluated and its contractility has been quantified. The IVC is typically used to obtain this information (Figure 4-43, probe position A). If the IVC cannot be seen well, the internal jugular veins provide an alternative means for volume assessment (Figures 4-27 and 4-28).

The leakiness of the tank refers to hemodynamic compromise resulting from loss of fluid from the core vascular circuit. It is assessed with the Extended Focused Assessment with Sonography for Trauma (E-FAST) examination (Figure 4-43, probe positions B, C, and D).[81,82] The traditional FAST examination identifies fluid collections in the abdominal and pelvic cavities. The E-FAST examination evaluates the thoracic cavity for fluid and pneumothorax.

A thoracic fluid collection (typically a pleural effusion or hemothorax, depending on the clinical scenario) can be identified by aiming the probe above the diaphragm from the standard right and left upper quadrant views (Figure 4-31). Finally, lung ultrasound can identify pulmonary edema, a sign often indicative of tank overload and tank leakiness with fluid accumulation in the lung parenchyma.[95-97] This examination is performed by placing the phased-array probe over the thorax in the anterior (Figure 4-43, probe position E) and lateral positions to look for ultrasound B-lines, or lung rockets (Figure 4-44).[98]

The third component is assessment for tank compromise. A tension pneumothorax can result in hypotension by severely limiting venous return to the heart from the superior and inferior vena cava. Pneumothorax can be diagnosed on bedside ultrasound by looking for the absence of lung sliding and the vertical comet tails seen in normal lungs.[99,100] When a pneumothorax is identified with ultrasound, emergency needle decompression can be performed rapidly in patients in shock, especially if chest radiography will be delayed.

Step 3—The Pipes. The third and final step in the RUSH examination is examination of the pipes, that is, the major arterial and venous structures (Figure 4-45). The first part of this examination is to assess the arterial side of the circulatory system. Vascular catastrophes, such as a ruptured abdominal aortic aneurysm or an aortic dissection, are life-threatening causes of hypotension that can be diagnosed accurately with bedside ultrasound (Figure 4-45, probe positions A-D; Figure 4-46).[101]

TABLE 4-7.
Ultrasound Resuscitation Protocols and Examination Components

Protocol	ACES	BEAT	BLEEP	Boyd ECHO	EGLS	Elmer/Noble	FATE	FAST	FALLS	E-FAST	FEEL RESUS	FEER	FREE	POCUS	RUSH: HIMAP	RUSH: Pump Tank Pipes	Trinity	UHP
Cardiac	1	1	1	1	2	1	1	2	3	2	1	1	1	3	1	1	1	3
IVC	2	2	2	2	3	2			4					4	2	2		
FAST-A/P	4				3		1		1					1	3	3	3	1
Aorta	3													5	4	7	2	2
Lungs-PTX					1	4			2	4				2	5	6		
Lungs-Effusion	5						2		3							4		
Lungs-Edema					4	5			1					6		5		
DVT														7		8		
Ectopic Pregnancy														8				

CARDIOVASCULAR EMERGENCIES

FIGURE 4-43.
RUSH Step 2: evaluation of the tank

Rapid Ultrasound in SHock (RUSH)
Step 2: Evaluation of the Tank

- Probe Position A: IVC Views
- Probe Position B: FAST / RUQ add pleural view
- Probe Position C: FAST / LUQ add pleural view
- Probe Position D: FAST / Pelvis
- Probe Position E: Lung Views

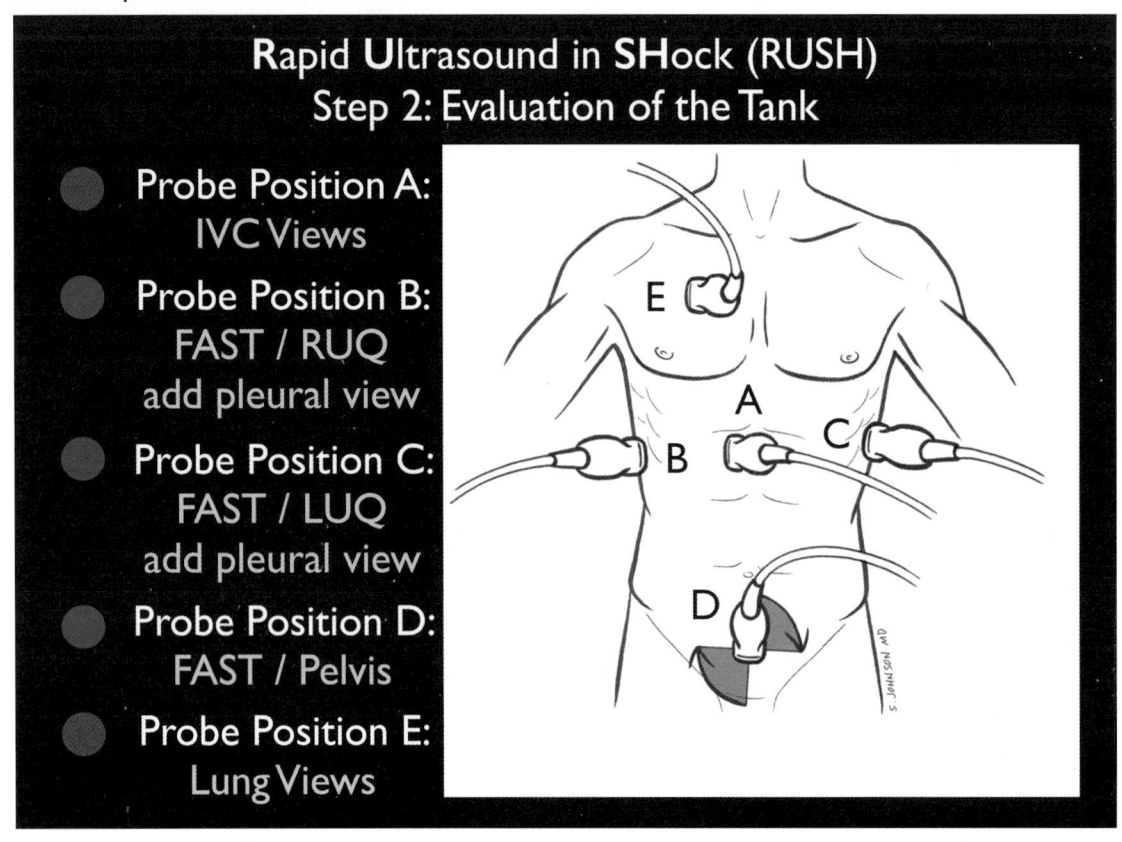

FIGURE 4-44.
Ultrasound B-lines, lung rockets

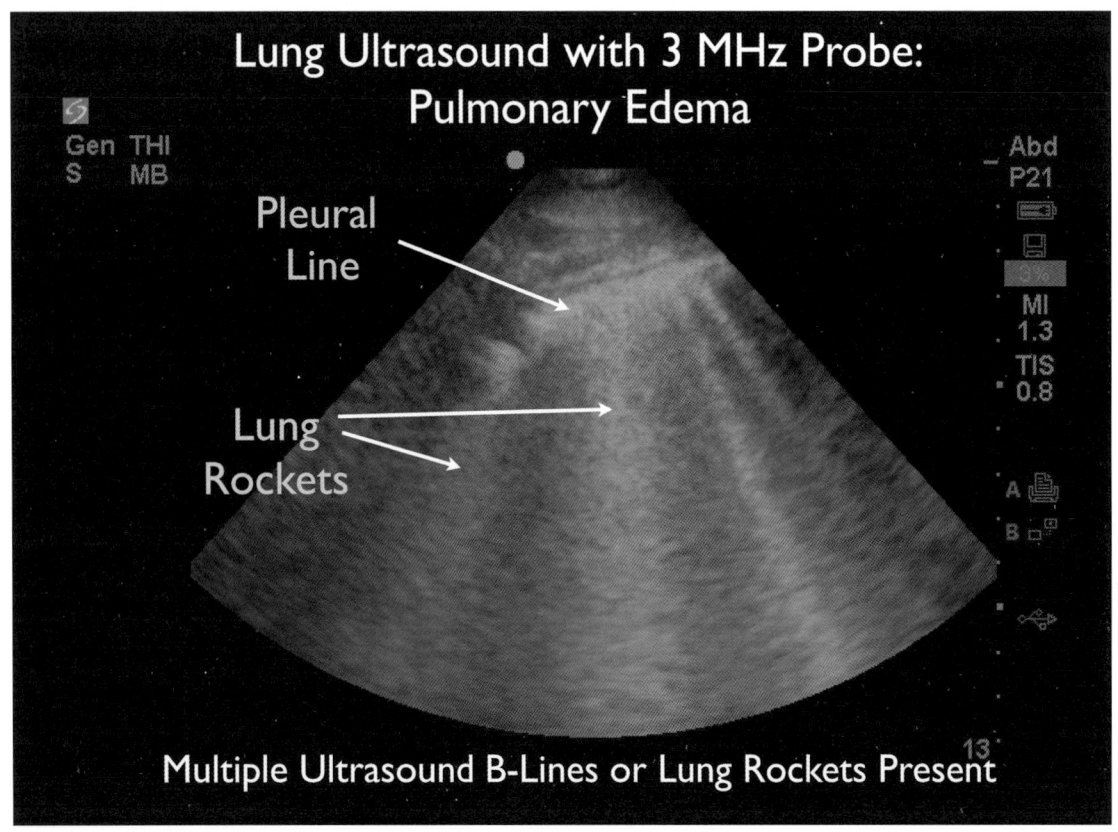

Lung Ultrasound with 3 MHz Probe: Pulmonary Edema

Pleural Line

Lung Rockets

Multiple Ultrasound B-Lines or Lung Rockets Present[13]

84

If right ventricular enlargement is identified on echo and a thromboembolic cause of shock is suspected, evaluation of the major venous structures is then indicated. In this scenario, the veins of the lower extremities should be assessed for deep venous thrombosis (DVT). The limited leg-compression DVT examination can be performed rapidly by evaluating a targeted portion of the proximal femoral and popliteal veins, where the majority of thrombi are located (Figure 4-45, probe positions E and F).[102,103]

Putting RUSH into Action

The RUSH protocol was designed to be performed expediently by specifically choosing the examination components most applicable to the patient's clinical context. While the entire protocol is extensive and incorporates multiple ultrasound elements, the clinician should generally begin with evaluation of the heart and IVC (and, if indicated, the internal jugular veins). The RUSH examination should be tailored based on clinical suspicion, as many patients can be assessed with an abbreviated examination. The need to incorporate other components, such as FAST or lung, aorta, and DVT examinations, can be determined as the clinical picture dictates. Table 4-8 demonstrates how using the RUSH examination at the bedside can assist in identifying the type of shock in the critically ill patient.

KEY POINTS

The Rapid Ultrasound in SHock protocol is a resuscitation ultrasound protocol that can improve the diagnosis, treatment, and monitoring of the patient in shock.

First, the cause of shock can be diagnosed more accurately. Second, an improved treatment plan can be formulated during the initial assessment to better match the patient's physiologic state. Third, the response to therapy can be monitored closely over time.

Evaluation of the pump is the first step in the RUSH examination. It has three components: evaluation of the heart for pericardial effusion and tamponade, assessment of left ventricular contractility, and detection of right ventricular strain.

Evaluation of the tank is the second step in the RUSH examination. It also has three components. The first is evaluation of tank fullness (the relative intravascular volume, or CVP), which is determined by assessment of the IVC and internal jugular veins. The second is assessment for tank leakiness, performed by looking for free fluid in the chest, abdomen, and pelvis through the E-FAST examination. Lung ultrasound can reveal B-lines or lung rockets, signs of pulmonary edema and tank leakiness secondary to overload. The third component is assessment of tank compromise: in the shock patient, detection of a pneumothorax on ultrasound can signal tension physiology requiring emergency needle decompression.

Evaluation of the pipes is the third step in the RUSH examination. It has two components. The first is evaluation for major arterial vascular pathology, such as an aneurysm or dissection of the abdominal and/or thoracic aorta. The second is evaluation for significant venous vascular

FIGURE 4-45.

RUSH Step 3: evaluation of the pipes

Rapid Ultrasound in SHock (RUSH)
Step 3: Evaluation of the Pipes

- Probe Position A: Suprasternal Aorta
- Probe Position B: Parasternal Aorta
- Probe Position C: Epigastric Aorta
- Probe Position D: Supraumbilical Aorta
- Probe Position E: Femoral DVT
- Probe Position F: Popliteal DVT

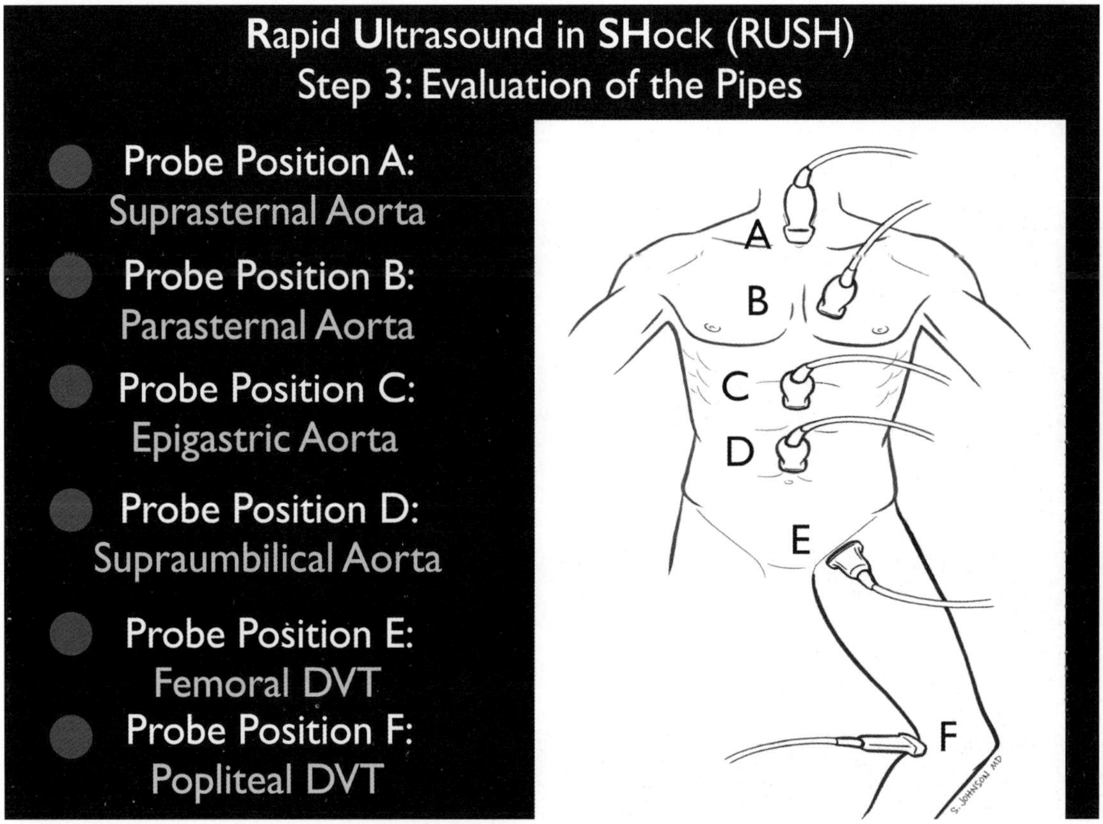

pathology, specifically DVT in the lower extremity, which should be considered in the shock patient with acute right ventricular enlargement.

Focused Echocardiography in Cardiac Arrest

In cardiac arrest, bedside focused echo can be used to guide management. The clinician should first look for pericardial effusion and cardiac tamponade; if either is found, immediate pericardiocentesis is indicated. The next step is assessment of cardiac contractions. If contractions are seen, the clinician should then look for coordinated movements of the cardiac valves.[83,84] Finally, identification of right ventricular enlargement could indicate a massive pulmonary embolus as the cause of arrest, in which case, fibrinolysis may be considered.

Specific protocols for sonography in the setting of cardiac arrest have been used clinically, and further research is underway.[104,105] These protocols integrate examination of the heart, the lungs, and the flow in the carotid artery. The subxiphoid view is often used for assessment of the heart during cardiac arrest (chest compressions can continue with minimal interruption). Assessment of Doppler flow in the carotid arteries, with and without chest compressions, indicates the adequacy of blood flow to the brain and can be used to augment simple pulse checks. A high-frequency probe should be used for this assessment.

Several studies have advocated the use of transesophageal echocardiography during cardiac arrest.[106-108] The images can be obtained without interruption of chest compressions and can concurrently seek the cause of the cardiac arrest, the quality of chest compressions, and the patient's response to medications. The current limiting factor for widespread adoption of transesophageal echocardiography in cardiac arrest is the high price of the probe. As the cost of the probe becomes more economical, this modality could move to the front line in cardiac arrest echocardiography.

If the bedside echo demonstrates cardiac standstill after prolonged advanced cardiovascular life support resuscitation, it is unlikely that an adult patient who has experienced cardiac arrest will have return of spontaneous circulation.[109-111] The absence of cardiac motion after trauma resuscitation is also associated with poor survival rates.[112]

KEY POINTS

Bedside echo can be helpful in the cardiac arrest patient first by allowing detection of pathology that might be amenable to rapid treatment such as cardiac tamponade, a hemodynamically significant pulmonary embolism, hemorrhage into the chest or abdomen, aortic pathology, or a tension pneumothorax.

Echo also facilitates evaluation of physiology in the arrest patient by determining if coordinated cardiac contractions are present.

Echo can help in determining when to stop resuscitation efforts. The presence of cardiac standstill after a reasonable

FIGURE 4-46.

Abdominal vascular emergencies

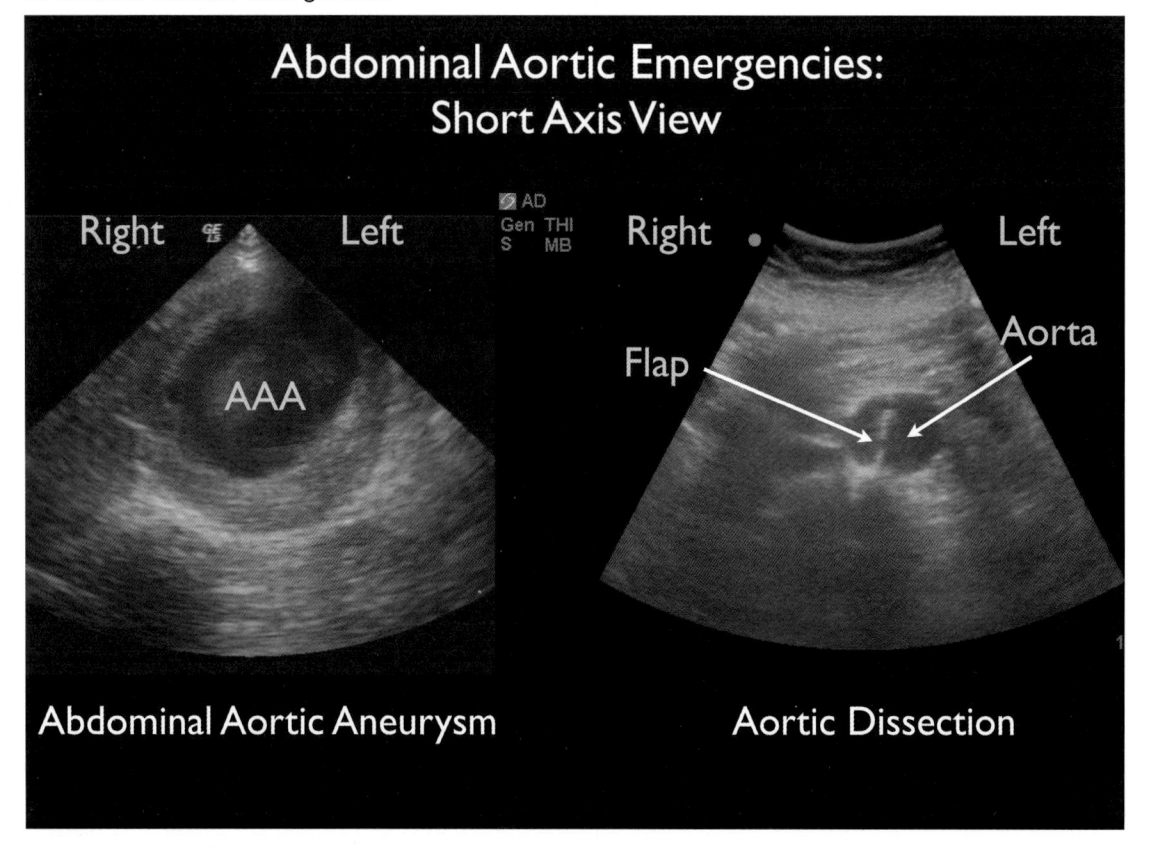

period of advanced cardiovascular life support treatment indicates very poor prognosis, suggesting that cessation of resuscitation efforts should be considered.

Echo evaluation of the cardiac arrest patient can be performed from the subxiphoid view, during periods of CPR as well as during pulse checks.

Look specifically for the presence of cardiac contractions leading to coordinated valvular activity. Doppler ultrasound of the carotid artery can be used to assess blood flow to the brain. If cardiac effusions and tamponade are found, pericardiocentesis can be performed if needed. Finally, acute right ventricular enlargement could be an indication for fibrinolysis in the cardiac arrest patient, especially if the arrest occurs in the emergency department or if the patient has a very short "down time."

Transesophageal echocardiography seems to be a better means of evaluating the patient in cardiac arrest and might be more widely used in the future.

Conclusion

Focused echocardiography allows the immediate diagnosis of a range of serious pathology in critically ill patients being assessed in an emergency department.[113] Pericardial effusion and cardiac tamponade can be detected rapidly with ultrasound. Cardiac contractility and volume status can also be assessed, providing a better guide to therapeutic management in the cardiac patient. Acute right heart enlargement indicating significant pulmonary embolus can also be diagnosed, with targeted therapy guided by this finding. The invasive cardiac procedures of pericardiocentesis and placement of a transvenous pacemaker can be performed more accurately using ultrasound. For emergency physicians caring for the sickest patients, learning the skill of focused bedside echo can be of great benefit in providing both timely and optimal care.

References

1. Moore CL, Copel JA. Current concepts: point of care ultrasonography. *N Engl J Med*. 2011;364:749-757.
2. American College of Emergency Physicians. Policy statement: emergency ultrasound guidelines. *Ann Emerg Med*. 2009;53:550-570.
3. Akhtar S, Theodoro D, Gaspari R, et al. Resident training in emergency ultrasound: consensus recommendations from the 2008 Council of Emergency Medicine Residency Directors conference. *Acad Emerg Med*. 2009;16:S32-S36.
4. Ultrasound position statement. Society for Academic Emergency Medicine. Available at www.saem.org. Accessed July 19, 2013.
5. Jang TB, Coates WC, Jiu YT. The competency based mandate for emergency bedside bedside sonography and a tale of two residency programs. *J Ultrasound Med*. 2012;31:515-521.
6. Labovitz AJ, Noble VE, Bierig M, et al. Focused cardiac ultrasound in the emergent setting: a consensus statement of the American Society of Echocardiography and the American College of Emergency Physicians. *J Am Soc Echocardiogr*. 2010;23:1225-1230.
7. Weekes AJ, Quirke DP. Emergency echocardiography. *Emerg Med Clin North Am*. 2011;29:759-787.
8. Reardon RF, Joing SA. Cardiac. In Ma OJ, Mateer JR, Blaivas M, editors. *Emergency Ultrasound*. New York: McGraw Hill; 2008:107-148.
9. Moore CL, Lin H. Echocardiography. In Cosby KS, Kendall JL, editors. *Practical Guide to Emergency Ultrasound*. Philadelphia: Lippincott Williams & Wilkins; 2006:93-122.
10. Taylor RA, Oliva I, Van Tonder R, et al. Point of care focused cardiac ultrasound for the assessment of thoracic aortic dimensions, dilation and aneurysmal disease. *Acad Emerg Med*. 2012;19:244-247.
11. Fojtik, JP, Costantino TG, Dean AJ. The diagnosis of aortic dissection by emergency medicine ultrasound. *J Emerg Med*. 2007;32:191-196.
12. Budhram G, Reardon R. Diagnosis of ascending aortic dissection using emergency department bedside echocardiogram. *Acad Emerg Med*. 2008;15:584.
13. Chen RS, Bivens MJ, Grossman SA. Diagnosis and management of valvular heart disease in emergency medicine. *Emerg Med Clin North Am*. 2011;29:801-810.
14. Wallace DJ, Allison M, Stone MB. Inferior vena cava percentage collapse during respiration is affected by the sampling location: an ultrasound study in healthy volunteers. *Acad Emerg Med*. 2010;17:96-99.
15. Kircher BJ, Himelman RB, Schiller NB. Noninvasive estimation of right atrial pressure from the inspiratory collapse of the inferior vena cava. *Am J Cardiol*. 1990;66:493-496.
16. Simonson JS, Schiller NB. Sonospirometry: a new method for noninvasive estimation of mean right atrial pressure based on two-dimensional echocardiographic measurements of the inferior vena cava during measured inspiration. *J Am Coll Cardiol*. 1988;11:557-564.
17. Randazzo MR, Snoey ER, Levitt, MA, Binder K. Accuracy of emergency physician assessment of left ventricular ejection fraction and central venous pressure using echocardiography. *Acad Emerg Med*. 2003;10:973-977.
18. Jardin F, Vieillard-Baron A. Ultrasonographic examination of the venae cavae. *Intens Care Med*. 2006;32:203-206.
19. Marik PA. Techniques for assessment of intravascular volume in critically ill patients. *J Intensive Care Med*. 2009;24:329-337.

TABLE 4-8.

Using the RUSH Protocol to Diagnose the Type of Shock

RUSH Protocol (Rapid Ultrasound in Shock)

RUSH Exam	Hypovolemic Shock	Cardiogenic Shock	Obstructive Shock	Distributive Shock
Pump	Hypercontractile heart Small heart size	Hypocontractile heart Dilated heart size	Pericardial effusion RV strain Hypercontractile heart	Hypercontractile heart (early sepsis) Hypocontractile heart (late sepsis)
Tank	Flat IVC Flat internal jugular vein Peritoneal fluid Pleural fluid	Distended IVC Distended internal jugular vein Lung rockets Pleural effusions Ascites	Distended IVC Distended internal jugular vein Absent lung sliding (pneumothorax)	Normal/small IVC Normal/small internal jugular vein Pleural fluid (empyema) Peritoneal fluid (peritonitis)
Pipes	Abdominal aortic aneurysm Aortic dissection	Normal	DVT	Normal

20. Blehar DJ, Dickman E, Gaspari R. Identification of congestive heart failure via respiratory variation of inferior vena cava diameter. *Am J Emerg Med.* 2009;27:71-75.
21. Nagdev AD, Merchant RC, Tirado-Gonzalez A, et al. Emergency department bedside ultrasonographic measurement of the caval index for noninvasive determination of low central venous pressure. *Ann Emerg Med.* 2010;55:290-295.
22. Schefold JC, Storm C, Bercker S, et al. Inferior vena cava diameter correlates with invasive hemodynamic measures in mechanically ventilated intensive care unit patients with sepsis. *J Emerg Med.* 2010;38:652-637.
23. Seif D, Mailhot T, Perera P, Mandavia D. Caval sonography in shock: a non-invasive method for evaluating intravascular volume in critically ill patients. *J Ultrasound Med.* 2012;31:1885-1890.
24. Rudski LG, Lai WW, Afilalo J, et al. Guidelines for the echocardiographic assessment of the right heart in adults: a report from the American society of echocardiography. *J Am Soc Echocardiogr.* 2010;23:685-713.
25. Barbier C, Loubieres Y, Schmit C, et al. Respiratory changes in the inferior vena cava diameter are helpful in predicting fluid responsiveness in ventilated septic patients. *Intens Care Med.* 2004;30:1740-1746.
26. Simon MA, Kliner DE, Girod JP, et al. Jugular venous distention on ultrasound: sensitivity and specificity for heart failure in patients with dyspnea. *Am J Emerg Med.* 2011;159:421-427.
27. Jang T, Aubin C, Naunheim R, Char D. Ultrasonography of the internal jugular vein in patients with dyspnea without jugular venous distention on physical examination. *Ann Emerg Med.* 2004;44:160-168.
28. Jang T, Aubin C, Naunheim R, et al. Jugular venous distention on ultrasound: sensitivity and specificity for heart failure in patients with dyspnea. *Ann Emerg Med.* 2011;29:1198-1202.
29. Blaivas M. Incidence of pericardial effusion in patients presenting to the emergency department with unexplained dyspnea. *Acad Emerg Med.* 2001;8:1143-1146.
30. Tayal VS, Kline JA. Emergency echocardiography to determine pericardial effusions in patients with PEA and near PEA states. *Resuscitation.* 2003;59:315-318.
31. Mandavia DP, Hoffner RJ, Mahaney K, Henderson SO. Bedside echocardiography by emergency physicians. *Ann Emerg Med.* 2001;38:377-382.
32. Grecu L. Cardiac tamponade. *Intern Anesth Clin.* 2012;50:59-77.
33. Shabetai R. Pericardial effusions: haemodynamic spectrum. *Heart.* 2004;90:255-256.
34. Russo AM, O'Connor WH, Waxman HL. Atypical presentations and echocardiographic findings in patients with cardiac tamponade occurring early and late after cardiac surgery. *Chest.* 1993;104:71-78.
35. Trojanos CA, Porembka DT. Assessment of left ventricular function and hemodynamics with transesophageal echocardiography. *Crit Care Clin.* 1996;12:253-272.
36. Goodman A, Perera P, Mailhot T, Mandavia D. The role of bedside ultrasound in the diagnosis of pericardial effusions and cardiac tamponade. *J Emerg Trauma Shock.* 2012;5:72-75.
37. Nabazivadeh SA, Meskshar A. Ultrasonic diagnosis of cardiac tamponade in trauma patients using the collapsibility index of the inferior vena cava. *Acad Radiol.* 2007;14:505-506.
38. Armstrong WF, Ryan T. *Feigenbaum's Echocardiography*, 7th edition. Philadelphia: Lippincott Williams & Wilkins; 2010.
39. Tsang T, Enriquez-Sarano M, Freeman WK. Consecutive 1127 therapeutic echocardiographically guided pericardiocenteses: clinical profile, practice patterns and outcomes spanning 21years. *Mayo Clin Proc.* 2002;77:429-436.
40. Salazar M, Mohar D, Bhardwaj R, et al. Use of contrast echocardiography to detect displacement of the needle during pericardiocentesis. *Echocardiography.* 2012;29:E60-E61.
41. Ainsworth CD, Salehian O. Echo-guided pericardiocentesis: let the bubbles show the way. *Circulation.* 2011;123:e210-e211.
42. Jones AE, Craddock PA, Tayal VS, et al. Diagnostic accuracy of identification of left ventricular function among emergency department patients with nontraumatic symptomatic undifferentiated hypotension. *Shock.* 2005;24:513-517.
43. Moore CL, Rose GA, Tayal VS, et al. Determination of left ventricular function by emergency physician echocardiography of hypotensive patients. *Acad Emerg Med.* 2002;9:186-193.
44. Joseph M, Disney P. Transthoracic echocardiography to identify or exclude cardiac cause of shock. *Chest.* 2004;126:1592-1597.
45. Aurigemma GR, Gaasch WH. Diastolic heart failure. *N Engl J Med.* 2004;51:1097-1105.
46. Brown SM, Pittman JE, Hirshberg EL, et al. Diastolic dysfunction and mortality in early sepsis and septic shock: a prospective observational echocardiographic study. *Crit Ultrasound J.* 2012;2:8.
47. Khouri SJ, Maly GT, Suh DD, Walsh TE. A practical approach to the echocardiographic evaluation of diastolic function. *Am Soc Echocardiogr.* 2004;17:290-297.
48. Lang RM, Bierig M, Devereux RB, et al. Recommendations for chamber quantification. *Eur J Echocardiogr.* 2006;7:79-108.
49. Weekes AJ, Tassone HM, Babcock A, et al. Comparison of serial qualitative and quantitative assessments of caval index and left ventricular systolic function during early fluid resuscitation of hypotensive emergency department patients. *Acad Emerg Med.* 2011;18:912-921.
50. Secko MA, Lazar JM, Salciccioli L, Stone MB. Can junior emergency physicians use E-point septal separation to accurately estimate left ventricular function in acutely dyspneic patients? *Acad Emerg Med.* 2011;18:1223-1226.
51. Ahmadpour H, Shah AA, Allen JW. Mitral E point septal separation: a reliable index of left ventricular performance in coronary artery disease. *Am Heart J.* 1983;106:21-28.
52. Silverstein JR, Laffely NH, Rifkin RD. Quantitative estimation of left ventricular ejection fraction from mitral valve E-point to septal separation and comparison to magnetic resonance imaging. *Am J Cardiol.* 2006;97:137-140.
53. Weekes AJ, Reddy A, Lewis MR, Norton JH. E-point septal separation compared to fractional shortening measurements of systolic function in emergency department patients. *J Ultrasound Med.* 2012;31:1891-1897.
54. St. John Sutton MG, Plappert T, Rahmouni H. Assessment of left ventricular systolic function by echocardiography. *Ultrasound Clin.* 2009;4:167-180.
55. Abraham J, Abraham TP. The role of echocardiography in hemodynamic assessment of heart failure. *Ultrasound Clin.* 2009;4:149-166.
56. Gifroni S, Olivotto I, Cecchini P, et al. Short term clinical outcome of patients with acute pulmonary embolism, normal blood pressure and echocardiographic right ventricular dysfunction. *Circulation.* 2000;101:2817-2822.
57. Becattini C, Agnelli G. Acute pulmonary embolism: risk stratification in the emergency department. *Intern Emerg Med.* 2007;2:119-129.
58. Nazeyrollas D, Metz D, Jolly D, et al. Use of transthoracic Doppler echocardiography combined with clinical and electrographic data to predict acute pulmonary embolism. *Eur Heart J.* 1996;17:779-786.
59. Jardin F, Duborg O, Bourdarias JP. Echocardiographic pattern of acute cor pulmonale. *Chest.* 1997;111:209-217.
60. Jardin F, Dubourg O, Gueret P, et al. Quantitative two dimensional echocardiography in massive pulmonary embolism: emphasis on ventricular interdependence and leftward septal displacement. *J Am Coll Cardiol.* 1987;10:1201-1206.
61. Rudoni R, Jackson R. Use of two-dimensional echocardiography for the diagnosis of pulmonary embolus. *J Emerg Med.* 1998;16:5-8.
62. Jackson RE, Rudoni RR, Hauser AM, et al. Prospective evaluation of two-dimensional transthoracic echocardiography in emergency department patients with suspected pulmonary embolism. *Acad Emerg Med.* 2000;7:994-998.
63. Miniati M, Monti S, Pratali L, et al. Value of transthoracic echocardiography in the diagnosis of pulmonary embolism: results of a prospective study in unselected patients. *Am J Med.* 2001;110:528-535.
64. Stein J. Opinions regarding the diagnosis and management of venous thrombo-embolic disease. ACCP Consensus Committee on pulmonary embolism. *Chest.* 1996;109:233-237.
65. Konstantinides S, Geibel A, Heusel G, et al. Heparin plus alteplase compared with heparin alone in patients with submassive pulmonary embolus. *N Engl J Med.* 2002;347:1143-1150.
66. Kucher N, Goldhaber SZ. Management of massive pulmonary embolism. *Circulation.* 2005;112:e28-32.
67. Jaff MR, McMurtry S, Archer S, et al. Management of massive and submassive pulmonary embolism, iliofemoral deep venous thrombosis and chronic thrombo-embolic pulmonary embolism: a scientific statement from the American Heart Association. *Circulation.* 2011;123:1788-1830.
68. Sharifi M, Bay C, Skrocki L, et al. Moderate pulmonary embolism treated with thrombolysis (MOPETT trial). *J Cardiol.* 2012;111:273-277.
69. Vieillard-Baron A, Page B, Augarde R, et al. Acute cor pulmonale in massive pulmonary embolism: incidence, echocardiographic pattern, clinical implications and recovery rate. *Intens Care Med.* 2001;27:1481-1486.
70. Mookadam F, Jiamsripong P, Goel R, et al. Critical appraisal on the utility of echocardiography in the management of acute pulmonary embolism. *Cardiol Rev.* 2010;18:29-37.
71. Riley D, Hultgren A, Merino D, Gerson S. Emergency department bedside echocardiographic diagnosis of massive pulmonary embolism with direct visualization of thrombus in the pulmonary artery. *Crit Ultrasound J.* 2011;3:155-160.
72. Madan A, Schwartz C. Echocardiographic visualization of acute pulmonary embolus and thrombolysis in the ED. *Am J Emerg Med.* 2004;22:294-300.
73. Atkinson PRT, McAuley DJ, Kendall RJ, et al. Abdominal and cardiac evaluation with sonography in shock (ACES): an approach by emergency physicians for use of ultrasound in patients with undifferentiated hypotension. *Emerg Med J.* 2009;26:87-91.
74. Gunst M, Gaemmaghami V, Sperry J. Accuracy of cardiac function and volume status estimates using the bedside echocardiographic assessment in trauma/critical care (BEAT). *J Trauma.* 2008;65:509-516.
75. Pershad J, Myers S, Plouman C, et al. Bedside limited echocardiography by the emergency physician is accurate during evaluation of the critically ill patient (BLEEP). *Pediatrics.* 2004;114:e667-71.
76. Boyd JH, Walley KR. The role of echocardiography in hemodynamic monitoring. *Curr Opin Crit Care.* 2009;15:239-243.

77. Lanctot YF, Valois M, Bealieu Y. EGLS: echo guided life support. An algorithmic approach to undifferentiated shock. *Crit Ultrasound J*. 2011;3;123-129.
78. Elmer J, Noble VA. An Evidence based approach for integrating bedside ultrasound into routine practice in the assessment of undifferentiated shock. *ICU Director*. 2010;1:163-174.
79. Lichtenstein DA, Karakitsos D. Integrating ultrasound in the hemodynamic evaluation of acute circulatory failure (FALLS-the fluid administration limited by lung sonography protocol). *J Crit Care*. 2012;27:533el-533el9.
80. Jensen MB, Sloth E, Larsen M, Schmidt MB. Transthoracic echocardiography for cardiopulmonary monitoring in intensive care (FATE). *Eur J Anaesthes*. 2004;21:700-707.
81. Rozycki G, Oschner MG, Schmidt JA, et al. A prospective use of surgeon's performed ultrasound as the primary adjunct modality for injured patient assessment. *J Trauma*. 1995;39:879-885.
82. Kirkpatrick AW, Sirois M, Laupland KB, et al. Hand-held thoracic sonography for detecting post-traumatic pneumothoraces: the Extended Focused Assessment with Sonography for Trauma (EFAST). *J Trauma*. 2004;57:288-295.
83. Breitkreutz R, Price S, Steiger HV, et al. Focused echocardiographic examination in life support and peri-resuscitation of emergency patients (FEEL-Resus): a prospective trial. *Resuscitation*. 2010;81:1527-1533.
84. Breitkreutz R, Walcher F, Seeger F. Focused echocardiographic evaluation in resuscitation management (FEER): concept of an advanced life support-conformed algorithm. *Crit Care Med*. 2007;35:S150-S161.
85. Ferrada P, Murthi S, Anand RJ, et al. Transthoracic focused rapid echocardiography examination: real-time evaluation of fluid status in critically ill trauma patients (FREE). *J Trauma*. 2010;70:56-64.
86. Liteplo A, Noble V, Atkinson P. My patient has no blood pressure: point of care ultrasound in the hypotensive patient-FAST and RELIABLE. *Ultrasound*. 2012;20:64-68.
87. Weingart SD, Duque D, Nelson B. Rapid Ultrasound for Shock and Hypotension (RUSH-HIMAPP). *EMedHome.com*; April 2009.
88. Perera P, Mailhot T, Riley D, Mandavia D. The RUSH exam: Rapid Ultrasound in SHock in the evaluation of the critically ill. *Emerg Med Clin North Am*. 2010;28:29-56.
89. Perera P, Mailhot T, Riley D, Mandavia D. The RUSH exam: Rapid Ultrasound in SHock in the evaluation of the critically ill (2012 update). *Ultrasound Clin*. 2012;255-278.
90. Seif D, Perera P, Mailhot T, et al. Bedside ultrasound in resuscitation and the Rapid Ultrasound in SHock protocol. *Crit Care Res Pract*. 2012;Article ID 503254.
91. Bahner DP. Trinity, A hypotensive ultrasound protocol. *J Diag Med Ultras*. 2002;18:193-198.
92. Rose JS, Bair AE, Mandavia DP. The UHP ultrasound protocol: a novel ultrasound approach to the empiric evaluation of the undifferentiated hypotensive patient. *Am J Emerg Med*. 2001;19:299-302.
93. Lichtenstein DA, Meziere GA. Relevance of lung ultrasound in the diagnosis of acute respiratory failure: the BLUE protocol. *Chest*. 2008;134:117-125.
94. Manson W, Hafez NM. The rapid assessment of dyspnea with ultrasound: RADIUS. *Ultrasound Clin*. 2011;6:261-276.
95. Volpicelli G, Caramello V, Cardinale L, et al. Bedside ultrasound of the lung for the monitoring of acute decompensated heart failure. *Am J Emerg Med*. 2008;26:585-591.
96. Soldati G, Copetti R, Sher S. Sonographic interstitial syndrome: the sound of lung water. *J Ultrasound Med*. 2009;28:163-174.
97. Liteplo AS, Marrill KA, Villen T, et al. Emergency thoracic ultrasound in the differentiation of the etiology of shortness of breath (ETUDES): sonographic B-lines and N-terminal pro-brain-type natriuretic peptide in diagnosing heart failure. *Acad Em Med*. 2009;16:201-210.
98. Volpicelli G, Noble VE, Liteplo A, Cardinale L. Decreased sensitivity of lung ultrasound limited to the anterior chest in emergency department diagnosis of cardiogenic pulmonary edema: a retrospective analysis. *Crit Ultrasound J*. 2010;2:47-52.
99. Lichtenstein DA, Menu Y. A bedside ultrasound sign ruling out pneumothorax in the critically ill. Lung sliding. *Chest*. 1995;108:1345-1348.
100. Lichtenstein D, Meziere G, Biderman P, et al. The comet-tail artifact: an ultrasound sign ruling out pneumothorax. *Intensive Care Med*. 1999;25:383-388.
101. Rubano E, Mehta N, Caputo W, et al. Systematic review: emergency department bedside ultrasonography for diagnosing suspected abdominal aortic aneurysm. *Acad Emerg Med*. 2013;20:128-138.
102. Bernardi E, Camporese G, Büller H, et al. Serial 2-point ultrasonography plus D-dimer vs. whole-leg color-coded Doppler ultrasonography for diagnosing suspected symptomatic deep vein thrombosis. *JAMA*. 2008;300:1653-1659.
103. Farahmand S, Farnia M, Shahriaran S, et al. The accuracy of limited B-mode compression technique in diagnosing deep venous thrombosis in lower extremities. *Am J Emerg Med*. 2011;29:687-690.
104. Hernandez C, Shuler K, Hannan H, et al. C.A.U.S.E.: cardiac arrest ultrasound exam: a better approach to managing patients in primary non-arrhythmogenic cardiac arrest. *Resuscitation*. 2008;76:198-206.
105. Haas M, Allendorfer J, Walcher F, et al. Focused examination of cerebral blood flow in peri-resuscitation: a new advanced life support compliant concept-an extension of the focused echocardiography evaluation in life support examination. *Crit Ultrasound J*. 2010;2:1-12.
106. Blaivas M. Transesophageal echocardiography during cardiopulmonary arrest in the emergency department. *Resuscitation*. 2008;78:135-140.
107. Wei J, Yang HS, Tsai SK, et al. Emergent bedside real-time three-dimensional echocardiography in a patient with cardiac arrest following a caesarean section. *Eur J Echo*. 2011;12:E16.
108. Memtsoudis SG, Rosenberger P, Loffler M, et al. The usefulness of transesophageal echocardiography during intraoperative cardiac arrest in noncardiac surgery. *Anesth Analg*. 2006;102:1653-1657.
109. Blaivas M, Fox JC. Outcome in cardiac arrest patients found to have cardiac standstill on bedside emergency department echocardiogram. *Acad Emerg Med*. 2001;8:616-621.
110. Salen P, Melniker L, Chooljian C, et al. Does the presence or absence of sonographically identified cardiac activity predict resuscitation outcomes of cardiac arrest patients? *Am J Emerg Med*. 2005;23:459-462.
111. Blyth L, Atkinson P, Gadd K, Lang E. Bedside focused echocardiography as predictor of survival in cardiac arrest: a systematic review. *Acad Emerg Med*. 2012;19:1119-1126.
112. Cureton EL, Yeung LY, Kwan RO, et al. The heart of the matter: utility of ultrasound of cardiac activity during traumatic arrest. *J Trauma Acute Care Surg*. 2012;73:102-110.
113. Nalin Shah B, Ahmadvazir S, Sihgh Pabla J, et al. The role of transthoracic echocardiography in the evaluation of the patient with acute chest pain. *Eur J Emerg Med*. 2012;19:277-283.

CARDIOVASCULAR EMERGENCIES

CHAPTER 5

Acute Coronary Syndrome: Modern Treatment of STEMI and NSTEMI

Tarlan Hedayati and Atman P. Shah

IN THIS CHAPTER

Initial anti-ischemic therapy
Revascularization therapy in STEMI
STEMI complications
Adjunctive therapy in ACS

Acute coronary syndrome (ACS) is a spectrum of ischemic myocardial disease that includes unstable angina (UA), non–ST-elevation myocardial infarction (NSTEMI), and ST-elevation myocardial infarction (STEMI). UA, NSTEMI, and STEMI represent the same pathophysiology but at increasing severity respectively. The diagnosis of ACS has already been addressed in preceding chapters of this textbook and, therefore, this chapter will focus on the emergency department management and treatment of ACS. At the time of the initial emergency department presentation, UA and NSTEMI may be indistinguishable and, therefore, are treated similarly. By definition, STEMI is identifiable immediately by electrocardiography. The treatment of STEMI is addressed in a separate chapter of this textbook. Next to each therapy discussed in this chapter, you will find the associated American College of Cardiology Foundation (ACCF) and American Heart Association (AHA) class of recommendation and the corresponding level of evidence. Briefly, Class I represents the highest or strongest level of recommendation, while Class III represents the presence of either no benefit or actual harm with therapy. "Level of evidence A" represents the most convincing evidence based on well-designed supporting research and trials, while "level of evidence C" represents a recommendation based on very limited data (Table 5-1).

Initial Anti-Ischemic Therapy

Nitrates

Patients with ACS can obtain relief of symptoms with the addition of nitrates, which reduce left ventricular (LV) preload, increase coronary blood flow, and decrease myocardial oxygen demand. Although nitrates may have a role in ACS that includes vasospasm and in patients who have concomitant hypertension or heart failure, there is no mortality benefit to their use.[1] Patients experiencing a right ventricular (RV) myocardial infarction (MI) tend to be dependent on preload to maintain adequate LV stroke volume and cardiac output. Therefore nitrates should generally be administered either very cautiously or not at all in suspected cases of RV MI because severe hypotension can result. Further, patients with bradyarrhythmias or tachyarrhythmias, hypotension, severe aortic stenosis, or 5′-phosphodiesterease inhibitor use (eg, sildenafil) in the past 24 to 48 hours should also avoid nitrates because administration of nitrates in these situations can lead to hemodynamic compromise.[2] Nitroglycerin therapy may be initiated using 0.4 mg sublingually every 5 minutes, typically up to 3 doses. After 3 doses, a continuous infusion of intravenous nitroglycerin may be more appropriate. Although transdermal nitroglycerin paste has been used for nitroglycerin administration in ACS, the paste is more unpredictable in its absorption and clinical effect, making this route of administration less desirable.

KEY POINTS

Patients with ACS and ongoing ischemic discomfort should receive sublingual nitroglycerin 0.4 mg every 5 minutes for a total of 3 doses (IC).

Patients with ACS/NSTEMI and persistent ischemia, heart failure, and/or hypertension should be started on intravenous nitroglycerin (IC).

Nitrates should not be given to patients with hypotension, bradycardia, tachycardia without clinical heart failure, and RV infarction and those having taken a 5'-phosphodiesterase inhibitor in the past 24 hours (eg, sildenafil) or 48 hours (eg, tadalafil) (IIIB).

Beta-Receptor Antagonists

Beta-blockers decrease the heart rate, systolic blood pressure, and myocardial contractility, thereby reducing oxygen demand and ischemia. Beta-blockers have been part of the medical treatment of ACS since the 1980s when patients suffering from an acute MI experienced reduced mortality when treated with metoprolol.[3] Further trials including ISIS-1[4] supported the early use of beta-blockers in the prefibrinolytic era. The COMMIT trial studied the effects of intravenous metoprolol followed by oral metoprolol in over 40,000 patients with STEMI.[5] The primary end points of the study were the composite of death, reinfarction, or cardiac arrest, as well as death from any cause during the treatment period. Although there were lower rates of recurrent MI and ventricular fibrillation in the treatment group, there was no effect on the primary combined end point. However, the administration of metoprolol was associated with a higher rate of cardiogenic shock, especially in patients who

TABLE 5-1.

Applying Classification of Recommendations and Level of Evidence. From: O'Gara PT, Kushner FG, Ascheim DD, et al. 2013 ACCF/AHA guideline for the management of ST-elevation myocardial infarction: a report of the American College of Cardiology Foundation/American Heart Association Task Force on Practice Guidelines. *J Am Col Cardiol.* 2013;61(4):e78-e140. Open archive.

	Size of Treatment Effect			
	Class I Benefit >>> Risk Procedure/Treatment **SHOULD** be performed/administered	**Class IIa** Benefit >> Risk Additional studies with focused objectives needed **IT IS REASONABLE** to perform procedure/administer treatment	**Class IIb** Benefit ≥ Risk Additional studies with broad objectives needed; additional registry data would be helpful Procedure/Treatment **MAY BE CONSIDERED**	**Class II** Risk ≥ Benefit Procedure/Treatment should **not** be performed/administered **SINCE IT IS NOT HELPFUL AND MAY BE HARMFUL**
LEVEL A Multiple populations evaluated* Data derived from multiple randomized clinical trials or meta-analyses	Recommendation that procedure or treatment is useful/ineffective Sufficient evidence from multiple randomized trials or meta-analyses	Recommendation in favor of treatment or procedure being useful/effective Some conflicting evidence from multiple randomized trials or meta-analyses	Recommendation's usefulness/efficacy less well established Greater conflicting evidence from multiple randomized trials or meta-analyses	Recommendation that procedure or treatment is not useful/effective and may be harmful Sufficient evidence from multiple randomized trials or meta-analyses
LEVEL B Limited populations evaluated Data derived from a single randomized trial or nonrandomized studies	Recommendation that procedure or treatment is useful/effective Evidence from single randomized trial or nonrandomized studies	Recommendation in favor of treatment or procedure being useful/effective Some conflicting evidence from single randomized trial or nonrandomized studies	Recommendation's usefulness/efficacy less well established Greater conflicting evidence from single randomized trial or nonrandomized studies	Recommendation that procedure or treatment is not useful/effective and may be harmful Evidence from single randomized trial or nonrandomized studies
LEVEL C Very limited populations evaluated Only consensus opinion of experts, case studies, or standard of care	Recommendation that procedure or treatment is useful/effective Only expert opinion, case studies, or standard or care	Recommendation in favor of treatment or procedure being useful/effective Only diverging expert opinion, case studies, or standard of care	Recommendation's usefulness/efficacy less well established Only diverging expert opinion, case studies, or standard of care	Recommendation that procedure or treatment is not useful/effective and may be harmful Only expert opinion, case studies, or standard of care
Suggested phrases for writing recommendations	Should, is recommended, is indicated, is useful/effective/beneficial	Is reasonable, can be useful/effective/beneficial, is probably recommended or indicated	May/might be considered, may/might be reasonable, usefulness/effectiveness is unknown/unclear/uncertain or not well established	Is not recommended, is not indicated, should not, is not useful/effective/beneficial, may be harmful

Estimate of Certainty (Precision) of Treatment Effect

were in heart failure, hemodynamically compromised, or stable but at risk for development of shock. Risk factors for developing shock included age above 70 years, female sex, more prolonged time since symptom onset, higher Killip classification (used to risk stratify patients with MI), systolic blood pressure less than 120, heart rate faster than 110, presence of an electrocardiographic (ECG) abnormality, and previous hypertension. Because many patients with STEMI could be in cardiogenic shock on admission and prior to revascularization, routine immediate administration of beta-blockers is not necessary.

KEY POINTS

Oral beta-blockers should be given within the first 24 hours to UA/NSTEMI and STEMI patients who are not in cardiogenic shock or do not have overt signs of heart failure, active asthma, reactive airway disease, or atrioventricular (AV) block (IA).[6,7]

Intravenous beta-blockers have achieved a secondary recommendation in patients who are hypertensive or have continuing ischemia in the setting of STEMI (IIA/B).[7,8]

Intravenous beta-blockers should *not* be given to patients who have contraindications to beta-blockade, signs of heart failure or low-output state, or other risk factors for cardiogenic shock (IIIB).

Calcium Channel Blockers

Calcium channel blockers (CCBs) can inhibit peripheral vasoconstriction and slow conduction through the AV node. Therefore, there is a potential benefit for CCBs, especially the nondihydropyridines verapamil and diltiazem. DAVIT (Danish Verapamil Infarction Trial) is the largest randomized trial to have evaluated CCB effects in patients with ACS. The results showed a trend toward lower rates of death or MI when verapamil was administered to patients with suspected ACS.[9] However, a later metaanalysis of over 19,000 patients showed no mortality benefit for CCBs in STEMI patients.[10] Nifedipine is contraindicated because of its association with hypotension.[11]

KEY POINTS

Oral nondihydropyridine CCBs can be given as initial therapy in UA/NSTEMI patients with continuing or frequently recurring ischemia and in whom beta-blockers are contraindicated, in the absence of clinically significant LV dysfunction or other contraindications (IB).[6]

Oral long-acting CCBs are recommended in persistently symptomatic patients who have already received full-dose nitrates and beta-blockers (IC).[6]

Renin-Angiotensin-Aldosterone System Inhibitors

Activation of the renin-angiotensin-aldosterone system (RAAS) is an essential component of the "flight or fight" response of the body to stress. Chronic activation of the RAAS system can lead to systemic hypertension, myocardial hypertrophy and fibrosis, and accelerated cardiovascular atherosclerosis.[12] The acute inflammatory state that is associated with STEMI can up-regulate the RAAS system. In STEMI patients, treatment with oral angiotensin-converting enzyme (ACE) inhibitors has resulted in decreased all-cause mortality by 19%, and the effect is even more pronounced in patients with an ejection fraction below 40%, hypertension, prior MI, and tachycardia.[13] In patients who cannot tolerate ACE inhibitors, the angiotensin-receptor blocker (ARB) valsartan was found to be noninferior to captopril in patients with STEMI.[14]

KEY POINTS

Oral ACE inhibitors (or ARBs if the patient is ACE-inhibitor intolerant) are indicated for all UA/NSTEMI and STEMI patients within the first 24 hours (IIA/B), with the greatest benefit for patients who have a low ejection fraction, anterior infarct, or heart failure (IA). There is no recommendation for emergent oral ACE inhibitor administration in the emergency department.

Intravenous ACE inhibitors should be avoided in the first 24 hours because of the increased risk of hypotension, unless they are needed for control of hypertension (IIIB).[6]

Oxygen

Oxygen therapy is a mainstay of therapy for all ACS patients, but there are few data to support its use in patients who are not hypoxemic. Supplemental oxygen might increase coronary vascular resistance. A Cochrane analysis revealed an increased risk of death for MI patients treated with supplemental oxygen compared to room air.[15] Current recommendations state that it is reasonable to administer oxygen at ACS presentation if the oxygen saturation is below 90% or the patient appears to be in respiratory distress (IC).[6,16]

Lipid-Lowering Agents

The use of HMG-CoA reductase inhibitors (statins) has proved beneficial in reducing adverse cardiovascular events in both primary and secondary prevention. In addition, the pleiotropic, anti-inflammatory effects of statins can enhance plaque stabilization and endothelial function during STEMI.[17] In clinical trials, atorvastatin, 80 mg, has been shown to reduce cardiac death and ischemic events in patients with ACS and STEMI.[18] However, there are no recommendations at this time supporting the use of statins in the emergency department at the time of presentation.

Analgesics

Morphine is the preferred agent for pain relief in patients with ACS who have had no relief with nitrates or who continue to have or develop pain after full-dose nitrates have been given (IIB). Blood pressure and respiratory rate should be monitored whenever morphine is used. The CRUSADE trial demonstrated increased adverse events, including MI and death, in ACS patients who received morphine regardless of age, blood pressure, ST changes on ECG, cardiac markers, concomitant nitroglycerin use, or presence or absence of heart failure. The current guidelines recommend morphine administration only if the patient continues to have pain despite maximal nitrate therapy (IIbB). Nonsteroidal anti-inflammatory drugs and cyclooxygenase II enzyme (COX-2) inhibitors are contraindicated in UA/NSTEMI and STEMI patients due to an associated increased risk of adverse cardiovascular events (III).[7]

Revascularization Therapy in STEMI

STEMI occurs when a ruptured plaque leads to platelet aggregation and thrombotic occlusion of an epicardial coronary artery. The resultant cessation of flow leads to myocardial injury and infarction.

Successful treatment of the STEMI patient depends on rapid recognition and implementation of therapeutic pathways to help disrupt the thrombotic occlusion and revascularize the occluded artery. Primary percutaneous coronary intervention (pPCI) remains the preferred method of revascularization when performed within 90 minutes of first medical contact (IA).[19] However, most hospitals are not pPCI-capable, and STEMI patients who present to these hospitals should be given fibrinolytic therapy.[20] If a patient presents to a non–pPCI-capable hospital and the anticipated time from first medical contact to balloon is less than 120 minutes including transfer, the patient should be transferred to a pPCI-capable hospital (IB).[21] If the anticipated time is greater than 120 minutes, the patient should be given fibrinolytic therapy (IB).[22] Figure 5-1 provides an overview of the management of STEMI.

Fibrinolysis in STEMI

Fibrinolytics convert plasminogen into plasmin, which then allows fibrinolysis and enhanced thrombus degradation to occur. The ease of use of fibrinolytics and the rapidity with which it can be administered have led to its implementation in the prehospital setting. In patients who present with STEMI, prehospital fibrinolytic therapy resulted in a nearly 50% reduction in 1-year mortality.[23] A metaanalysis of six trials studying the effects of prehospital fibrinolytics reported no reduction in longer-term mortality at one or two years but did report a 60-minute reduction in the time to fibrinolytic administration and a decrease in all-cause hospital mortality (relative risk reduction of 17%).[24] Recent trials, including the CAPTIM, WEST, USIC, and Swedish Registry of Cardiac Intensive Care, report decreased mortality in STEMI patients treated with prehospital fibrinolytics.[25-28] Despite the promising data, the cost of training paramedics and providing equipment has precluded its adoption in the United States.

Several large trials have reported that STEMI patients who present within 12 hours of symptom onset have a survival benefit with the administration of fibrinolytics, in the absence of contraindications (Table 5-2) as compared to medical therapy (IA). Patients who present between 12 and 24 hours after symptom onset with ECG and clinical evidence of ongoing instability should also be given fibrinolytics in the absence of contraindications (IIA/C).[29] Dosages and coronary artery patency

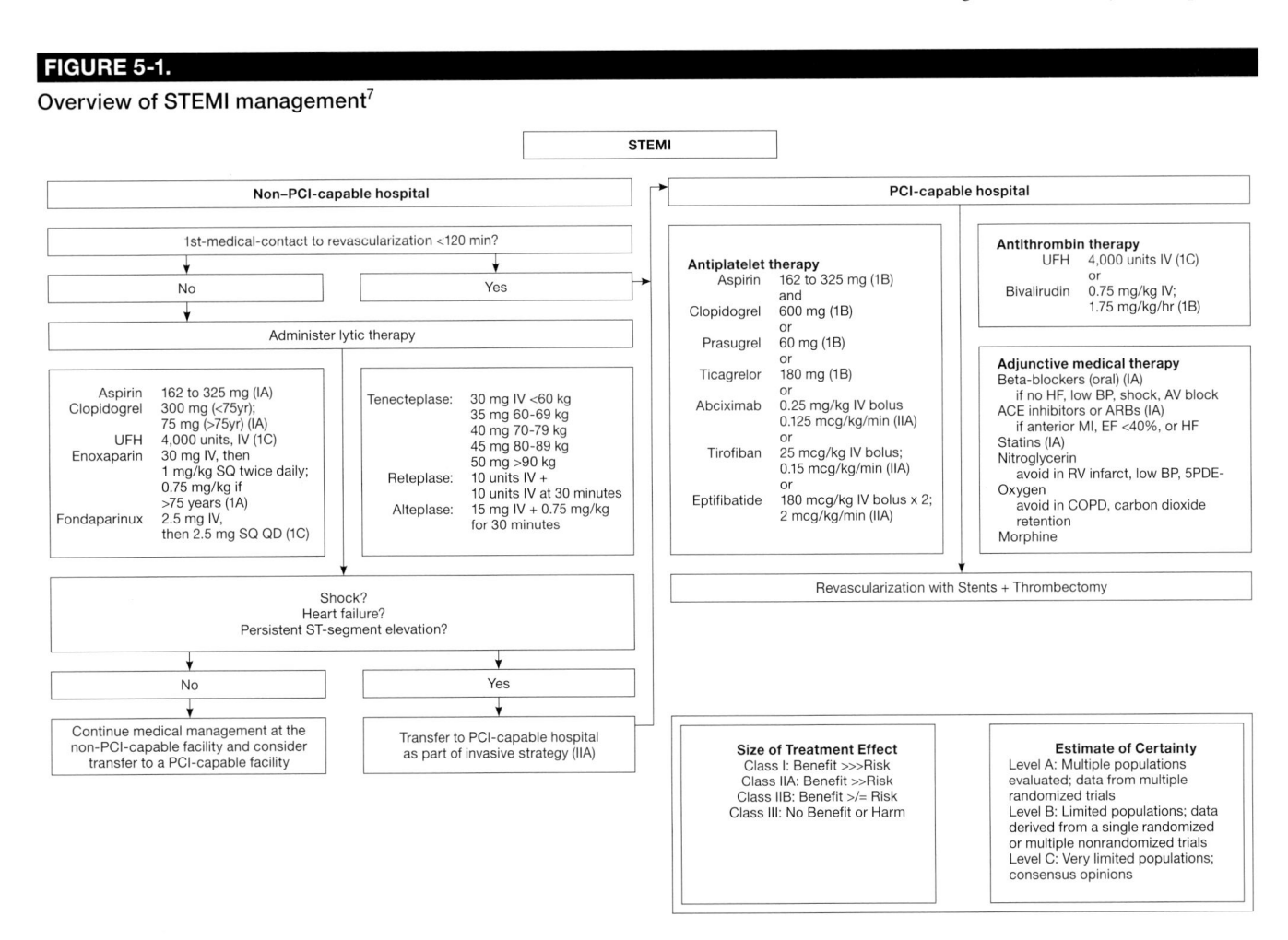

FIGURE 5-1.

Overview of STEMI management[7]

```
                              STEMI
        ┌───────────────────────┴───────────────────────┐
Non–PCI-capable hospital                      PCI-capable hospital

1st-medical-contact to revascularization <120 min?
        ┌──────────┴──────────┐
       No                    Yes
        │                     │
Administer lytic therapy

Aspirin      162 to 325 mg (IA)
Clopidogrel  300 mg (<75yr);
             75 mg (>75yr) (IA)
UFH          4,000 units, IV (1C)
Enoxaparin   30 mg IV, then
             1 mg/kg SQ twice daily;
             0.75 mg/kg if
             >75 years (1A)
Fondaparinux 2.5 mg IV,
             then 2.5 mg SQ QD (1C)

Tenecteplase:  30 mg IV <60 kg
               35 mg 60-69 kg
               40 mg 70-79 kg
               45 mg 80-89 kg
               50 mg >90 kg
Reteplase:     10 units IV +
               10 units IV at 30 minutes
Alteplase:     15 mg IV + 0.75 mg/kg
               for 30 minutes

Shock?
Heart failure?
Persistent ST-segment elevation?
     ┌──────┴──────┐
    No            Yes
     │             │
Continue medical management at the    Transfer to PCI-capable hospital
non-PCI-capable facility and consider   as part of invasive strategy (IIA)
transfer to a PCI-capable facility

Antiplatelet therapy
Aspirin      162 to 325 mg (1B)
             and
Clopidogrel  600 mg (1B)
             or
Prasugrel    60 mg (1B)
             or
Ticagrelor   180 mg (1B)
             or
Abciximab    0.25 mcg/kg IV bolus
             0.125 mcg/kg/min (IIA)
             or
Tirofiban    25 mcg/kg IV bolus;
             0.15 mcg/kg/min (IIA)
             or
Eptifibatide 180 mcg/kg IV bolus x 2;
             2 mcg/kg/min (IIA)

Antithrombin therapy
UFH          4,000 units IV (1C)
             or
Bivalirudin  0.75 mg/kg IV;
             1.75 mg/kg/hr (1B)

Adjunctive medical therapy
Beta-blockers (oral) (IA)
   if no HF, low BP, shock, AV block
ACE inhibitors or ARBs (IA)
   if anterior MI, EF <40%, or HF
Statins (IA)
Nitroglycerin
   avoid in RV infarct, low BP, 5PDE-
Oxygen
   avoid in COPD, carbon dioxide
   retention
Morphine

Revascularization with Stents + Thrombectomy
```

Size of Treatment Effect
Class I: Benefit >>>Risk
Class IIA: Benefit >>Risk
Class IIB: Benefit >/= Risk
Class III: No Benefit or Harm

Estimate of Certainty
Level A: Multiple populations evaluated; data from multiple randomized trials
Level B: Limited populations; data derived from a single randomized or multiple nonrandomized trials
Level C: Very limited populations; consensus opinions

rates of commonly used fibrinolytics are shown in Table 5-3. Of note, while the patency rate of tenecteplase is higher than that of other fibrinolytics, it is associated with clinical equivalency with decreased bleeding when compared with alteplase.[33]

Fibrinolytics can increase the levels of thrombin through a feedback loop and, therefore, anticoagulation is recommended to improve vessel patency and prevent reocclusion.[34] Choices in anticoagulation therapy and dosages are presented later in this chapter.

Fibrinolytic therapy restores normal flow in only one-half of STEMI patients with even less success in elderly patients and those in cardiogenic shock.[35] Patients who demonstrate shock, severe heart failure, and persistent ST-segment elevation following fibrinolytic therapy should be transferred to a pPCI-capable hospital for rescue PCI.[36] Even after successful fibrinolysis, it is recommended that patients be transferred to a pPCI hospital for angiography.[37]

Given that almost all patients who receive fibrinolytics should be transferred to a pPCI-capable hospital for angiography, two large studies investigated the role of facilitated PCI (fibrinolysis with immediate transfer to a pPCI hospital) within 120 minutes. These studies failed to show a benefit for the strategy of full- or half-dose lytics with planned PCI within 90 to 120 minutes as compared to pPCI alone.[38,39]

KEY POINTS

Fibrinolytics should be administered to a STEMI patient who presents to a non–PCI-capable hospital if the anticipated first medical contact-to-balloon time exceeds 120 minutes if the patient were transferred to a pPCI-capable center.

Patients should be transferred to a pPCI-capable center if they demonstrate shock, recurrent angina, heart failure, or persistent ST-segment elevation.

Guidelines suggest the transfer of all STEMI patients treated with fibrinolytics to a pPCI center for further care.

Primary Percutaneous Coronary Intervention in STEMI

The occluded coronary artery can be treated with pPCI.

TABLE 5-2.

Absolute and Relative Contraindications to Fibrinolytic Therapy. Adapted from: O'Gara PT, Kushner FG, Ascheim DD, et al. 2013 ACCF/AHA guideline for the management of ST-elevation myocardial infarction: a report of the American College of Cardiology Foundation/American Heart Association Task Force on Practice Guidelines. *J Am Col Cardiol.* 2013;61(4):e78-e140. Open archive.

Absolute Contraindications	Any prior intracerebral hemorrhage
	Arteriovenous malformation, malignant neoplasm
	Ischemic stroke within 3 months (except within 4.5 hours)
	Suspected aortic dissection
	Active bleeding
	Significant head/facial trauma
	Severe uncontrolled hypertension
	Intracranial/intraspinal surgery within 2 months
	If streptokinase is used, prior treatment within 6 months
Relative Contraindications	History of poorly controlled hypertension or systolic blood pressure above 180 or diastolic blood pressure above 110
	Prior stroke more than 3 months ago
	Dementia
	Other intracranial pathology
	Traumatic or prolonged (>10 min) cardiopulmonary resuscitation
	Major surgery within 3 weeks
	Recent (within 2 to 4 weeks) internal bleeding
	Noncompressible vascular puncture
	Pregnancy
	Active peptic ulcer
	Oral anticoagulant therapy

The procedure can involve an angioplasty balloon, a mechanical thrombus aspiration catheter, and a stent, which results in physical disruption of the occlusive thrombus and scaffolding of the culprit artery to maintain adequate coronary blood flow (Figure 5-2).

Compared to fibrinolytic therapy, pPCI results in higher rates of infarct artery patency and lower rates of nonfatal MI ($P<.01$), recurrent ischemia ($P<.01$), total stroke ($P<.01$), hemorrhagic stroke ($P<.01$), and short- and long-term death ($P<.01$).[40] Therefore, pPCI should be performed in patients who present with STEMI within 12 hours of symptom onset (IA),[41] who have contraindications to fibrinolytic therapy (IB),[42] who present with cardiogenic shock (IB),[43] or who present within 24 hours after symptom onset (IIA/B).[44]

KEY POINT

Primary PCI is superior to fibrinolytic therapy for STEMI with a goal of 90 minutes between first medical contact and revascularization.

STEMI Complications

Profound infarction can lead to massive structural damage to the heart and mechanical complications such as papillary muscle rupture and severe mitral regurgitation, left ventricular free wall rupture, and ventricular septal rupture. These are best diagnosed with transthoracic echocardiography and necessitate immediate cardiothoracic surgical evaluation.

Other complications such as bradycardia, ventricular tachycardia, and RV infarction may be managed in the emergency department (Figure 5-3).

Adjunctive Therapy in ACS

Antiplatelet Therapy

Patients with ACS should be started on dual antiplatelet therapy, including aspirin and a $P2Y_{12}$ receptor inhibitor.

Aspirin

Aspirin decreases platelet aggregation by irreversibly inhibiting cyclooxygenase-1, thereby blocking production of thromboxane 2, which is also a potent vasoconstrictor. Multiple studies have shown and confirmed a 50% to 70% reduction in the risk of death from cardiac causes and fatal and nonfatal MI in patients treated with aspirin. This benefit to aspirin therapy has been shown as compared to placebo or to other medications in both UA/NSTEMI and STEMI.[6,45-51] The ACCF/AHA guidelines recommend a dose of 162 to 325 mg orally initially (IA).[52] Physicians should be sure to ask patients if aspirin was taken at home or given by EMS and at what dosage. In patients with aspirin hypersensitivity or major gastrointestinal intolerance, a loading dose of a $P2Y_{12}$ ADP receptor inhibitor may be used instead (IB).[52]

$P2Y_{12}$ ADP Inhibitors

The $P2Y_{12}$ ADP receptor inhibitors (eg, clopidogrel, prasugrel, ticagrelor) block platelet activation and aggregation. Their mechanism of action is independent of aspirin's mechanism of action, and the effect of a combination of aspirin and a $P2Y_{12}$ ADP inhibitor is more powerful than that of aspirin alone.[51,53,54] The $P2Y_{12}$ inhibitors currently available and FDA approved are clopidogrel, prasugrel, and ticagrelor.

Clopidogrel. Of the three $P2Y_{12}$ inhibitors that are FDA approved and currently in use, clopidogrel is the oldest and

FIGURE 5-2.

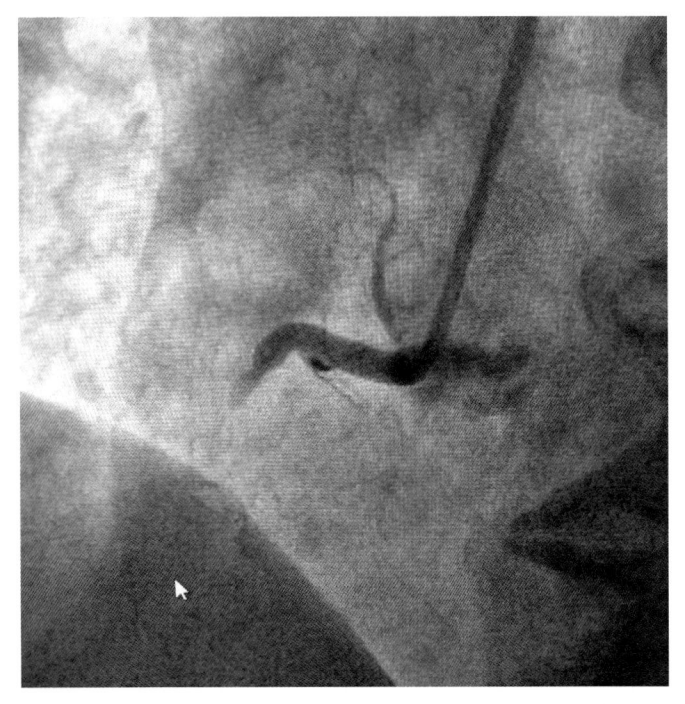

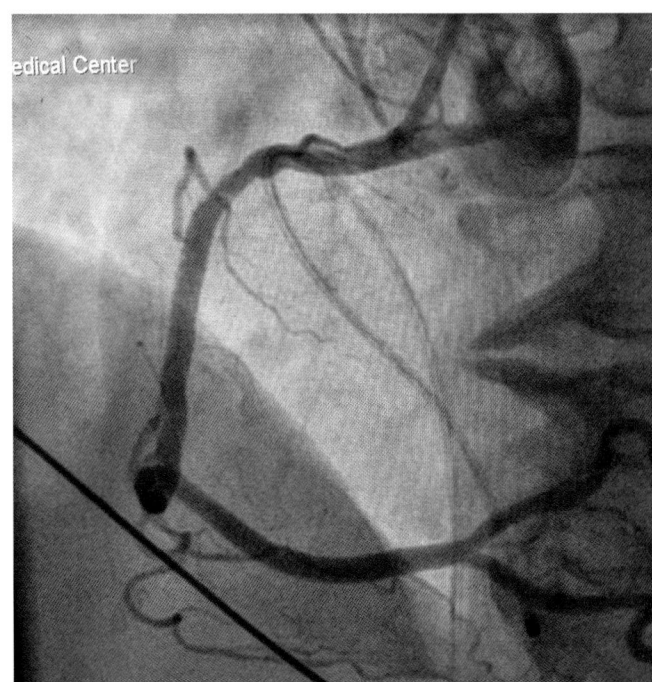

Cineangiographic images of occluded (left) and opened (right) right coronary artery (RCA) during STEMI

best studied. In patients with UA/NSTEMI, the ACCF/AHA guidelines recommend a loading dose of clopidogrel of 300 to 600 mg (IB).[6,45,46,52,55] This recommendation is based on multiple studies, including the CURE trial with 12,562 patients, which demonstrated a 20% decrease in the incidence of cardiovascular death, MI, or stroke in low- and high-risk UA/NSTEMI patients on clopidogrel compared to those taking placebo.[53,54] This benefit also extended to a subgroup of patients that were slated for PCI, demonstrating an overall 31% reduction in cardiovascular events at 1 year.[56] However, there was also an increased risk of non–life-threatening bleeding reported in patients on clopidogrel. The CREDO trial, looking at high-risk ACS patients referred for PCI, compared clopidogrel, 300 mg loading dose, to placebo 3 to 24 hours before PCI, with daily clopidogrel maintenance therapy for all patients post-PCI for 28 days. Although there appeared to be a greater number of improved results in the clopidogrel-loading group for the composite end point of death/MI/urgent target vessel revascularization, the numbers did not reach statistical significance.[57] Increasing the loading dose of clopidogrel from 300 mg to 600 mg in the HORIZONS-AMI trial of PCI-bound STEMI patients demonstrated not only significantly decreased rates of the primary end points of death (3.1% vs 1.9%, P=.03), reinfarction (2.3% vs 1.3%, P=.02), and stent thrombosis (2.8% vs 1.7%, P=.04) at 30 days but also showed no significant difference in rates of major or minor bleeding.[58,59] Corroborating results were found in the ARMYDA 6 trial. This helped establish the current loading dose for clopidogrel of 600 mg orally in PCI-bound STEMI patients.

There is evidence that some patients demonstrate a "clopidogrel resistance," putting them at risk for recurrent thrombosis despite long-term dual antiplatelet therapy. This clopidogrel resistance is thought to be caused by genetic polymorphisms in the liver cytochrome P450 (CYP) system responsible for the two-step enzymatic conversion of the clopidogrel pro-drug to its active metabolite. Commercially available genetic tests can identify those with the loss-of-function CYP alleles, but these tests are expensive, not routinely covered by insurance companies, and have not been studied to determine their clinical utility.[60-62]

Finally, there has been some suggestion that routine use of proton-pump inhibitors (PPIs) could interfere with and inhibit the conversion of clopidogrel to its active metabolite, as they are also metabolized in varying degrees by the CYP.[63] PPIs were often started in conjunction with thienopyridine therapy in an effort to reduce the gastrointestinal complications associated with dual antiplatelet therapy.[64] In fact, the 2007 ACCF/AHA UA/NSTEMI guidelines had recommended adding a PPI to dual antiplatelet therapy. Since then, the FDA has released an advisory warning based on a few studies about the risk of adverse cardiovascular events associated with concomitant use of clopidogrel and the PPI omeprazole.[65,66] As a result, the recommendation for routine PPI use with thienopyridines was removed from subsequent guidelines. More studies are needed in order to make a clear recommendation regarding the use of clopidogrel and PPIs in the future.

Prasugrel. Prasugrel is a newer thienopyridine that irreversibly blocks the $P2Y_{12}$ receptor but is more potent and faster than clopidogrel at platelet inhibition. In the TRITON-TIMI 38, a large industry-sponsored, randomized, double-blinded study comparing prasugrel with clopidogrel in 13,608 moderate- or high-risk ACS patients (10,074 with UA/STEMI), patients using prasugrel had a significantly lower incidence of the composite of cardiovascular death and nonfatal MI/stroke (9.9% vs 12.1%), as well as reduced rates of stent rethrombosis (2.4% to 1.1%). However, prasugrel was also associated with significantly

FIGURE 5-3.

Management of STEMI complications in the emergency department

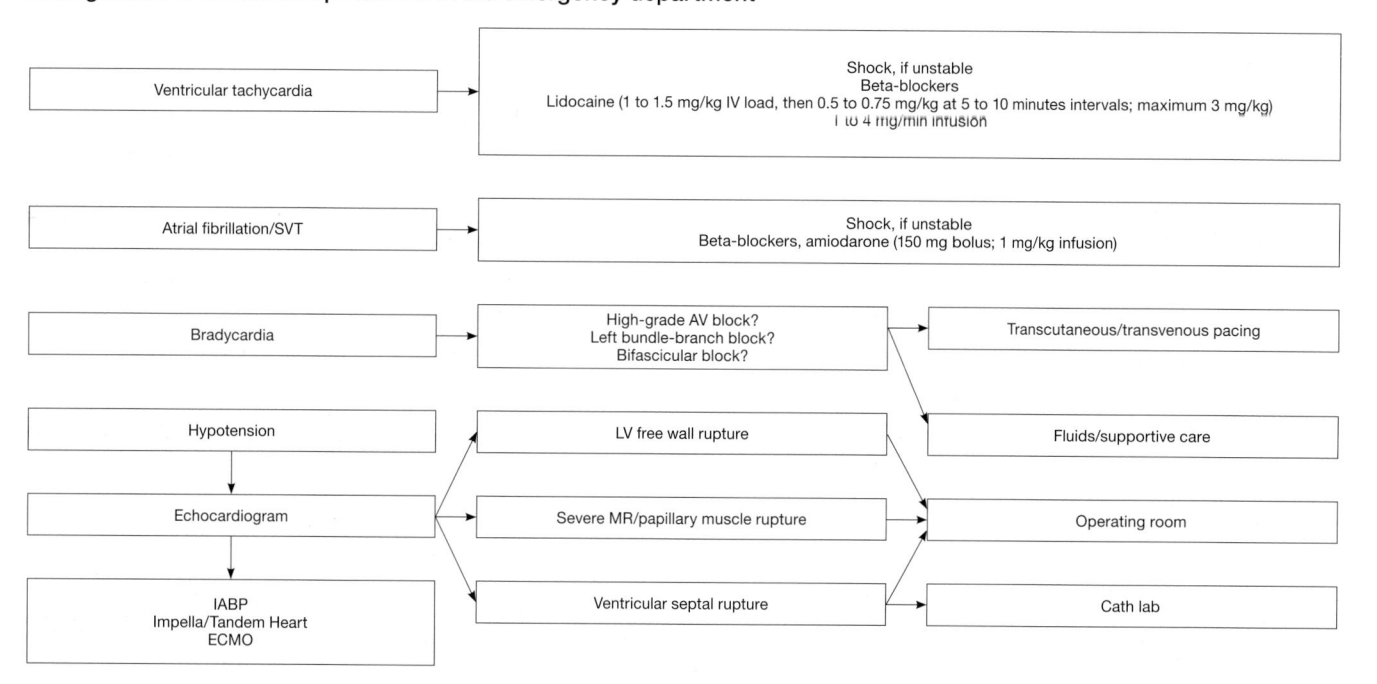

Condition	Assessment	Treatment
Ventricular tachycardia		Shock, if unstable; Beta-blockers; Lidocaine (1 to 1.5 mg/kg IV load, then 0.5 to 0.75 mg/kg at 5 to 10 minutes intervals; maximum 3 mg/kg) 1 to 4 mg/min infusion
Atrial fibrillation/SVT		Shock, if unstable; Beta-blockers, amiodarone (150 mg bolus; 1 mg/kg infusion)
Bradycardia	High-grade AV block? Left bundle-branch block? Bifascicular block?	Transcutaneous/transvenous pacing
Hypotension → Echocardiogram → IABP Impella/Tandem Heart ECMO	LV free wall rupture	Fluids/supportive care
	Severe MR/papillary muscle rupture	Operating room
	Ventricular septal rupture	Cath lab

higher risk for major bleeding and for life-threatening bleeding.[67] In a post-hoc analysis of the TRITON-TIMI 38 study, three subgroups of ACS patients were identified who did not have a favorable net benefit from prasugrel use and, therefore, should not receive the drug and they are as follows: patients with a history of stroke or transient ischemic attack, patients older than 75 years, and patients with a body weight below 60 kg[67] (IIIB). These findings prompted the FDA to release an advisory in 2009 warning against the use of prasugrel in the aforementioned populations.

Current ACCF/ACC guidelines recommend prasugrel, 60 mg orally, as an alternative to clopidogrel in PCI-bound STEMI patients *at the time of PCI*. It is not recommended for use in patients prior to catheterization. It has not been studied in STEMI patients undergoing fibrinolysis, and therefore it is not recommended in this circumstance.

Like clopidogrel, prasugrel is a pro-drug that requires conversion to its active metabolite. However, in contrast to clopidogrel's two-step process, prasugrel requires only a one-step conversion through the CYP path. Observational studies have not shown a similar increase in cardiovascular events in patients on prasugrel with the loss-of-function allele.[68]

Ticagrelor. Ticagrelor is an oral, nonthienopyridine $P2Y_{12}$-receptor blocker that is even more potent and faster acting than clopidogrel. It is not a pro-drug, does not require conversion, and is therefore unaffected by the CYP loss-of-function allele. It received FDA approval in July 2011.

In the PLATO study, a manufacturer-sponsored, double-blinded trial of 18,624 ACS patients randomized to ticagrelor or clopidogrel, the 1-year primary end point of MI, stroke, or death from vascular causes was significantly lower in the ticagrelor group than the clopidogrel group (9.8% vs 11.7%), as were rates of MI, death from vascular causes, and death from all causes. The rate of major bleeding did not differ significantly between the groups.[69]

The ACCF/AHA guidelines recommend the use of loading-dose ticagrelor, 180 mg orally, as an alternative to clopidogrel in patients with UA/NSTEMI and PCI-bound STEMI as part of dual antiplatelet therapy (IB) and in patients unable to take aspirin (IC).[52] Ticagrelor has not been studied in STEMI patients undergoing fibrinolysis and its use is therefore not recommended in this situation.

KEY POINTS

In patients with UA/NSTEMI managed conservatively, a loading dose of clopidogrel, 300 to 600 mg, or ticagrelor, 180 mg orally, (IB) is recommended, as soon as possible *after admission*.[6,45,45,52,55]

In patients with UA/NSTEMI or STEMI undergoing pPCI, a loading dose of clopidogrel, 600 mg orally, or ticagrelor, 180 mg orally, is recommended as early as possible or at the time of PCI (IA).[7] Ticagrelor is preferred to clopidogrel in this early-invasive group (IIB). However, pPCI should not be delayed in an effort to administer these medications in the emergency department unless the medications are not available in the cardiac catheterization laboratory.

In patients with STEMI undergoing fibrinolysis, a loading dose of clopidogrel, 300 mg orally, is recommended for patients younger than 75 years; a dose of 75 mg is recommended for patients older than 75 years (IA).[7]

Glycoprotein IIb-IIIa Receptor Antagonist

The platelet glycoprotein IIb-IIIa (GpIIb-IIIa) receptor is a key mediator of platelet aggregation and adhesion. Three GpIIb-IIIa receptor antagonists are currently available for use: abciximab, eptifibatide, and tirofiban. Although studies of oral GpIIb-IIIa receptor antagonists have not reduced adverse cardiovascular events in ACS/NSTEMI patients,[70] randomized trials of intravenous GpIIb-IIIa receptor antagonists have demonstrated significant reductions in ischemic complications in patients with ACS/NSTEMI compared to standard therapy.[71-73] GpIIb-IIIa receptor antagonists have the strongest clinical benefit when used immediately prior to PCI.[74] However, these studies were in the absence of widespread dual antiplatelet agent use. Two large recent trials, the EARLY ACS and the ACUITY trials, studied the role of early "upstream" GpIIb-IIIa receptor antagonism in patients with ACS who had received clopidogrel. Neither trial showed a reduction in adverse cardiovascular events in patients treated with a GpIIb-IIIa receptor antagonist, but administration did result in increased bleeding.[75,76]

Intravenous GpIIb-IIIa receptor antagonists were studied

TABLE 5-3.

Fibrinolytic Dosage and Associated Coronary Patency Rate

Fibrin-Specific Agent	Dose	Patency Rate
Tenecteplase	Single intravenous bolus: 30 mg for patients weighing less than 60 kg 35 mg for patients weighing 60 to 69 kg 40 mg for patients weighing 70 to 79 kg 45 mg for patients weighing 80 to 89 kg 50 mg for patients weighing more than 90 kg	85%[30]
Reteplase	10 units IV + 10 units IV at 30 min	84%[31]
Alteplase	15 mg bolus, 0.75 mg/kg for 30 minutes (maximum 50 mg), then 0.5 mg/kg for 60 minutes (maximum 35 mg; total dose not to exceed 100 mg)	73% to 84%[32]

in STEMI patients prior to the clopidogrel and P2Y$_{12}$ receptor antagonists. Routine "upstream" use of GpIIb-IIIa receptor antagonists has not resulted in superior clinical outcomes, but may be of some benefit in the cardiac catheterization lab to treat patients with a large thrombus burden (IIA/B).[77]

GpIIb-IIIa inhibitors should not be given to patients in whom PCI is not planned, a Class III recommendation by the ACCF/AHA.

KEY POINT

At this time, GpIIb-IIIa receptor antagonists do not need to be administered upstream in the emergency department in either UA/NSTEMI or STEMI patients.

Anticoagulant Therapy

Anticoagulant therapy should be initiated in all ACS patients as soon as possible after presentation. There are currently four options available in the United States: unfractionated heparin (UFH), enoxaparin, fondaparinux, and bivalirudin.

Unfractionated Heparin

Heparin helps reduce thrombus propagation by binding to antithrombin and, thereby, making it a fast-acting thrombin and factor Xa inhibitor. Benefits of heparin, compared to other anticoagulants, are its reversibility with protamine, ease of monitoring, and cost-effectiveness. Complications include variability in efficacy because of protein-binding, autoimmune heparin-induced thrombocytopenia, and bleeding. UFH with aspirin has been shown to be associated with lower rates of MI or death than aspirin monotherapy, with a relative risk of MI or death of 0.5.[78] The ACCF/AHA guidelines recommend a weight-based dosing of 60 units/kg bolus followed by a 12-units/kg/hour infusion in ACS patients.

Low-Molecular-Weight Heparins

Low molecular weight heparins (LMWHs), such as enoxaparin and fondaparinux, inactivate factor Xa. Enoxaparin also inhibits factor IIa, inhibiting both the action and the production of thrombin. Enoxaparin is the most studied LMWH in the setting of ACS. Multiple studies including the early ESSENCE and TIMI 11B trials have shown that, when compared to UFH, enoxaparin is associated with significantly lower incidence of the composite end point of death, MI, or recurrent ischemia, with similar bleeding risk profiles during hospitalization.[79,80] In the ESSENCE trial, the composite end point was 23.3% for LMWH compared to 19.8% for UFH at 30 days (P <.02), with a risk of major bleeding at 30 days of 6.5% for LMWH and 7% for UFH (P=.57) In fact, the superiority of enoxaparin over UFH is even more pronounced in higher-risk UA/NSTEMI patients.[80,81] In fibrinolysis-treated STEMI patients, enoxaparin can be given as a 30-mg IV bolus, followed by 1 mg/kg subcutaneously after 15 minutes in patients younger than 75 years. Patients older than 75 years need no intravenous bolus and can be given 0.75 mg/kg subcutaneously (IA). There is no role for enoxaparin in STEMI patients that are PCI-bound.

Fondaparinux is a subcutaneously administered factor Xa inhibitor that does not inhibit thrombin.[82] It requires antithrombin for its mechanism of action. It has been studied and used for the prevention of deep venous thrombosis and for the treatment of acute pulmonary embolism. In the OASIS trial, treatment of ACS/NSTEMI patients with fondaparinux resulted in similar rates of ischemic events but lower rates of major bleeding when compared to patients on enoxaparin. However, use of fondaparinux was associated with a significant increase in catheter-related thrombus in patients who proceeded to angiography[83] and therefore a second antithrombin needs to be used during PCI if fondaparinux has been initiated.[84] Fondaparinux may be used in patients with UA/NSTEMI (IB) and may be preferred to unfractionated heparin (IIaB).[52]

Bivalirudin

Bivalirudin is an intravenous direct thrombin inhibitor that has been well studied in the setting of ACS. In the ACUITY trial of 13,819 patients, bivalirudin was noninferior in terms of 30-day ischemic end points compared to heparin and a GpIIb-IIIa receptor antagonist in ACS/NSTEMI patients who were treated with early angiography and intervention (7.8% vs 7.3%). However, bivalirudin was associated with a significant lower rate of major bleeding (3% in bivalirudin arm vs 5.7% in the heparin + GpIIb-IIIa arm).[85] In the HORIZONS-AMI trial, the use of bivalirudin compared to UFH and GpIIb-IIIa receptor antagonists resulted in decreased major bleeding (6.9% in the bivalirudin arm vs 10.5% in the GpIIb-IIIa arm), but an increased rate (over 4%) in early stent thrombosis.[86] These results remained consistent at 30-day, 1-year, and 3-year follow-ups. Therefore, bivalirudin may be given in emergency department patients selected for cardiac catheterization (IB).[52]

KEY POINTS

Patients with UA/NSTEMI should receive:

UFH, 60 units/kg bolus, then 12 units/kg/hour infusion (IA), or

Enoxaparin, 1 mg/kg SQ (IA), which is preferred over UFH if the patient is to be managed conservatively (IIaB), or

Fondaparinux, 2.5 mg SQ (IB), which is preferred over UFH if the patient is to be managed conservatively (IIaB), or

Bivalirudin, 0.1 mg/kg bolus, then 0.25 mg/kg/hour infusion in patients with a creatinine clearance less than 30 mL/min, which may be used as an alternative to UFH or enoxaparin for patients destined for cardiac catheterization (IB).

Patients with STEMI undergoing PCI should receive:

UFH, 70 to 100 units/kg bolus (IC), or

Bivalirudin, 0.75 mg/kg IV bolus, then 1.75 mg/kg/h infusion (IB).

Note: Fondaparinux should not be used because of its associated risk of catheter thrombosis (IIIB).

Patients with STEMI undergoing fibrinolysis should receive:

UFH, 60 units/kg bolus and 12 units/kg/hour infusion (IC), or

Enoxaparin, 30 mg IV bolus, followed by 1 mg/kg SQ

after 15 minutes in patients younger than 75 years old. Patients older than 75 years need no bolus and 0.75 mg/kg SQ (IA), or

Fondaparinux, 2.5 mg IV, then 2.5 mg SQ (IB).

Conclusion

The management of UA/NSTEMI and STEMI is a dynamic and ever-changing landscape, as evidenced by the frequent publication of updated guidelines, in an attempt to keep up with emerging research and data. The approach to ACS should be individualized to each patient and care must be taken to remember that guidelines are simply just that—a scaffolding upon which to build good patient care. Practitioners will need to consider individual patient's needs in their approach to the management of this disease process.

References

1. ISIS-4: a randomised factorial trial assessing early oral captopril, oral mononitrate, and intravenous magnesium sulphate in 58,050 patients with suspected acute myocardial infarction. ISIS-4 (Fourth International Study of Infarct Survival) Collaborative Group. *Lancet.* 1995;345(8951):669-85.
2. Cheitlin MD, Hutter AM Jr, Brindis RG, et al. ACC/AHA expert consensus document: use of sildenafil (Viagra) in patients with cardio- vascular disease. *Circulation.* 1999;99:168-177. Erratum in: *J Am Coll Cardiol.* 1999;34(6):1850.
3. Hjalmarson A, Elmfeldt D, Herlitz J, et al. Effect on mortality of metoprolol in acute myocardial infarction. A double blind randomized trial. *Lancet.* 1981;2(8252):823-827.
4. First International Study of Infarct Survival Collaborative Group. Randomised trial of intravenous atenolol among 16 027 cases of suspected acute myocardial infarction: ISIS-1. *Lancet.* 1986;2(8498):57-66.
5. Chen ZM, Pan HC, Chen YP, et al. Early intravenous then oral metoprolol in 45,852 patients with acute myocardial infarction: randomised placebo-controlled trial. *Lancet.* 2005;366(9497):1622-1632.
6. Anderson JL, Adams CD, et al. ACC/AHA 2007 guidelines for the management of patients with unstable angina/non ST-elevation myocardial infarction: a report of the American College of Cardiology/American Heart Association Task Force on Practice Guidelines (Writing Committee to Revise the 2002 Guidelines for the Management of Patients With Unstable Angina/Non ST-Elevation Myocardial Infarction). *J Am Coll Cardiol.* 2007;50:e1-e157.
7. O'Gara PT, Kushner FG, Ascheim DD, et al. 2013 ACCF/AHA guideline for the management of ST-elevation myocardial infarction: a report of the American College of Cardiology Foundation/American Heart Association Task Force on Practice Guidelines. *J Am Col Cardiol.* 2013;61(4):e78-e140.
8. Roberts R, Rogers WJ, Mueller HS, et al. Immediate versus deferred beta-blockade following thrombolytic therapy in patients with acute myocardial infarction: results of the Thrombolysis In Myocardial Infarction (TIMI) II-B Study. *Circulation.* 1991;83:422-237.
9. The Danish Study Group on Verapamil in Myocardial Infarction (DAVIT). Verapamil in acute myocardial infarction. *Eur Heart Journal.* 1984;5(7):516-528.
10. Held PH, Yusuf S, Furberg CD. Calcium channel blockers in acute myocardial infarction and unstable angina: an overview. *BMJ.* 1989;299:1187–1192.
11. Furberg CD, Psaty BM, Meyer JV. Nifedipine: dose-related increase in mortality in patients with coronary heart disease. *Circulation.* 1995;92:1326-1331.
12. Schrier RW, Abraham WT. Hormones and hemodynamics in heart failure. *N Engl J Med.* 1999;341(8):577-585.
13. Pfeffer MA, Braunwald E, Moye LA, et al. Effect of captopril on mortality and morbidity in patients with left ventricular dysfunction after myocardial infarction. Results of the survival and ventricular enlargement trial: The SAVE Investigators. *N Engl J Med.* 1992;327(10):669-677.
14. Pfeffer MA, McMurray JJV, Velazquez EJ, et al. Valsartan, captopril or both in myocardial infarction complicated by heart failure, left ventricular dysfunction, or both. *N Engl J Med.* 2003;349:1893-1906.
15. McNulty PH, King N, Scott S, et al. Effects of supplemental oxygen administration on coronary blood flow in patients undergoing cardiac catheterization. *Am J Physiol Heart Circ Physiol.* 2005;288:H1057–H1062.
16. Antman EM, Anbe DT, Armstrong PW, et al. ACC/AHA guidelines for the management of patients with ST-elevation myocardial infarction: a report of the American College of Cardiology/American Heart Association Task Force on Practice Guidelines (Committee to Revise the 1999 Guidelines for the Management of Patients with Acute Myocardial Infarction). *J Am Coll Cardiol.* 2004;44:e1-e211.
17. Pucci A, Sheiban I, Formato L, et al. In vivo coronary plaque histology in patients with stable and acute coronary syndrome: relationships with hyperlipidemic status and statin treatment. *Atherosclerosis.* 2007;194(1):189-195.
18. Cannon CP, Braunwald E, McCabe CH, et al. Intensive versus moderate lipid lowering with statins after acute coronary syndromes. *N Engl J Med.* 2004;350:1495-1504.
19. Andersen HR, Nielsen TT, Rasmussen K, et al. A comparison of coronary angioplasty with fibrinolytic therapy in acute myocardial infarction. *N Engl J Med.* 2003;349:733-742.
20. Pinto DS, Kirtane AJ, Nallamothu BK, et al. Hospital delays in reperfusion for ST-elevation myocardial infarction: implications when selecting a reperfusion strategy. *Circulation.* 2006;114(19):2019-2025.
21. Andersen HR, Nielsen TT, Vesterlund T, et al. Danish multicenter randomized study on fibrinolytic therapy versus acute coronary angioplasty in acute myocardial infarction: rationale and design of the DANish trial in Acute Myocardial Infarction -2 (DANAMI-2). *Am Heart J.* 2003;146:234-241.
22. Nallamothu BK, Bates ER. Percutaneous coronary intervention versus fibrinolytic therapy in acute myocardial infarction: is timing (almost) everything? *Am J Cardiol.* 2003;92:824-826.
23. Rawles J. Halving of mortality at 1 year by domiciliary thrombolysis in the Grampian Region Early Anistreplase Trial (GREAT). *J Am Coll Cardiol.* 1994;231:1-5.
24. Morrison LH, Verbeek PR, McDonald AC, Sawadsky BV, Cook DJ. Mortality and prehospital thrombolysis for acute myocardial infarction: a meta-analysis. *JAMA.* 2000;283(20):2686-2692.
25. Bonnefoy E, Steg PG, Boutitie F, et al. Comparison of primary angioplasty and prehospital fibrinolysis in acute myocardial infarction (CAPTIM) trial: a 5 year follow-up. *Eur Heart J.* 2009;30:1598-1606.
26. Welsh RC, Travers A, Senaratne M, et al. Feasibility and applicability of paramedic based prehospital fibrinolysis in a large North American center. *Am Heart J.* 2006;152:1007-1014.
27. Danchin N, Blanchard D, Steg PG, et al. Impact of prehospital thrombolysis for acute myocardial infarction on 1-year outcome: results from the French Nationwide USIC 2000 Registry. *Circulation.* 2004;110:1909-1915.
28. Bjorklund E, Stenestrand U, Lindback J, et al. Pre-hospital thrombolysis delivered by paramedics is associated with reduced time delay and mortality in ambulance transported real life patients with STEMI. *Eur Heart J.* 2006;27:1146-1152.
29. Fibrinolytic Therapy Trialists' (FTT) Collaborative Group. Indications for fibrinolytic therapy in suspected acute myocardial infarction: collaborative overview of early mortality and major morbidity results from all randomized trials of more than 1000 patients. *Lancet.* 1994;343:311-322.
30. Cannon CP, McCabe CH, Gibson CM, et al. TNK-tissue plasminogen activator in acute myocardial infarction: results of the Thrombolysis in Myocardial Infarction (TIMI) 10A dose-ranging trial. *Circulation.* 1997;95:351-356.
31. Bode C, Smalling RW, Berg G, et al., RAPID II Investigators. Randomized comparison of coronary thrombolysis achieved with double-bolus reteplase (recombinant plasminogen activator) and front- loaded, accelerated alteplase (recombinant tissue plasminogen activator) in patients with acute myocardial infarction. *Circulation.* 1996;94:891-898.
32. The GUSTO Angiographic Investigators. The effects of tissue plasminogen activator, streptokinase, or both on coronary-artery patency, ventricular function, and survival after acute myocardial infarction. *N Engl J Med.* 1993;329:1615-1622. Erratum in: *N Engl J Med.* 1994;330:516.
33. Sinnaeve PA, Alexander JB, Belmans AC, et al. One year follow-up of the ASSENT-2 trial: a double blind, randomized comparison of single-bolus tenecteplase and front loaded alteplase in 16949 patients with STEMI. *Am Heart J.* 2003;146:27-32.
34. Eisenberg PR. Role of heparin in coronary thrombolysis. *Chest.* 1992;101:131-139.
35. Simes RJ, Topol EJ, Homes DR, GUSTO-1 Investigators et al. Link between the angiographic substudy and mortality outcomes in a large randomized trial of myocardial reperfusion. Importance of early and complete infarct artery reperfusion. *Circulation.* 1995;91:1923-1928.
36. Hochman JS, Sleeper LA, White HD, et al. One-year survival following early revascularization for cardiogenic shock. *JAMA.* 2001;285:190-192.
37. Cantor WJ, Fitchett D, Borgundvaag B, et al. Routine early angioplasty after fibrinolysis for acute myocardial infarction. *N Engl J Med.* 2009;360:2705-2718.
38. Primary versus tenecteplase-facilitated percutaneous coronary intervention in patients with ST-segment elevation acute myocardial infarction (ASSENT-4 PCI): randomized trial. *Lancet.* 2006;367:569-578.
39. Ellis SG, Tendera M, de Belder MA, et al. Facilitated PCI in patients with ST-elevation myocardial infarction. *N Engl J Med.* 2008;358:2205-2217.
40. Keeley EC, Boura JA, Grines CL. Primary angioplasty versus intravenous thrombolytic therapy for acute myocardial infarction: a quantitative review of 23 randomized trials. *Lancet.* 2003;361:13-20.
41. Zijlstra F, Hoorntje JC, de Boer MJ, et al. Long-term benefit of primary angioplasty as compared with thrombolytic therapy for acute myocardial infarction. *N Engl J Med.* 1999;341:1413-1419.

42. Grzybowski M, Clements EA, Parsons L, et al. Mortality benefit of immediate revascularization of acute ST segment elevation myocardial infarction in patients with contraindications to thrombolytic therapy: a propensity analysis. *JAMA*. 2003;290:1891-1898.
43. Hochman JS, Sleeper LA, Webb JG, et al. for the SHOCK Investigators. Early revascularization in acute myocardial infarction complicated by cardiogenic shock. *N Engl J Med*. 1999;341:625-634.
44. Gierlotka M, Gasior M, Wilczek K, et al. Reperfusion by primary percutaneous coronary intervention in patients with ST-segment elevation myocardial infarction within 12 to 24 hours of the onset of symptoms. *Am J Cardiol*. 2011;107:501-508.
45. Wright RS, Anderson JL, Adams CD, et al. 2011 ACCF/AHA focused update of the guidelines for the management of patients with unstable angina/non–ST-elevation myocardial infarction (updating the 2007 guideline): a report of the American College of Cardiology Foundation/American Heart Association Task Force on Practice Guidelines. *J Am Coll Cardiol*. 2011;57(19):1920-1959.
46. Brindis RG, et al. 2014 ACC/AHA guideline for the management of patients with non–ST-elevation acute coronary syndromes: a report of the American College of Cardiology/American Heart Association Task Force on Practice Guidelines. *Circulation*. 2014.
47. Theroux P, Ouimet H, et al. Aspirin, sulfinpyrazone or both in unstable angina: results of a Canadian multicenter trial. *N Engl J Med*. 1985;313:1369-1375.
48. Antithrombotic Trialists' Collaboration. Collaborative meta-analysis of randomized trials of antiplatelet therapy for prevention of death, myocardial infarction, and stroke in high risk patients. *BMJ*. 2002;324(7330):141.
49. Théroux P, Ouimet H, McCans J, et al. Aspirin, heparin or both to treat unstable angina. *N Engl J Med*. 1988;319(17):1105-1111.
50. Cairns JA, Gent M, Singer J, et al. Aspirin, sulfinpyrazone, or both in unstable angina; results of a Canadian multicenter trial. *N Engl J Med*. 1985;313(22):1369-1375.
51. Lewis HD, Davis JW, Archibald DG, et al: Protective effects of aspirin against acute myocardial infarction and death in men with unstable angina. *N Engl J Med*. 1983;309:396-403.
52. Jneid H, Anderson JL, Wright RS, et al. 2012 ACCF/AHA focused update of the guideline for the management of patients with unstable angina/Non-ST-elevation myocardial infarction (updating the 2007 guideline and replacing the 2011 focused update): a report of the American College of Cardiology Foundation/American Heart Association Task Force on practice guidelines. *Circulation*. 2012;126(7):875-910.
53. Mehta SR, Yusuf S; Clopidogrel in Unstable angina to prevent Recurrent Events (CURE) Study Investigators. The Clopidogrel in Unstable angina to prevent Recurrent Events (CURE) trial programme; rationale, design and baseline characteristics including a metaanalysis of the effects of thienopyridines in vascular disease. *Eur Heart J*. 2000;21(24):2033-2041.
54. Yusuf S, Zhao F, Mehta SR, et al. Effects of clopidogrel in addition to aspirin in patients with acute coronary syndromes without ST-segment elevation. *N Engl J Med*. 2001;345(7):494-502.
55. Mehta SR, Tanguay JF, Eikelboom JW, et al. Double-dose versus standard-dose clopidogrel and high dose versus low-dose aspirin in individuals undergoing percutaneous coronary intervention for acute coronary syndromes (CURRENT-OASIS 7): a randomized factorial trial. *Lancet*. 2010;376(9748):1233-1243.
56. Mehta SR, Yusuf S, Peters RJ, et al. Effects of pretreatment with clopidogrel and aspirin followed by long-term therapy in patients undergoing percutaneous coronary intervention: the PCI-CURE study. *Lancet*. 2001;358(9281):527-533.
57. Steinhubl SR, Berger PB, Mann III JT. Early and sustained dual oral antiplatelet therapy following percutaneous coronary intervention: a randomized controlled trial. *JAMA*. 2002;288(19):2411-2420.
58. Dangas G, Mehran R, Guagliumi G, et al. Role of clopidogrel loading dose in patients with ST-segment elevation myocardial infarction undergoing primary angioplasty: Results from the HORIZONS-AMI (harmonizing outcomes with revascularization and stents in acute myocardial infarction) trial. *J Am Coll Cardiol*. 2009;54(15):1438-1446.
59. Patti G, Bárczi G, Orlic D, et al. Outcome comparison of 600- and 300-mg loading doses of clopidogrel in patients undergoing primary percutaneous coronary intervention for ST-segment elevation myocardial infarction: Results from the ARMYDA-6 MI (Antiplatelet therapy for Reduction of Myocardial Damage during Angioplasty-Myocardial Infarction) randomized study. *J Am Coll Cardiol*. 2011;58(15):1592-1599.
60. Varenhorst C, James S, Erlinge D, et al. Genetic variation of CYP2C19 affects both pharmacokinetic and pharmacodynamic responses to clopidogrel but not prasugrel in aspirin-treated patients with coronary artery disease. *Eur Heart J*. 2009;30(14):1744-1752.
61. Roberts JD, Wells GA, Le May MR, et al. Point-of-care genetic testing for personalisation of antiplatelet treatment (RAPID GENE): a prospective, randomised, proof-of-concept trial. *Lancet*. 2012;379(9827):1705-1711.
62. Beitelshees AL. Personalised antiplatelet treatment: A RAPIDly moving target. *Lancet*. 2012;379(9827):1680-1682.
63. Ho PM, Maddox TM, Wang L, et al. Risk of adverse outcomes associated with concomitant use of clopidogrel and proton pump inhibitors following acute coronary syndrome. *JAMA*. 2009;301:937-944.
64. Bhatt DL, Scheiman J, Abraham NS, et al. ACCF/ACG/AHA 2008 expert consensus document on reducing the gastrointestinal risks of antiplatelet therapy and NSAID use: a report of the American College of Cardiology Foundation Task Force on Clinical Expert Consensus Documents. *Circulation*. 2008;118:1894-1909.
65. Gilard M, Arnaud B, Cornily JC, et al. Influence of omeprazole on the antiplatelet action of clopidogrel associated with aspirin: the randomized, double-blind OCLA (Omeprazole CLopidogrel Aspirin) study. *J Am Coll Cardiol*. 2008;51:256-260.
66. Sibbing D, Morath T, Stegherr J, et al. Impact of proton pump inhibitors on the antiplatelet effects of clopidogrel. *Thromb Haemost*. 2009;101:714-719.
67. Wiviott SD, Braunwald E, et al. Prasugrel versus clopidogrel in patients with acute coronary syndromes. *N Engl J Med*. 2007;357:2001-2015.
68. O'Donoghue ML, Braunwald E, Antman EM, et al. Pharmacodynamic effect and clinical efficacy of clopidogrel and prasugrel with or without a proton-pump inhibitor: an analysis of two randomised trials. *Lancet*. 2009;374(9694):989-997.
69. Wallentin L et al. for the PLATO Investigators. Ticagrelor versus clopidogrel in patients with acute coronary syndromes. *N Engl J Med*. 2009;361:1045.
70. Cannon CP, McCabe CH, Wilcox RG, et al. Oral Glycoprotein IIb/IIIa Inhibition with Orbofiban in patients with unstable Coronary Syndromes (OPUS-TIMI 16) trial. *Circulation*. 2000;102:149-156.
71. CAPTURE Study Investigators. Randomised placebo-controlled trial of abciximab before and during coronary intervention in refractor unstable angina: the CAPTURE Study. *Lancet*. 1997;349:1429-1435.
72. Lincoff AM, Califf RM, Moliterno DJ, et al. Complementary clinical benefits of coronary-artery stenting and blockade of platelet glycoprotein IIb/IIIa receptors: evaluation of platelet IIb/IIIa Inhibition in Stenting Investigators. *N Engl J Med*. 1999;341:319-327.
73. PRISM-PLUS Study Investigators. Inhibition of the platelet glycoprotein IIb/IIIa receptor with tirofiban in unstable angina and non-Q-wave myocardial infarction: Platelet Receptor Inhibition in Ischemic Syndrome Management in Patients Limited by Unstable Signs and Symptoms (PRISM-PLUS) Study Investigators. *N Engl J Med*. 1998;338:1488-1497.
74. Boersma E, Simoons ML. Reperfusion strategies in acute myocardial infarction. *Eur Heart J*. 1997;18:1703-1711.
75. Giugliano RP, White JA, Bode C, et al. Early versus delayed, provisional eptifibatide in acute coronary syndromes. *N Engl J Med*. 2009;360:2176-2190.
76. Stone GW, Bertrand ME, Moses JW, et al. Routine upstream initiation vs deferred selective use of glycoprotein IIb/IIIa inhibitors in acute coronary syndromes: the ACUITY Timing trial. *JAMA*. 2007;297:591-602.
77. Shimada YJ, Nakra NC, Fox JT, et al. Meta-analysis of prospective randomized controlled trials comparing intracoronary versus intravenous abciximab in patients with ST-elevation myocardial infarction undergoing primary percutaneous coronary intervention. *Am J Cardiol*. 2012;109:624-628.
78. Théroux P, Waters D, Qiu S, McCans J, de Guise P, Juneau M. Aspirin versus heparin to prevent myocardial infarction during the acute phase of unstable angina. *Circulation*. 1993;88(5, pt 1):2045-2048.
79. Antman EM, Cohen M, Radley D, et al. Assessment of the treatment effect of enoxaparin for unstable Angina/Non-Q-wave myocardial infarction: TIMI 11B-ESSENCE meta-analysis. *Circulation*. 1999;100(15):1602-1608.
80. Antman EM, McCabe CH, Gurfinkel EP, et al. Enoxaparin prevents death and cardiac ischemic events in unstable angina/non-Q-wave myocardial infarction: results of the Thrombolysis In Myocardial Infarction (TIMI) 11B trial. *Circulation*. 1999;100(15):1593-1601.
81. de Lemos JA, Rifai N, Morrow DA, et al. Elevated baseline myoglobin is associated with increased mortality in acute coronary syndromes, even among patients with normal baseline troponin I: a TIMI 11B substudy. *Circulation*.1999;100(suppl I):I372-I373.
82. Warkentin TE, Pai M, Sheppard JI, et al. Fondaparinux treatment of acute heparin-induced thrombocytopenia confirmed by the serotonin-release assay: a 30 month, 16 patient case series. *J Thromb Haem*. 2011;9(12):2389-2396.
83. The Fifth Organization to Assess Strategies in Acute Ischemic Syndromes Investigators. Comparison of Fondaparinux and Enoxaparin in Acute Coronary Syndromes. *N Engl J Med*. 2006;354:1464-1476.
84. Yusuf S, Mehta SR, Chrolavicius S, et al. Effects of fondaparinux on mortality and reinfarction in patients with acute ST-segment elevation myocardial infarction: the OASIS-6 randomized trial. *JAMA*. 2006;295:1519-1530.
85. Stone GW, McLaurin BT, Cox DA, et al. Bivalirudin for patients with acute coronary syndromes. *N Engl J Med*. 2006;355(21):2203-2216.
86. Stone GW, Witzenbichler B, Guagliumi G, et al. Bivalirudin during primary PCI in acute myocardial infarction. *N Engl J Med*. 2008;358:2218-2230.

CARDIOVASCULAR EMERGENCIES

CHAPTER 6

Cardiogenic Shock

Semhar Z. Tewelde

IN THIS CHAPTER

Epidemiology

Etiology

Prediction scores and risk factors

Pathophysiology

Assessment and resuscitation

Stabilization and hemodynamic monitoring

Reperfusion

Medical management

Inotropes and vasopressors

Circulatory support devices

Other mechanical devices

Therapeutic hypothermia

Novel therapy

Cardiogenic shock is a life-threatening emergency that requires rapid diagnosis and prompt initiation of therapy. Emergency physicians are often the first health care providers to assess patients in cardiogenic shock and thereby constitute a critical element in formulating a timely diagnosis and successful treatment. Cardiogenic shock can be defined as cardiac function that is inadequate to meet the resting metabolic demands of the body. The deficient supply of oxygen to vital organs leads to end-organ dysfunction, which can manifest as altered mental status, oliguria, and cool extremities. Cardiogenic shock also can be defined by hemodynamic parameters as follows: persistent hypotension (systolic blood pressure <80 mm Hg or mean arterial pressure 30 mm Hg lower than baseline), reduction in cardiac index (<1.8 L/min/m^2 without support devices or <2 L/min/m^2 with support devices), and elevated filling pressure (left ventricular end-diastolic pressure >18 mm Hg or right ventricular end-diastolic pressure >10 mm Hg).[1,2] Obtaining these objective parameters requires invasive right heart catheterization with a pulmonary artery catheter; however, with the advent of noninvasive means of assessing cardiac function (eg, echocardiography), the diagnosis of cardiogenic shock is now more frequently based on clinical parameters. In a very basic sense, cardiogenic shock can be defined as systemic hypoperfusion with hypotension resulting from inadequate cardiac output that is unresponsive to volume resuscitation and/or vasopressor administration.

Epidemiology

The most common cause of cardiogenic shock is acute myocardial infarction (AMI). Left ventricular failure (>40% myocardial injury) complicates 5% to 8% of cases of ST elevation myocardial infarction (STEMI) and about 2.5% of cases of non-STEMI (NSTEMI).[2-4] However, the incidence of cardiogenic shock is declining, falling from 12.9% to 5.5% over the previous decade, because of increasing rates of percutaneous coronary intervention (PCI) for AMI.[5] Early revascularization has improved morbidity and mortality rates substantially. About 50,000 cases of cardiogenic shock are documented each year in the United States.[5] These statistics should be interpreted with caution, however, because they do not include patients who die of cardiogenic shock before arriving at the hospital and therefore probably underestimate the condition's true incidence.

KEY POINT

The most common presentation involving cardiogenic shock is acute left ventricular failure following ST-elevation myocardial infarction.

Etiology

Although myocardial infarction (MI) is the most common culprit in cardiogenic shock, any cause of left or right ventricular dysfunction can lead to this condition. Mechanical, infectious, toxic, valvular, and obstructive abnormalities can all cause the release of cardiac biomarkers in the absence of coronary artery disease (Table 6-1).[6] Foremost among these are mechanical complications.

Mechanical abnormalities following MI typically emerge within 7 days after injury. Ventricular septal rupture (VSR), with an incidence of 3.9%, is the most common.[2,7] VSR is associated with transmural infarct; a few cases have occurred after early reperfusion. Rupture produces a left-to-right shunt and volume overload, with increased pulmonary blood flow, often accompanied by a loud systolic murmur and thrill. The mortality rate for VSR is 24% in 24 hours and 82% within 2 months.[2,7] Guidelines issued by the American College of Cardiology and the American Heart Association (ACC/AHA) recommend immediate operative intervention for VSR regardless of the patient's clinical status.

Left ventricular free wall rupture is the second most common complication, affecting 1% to 3%.[2,7] Left ventricular rupture is the most common cause of death among patients older than 75 years who are undergoing fibrinolysis, occurring in 54%.[2] Urgent pericardiocentesis followed by surgical repair provides the optimal chance for survival.

The third most common complication is mitral regurgitation from papillary muscle rupture, which occurs following infarct and leads to 70% of deaths.[2] Papillary muscle dysfunction without dehiscence can be managed medically with afterload reducers and vasodilators; however, if regurgitation is severe, early surgery is preferred.

Right ventricular failure can result purely from right coronary artery occlusion or from deterioration of the left ventricle, VSR, or papillary muscle rupture, leading to increased afterload, displacement of the intraventricular septum to the right, and pulmonary hypertension. The management of right ventricular dysfunction is complex. Optimizing volume status, reducing right ventricular afterload with pulmonary vasodilators, and providing inotropic support are often all required.

Prediction Scores and Risk Factors

No uniform criteria exist for predicting the conditions under which cardiogenic shock will develop. In the GUSTO-I and GUSTO-II trials, 85% to 95% of cases of shock were predicted by patient age, systolic blood pressure, heart rate, or Killip class at the time of emergency department presentation.[8] Sleeper et al published a shock severity scoring system from the original SHOCK trial data (Table 6-2).[9] More than 20 years ago, Tan and associates explored the concept of cardiac power—the product of cardiac output and mean arterial pressure—as a prognostic indicator in cardiogenic shock.[10,11] Cardiac power output is calculated by dividing the cardiac power by 451, roughly accounting for systemic flow and physiologically appropriate blood pressure. In the standard sized adult, the cardiac power output is about 1 watt. When a person exercises or is under stress, the cardiac power output can be as high as about 6 watts. Data collected from the SHOCK trial and multivariate

TABLE 6-1.
Causes of Cardiogenic Shock

Ischemia
STEMI/NSTEMI
Mechanical complications of acute myocardial infarction
Left ventricular free wall rupture
Mitral regurgitation secondary to papillary muscle rupture
Ventricular septal rupture
Valvular
Mitral and aortic stenosis or regurgitation
Nonischemic
Myocardial contusion
Myocarditis/pericarditis
Takotsubo cardiomyopathy
Infectious
Sepsis
Obstructive
Hypertrophic obstructive cardiomyopathy
Left atrial myxoma
Massive pulmonary embolism
Pericardial effusion with tamponade
Toxic
Acute overdose (beta-blockers, calcium channel blockers, digoxin)

TABLE 6-2.
Predictors of Mortality in Cardiogenic Shock. Adapted from: Sleeper LA, Reynolds HR, White HD, et al. A severity scoring system for risk assessment of patients with cardiogenic shock: a report from the SHOCK Trial and Registry. *Am Heart J.* 2010;160:443-450.

Advanced age
Shock on admission
Clinical evidence of end-organ hypoperfusion
Noninferior MI
Prior CABG
Anoxic brain injury
Creatinine 1.9 mg/dL or higher
Left ventricular ejection fraction less than 28%

analysis show that cardiac power output is the strongest independent hemodynamic correlate with in-hospital death.[12] Other risk factors for the development of cardiogenic shock include anterior MI, left bundle-branch block, multivessel coronary artery disease, diabetes, and hypertension.

Pathophysiology

Cardiogenic shock is the result of multiple derangements in the circulatory system.[13] Left ventricular pump failure is often the primary insult, succeeded by neurohormonal and cytokine activation with inadequate myocardial compensation.[2] Classically, hypotension ensues, resulting in decreased cardiac output, which decreases coronary perfusion, increases catecholamine release, and causes peripheral vasoconstriction. The vasoconstriction further impairs myocardial function by increasing afterload. The combination of low cardiac output and elevated systemic vascular resistance leads to hypoperfusion of extremities and vital organs—the hallmark of cardiogenic shock. Furthermore, activation of the neurohormonal and cytokine cascades leads to pulmonary vascular overload, elevated levels of nitric oxide, and inappropriate vasodilation of the peripheral vasculature.[5]

The time between myocardial insult and the onset of cardiogenic shock is variable; however, it usually emerges following hospital admission. In the SHOCK registry, the median time for development of shock was approximately 6 hours after hospital presentation.[14] Only 10% to 15% of patients with STEMI exhibited clinical signs of shock at the time of hospital admission.[2] In the GUSTO-IIb trial, shock emerged at about 76 hours in patients with NSTEMI and at 9.6 hours in patients with STEMI.[15] More perplexing is the variability in patient presentation. In the SHOCK registry only 64% of patients had classic physical examination findings of shock (eg, pulmonary congestion and hypotension).[2]

Cardiogenic shock is a complex and quickly degenerating clinical spiral of multiorgan dysfunction resulting from a massively weakened myocardium. An aggressive management plan is necessary to interrupt the vicious cycle, requiring a multidisciplinary approach involving the emergency physician as well as the intensivist, cardiologist, and cardiothoracic surgeon. Initial resuscitation, medical management, and stabilization with pharmacologic and circulatory support devices are discussed below.

Assessment and Resuscitation

Establishing an accurate diagnosis in the hemodynamically unstable patient is critical; therefore, every patient with undifferentiated shock should be approached algorithmically (Table 6-3). Because many patients present in extremis, it is vital to rapidly obtain all available history from the family and emergency medical service personnel. If the patient is capable of providing a history, information about chest pain, anginal equivalents, (eg, dyspnea), syncope, diaphoresis, orthopnea, exertional capacity, and recent hospitalizations should be elicited. Before performing a detailed physical examination, as for any patient, airway, breathing, and circulation (the ABCs) should be assessed. Emergent intubation should be strongly considered for any critically ill patient. Early intubation not only protects the airway in a patient who may clinically deteriorate, it also diverts energy consumption away from breathing and toward necessary vital organs. However, the initiation of mechanical ventilation can inadvertently lower preload and worsen cardiogenic shock; thus, it is paramount to optimize the patient's fluid status prior to intubation.[16] When beginning mechanical ventilation, use the lowest tidal volume and positive end-expiratory pressure to achieve an oxygen saturation above 92%.[17] Care should be taken to avoid hypercapnia because it can worsen pulmonary arterial pressure and right ventricular failure.[2] Circulation can be assessed quickly by inspection of the skin and vital signs. A rapid, weak pulse can indicate hypoperfusion secondary to cardiogenic shock; this hypoperfusion is often also manifested by other abnormal vital signs such as tachycardia, hypotension, or tachypnea. The physical examination is invaluable and can reveal clinical manifestations of cardiogenic shock as follows: agitation or alteration of mental status, weak heart sounds or a bounding murmur, jugular venous distention, pulmonary rales, cyanosis, clammy skin, or poor capillary refill.[18] Circulation can also be assessed in terms of tissue perfusion (warm versus cold) and volume status (dry versus wet). "Warm" indicates

TABLE 6-3.

Shock Algorithm: Undifferentiated Hypotensive Patient

1. First consider a differential diagnosis: **SHOCKD** mnemonic
Spinal or neurogenic shock
Hypovolemic/hemorrhagic shock
Obstructive (pulmonary embolism/tamponade/tension pneumothorax)
Cardiogenic shock
Kortisol deficiency
Distributive shock (sepsis/anaphylaxis)
2. Obtain history/physical examination/bedside ultrasonography/ECG with simultaneous normal saline fluid bolus (500-1,000 mL IV)
3. Basic management strategy based on potential etiology
Evidence of ACS ↦ Emergent revascularization
Nonischemic cause of cardiogenic shock ↦ Specific therapy (indicated by cause)
Mechanical/valvular pathology ↦ Cardiothoracic surgeon consultation
Nonstructural pathology ↦ Stabilization of hemodynamics
4. Advanced management considerations
Emergent coronary revascularization (fibrolytic and PCI)
Inotropes and vasopressors
IABP/LVAD/ventricular assist device
ECMO

adequate perfusion, while "cold" refers to patients with inadequate perfusion. The "wet" patient has pulmonary edema; the "dry" patient lacks this finding. Patients who present as "cold and wet" (ie, hypoperfused with pulmonary edema) have the highest risk of death and the worst prognosis.[19]

Stabilization and Hemodynamic Monitoring

In the unstable patient with cardiogenic shock, it is essential to simultaneously initiate oxygen therapy, establish central intravenous access, and begin arterial and cardiac monitoring. An electrocardiogram (ECG) should be obtained emergently to assess for STEMI and acute coronary syndrome (ACS) (Table 6-4).[20,21] If evidence of STEMI is seen, the patient should be transferred for immediate revascularization to a facility with PCI capability. If no facility with that capability is located within the recommended door-to-balloon-time of 90 minutes, fibrinolytic therapy administered in conjunction with cardiology consultation is a second-line option. The ECG might provide insight to other causes of cardiogenic shock. Low voltage, tachycardia, and electrical alternans suggest cardiac tamponade.[22] Right heart strain and tachycardia with inferior and anterior T-wave inversion suggest pulmonary embolism. A chest radiograph should also be obtained to note the presence or absence of vascular congestion.[23] Routine blood work to include cardiac biomarkers, chemistry, CBC, coagulation profile, arterial blood gas analysis, and lactate concentration should be obtained and analyzed.

> **KEY POINT**
>
> Concurrent resuscitation, stabilization, rapid diagnosis, and appropriate consultation are essential in managing the course of cardiogenic shock.

Although the ACC/AHA guidelines call for the insertion of a pulmonary artery catheter when managing a patient with cardiogenic shock, the use of these devices in this clinical scenario continues to decline and is not recommended in the emergency department. This decrease in use might be related to the potential for poor patient outcome[24] and to the fact that noninvasive adjuncts such as echocardiography can provide hemodynamic data similar to those obtained from pulmonary artery catheter readings, without introducing complications.[25] Evaluating the heart and inferior vena cava can provide important supplemental information to the physical examination findings in looking for circulatory abnormalities. With the advent of bedside ultrasonography, this assessment has become simple and indispensable. With minimal training, emergency physicians can identify poor ejection fraction, global wall motion abnormalities, pericardial effusion/tamponade, and right ventricular dilation and assess volume.[26] This skill set allows emergency physicians to identify or at least narrow the field of potential causes of cardiogenic shock and tailor therapy accordingly.

> **KEY POINT**
>
> The advent of bedside echocardiography allows emergency physicians to promptly assess left ventricular ejection fraction, structural abnormalities, and noncardiac causes of undifferentiated shock.

Reperfusion

MI is the most common cause of cardiogenic shock, and reperfusion is the cornerstone of its treatment. The SHOCK trial did not demonstrate a difference in 30-day mortality rates between revascularized patients and those receiving medical therapy; however, a survival benefit at 6 months was noted in those who underwent PCI or coronary artery bypass grafting (CABG) compared with those who were medically treated (50.3% versus 63.1% [$P=.03$]).[14] PCI is associated with a more predictable and lower re-occlusion rate than fibrinolysis (2% versus 20%, respectively).[17] There is a clear mortality benefit with PCI or CABG versus fibrinolysis in cardiogenic shock. However, PCI must occur within 120 minutes after symptom onset to provide substantial benefit.[27] After this time, little myocardium is salvageable, so only minimal improvement is likely. Thus, early fibrinolysis conveys greater benefit than late PCI.[28,29]

Statins confer benefit for myocardial perfusion when initiated early in patients with ACS.[30] They have also been shown to decrease platelet adhesion, endothelial function, inflammation, and thrombosis. The AMIS plus registry showed that administration of lipid-lowering medication and PCI were associated with lower mortality rates among patients with ACS and lower rates of in-hospital cardiogenic shock.[31] Early institution of lipid-lowering medication does not seem to confer any risk and might, in fact, be beneficial. This early use should occur in the initial 24 hours of management, although not necessarily in the early resuscitation phase in the emergency department.

Medical Management

The approach to critically ill patients in cardiogenic shock is challenging. The hallmark of cardiogenic shock is systemic hypotension leading to hypoxia, lactic acidosis, and further myocardial depression; these conditions decrease the patient's responsiveness to vasoactive agents. Despite vascular congestion in the setting of hypotension and inadequate tissue perfusion, fluid boluses with assessment of inferior vena cava diameter should be first-line medical therapy. In the setting of right ventricular infarct, patients are extremely preload dependent and often require aggressive fluid boluses to maintain adequate perfusion.[32] Correction of hypoxemia, hyperglycemia, venous oxygen saturation, and lactic acidosis are also essential in medical management. Vasodilators, including nitroglycerin and nitroprusside, are generally avoided in patients with cardiogenic

TABLE 6-4.

ECG Abnormalities in Cardiogenic Shock

STEMI: ST-segment elevation or new left bundle-branch block
ACS: Hyperacute or inverted T waves with or without ST-segment depression

shock because of their propensity to cause hypotension. Beta- and calcium channel blockers should not be administered because of their negative inotropic and blood-pressure–lowering effects.[33]

Inotropes and Vasopressors

When reperfusion is not clinically indicated, the management of hypotension resulting from cardiogenic shock proves to be a challenging task. Overzealous fluid administration "floods the lungs" with pulmonary edema and does not always translate into improved mean arterial pressure. The goal of an initial fluid bolus is to determine if fluids alone will restore cardiac output and prevent end-organ dysfunction. In many cases, fluids alone do not improve hemodynamics, so adjunctive pharmacologic therapy is used to assist native hemodynamics. Both inotropes and vasopressors elevate stroke work, increase myocardial oxygen consumption, and deplete energy reserves (Table 6-5).[34] However, accepting these "necessary evils" with the goal of augmented perfusion is the initial step in recovery.

Current guidelines recommend treatment of cardiogenic shock that does not respond to fluids with the administration of inotropes such as dobutamine unless hypotension is present, with blood pressure lower than 90 mm Hg.[35] Dobutamine augments diastolic coronary blood flow to ischemic areas and increases myocardial contractility, thus increasing cardiac output and lowering left ventricular filling pressure. Levosimendan, another potent inodilator similar to dobutamine, is another new alternative.[36] For patients taking long-acting beta-blockers, therapy with milrinone is recommended, owing to its mechanism of action distal to the beta-adrenergic receptor. For hypotensive patients, vasopressors such as dopamine or norepinephrine are initiated to restore perfusion. Norepinephrine is often preferred to dopamine given dopamine's adverse side effects (eg, increased myocardial oxygen demand and arrhythmogenic effects).[37] The largest randomized controlled trial of vasopressors was the SOAP-2 trial, which compared dopamine and norepinephrine. Norepinephrine was associated with a reduced mortality rate and dopamine with a higher arrhythmia burden. If clinical deterioration continues despite the use of traditional inotropes and vasopressors, other agents such as epinephrine may be used until a circulatory support device can be inserted.

Circulatory Support Devices

The ability to maintain hemodynamic support is a primary objective in the management of cardiogenic shock. Blood flow and perfusion must be restored to prevent permanent brain injury. Mechanical circulatory devices can sustain life and are an important adjunct to PCI in rapidly deteriorating patients. Although ACC/AHA guidelines call for the use of the intraaortic balloon pump (IABP), this has not been shown to improve survival rates among patients with cardiogenic shock.[38,39] However, these mechanical assist devices do provide the time that is necessary for native hemodynamic recovery after myocardial stunning and can serve as a bridge to more permanent circulatory devices or cardiac transplantation. The alternative to implantation of assist devices is death; therefore, randomized trials are unlikely to be conducted and clinical experience will continue to guide therapy.

> **KEY POINT**
>
> The advent of bedside echocardiography allows the emergency physician to promptly assess left ventricular ejection fraction, structural abnormalities, and noncardiac causes of undifferentiated shock.

Developed in 1968, the IABP was initially the only widely available and most often used percutaneous assist device. It can be placed quickly and has a low complication rate. The IABP is

TABLE 6-5.

Inotropes and Vasopressors

Inotropes	Mechanism	Notes
Improve cardiac output		
Dobutamine	Cardiac beta$_1$- and peripheral alpha$_2$- and beta$_2$-adrenoreceptor agonist	Can exacerbate hypotension
Milrinone	Phosphodiesterase-3 inhibitor, potentiates cAMP	Useful in patients on beta-blockers
Levosimendan	Increases sensitivity to calcium	Not available in United States
Vasopressors		
Increase blood pressure		
Norepinephrine	Alpha$_1$- and beta$_1$-adrenoreceptor agonist	Decreased mortality in subset
Dopamine	5 to 10 mcg/kg/min beta$_1$-agonist, 10 to 20 mcg/kg/min alpha$_1$-agonist	Increased arrhythmogenicity
Epinephrine	Alpha$_1$-, beta$_1$-, and beta$_2$-agonist	
Phenylephrine	Pure alpha-agonist	

inserted into the descending aorta between the arch and renal arteries. The device works by aortic counterpulsation. During diastole, the balloon inflates and leads to both antegrade and retrograde displacement of blood, improving mean arterial pressure and both systemic and coronary perfusion. When the balloon deflates, end-diastolic pressure and left ventricular afterload are reduced. Overall, cardiac output increases and left ventricular work and myocardial oxygen consumption both decrease. For patients with acute MI, ACC/AHA guidelines have a class I recommendation for the use of an IABP for stabilization as well as to manage acute valvular dysfunction, intractable arrhythmias with hemodynamic instability, and refractory postinfarction angina. Despite these indicated uses, an IABP is used in only 20% to 40% of patients with cardiogenic shock complicating STEMI.[40] The recent SHOCK II trial demonstrated a lack of clear mortality benefit after IABP placement and thus challenges current guidelines.[24] Limitations of the IABP include minimal hemodynamic augmentation (the device increases cardiac output by only 0.5 L/min); reliance on a stable electrical rhythm; and mechanical obstruction, possibly leading to limb ischemia, thrombosis, or embolism.

A cardiologist, without surgery, can place left ventricular assist devices (LVADs) such as the Tandem Heart and the Impella pump percutaneously. These devices can improve systemic blood pressure, reduce wall stress, and improve coronary blood flow.[41] The Tandem Heart is a short-term centrifugal pump that is inserted through the right femoral vein and then advanced to the right atrium. A transatrial septal perforation introduces the tip of the cannula into the left atrium. A femoral artery cannula provides left heart bypass. The Tandem Heart augments the cardiac index and decreases pulmonary wedge pressure, but when it was compared with the IABP in trials, no survival benefit was reported.[42] The catheter-based Impella 2.5 is a pump that is placed, via the femoral artery, across the aortic valve. Similar to the Tandem Heart, this device is intended for short-term use and greatly improves the cardiac index and hemodynamic parameters. Also like the Tandem Heart, in comparison with the IABP, the Impella pump does not confer a survival advantage.[43] Various studies have shown that LVADs improve cardiac index, increase mean arterial pressure, and reduce capillary wedge pressure, but these findings do not translate into survival benefit. Complications associated with these devices include limb ischemia, sepsis, septal defects, and bleeding.

Other Mechanical Devices

Extracorporeal membrane oxygenation (ECMO) is delivered with a device consisting of a centrifugal pump, membrane oxygenator, and heparin-coated circuit. ECMO provides cardiac and pulmonary support. It can be used to sustain perfusion in shock, to improve hypoxia, and as a rescue device in cardiopulmonary resuscitation.[44] Typically, peripheral femoral arterial and venous cannulation is established with the Seldinger technique. The arterial cannula is advanced to the aorto-iliac junction, and the venous cannula is advanced into the lower right atrium. The entire circuit takes about 10 minutes to assemble. This approach allows rapid stabilization of hemodynamics and correction of metabolic derangement. The potential for myocardial recovery, long-term reliance on an LVAD, or cardiac transplant can then be assessed. ECMO provides an effective bridge to further therapy but does not adequately unload the left ventricle and therefore is not definitive care. Limitations in its use also include limb ischemia, bleeding, infection, thromboembolism, and pulmonary edema. Pagani et al[45] reported a 1-year survival rate of 43% with ECMO in patients with cardiogenic shock complicated by cardiac arrest or hemodynamic instability.

If the treatment strategies described above do not lead to recovery of the native heart, several surgically implanted ventricular assist devices, intended for long-term use, can be implanted in a patient with cardiogenic shock. During the past 10 years, studies of rotary pumps such as the HeartMate, HeartWare, DuraHeart, and the Jarvik have demonstrated mechanical reliability and low complication rates. These devices offer a proven rescue strategy for patients with cardiogenic shock who are not candidates for transplantation.[46,47]

The use of a total artificial heart as a bridge to transplantation remains controversial, but it is advantageous in that it provides biventricular support and an option for patients who are not candidates for ventricular assist devices.[48] In this treatment option, the native heart is excised and then prosthetic ventricles are sewn into place. A portable external pump driver allows patients to live at home while awaiting transplantation. This option is used only when the heart will not recover with isolated left ventricular support using cardiopulmonary bypass.[49]

Therapeutic Hypothermia

The results of two randomized, controlled trials, published in the *New England Journal of Medicine*, outlined the neurologic benefit of therapeutic hypothermia in cardiac arrest patients with ventricular fibrillation as the initial rhythm.[50,51] As a result of these findings, current ACC/AHA guidelines recommend therapeutic hypothermia after cardiac arrest and return of spontaneous circulation in patients who remain comatose. Ventricular fibrillation often is the final pathway in patients with ACS and cardiogenic shock. The rationale for the use of therapeutic hypothermia in cardiogenic shock lies in the prevention of reperfusion injury.[52] In laboratory studies, hypothermia has been shown to decrease heart rate, increase systemic vascular resistance, and improve cardiac output. Unlike inotropic drugs, hypothermia increases the maximal force developed by the heart, although the speed of force development is unchanged or decreased.[53] Cooling in patients with cardiogenic shock has not been studied by randomized, controlled trials, but current data suggest recovery of systolic function over time with therapeutic hypothermia.[54]

Novel Therapy

The hallmark manifestations of cardiogenic shock, hypotension and end-organ hypoperfusion, are worsened by cytokine activation and can trigger vasodilatory shock and lactic acidosis. Vasopressors and inotropes are ineffective antidotes and can contribute to loss of vascular tone. Argenziano and colleagues showed that patients with vasodilatory shock after LVAD implantation had low levels of autologous vasopressin and that shock resolved when intravenous vasopressin was given.[55,56] The beneficial effects of vasopressin are now well established; it has no role in normotensive patients. Low-dose vasopressin therapy is an adjunctive strategy to consider for cardiogenic shock patients on LVAD rescue complicated by hypotension.

Conclusion

Cardiogenic shock leads to four possible scenarios: functional recovery after treatment, inadequate recovery necessitating implantation of a longer-term ventricular assist device, urgent cardiac transplantation, or death despite appropriate therapy. Improved survival among patients with cardiogenic shock requires early diagnosis, aggressive emergent care, and a multidisciplinary approach. Resuscitation and stabilization require early reperfusion; optimization of hemodynamics with early intubation; optimal fluid management; minimal use of inotropes/vasopressors; and the provision for IABP, short-term LVAD, or ECMO until the patient can be transferred to a quaternary care facility. In patients whose cardiac reserve proves inadequate for recovery, a long-term ventricular assist device can provide several years of good quality of life and does not preclude cardiac transplantation. Questions regarding circulatory support devices have not been fully resolved, but with improved devices, availability, and expertise, the morbidity and mortality rates associated with cardiogenic shock should continue to decline.

References

1. Awad HH, Anderson FA Jr, Gore JM, et al. Cardiogenic shock complicating acute coronary syndromes: insights from the Global Registry of Acute Coronary Events. *Am Heart J*. 2012;163(6):963-971.
2. Hasdai D, Topol EJ, Califf RM, et al. Cardiogenic shock complicating acute coronary syndromes. *Lancet*. 2000;356(9231):749-756.
3. Babaev A, Frederick PD, Pasta DJ, et al. Trends in management and outcomes of patients with acute myocardial infarction complicated by cardiogenic shock. *JAMA*. 2005;294(4):448-454.
4. Brodie BR, Stuckey TD, Hansen C, et al. Comparison of late survival in patients with cardiogenic shock due to right ventricular infarction versus left ventricular pump failure following primary percutaneous coronary intervention for ST-elevation acute myocardial infarction. *Am J Cardiol*. 2007;99(4):431-435.
5. Westaby S, Kharbanda R, Banning AP. Cardiogenic shock in ACS. Part 1: prediction, presentation and medical therapy. *Nat Rev Cardiol*. 2011;9(3):158-171.
6. Hochman JS, Buller CE, Sleeper LA, et al. Cardiogenic shock complicating acute myocardial infarction—etiologies, management and outcome: a report from the SHOCK Trial Registry. SHould we emergently revascularize Occluded Coronaries for cardiogenic shocK? *J Am Coll Cardiol*. 2000;36(3 suppl A):1063-1070.
7. Holmes DR Jr, Berger PB, Hochman JS, et al. Cardiogenic shock in patients with acute ischemic syndromes with and without ST-segment elevation. *Circulation*. 1999;100(20):2067-2073.
8. A clinical trial comparing primary coronary angioplasty with tissue plasminogen activator for acute myocardial infarction. The Global Use of Strategies to Open Occluded Coronary Arteries in Acute Coronary Syndromes (GUSTO IIb) Angioplasty Substudy Investigators. *N Engl J Med*. 1997;336(23):1621-1628.
9. Sleeper LA, Reynolds HR, White HD, et al. A severity scoring system for risk assessment of patients with cardiogenic shock: a report from the SHOCK Trial and Registry. *Am Heart J*. 2010;160(3):443-450.
10. Tan LB. Cardiac pumping capability and prognosis in heart failure. *Lancet*. 1986;2(8520):1360-1363.
11. Tan LB, Bain RJ, Littler WA. Assessing cardiac pumping capability by exercise testing and inotropic stimulation. *Br Heart J*. 1989;62(1):20-25.
12. Mendoza DD, Cooper HA, Panza JA. Cardiac power output predicts mortality across a broad spectrum of patients with acute cardiac disease. *Am Heart J*. 2007;153(3):366-370.
13. Shpektor A. Cardiogenic shock: the role of inflammation. *Acute Card Care*. 2010;12(4):115-118.
14. Hochman JS, Sleeper LA, Godfrey E, et al. SHould we emergently revascularize Occluded Coronaries for cardiogenic shocK: an international randomized trial of emergency PTCA/CABG-trial design. The SHOCK Trial Study Group. *Am Heart J*. 1999;137(2):313-321.
15. Holmes DR Jr, Bates ER, Kleiman NS, et al. Contemporary reperfusion therapy for cardiogenic shock: the GUSTO-I trial experience. The GUSTO-I Investigators. Global Utilization of Streptokinase and Tissue Plasminogen Activator for Occluded Coronary Arteries. *J Am Coll Cardiol*. 1995;26(3):668-674.
16. Patel AK, Hollenberg SM. Cardiovascular failure and cardiogenic shock. *Semin Respir Crit Care Med*. 2011;32(5):598-606.
17. Reynolds HR, Hochman JS. Cardiogenic shock: current concepts and improving outcomes. *Circulation*. 2008;117(5):686-697.
18. Vazquez R, Gheorghe C, Kaufman D, Manthous CA. Accuracy of bedside physical examination in distinguishing categories of shock: a pilot study. *J Hosp Med*. 2010;5(8):471-474.
19. Nohria A, Tsang SW, Fang JC, et al. Clinical assessment identifies hemodynamic profiles that predict outcomes in patients admitted with heart failure. *J Am Coll Cardiol*. 2003;41(10):1797-1804.
20. Zehender M, Kasper W, Kauder E, et al. Right ventricular infarction as an independent predictor of prognosis after acute inferior myocardial infarction. *N Engl J Med*. 1993;328(14):981-988.
21. Sugiura T, Nagahama Y, Takehana K, et al. Prognostic significance of precordial ST-segment changes in acute inferior wall myocardial infarction. *Chest*. 1997;111(4):1039-1044.
22. Eisenberg MJ, de Romeral LM, Heidenreich PA, et al. The diagnosis of pericardial effusion and cardiac tamponade by 12-lead ECG: a technology assessment. *Chest*. 1996;110(2):318-324.
23. Collins SP, Lindsell CJ, Storrow AB, et al. Prevalence of negative chest radiography results in the emergency department patient with decompensated heart failure. *Ann Emerg Med*. 2006;47(1):13-18.
24. Thiele H, Schuler G, Neumann FJ, et al. Intraaortic balloon counterpulsation in acute myocardial infarction complicated by cardiogenic shock: design and rationale of the Intraaortic Balloon Pump in Cardiogenic Shock II (IABP-SHOCK II) trial. *Am Heart J*. 2012;163(6):938-945.
25. Labovitz AJ, Noble VE, Bierig M, et al. Focused cardiac ultrasound in the emergent setting: a consensus statement of the American Society of Echocardiography and American College of Emergency Physicians. *J Am Soc Echocardiogr*. 2010;23(12):1225-1230.
26. Mandavia DP, Hoffner RJ, Mahaney K, et al. Bedside echocardiography by emergency physicians. *Ann Emerg Med*. 2001;38(4):377-382.
27. Jennings RB, Reimer KA. Factors involved in salvaging ischemic myocardium: effect of reperfusion of arterial blood. *Circulation*. 1983;68(2 Pt 2):I25-I36.
28. Indications for fibrinolytic therapy in suspected acute myocardial infarction: collaborative overview of early mortality and major morbidity results from all randomised trials of more than 1000 patients. Fibrinolytic Therapy Trialists' (FTT) Collaborative Group. *Lancet*. 1994;343(8893):311-322.
29. Effectiveness of intravenous thrombolytic treatment in acute myocardial infarction. Gruppo Italiano per lo Studio della Streptochinasi nell'Infarto Miocardico (GISSI). *Lancet*. 1986;1(8478):397-402.
30. Garot P, Bendaoud N, Lefèvre T, et al. Favourable effect of statin therapy on early survival benefit at the time of percutaneous coronary intervention for ST-elevation myocardial infarction and shock. *EuroIntervention*. 2010;6(3):350-355.
31. Aronow HD, Topol EJ, Roe MT, et al. Effect of lipid-lowering therapy on early mortality after acute coronary syndromes: an observational study. *Lancet*. 2001;357(9262):1063-1068.
32. Forrester JS, Diamond G, McHugh TJ, et al. Filling pressures in the right and left sides of the heart in acute myocardial infarction. A reappraisal of central-venous-pressure monitoring. *N Engl J Med*. 1971;285(4):190-193.
33. Edwards J, Goodman SG, Yan RT, et al. Has the ClOpidogrel and Metoprolol in Myocardial Infarction Trial (COMMIT) of early beta-blocker use in acute coronary syndromes impacted on clinical practice in Canada? Insights from the Global Registry of Acute Coronary Events (GRACE). *Am Heart J*. 2011;161(2):291-297.
34. Valente S, Lazzeri C, Vecchio S, et al. Predictors of in-hospital mortality after percutaneous coronary intervention for cardiogenic shock. *Int J Cardiol*. 2007;114(2):176-182.
35. Antman EM, Anbe DT, Armstrong PW, et al. ACC/AHA guidelines for the management of patients with ST-elevation myocardial infarction—executive summary: a report of the American College of Cardiology/American Heart Association Task Force on Practice Guidelines (Writing Committee to Revise the 1999 Guidelines for the Management of Patients With Acute Myocardial Infarction). *Circulation*. 2004;110(5):588-636.
36. Buerkem B, Lemm H, Drohe K, et al. Levosimendan in the treatment of cardiogenic shock. *Minerva Cardioangiol*. 2010;58(4):519-530.
37. De Backer D, Aldecoa C, Nijmi H, et al. Dopamine versus norepinephrine in the treatment of septic shock: a meta-analysis. *Crit Care Med*. 2012;40(3):725-730.
38. Thiele H, Zeymer U, Neumann FJ, et al. Intraaortic balloon support for myocardial infarction with cardiogenic shock. *N Engl J Med*. 2012;367(14):1287-1296.
39. O'Connor CM, Rogers JG. Evidence for overturning the guidelines in cardiogenic shock. *N Engl J Med*. 2012;367(14):1349-1350.
40. Sjauw KD, Engström AE, Vis MM, et al. Efficacy and timing of intra-aortic counterpulsation in patients with ST-elevation myocardial infarction complicated by cardiogenic shock. *Neth Heart J*. 2012;20(10):402-409.

41. Naidu SS. Novel percutaneous cardiac assist devices: the science of and indications for hemodynamic support. *Circulation.* 2011;123(5):533-543.
42. Burkhoff D, Cohen H, Brunckhorst C, et al. A randomized multicenter clinical study to evaluate the safety and efficacy of the TandemHeart percutaneous ventricular assist device versus conventional therapy with intraaortic balloon pumping for treatment of cardiogenic shock. *Am Heart J.* 2006;152(3):469 e1-8.
43. Thiele H, Sick P, Boudriot E, et al. Randomized comparison of intra-aortic balloon support with a percutaneous left ventricular assist device in patients with revascularized acute myocardial infarction complicated by cardiogenic shock. *Eur Heart J.* 2005;26(13):1276-1283.
44. Cove ME, MacLaren G. Clinical review: mechanical circulatory support for cardiogenic shock complicating acute myocardial infarction. *Crit Care.* 2010;14(5):235.
45. Pagani FD, Aaronson KD, Swaniker F, et al. The use of extracorporeal life support in adult patients with primary cardiac failure as a bridge to implantable left ventricular assist device. *Ann Thorac Surg.* 2001;71(3 suppl):S77-S85.
46. Leshnower BG, Gleason TG, O'Hara ML, et al. Safety and efficacy of left ventricular assist device support in postmyocardial infarction cardiogenic shock. *Ann Thorac Surg.* 2006;81(4):1365-1371.
47. Slaughter MS, Tsui SS, El-Banayosy A, et al. Results of a multicenter clinical trial with the Thoratec Implantable Ventricular Assist Device. *J Thorac Cardiovasc Surg.* 2007;133(6):1573-1580.
48. Slepian MJ, Copeland JG. The total artificial heart in refractory cardiogenic shock: saving the patient versus saving the heart. *Nat Clin Pract Cardiovasc Med.* 2008;5(2):64-65.
49. Copeland JG, Smith RG, Arabia FA, et al. Cardiac replacement with a total artificial heart as a bridge to transplantation. *N Engl J Med.* 2004;351(9):859-867.
50. Bernard SA, Gray TW, Buist MD, et al. Treatment of comatose survivors of out-of-hospital cardiac arrest with induced hypothermia. *N Engl J Med.* 2002;346:557-563.
51. Hypothermia after Cardiac Arrest Study Group. Mild therapeutic hypothermia to improve the neurologic outcome after cardiac arrest. *N Engl J Med.* 2002;346:549-556.
52. Callaway CW. Induced hypothermia after cardiac arrest improves cardiogenic shock. *Crit Care Med.* 2012;40(6):1963-1964.
53. Stegman BM, Newby LK, Hochman JS, et al. Post-myocardial infarction cardiogenic shock is a systemic illness in need of systemic treatment: is therapeutic hypothermia one possibility? *J Am Coll Cardiol.* 2012;59(7):644-647.
54. Zobel C, Adler C, Kranz A, et al. Mild therapeutic hypothermia in cardiogenic shock syndrome. *Crit Care Med.* 2012;40(6):1715-1723.
55. Argenziano M, Choudhri AF, Oz MC, et al. A prospective randomized trial of arginine vasopressin in the treatment of vasodilatory shock after left ventricular assist device placement. *Circulation.* 1997;96(9 suppl):II-286-II-290.
56. Argenziano M, Chen JM, Cullinane S, et al. Arginine vasopressin in the management of vasodilatory hypotension after cardiac transplantation. *J Heart Lung Transplant.* 1999;18(8):814-817.

CHAPTER 7

Acute Heart Failure

Natasha B. Wheaton and Peter S. Pang

IN THIS CHAPTER

Pathophysiology

Diagnosis

Initial stabilization of patients

Management of hypertensive and normotensive patients

Patient disposition

Acute heart failure (AHF) imposes a substantial public health burden because of its high mortality rate, morbidity rate, and financial cost. In the United States, AHF is the most common reason for hospitalization and rehospitalization among patients older than 65 years of age, accounting for more than 1 million admissions per year.[1-3] The diagnosis of AHF has great significance, as nearly one third of these patients will be dead or rehospitalized within 90 days after discharge.[4] AHF admissions are associated with a huge financial cost, estimated to exceed $20 billion per year.[2,5] The impact of this syndrome is also likely to increase as the population ages. AHF admissions have tripled over the past three decades for a multitude of reasons, including the aging of the population, an increase in the number of comorbid conditions contributing to heart failure (HF), an increase in the survival rate after myocardial infarction, and an overall decrease in the rate of sudden cardiac death.[6,7] Over 90% of the attributable risk associated with the development of HF is linked to comorbid hypertension, diabetes, and coronary artery disease. Although the number of AHF admissions has not changed in the past 10 years, the number of readmissions of Medicare recipients experiencing AHF has decreased while the number of those younger than 65 has increased.[1,8] As the incidence of associated comorbidities increases, the incidence of HF and AHF will increase proportionally.[3,6,9] Efforts to reduce the burden of AHF with novel therapies have largely failed, and even the evidence in support of early pharmacologic management in AHF is poor.[5,7]

Emergency physicians have a key role in the management of AHF, as nearly 80% of all AHF admissions originate in the emergency department.[10] With the recent focus on readmissions as a national quality measure, decisions made in the emergency department have potentially large downstream consequences. With the goal of providing meaningful guidance to clinicians, this chapter presents an evidenced-based, practical approach to the management of AHF in the emergency department.

Defining Acute Heart Failure

There is no universally recognized definition of AHF.[5] Based on expert consensus, we define AHF as follows: traditional signs and symptoms of HF requiring urgent or emergent therapy.[11] The heterogeneity of the AHF patient population in terms of etiology, precipitants, comorbidities, pathophysiologic processes, and clinical presentation hinders a simple definition. Understanding this heterogeneity is the first step toward comprehensive AHF management. Although the hypertensive patient with acute pulmonary edema often comes to mind when one thinks of a classic AHF presentation, in reality, the clinical presentation is variable. Approximately 50% of patients hospitalized with HF have normal systolic function (HF with preserved ejection fraction [EF]), and the other 50% have reduced systolic function (HF with reduced EF).[12] These patient groups present with unique clinical characteristics (or phenotypes), although there is overlap.[4] Ideally, acute treatment should be tailored to the patient's underlying myocardial substrate and function. Although evidence-based therapies differ for chronic HF patients depending on whether they have preserved or reduced EF,[7] robust data substantiating and guiding differential treatment in AHF are lacking.

KEY POINTS

The term *acute heart failure* encompasses a heterogeneous group of patients with multiple comorbid conditions and unique clinical presentations.

About half of patients with AHF have HF with preserved EF.

Whether AHF represents a unique entity with a distinct pathophysiology or heralds disease progression remains a topic of debate. Nonetheless, outcomes and long-term prognosis in HF worsen with each hospitalization (Figure 7-1); patients admitted with AHF have worse outcomes than chronic HF patients who are not admitted.[13]

Pathophysiology

Elevated left ventricular filling pressures with or without a marked decrease in cardiac output are a common feature of AHF. The mechanisms leading to this finding are highly variable. In AHF, patients experience some form of cardiac impairment caused by abnormal forward flow (systolic dysfunction), impaired myocardial relaxation (diastolic dysfunction), or both. In addition to nonadherence to medications or diet, precipitating events most commonly include respiratory processes (eg, pneumonia or exacerbation of chronic obstructive pulmonary disease), acute coronary syndrome (ACS), arrhythmias, and uncontrolled hypertension.[14]

Traditionally, patients with AHF were thought to suffer from total body volume overload and reduced systolic dysfunction. However, as previously stated, nearly half of AHF patients have preserved EF. Certain cases of AHF may result more from volume distribution than from total volume overload.[15,16] The classic example is the patient with "flash" pulmonary edema. Unlike patients with total body volume overload, who typically experience a slow, progressive worsening of their signs and symptoms, patients with flash pulmonary edema typically feel relatively well immediately prior to decompensation without overt weight gain or peripheral edema. This construct of volume redistribution forms the basis for recommended management of the hypertensive AHF patient.

Each AHF episode likely causes myocardial and/or renal damage, leading to worsening systemic illness, functional capacity, and, finally, death.[17] It is hoped that offering patients

FIGURE 7-1.

All-cause mortality after each subsequent hospitalization for HF. From: Setoguchi S, Stevenson LW, Schneeweiss S. Repeated hospitalizations predict mortality in the community population with heart failure. *Am Heart J*. 2007;154:260-266. Copyright 2007, with permission from Elsevier.

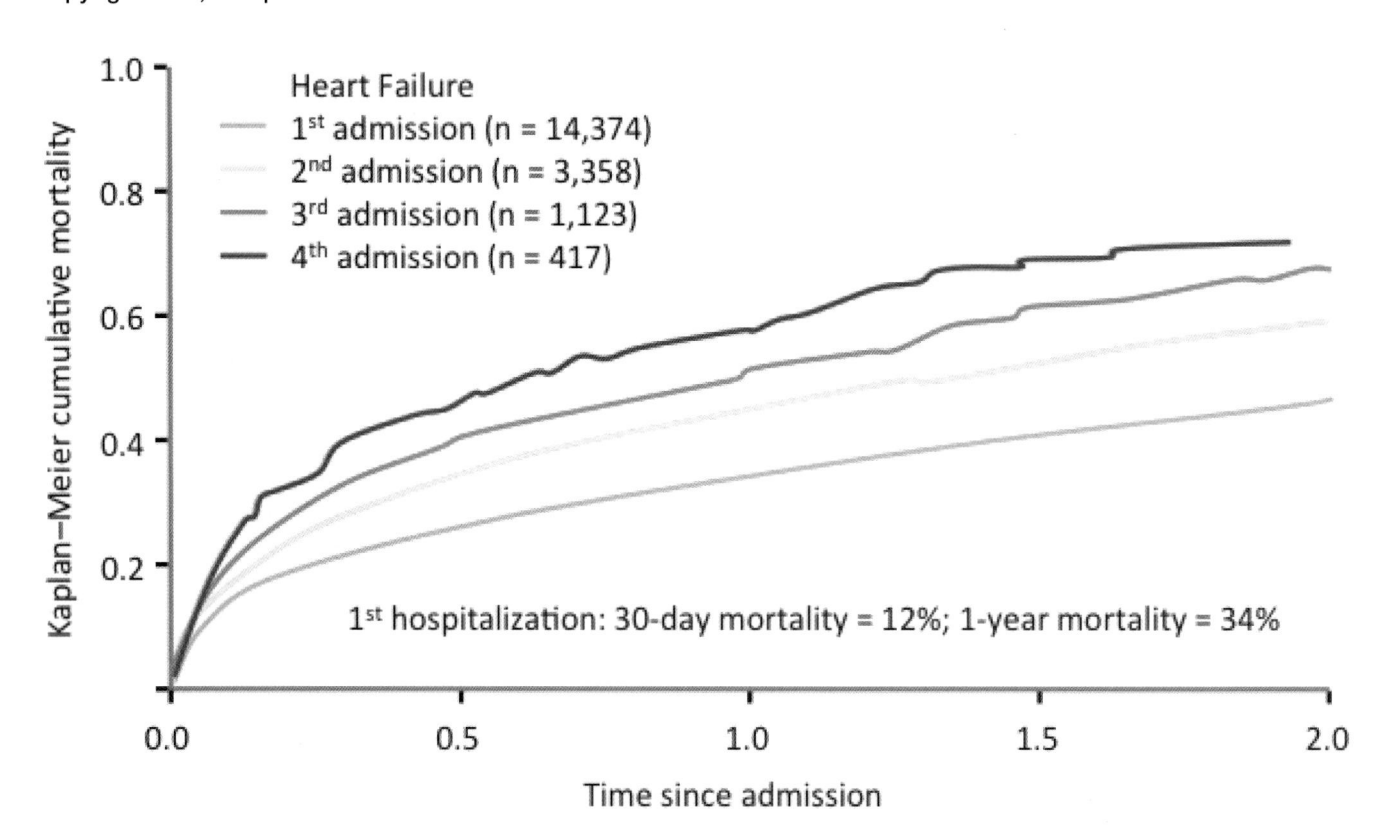

prevention or protection against such damage through early tailored interventions might alter the natural course of their disease, but data on the effect of acute interventions on overall long-term outcomes are sparse.[7,18] However, a recent study of a novel investigational agent, relaxin, has re-invigorated this hypothesis.[18,19]

Clinical Presentation

Dyspnea is the most common presenting symptom. Although typical signs and symptoms of HF are common, the presenting vital signs, precipitants, and etiology of HF differ substantially among patients (Table 7-1).[12,20-22]

> **KEY POINT**
>
> Dyspnea is the most common presenting symptom of AHF.

Patients with preserved EF tend to be older and female and to have a history of hypertension rather than coronary artery disease (CAD). The onset of their symptoms tends to be more acute (over 24 to 72 hours), and they tend to present with hypertension.[12,23] These patients often have a systolic blood pressure (SBP) above 140 mm Hg. Initial treatment includes blood pressure control rather than monotherapy with a diuretic.[23]

Patients with a reduced EF are relatively younger and male, with a history of CAD. Typically, symptom onset is subacute, occurring over days to weeks. Normotension or even hypotension with signs of hypoperfusion is the dominant presenting phenotype.[23] Diuresis is first-line therapy. Importantly, patients with advanced HF may appear more gravely ill by numbers (ie, SBP in 80s); however, the clinical context is critical. For patients with severely reduced EF, a low blood pressure might be "normal," so hemodynamic management must be provided with great care.[23,24]

> **KEY POINTS**
>
> Patients with preserved EF tend to be older and female, have a history of hypertension, and present with elevated blood pressure.
>
> Patients with reduced EF tend to be younger and male, to have a history of coronary artery disease, to present with symptoms that typically have been ongoing for several days to weeks, and to have a normal blood pressure.

Despite different causes and clinical phenotypes of AHF, both groups of patients can present in extremis. Although acute pulmonary edema patients appear more acutely ill, those with severe volume overload and borderline hypotension along with reduced EF are often more challenging to manage acutely.

Diagnosis

Heart failure is a clinical diagnosis. Ancillary testing such as chest radiograph, laboratory tests, and bedside ultrasound aid in diagnosis.

History

Although most AHF patients present with dyspnea, others describe more insidious symptoms such as fatigue.[25] The circumstances of their dyspnea as well as changes in exercise capacity should be explored (many patients with chronic HF have limited exercise capacity at baseline). Paroxysmal nocturnal dyspnea (PND) is particularly suggestive of AHF.[26] Signs and symptoms of fluid overload, including increasing abdominal distention, lower extremity edema, and weight gain, should be assessed carefully. Most patients, up to 75%, have a known history of HF. After diagnosis, identification and treatment of the precipitant leading to decompensation, including infectious causes, arrhythmias, ACS, medication, and dietary noncompliance, are important.

> **KEY POINT**
>
> Search for a precipitating event in a patient presenting with AHF.

Physical Examination

The physical examination begins with an evaluation of the patient's overall appearance in conjunction with his or her vital signs. Hypertension, hypotension, and other abnormal vital signs are important clues to potential precipitants. The physician should take note of the patient's breathing pattern, respiratory effort, skin color, and mental status.

Jugular venous distention (JVD) is the hallmark physical examination finding of AHF, although it has only 79% specificity and 70% sensitivity for increased left ventricular pressure with poor inter-rater reliability.[27] If JVD is difficult to visualize, the hepatojugular reflux may be assessed. Auscultation for extra heart sounds might yield an S_3, which is specific for HF but not very sensitive. Murmurs might be indicative of new or worsening valvular disease, and pulse irregularity raises the concern for arrhythmia. The pulmonary examination might reveal rales and decreased breath sounds representing pleural effusion. Coarse wheezing (known as "cardiac wheeze") from small airway bronchospasm and decreased airflow caused by fluid accumulation may also be auscultated. Finally, the presence of peripheral edema as well as the adequacy of perfusion should be examined by noting skin color, temperature, and capillary refill. For bed-bound patients, dependent peripheral edema might be more sacral than peripheral.

Ancillary Tests

We recommend the following ancillary tests to facilitate management, rule out potential contributing causes, and aid with disposition and prognosis: chest radiograph, ECG, and the specific laboratory tests discussed in detail below.

Chest Radiograph

A chest radiograph can exclude other diagnoses such as pneumothorax and pneumonia and often reveals or suggests pulmonary congestion. A classic bilateral butterfly alveolar pattern, small parallel linear lines at the lung periphery known as Kerley B lines, or even subtle perivascular cuffing can be seen. The pulmonary vasculature might be more prominent than usual in the upper lung fields (often referred to as "cephalization").

Chest radiographic findings appear to be related to pulmonary capillary wedge pressure (Table 7-2), although in clinical practice the findings do not always appear in sequence.[28] When present, pleural effusions are generally bilateral; however, when they are unilateral, 90% occur on the right. Cardiomegaly is common. A "boot-shaped" heart suggests pericardial effusion as the cause of dyspnea. Occasionally, the radiograph suggests enlargement of a specific heart chamber, implicating a contributing cause of AHF. For example, an enlarged left atrium might indicate mitral valve disease, and enlarged bilateral atria could indicate an infiltrative cause such as amyloidosis or sarcoidosis. Chest radiographs are specific but not sensitive—up to 18% of patients presenting with AHF have a normal chest radiograph. This is particularly true in patients with long-standing chronic HF.[29]

KEY POINT

A normal chest radiograph does *not* rule-out AHF.

Electrocardiogram

The electrocardiogram (ECG) can support the diagnosis of AHF as well as suggest a precipitant. A completely normal ECG is uncommon; therefore, a normal tracing should call the diagnosis into question. Left ventricular hypertrophy on the ECG increases the likelihood of HF, especially in the setting of strain, defined as a down-sloping convex ST segment with an inverted asymmetric T wave opposite the QRS axis in lead V_5 or V_6.[23,30] Always evaluate for evidence of ischemia on the ECG as a cause of AHF.

Atrial arrhythmias are the most common arrhythmias in AHF, with atrial fibrillation being the most common.[31] Atrial fibrillation with rapid ventricular response can result from or cause AHF. In a previously stable patient with a history of HF and atrial fibrillation, treatment of the AHF alone often reduces the heart rate.[32]

TABLE 7-1.

Characteristics of Patients With Reduced versus Preserved Systolic Function. Adapted and reproduced with permission from: Fonarow GC, Stough WG, Abraham WT, et al. Characteristics, treatments, and outcomes of patients with preserved systolic function hospitalized for heart failure: a report from the OPTIMIZE-HF Registry. *J Am Coll Cardiol.* 2007;50:771.

Characteristics at Admission	Patients With Left Ventricular Systolic Dysfunction (n=20,118)	Patients With Preserved Systolic Function (n=21,149)
Demographics		
Mean age (years)	70.4±14.3	75.1±13.1
Male	62%	38%
Caucasian	71%	77%
African American	21%	15%
Medical history		
Diabetes, insulin-treated	15%	17%
Diabetes, non–insulin-treated	24%	26%
Hypertension	66%	76%
Hyperlipidemia	34%	32%
Atrial arrhythmia	28%	33%
Vital signs on admission		
Median body weight (kg [25th, 75th percentile])	78.5 [65.8, 94]	78.9 [64, 97.5]
Mean heart rate (beats/min)	89±22	85±21
Mean SBP (mm Hg)	135±31	149±33
Mean diastolic blood pressure (mm Hg)	77±19	76±19
Etiology		
Ischemic	54%	38%
Hypertensive	17%	28%
Idiopathic	18%	21%

Acute Heart Failure

KEY POINTS

Atrial fibrillation is the most common arrhythmia seen in AHF.

Always assess for ischemia and arrhythmias as precipitants of AHF by ECG.

Lung Ultrasonography

Ultrasonography plays a key role in bedside evaluations, especially for unstable patients. Ultrasonography can be used to evaluate for pulmonary edema by screening for B lines, formerly known as "lung comets" (Figure 7-2).[33] In a small study conducted on patients in an intensive care unit (ICU), B lines were found in 100% of patients with pulmonary edema and were

TABLE 7-1. *(CONTINUED)*

Characteristics at Admission	Patients With Left Ventricular Systolic Dysfunction (n=20,118)	Patients With Preserved Systolic Function (n=21,149)
Findings on admission		
Acute pulmonary edema	3%	2%
Chest pain	23%	24%
Uncontrolled hypertension	9%	12%
Dyspnea at rest	44%	44%
Dyspnea on exertion	63%	62%
Rales	63%	65%
Lower extremity edema	62%	68%
Jugular venous pulsation	33%	26%
Left ventricular EF (mean)	24.3%±7.7%	54.7%±10.2%
Laboratory values		
Mean serum sodium (mEq/L)	137.7±4.6	137.9±4.8
Median serum creatinine (mg/dL [25th, 75th percentile])	1.4 [1.1, 1.9]	1.3 [1, 1.8]
Mean serum hemoglobin (g/dL)	12.5±2	11.9±2
Median BNP (pg/mL [25th, 75th percentile])	1,170 [603, 2,280]	601.5 [320, 1,190]
Median troponin I (ng/mL [25th, 75th percentile])	0.1 [0.1, 0.3]	0.1 [0.0, 0.3]
Medications on admission		
ACE inhibitor	45%	36%
ARB	11%	13%
Amlodipine	5%	10%
Aldosterone antagonist	10%	5%
Beta-blocker	56%	52%
Loop diuretic	63%	58%
Digoxin	30%	17%
Aspirin	42%	38%
Antiarrhythmic	13%	8%
Hydralazine	3%	3%
Nitrate	22%	21%
Statin[a]	40%	39%

[a]Statin use among patients with coronary artery disease, cerebrovascular disease/transient ischemic attack, diabetes, hyperlipidemia, or peripheral vascular disease.

absent in 24 of 26 patients with chronic obstructive pulmonary disease, translating to 100% sensitivity and 98% specificity. Additionally, B lines correlated closely with amino-terminal pro-B-type natriuretic peptide (NT-proBNP) levels.[34]

KEY POINT

Assess for B-lines with lung ultrasonography to facilitate the diagnosis of pulmonary edema versus other causes of shortness of breath.

Bedside Echocardiography

The use of simple bedside echocardiography has been adopted by emergency physicians for the detection of pericardial effusions in the undifferentiated hypotensive patient as well as for the detection of cardiac activity during cardiac arrest. Emergency physicians use limited bedside echocardiography for simple EF measurements, supporting a diagnosis of AHF in the patient with undifferentiated dyspnea.[35]

Laboratory Evaluation

Laboratory tests are not essential for the diagnosis of AHF; however, they are a key adjunct to management, aid with disposition and prognosis, and provide important clues regarding the precipitant or consequences of AHF. Natriuretic peptide testing is recommended in current guidelines.[5] The Breathing Not Properly multinational study demonstrated a diagnostic accuracy of 83.4% for HF, with a B-type natriuretic peptide (BNP) threshold of 100 pg/mL, and a negative predictive value of 96%, with BNP levels below 50 pg/mL.[36] Similarly, the PRIDE study demonstrated the diagnostic value of NT-proBNP; a value below 300 pg/mL had a 99% negative predictive value for the diagnosis of AHF. Age, sex, type of HF (systolic versus diastolic), body mass index, and renal function confound interpretation of these markers. Systemic illnesses such as sepsis, cirrhosis, hyperthyroidism, pulmonary embolism, and severe lung disease can elevate these biomarkers and should be considered when evaluating an elevated BNP or NT-proBNP.[37] Overall, natriuretic peptides facilitate the evaluation of patients with undifferentiated dyspnea but must be interpreted with an understanding of the underlying test characteristics. Prognostically, natriuretic peptides have been shown to have a strong independent predictive value for both morbidity and mortality.[37] Lower values might suggest patients who could be considered for early discharge or observation unit strategies.[38]

KEY POINTS

Natriuretic peptides facilitate the diagnosis, prognosis, and treatment of AHF.

Renal dysfunction, obesity, and other systemic illnesses such as sepsis can affect BNP levels.

A basic metabolic panel and complete blood count should be ordered for all patients in whom AHF is suspected. Electrolyte abnormalities are common, often as a result of diuretic use as well as underlying renal dysfunction. Electrolyte derangements can affect myocardial function as well as promote arrhythmias. Renal dysfunction is highly prevalent in patients with AHF, with nearly 90% having some form of mild dysfunction, as defined by the National Kidney Foundation.[39] Interaction between the heart and kidney is now a well-recognized phenomenon, with various pathophysiologic mechanisms influencing the effect of one organ on the other.[40] Anemia can complicate AHF both by decreasing myocardial oxygen delivery and by increasing myocardial stress. It is also an independent predictor of mortality in patients with chronic HF.

Most patients with AHF, up to 60%, have underlying CAD. Therefore, myocardial ischemia should always be considered in patients presenting with AHF as either a cause or a result of decompensation. In addition, troponin should be measured, and often repeated, and interpreted in context with both ECG changes and clinical presentation. Patients with troponin elevation have worse outcomes than their matched cohort, although it is unclear if a low-grade troponin "leak" should change management.[41,42] Some studies suggest improved outcomes with aggressive management of CAD, but this approach has not been well studied prospectively.[43,44] In part, the lack of clear guidance stems from our incomplete understanding of how to manage CAD in general and troponin release specifically in AHF.[41,45]

KEY POINT

Troponin release in AHF without ACS indicates a higher-risk sub-group.

Other laboratory values have important prognostic value (Table 7-3). Hyponatremia is associated with an increased length of hospital stay as well as a worse prognosis overall, although it is unclear whether normalizing this value improves outcomes.[58,59] Similarly, falling glomerular filtration rate, rising creatinine, and rising blood urea nitrogen are findings that

TABLE 7-2.

Correlation Between Pulmonary Capillary Wedge Pressure and Radiologic Findings[28]

Pulmonary Capillary Wedge Pressure	Radiologic Findings
5 to 12 mm Hg	Normal
12 to 17 mm Hg	Cephalization
17 to 20 mm Hg	Kerley B lines, pleural effusions
Above 25 mm Hg	Pulmonary edema

portend a poor prognosis and often indicate a worsening of the overall course of disease.[60] Metra and colleagues suggested that it is the combination of pulmonary vascular congestion and renal dysfunction that identifies the truly high-risk patient, rather than renal dysfunction alone. Mild renal dysfunction may be a necessary result of reducing pulmonary congestion and, by itself, might not be an adverse marker.[61] Interpretation requires the clinical context.

KEY POINT

Hyponatremia portends a poor prognosis in patients with AHF.

Initial Management

Treatment of any life-threatening condition comes first. The initial approach to patients presenting to an emergency department in AHF is summarized in Table 7-4. Other chapters in this book discuss the management of ST-elevation myocardial infarction with resultant AHF and critical aortic stenosis presenting as AHF.

Time to Treatment

Retrospective analyses suggest that earlier treatment leads to improved outcomes.[55,62] Prospective studies are needed. However, the concept of preventing or protecting the heart or kidneys from injury supports the hypothesis for early treatment.

Initial Stabilization

Diagnosis and management commonly occur in parallel, despite their stepwise discussion in this text. Although immediate, life-threatening conditions are uncommon, AHF patients can present in acute respiratory distress or frank respiratory failure requiring immediate intubation. In these cases, the fundamentals of emergency care apply, with focus on the ABCs of resuscitation (airway, breathing, circulation) to initially stabilize and resuscitate the patient.

For patients with severe respiratory distress who do not require immediate intubation and have an appropriate mental

FIGURE 7-2.
Lung ultrasound findings (B lines or comet tails) in a patient with pulmonary edema. Image courtesy of Luna Gargani, MD.

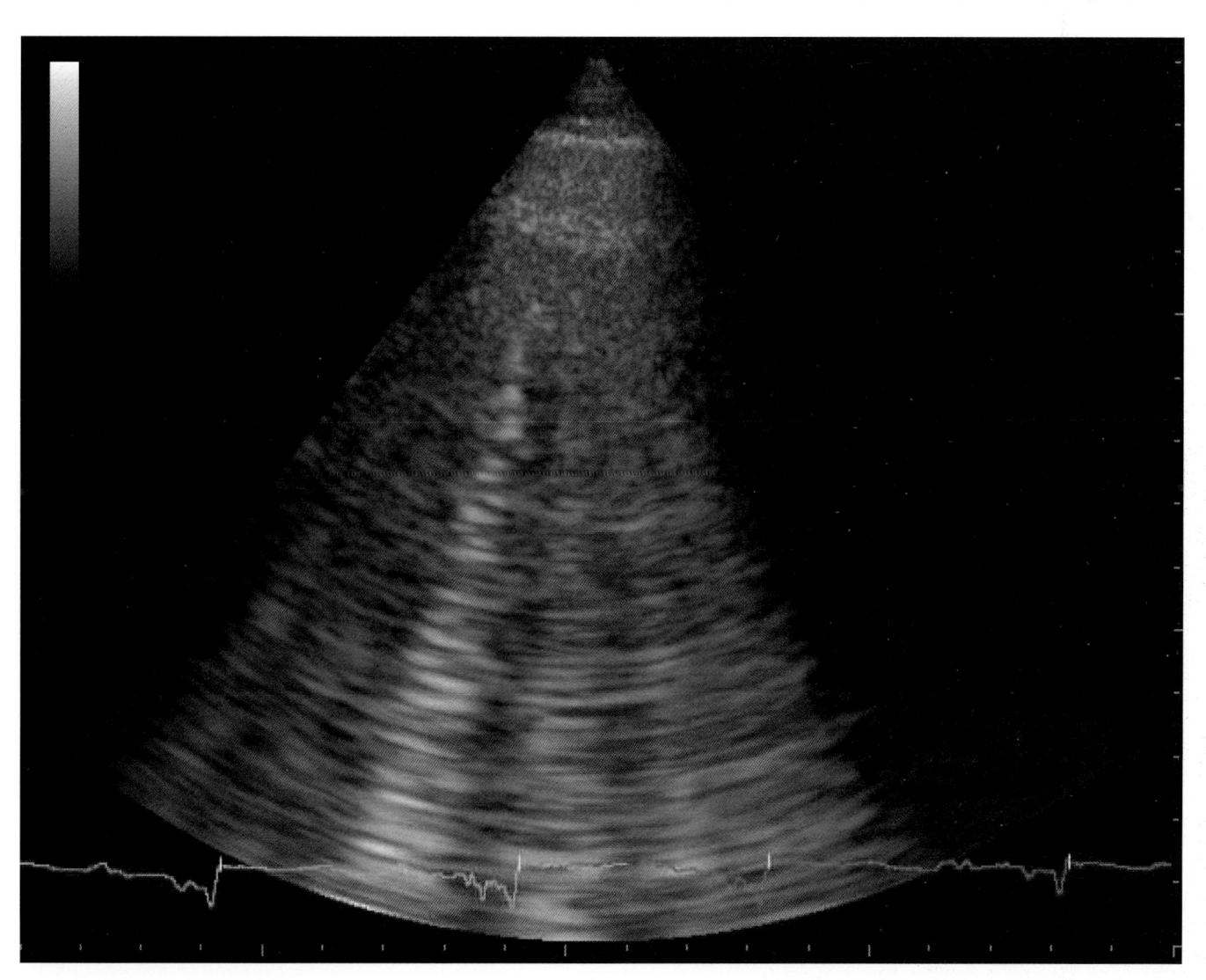

status, noninvasive ventilation (NIV) is recommended. Positive-pressure ventilation has proven benefits in AHF and is supported by the current Cochrane review.[63] Although small studies suggest an association between myocardial infarction and the use of bilevel positive airway pressure (BiPAP), the large 3CPO trial demonstrated no safety differences between continuous positive airway pressure (CPAP) and BiPAP compared with conventional treatment in respect to rates of myocardial infarction, critical care admission, and overall 7-day mortality.[64] Although there was no difference between NIV and face-mask oxygen in the 3CPO trial in terms of intubation rates, critical care admission rates, or length of stay, meta-analyses lead us to continue to recommend the use of NIV as early therapy for patients with respiratory distress who have no other contraindication. The 2005 Cochrane review examining 21 studies encompassing 1,017 patients found a decrease in intubation rates as well as in overall mortality when comparing NIV with conventional therapy.[63] The number needed to treat in order to decrease mortality was 13 and to decrease intubation, 8. Additionally, similar to the 3CPO trial, this review found no increase in myocardial infarction rates with the use of NIV compared with conventional therapy.

KEY POINT

The use of NIV is recommended for patients with respiratory distress and often obviates the need for intubation.

Appropriate use of NIV (either CPAP or BiPAP) in the setting of cardiogenic pulmonary edema decreases the work of breathing, reduces respiratory distress, improves left ventricular function by reducing preload, and decreases the need for intubation. Current European Society of Cardiology (ESC) guidelines recommend the use of CPAP with an initial peak end-expiratory pressure (PEEP) of 5 to 7.5 mm Hg, fraction of inspired oxygen above 40%, and titration of PEEP as needed to 10 mm Hg.[65] Contraindications to NIV include an unprotected airway, an altered sensorium, and lack of patient cooperation. Caution should be used in patients with cardiogenic shock and right ventricular failure. Occasionally, hypoxia refractory to NIV mandates intubation. Aggressive medical therapy with vasodilators in conjunction with NIV immediately on arrival at the emergency department often obviates the need for endotracheal intubation.

Once patients are stabilized, focus should turn to cardiovascular status. Patients should be placed on a cardiac monitor. Unstable rhythms should be addressed by electric or medical cardioversion, as outlined by advanced cardiovascular life support (ACLS) protocols. Significant abnormalities of blood pressure and perfusion should be addressed. Hypertensive patients should receive aggressive vasodilator therapy, although patients with significant hypotension and signs of hypoperfusion may require inotropic support. It is important to remember that hypoperfusion can result from overdiuresis. In this case, careful

TABLE 7-3.

Prognostic Indicators as Potential Targets of Therapy in AHF[a]. Adapted with permission from: Gheorghiade M, Zannad F, Sopko G, et al. Acute heart failure syndromes: current state and framework for future research. *Circulation.* 2005;112:3962.

Systolic blood pressure	Admission and early postdischarge SBP inversely correlates with postdischarge mortality. The higher the blood pressure, the lower both inhospital and postdischarge mortality rates. However, the readmission rate of approximately 30% is independent of the SBP at time of admission.[4]
Coronary artery disease	Extent and severity of CAD appear to be predictors of poor prognosis.[43]
Troponin release	Results in a three-fold increase in inhospital mortality, a two-fold increase in postdischarge mortality, and a three-fold increase in the rehospitalization rate.[42,46,47]
Ventricular dyssynchrony	Increase in QRS duration occurs in approximately 40% of patients with reduced systolic function and is a strong predictor of early and late postdischarge mortality and rehospitalization.[48]
Renal impairment	Associated with a two- to three-fold increase in postdischarge mortality. Worsening renal function during hospitalization or soon after discharge is also associated with an increase in inhospital and postdischarge mortality.[49-51]
Hyponatremia	Defined as serum sodium less than 135 mmol/L, occurs in approximately 25% of patients, and is associated with a two- to three-fold increase in postdischarge mortality.[52]
Clinical congestion at time of discharge	An important predictor of postdischarge mortality and morbidity.[53,54]
Ejection fraction	Considered an adverse prognostic marker. Similar postdischarge event rates and mortality between reduced and preserved EF.[12]
BNP/NT-proBNP	Elevated natriuretic peptides associated with increased resource utilization and mortality.[55]
Functional capacity at time of discharge	Predischarge functional capacity, defined by the 6-minute walk test, is emerging as an important predictor of postdischarge outcomes.[56,57]

[a]Not an all-inclusive list.

administration of small fluid boluses might actually be indicated, although this should be done only after careful examination confirms the absence of volume overload.

> **KEY POINT**
>
> Unstable arrhythmias should be addressed early using ACLS guidelines.

After initial stabilization, assuming no other precipitant takes precedence (eg, ST-elevation myocardial infarction or atrial fibrillation with rapid ventricular response), the patient should be classified into one of three categories: 1) hypertensive AHF, 2) normotensive AHF, or 3) hypotensive AHF (Figure 7-3). Despite this recommendation, prospective evidence is lacking and remains an area of ongoing research.

> **KEY POINT**
>
> Categorize AHF presentations as hypertensive, normotensive, or shock.

Hypertensive AHF

Hypertensive AHF (Figure 7-4) is broadly defined as SBP above 140 mm Hg. In addition to early NIV for patients with respiratory distress, aggressive blood pressure control with a vasodilator such as nitroglycerin is recommended. Higher doses of nitrates with relatively lower doses of diuretics yield better outcomes for these patients, compared with a higher-dose diuretic/lower-dose nitrate strategy.[66]

> **KEY POINT**
>
> In the management of hypertensive AHF, vasodilation is critical, followed by judicious diuresis.

Nitroglycerin is first-line recommended therapy and can be given sublingually, transdermally, or intravenously. Sublingual administration is the fastest route of delivery on immediate presentation, unless a prehospital call prompts preparation of intravenous nitrates. At lower doses, nitrates primarily cause vasodilation, leading to decreased left ventricular filling pressures, alleviating pulmonary congestion and decreasing myocardial oxygen consumption. At higher doses, nitrates cause arterial dilation, including the coronary circulation, and thus improve coronary perfusion.[67]

Nesiritide is a reasonable second-line vasodilator, although there is no contraindication to its use as first-line therapy for AHF patients with hypertension in the emergency department. Nesiritide is an intravenous recombinant form of human BNP that acts as both a venous and an arterial dilator. Invasive hemodynamic studies of nesiritide demonstrate a clear improvement in left ventricular filling pressures. Although the initial reports of nesiritide were favorable in the Vasodilation in the Management of Acute Congestive HF study, subsequent metaanalysis suggested an increase in worsening renal function and mortality.[66,68-70] However, this metaanalysis was contradicted by the ASCEND-HF trial, which demonstrated nesiritide's safety.[71] In this trial, nesiritide infusion, in addition to standard therapy, was compared with placebo plus standard therapy in more than 7,000 patients. No increase in mortality or worsening renal function was observed with nesiritide compared with placebo.

TABLE 7-4.

Initial Management for Acute Heart Failure[a]

1. Treat immediate life-threatening conditions.	Immediate resuscitative or life-saving measures may precede or parallel diagnostic evaluation (ie, unstable arrhythmia, flash pulmonary edema, ST-elevation myocardial infarction)
2. Establish the diagnosis.	Based on medical history, signs (JVD, S_3, edema), symptoms (dyspnea), biomarkers (eg, BNP)
3. Determine clinical profile.	Key components include heart rate, blood pressure, jugular venous pressure, presence of pulmonary congestion, ECG, chest radiograph, renal function, troponin, BNP, pulse oximetry, history of CAD
4. Determine and manage the precipitant.	Management of precipitants, such as ischemia, hypertension, arrhythmias, acute valvular pathologies, worsening renal function, uncontrolled diabetes, and/or infection, is critical to ensure maximal benefits from HF management.
5. Alleviate symptoms (eg, dyspnea).	Usually a diuretic with or without other vasoactive agents.
6. Protect and preserve myocardial and renal function.	Avoid hypotension or increase in heart rate. Use of inotropes should be restricted to patients with low-output state (low blood pressure or organ hypoperfusion). Risk for myocardial injury is greater in those with underlying CAD.
7. Determine patient disposition.	Majority are admitted to telemetry, with a small but significant number discharged home. Robust evidence to support risk stratification and disposition in terms of admission to the hospital or safe discharge with close outpatient followup is lacking.

[a]These steps usually occur in parallel, not series.

However, ASCEND-HF failed to achieve its prespecified primary efficacy end point of dyspnea improvement. Although a statistically significant improvement in dyspnea was seen, its clinical significance has been questioned. Therefore, nesiritide may be an acceptable alternative to nitrate therapy.

One advantage of nesiritide over intravenous nitrates is its proven safety for use outside intensive care units.[72] Given the national focus on readmissions, the ability to administer an intravenous vasodilator to certain patients in an observation unit is appealing.[38] Robust evidence supporting the safety of intravenous nesiritide now exists; similarly strong safety or efficacy data for nitroglycerin do not.[73] Nevertheless, we currently recommend nitroglygerin as the first-line agent. The value of prospective research and the potential pitfalls of metaanalyses, no matter how well conducted, highlight key lessons from nesiritide development. At present, no AHF therapy meets the criteria for Class I, Level A evidence.[5]

Sodium nitroprusside is less commonly used as a vasodilating agent in AHF because of its invasive monitoring and central line requirements as well as its potential deleterious side effects

FIGURE 7-3.
Algorithm for management of patients presenting with AHF. From: Collins S, Storrow AB, Kirk JD, et al. Beyond pulmonary edema: diagnostic, risk stratification, and treatment challenges of acute heart failure management in the emergency department. *Ann Emerg Med.* 2008;51:45-57. Copyright 2008. Used with permission.

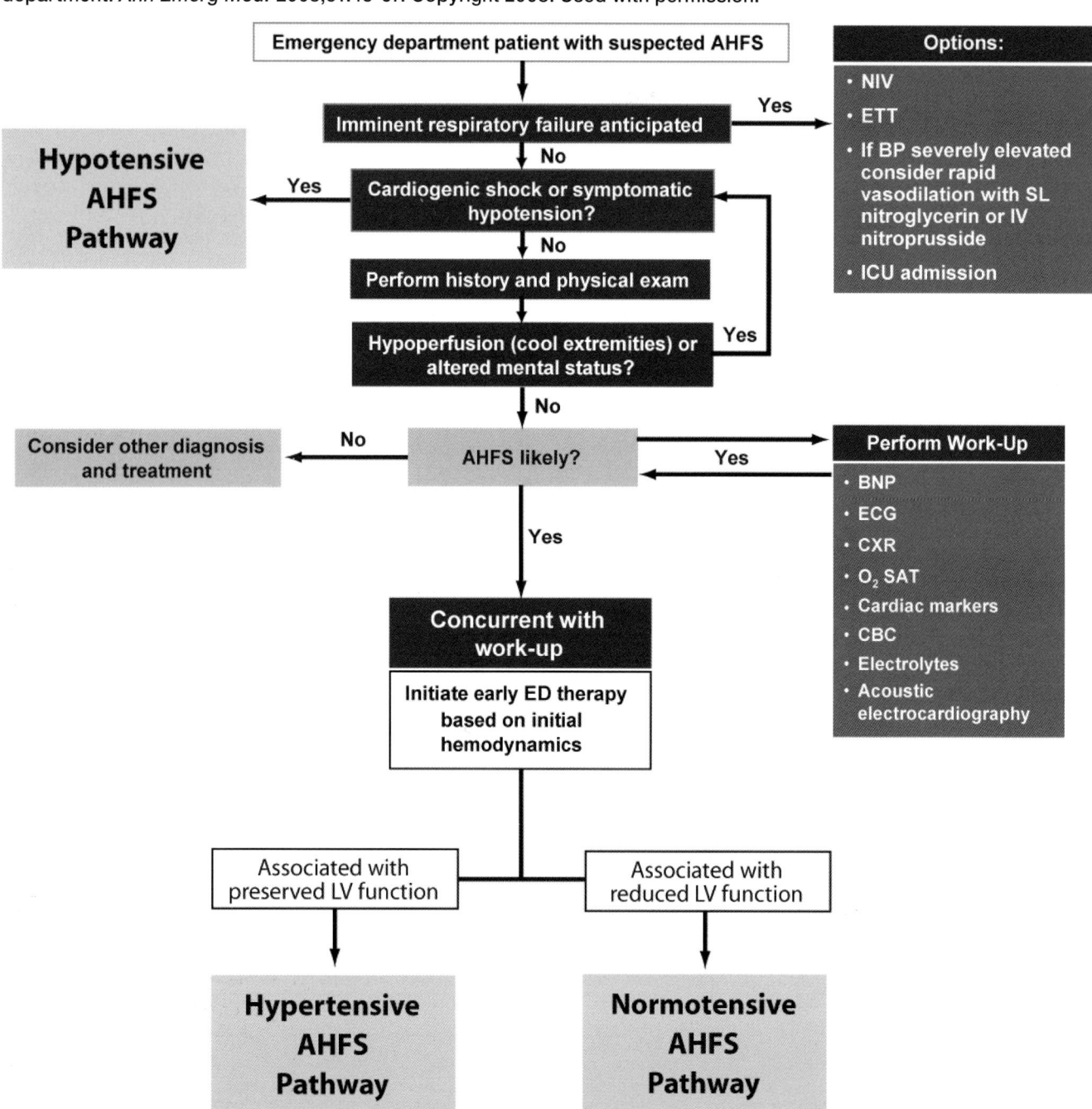

Acute Heart Failure

such as cyanide toxicity. Still, it is highly effective, affecting both the venous and arterial circulation, with the additional benefit of a rapid onset and short half-life. However, its pharmacokinetic properties can lead to "overshooting" resulting in severe hypotension.[74] Nitroprusside is associated with cyanide toxicity (especially in patients with renal dysfunction) and hypoxia in patients with chronic obstructive pulmonary disease due to perfusion-ventilation mismatch. It also can cause hemodynamic alterations that ultimately result in coronary steal syndrome in patients with underlying CAD.[74] In experienced hands, it is a safe and effective agent.

Other afterload-reducing medications such as hydralazine and angiotensin-converting enzyme (ACE) inhibitors are sometimes used in patients with hypertensive AHF. However, it is worth re-emphasizing that these therapies, like nitroglycerin, lack robust evidence. Additionally, many studies examining traditional AHF therapies were not performed in the emergency department setting. Of note, specific medical societies have published guidelines or clinical policy statements (eg, American College of Emergency Physicians versus ESC) with differing recommendations regarding the use of early ACE inhibitors, which highlights the lack of definitive evidence and consensus in this area.[65,75] With regard to hydralazine, there is a lack of evidence supporting its safe and effective use in AHF, and we therefore do not recommend its use for this condition.

Finally, beta-blockers and calcium channel blockers are generally contraindicated in the setting of AHF because of their negative effect on cardiac contractility. More recent studies of dihydropyridine calcium channel blockers have been conducted and may lead to a change in these recommendations in the future.

KEY POINT

Most blood pressure medications, including ACE inhibitors, hydralazine, and calcium channel blockers, have not been well studied in the setting of AHF.

Normotensive AHF

Patients presenting with normotensive AHF, defined as SBP between 90 and 140 mm Hg, are often younger male patients with a history of CAD, reduced EF, and underlying HF.[23] As a general rule, these presentations tend to be more insidious. Clinically, the patients appear less acutely ill in the emergency department, although, paradoxically, their postdischarge outcomes are worse.[4] The mainstay of emergency department treatment for these patients is diuresis (Figure 7-5).

KEY POINT

For patients with normotensive AHF, the primary therapy is

FIGURE 7-4.
Treatment algorithm for management of patients with hypertensive AHF. From: Collins S, Storrow AB, Kirk JD, et al. Beyond pulmonary edema: diagnostic, risk stratification, and treatment challenges of acute heart failure management in the emergency department. *Ann Emerg Med.* 2008;51:45-57. Copyright 2008. Used with permission.

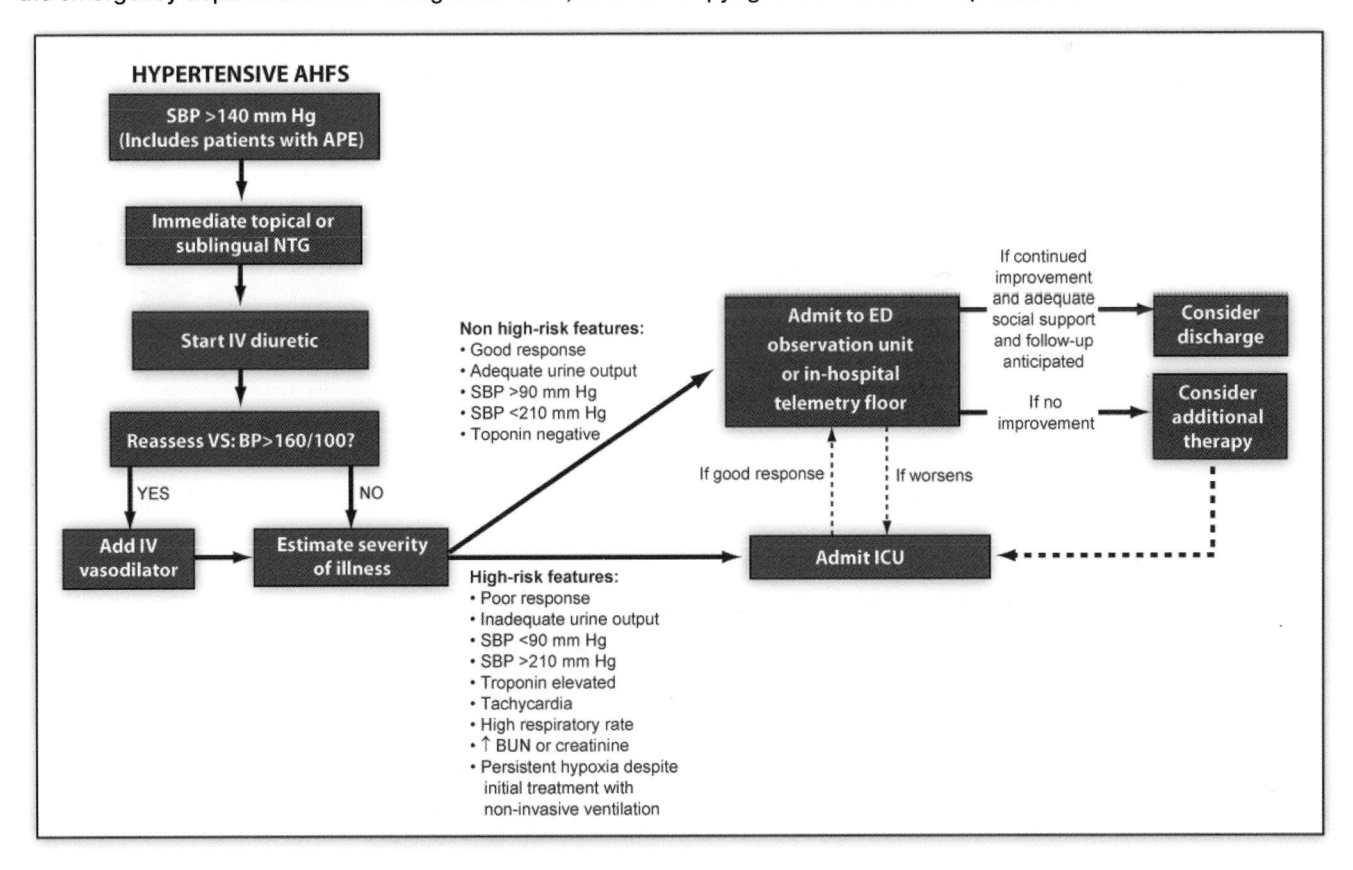

diuresis.

Intravenous administration of loop diuretics promotes natriuresis and results in improved signs and symptoms.[76] Intravenous formulations have a quicker onset of action and a better pharmacokinetic profile in the setting of volume overload than do oral formulations. The DOSE trial (Diuretic Strategies in Acute Decompensated Heart Failure) set out to examine the most effective dose and strategy of administering loop diuretics to patients presenting with acute decompensated HF.[77] The authors found that continuous infusions are equivalent to intravenous boluses in terms of symptom relief as well as effect on renal function. They also tested whether higher- or lower-dose diuretics were more efficacious. The benefits of high-dose intravenous diuresis (defined as 2.5 times the total oral dose given over a 24-hour period) included better dyspnea relief, improved net fluid loss, and greater decrease in BNP. However, worsening renal function was observed in the higher-dose group compared with the lower-dose group. This was a transient finding and, while no longer-term adverse outcomes were seen, the study was not designed to assess the longer-term safety of intravenous loop diuretics. Metra and colleagues found that the continued presence of clinically evident congestion was the principal driver of worse outcomes rather than renal dysfunction alone.[61] In other words, failure to decongest seemed to lead to worse outcomes as opposed to worsening renal function itself. Frequent reassessment of the patient, with close attention to urine output and vital signs, is key.

The ESC guidelines suggest an intravenous bolus dose of furosemide, 20 to 40 mg; bumetanide, 0.5 to 1 mg; or torsemide, 10 to 20 mg.[65] We recommend the high-bolus dose per the DOSE-AHF trial, defined as 2.5 times the total oral dose, divided three times daily and given intravenously.

KEY POINT

For diuresis, give 2.5 times the patient's home dose of oral diuretic intravenously, divided into three doses per day.

Hypotensive AHF

Despite the traditionally held view that most AHF patients have a severely reduced EF and low blood pressure, less than 5% of patients actually present with low blood pressure.[24,78] Although low blood pressure mandates prompt assessment, some of these patients may be at baseline, as severe systolic dysfunction limits the height of their SBP.[24] Hypotensive patients with AHF are difficult to manage. For patients with cardiogenic shock, immediate resuscitation should begin with aggressive hemodynamic support, including inotropes and vasopressors, as necessary. For patients with known advanced or end-stage HF, careful and judicious management is required (Figure 7-6). If possible, a call to the patient's cardiologist is warranted.

KEY POINTS

Hypotension in the setting of AHF could be normal depending on the patient's baseline blood pressure and whether clinical signs of hypoperfusion are present.

FIGURE 7-5.
Treatment algorithm for management of patients with normotensive AHF. From: Collins S, Storrow AB, Kirk JD, et al. Beyond pulmonary edema: diagnostic, risk stratification, and treatment challenges of acute heart failure management in the emergency department. *Ann Emerg Med.* 2008;51:45-57. Copyright 2008. Used with permission.

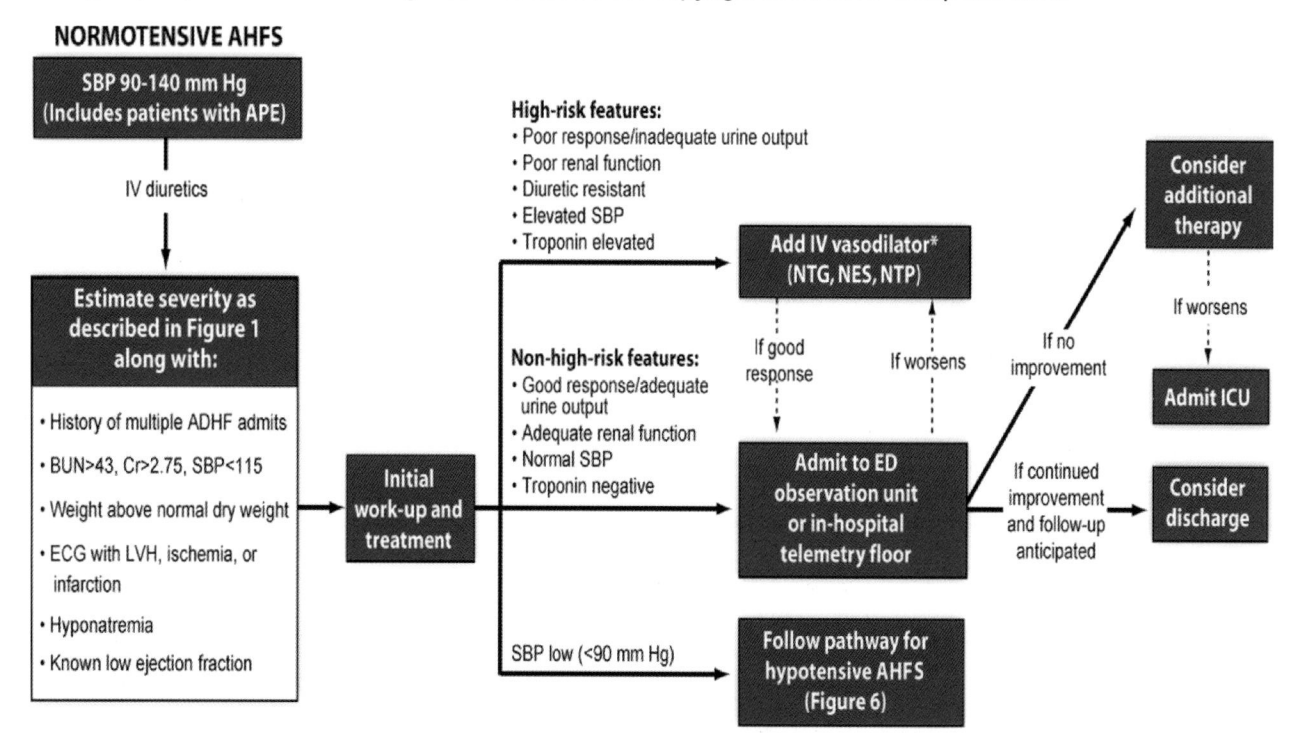

However, hypotension could also be a sign of worsening HF or cardiogenic shock. Rarely, hypotension may also result from overdiuresis.

Use inotropes only in the setting of low blood pressure (generally SBP below 90 mm Hg) and signs of hypoperfusion, after other therapies have not led to improvement, *not* based on blood pressure alone.

Diuresis can be difficult to achieve because of worsening hypotension and hypoperfusion as well as diuretic resistance. Such patients often require higher levels of care such as ICU admission. Although it seems paradoxical, some of these patients need vasodilation to decrease renal congestion and improve renal perfusion. This treatment decision should be made in consultation with a cardiologist. Inotropic options include dobutamine, dopamine, norepinephrine, and milrinone (Table 7-5). Dobutamine is the inotrope of choice in the emergency department, in part because of familiarity.[23,24,79] Although these medications improve patient hemodynamics, multiple studies demonstrate significant side effects, including increased rates of arrhythmia and mortality.[5,80] Thus, use of inotropes is suggested only for patients with HF and a reduced EF with signs of hypoperfusion, including decreased mentation, poor urine output, or cool extremities, after other therapeutic attempts have failed.[5,80,81]

KEY POINT

The combination of AHF and hypotension is an uncommon presentation and is the most challenging patient type to manage.

There are no definitive guidelines regarding which inotropes are recommended for patients in hypotensive HF with clinical signs of shock.[81] Felker and associates highlighted the increased mortality with inotropes and thus they are not routinely recommended.[80] Nevertheless, some patients require them to sustain life. If the AHF patient is hypotensive with signs of shock, the ESC currently recommends dobutamine (Class IIa) and dopa-

FIGURE 7-6.
Algorithm for management of patients with hypotensive (shock) AHF. From: Collins S, Storrow AB, Kirk JD, et al. Beyond pulmonary edema: diagnostic, risk stratification, and treatment challenges of acute heart failure management in the emergency department. *Ann Emerg Med.* 2008;51:45-57. Copyright 2008. Used with permission.

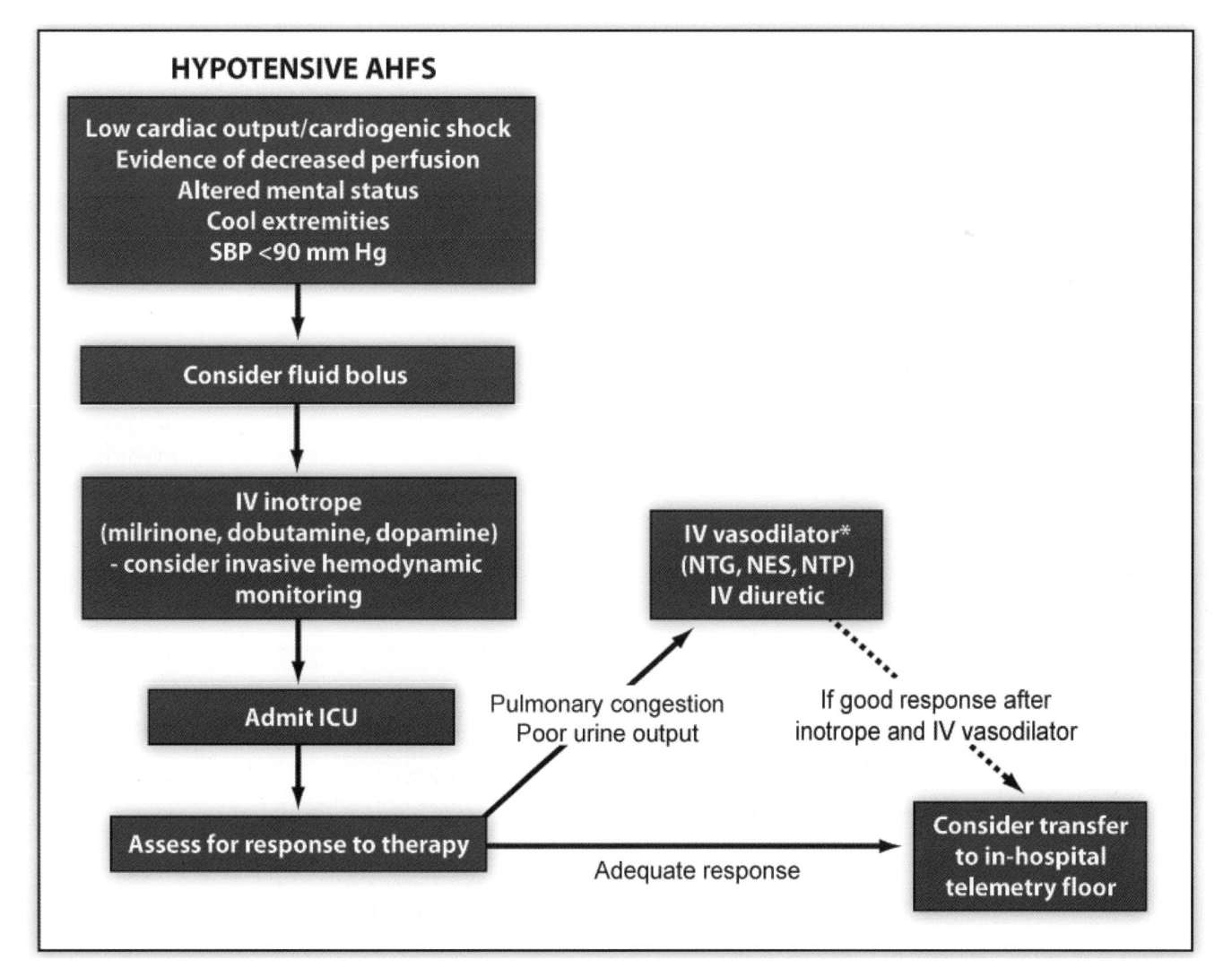

mine (Class IIb) as first-line agents, followed by milrinone.[65] Small studies comparing dobutamine and milrinone have found similar clinical outcomes.[82]

Dobutamine is a nonselective beta₁- and beta₂-adrenergic receptor agonist that decreases afterload and increases cardiac output. The recommended initial dose of dobutamine is an infusion of 2 or 3 mcg/kg/min, with further titration as needed, up to a maximum dose of 15 mcg/kg/min.[65] The most recent American College of Cardiology Foundation/American Heart Association guidelines support the use of inotropes (Class IIb) for patients with severe systolic dysfunction, low blood pressure, and evidence of low cardiac output, highlighting dopamine, dobutamine, and milrinone as potential options.[5] One agent is not preferentially listed over another, and the level of evidence is Class C (expert consensus).

KEY POINT

Dobutamine or dopamine is recommended as first-line therapy, when needed, for patients in cardiogenic shock or severe HF with evidence of hypoperfusion.

Dopamine can also be considered a first-line agent for patients with hypotension. At lower doses, dopamine acts as a dilator in the renal vasculature, contributing to diuresis and natriuresis. At higher doses, it acts as an inotropic and chronotropic agent, increasing heart rate and blood pressure.[83-85] At even higher doses, it acts as a vasoconstrictor, which can worsen perfusion of specific tissues. Initial recommended dosing is 2 mcg/kg/min, up to a maximum of 15 mcg/kg/min. In 2010, De Backer and colleagues documented worsening outcomes, including death, in the subgroup of patients with cardiogenic shock who were treated with dopamine, compared with those treated with norepinephrine.[86] The authors postulated that increased cardiac ischemia as a result of higher heart rates in the dopamine group was the reason. Based on these data, norepinephrine should be considered for cardiogenic shock, even though it has not been well compared with other inotropes for cardiogenic shock. Initial dosing is 2 mcg/kg/min, with titration up to 20 mcg/kg/min. Norepinephrine might cause less heart rate derangement than dopamine, an important consideration in patients with cardiogenic shock secondary to HF.[86]

Milrinone is a phosphodiesterase inhibitor, which, like other inotropes, is recommended only for patients with shock or borderline shock who have not responded to other treatment.[80,81] This recommendation is based on data showing an increase in the postdischarge mortality rate for patients with CAD as well as increased rates of arrhythmia overall.[87] The data also show no improvement in the hospital mortality rate, or 60-day mortality, or readmission rates. The initial dosing of milrinone is a bolus of 50 mcg/kg given over 10 minutes, followed by an infusion of 0.375 to 0.75 mcg/kg/min (not to exceed 1.13 mg/kg/day).

Other Pharmacologic Considerations

The use of morphine is controversial. Similar to other AHF medications in the emergency department setting, evidence for or against its use is largely based on small studies or secondary analyses.[5,88,89] No definitive prospective trials have been published showing benefit or harm from its administration. Consistent with ESC guidelines, morphine may be considered for judicious use among patients with hypertensive AHF, especially those receiving NIV.[65]

KEY POINT

Morphine should be used judiciously, if at all. Retrospective data suggest harm.

Disposition

Heart failure is the primary cause of hospital admission and readmission for Medicare beneficiaries.[1] A proportion of HF readmissions may be "unnecessary," thus the appeal to improve quality while reducing costs has led to national quality measures regarding readmission.[90] The disposition of patients with AHF after initial management is a critical decision with substantial downstream implications. Presently, most AHF patients presenting to an emergency department are admitted to the hospital, resulting in large financial costs, although many patients require hospitalization.[91] This is, in part, driven by the absence of easy-to-use, well-validated risk-stratification criteria for use in the emergency department setting, combined with the fact that these patients have a very high postdischarge rehospitalization and mortality rate, affecting one third of patients within 90 days.[4] Large database analyses performed by Lee and colleagues suggested that patients discharged from the emergency department actually have a worse mortality rate than those admitted, highlighting the need for effective disposition decision rules.[92]

TABLE 7-5.

Inotrope Mechanism of Action and Dosing

Medication	Mechanism of Action	Dosing
Dobutamine	Nonselective beta₁- and beta₂-receptor agonist	2 to 20 mcg/kg/min
Dopamine	Dopamine receptor agonist	2 to 15 mcg/kg/min
Milrinone	Phosphodiesterase inhibitor	5 to 15 mcg/kg given over 10 minutes followed by an infusion of 0.375 to 0.75 mcg/kg/min. Lower doses have also been recommended.

KEY POINT

Disposition is a difficult decision with significant implications for health care utilization; however, there are no robust guidelines to guide practitioners in their disposition decisions for patients with AHF in the emergency department.

Identifying high-risk patients is often easier than identifying lower-risk patients eligible for discharge or admission to the observation unit.[91] Importantly, a patient cannot be deemed low risk simply because he or she lacks high-risk features; however, it is true that patients are likely lower risk in the absence of higher-risk features. Targeted research needs to be performed to identify which patients are truly low risk and appropriate for discharge home or observation unit management with coordinated outpatient care.[93,94]

Conclusion

After initial stabilization, we recommend AHF patients be classified into hypertensive, normotensive, and hypotensive groups to facilitate initial treatment decisions. Significant overlap between these phenotypes highlights the need for tailoring initial management and frequent reassessment. Pharmacologic treatment of the hypertensive AHF patient should focus on blood pressure control, initially with nitrates in most cases, followed by judicious diuresis. Treatment of the normotensive AHF patient should begin with aggressive diuresis. Both populations may benefit from NIV if in respiratory distress. Evaluation and management of the hypotensive AHF patient is challenging. Inotropes should be used only if no other options are possible, given their association with worse longer-term outcomes.

Heterogeneity of patient presentation, cardiac substrate and function, comorbid conditions, and psychosocial and socioeconomic factors, as well as the lack of evidence-based acute therapeutic recommendations, highlight the difficulties of AHF management. Despite empirical evidence that current treatment "works," the high postdischarge morbidity and mortality rates demonstrate the need for further improvement. Furthermore, the societal burden of HF will increase as the population ages. Future research directed towards phenotypically targeted, outcome-driven acute treatment options and decision rules to aid practitioners in the disposition of these high-risk patients are needed.

References

1. Jencks SF, Williams MV, Coleman EA. Rehospitalizations among patients in the Medicare fee-for-service program. *N Engl J Med.* 2009;360:1418-1428.
2. Fang J, Mensah GA, Croft JB, Keenan NL. Heart failure-related hospitalization in the U.S., 1979 to 2004. *J Am Coll Cardiol.* 2008;52:428-434.
3. Roger VL, Go AS, Lloyd-Jones DM, et al. Heart disease and stroke statistics--2012 update: a report from the American Heart Association. *Circulation.* 2012;125(1):e2-e220.
4. Gheorghiade M, Abraham WT, Albert NM, et al. Systolic blood pressure at admission, clinical characteristics, and outcomes in patients hospitalized with acute heart failure. *JAMA.* 2006;296:2217-2226.
5. Hunt SA, Abraham WT, Chin MH, et al. 2009 Focused update incorporated into the ACC/AHA 2005 Guidelines for the Diagnosis and Management of Heart Failure in Adults A Report of the American College of Cardiology Foundation/American Heart Association Task Force on Practice Guidelines Developed in Collaboration With the International Society for Heart and Lung Transplantation. *J Am Coll Cardiol.* 2009;53(15):e1-e90.
6. Heidenreich PA, Trogdon JG, Khavjou OA, et al. Forecasting the future of cardiovascular disease in the United States: a policy statement from the American Heart Association. *Circulation.* 2011;123:933-944.
7. Pang PS, Komajda M, Gheorghiade M. The current and future management of acute heart failure syndromes. *Eur Heart J.* 2010;31:784-793.
8. Hall MJ, Levant S, DeFrances CJ. *Hospitalization for Congestive Heart Failure: United States, 2000-2010.* NCHS Data Brief No. 108. Hyattsville, MD: National Center for Health Statistics; 2012.
9. Levy D, Larson MG, Vasan RS, et al. The progression from hypertension to congestive heart failure. *JAMA.* 1996;275:1557-1562.
10. ADHERE Scientific Advisory Committee. *Acute Decompensated Heart Failure National Registry (ADHERE®) Core Module Q1 2006 Final Cumulative National Benchmark Report.* Scios, Inc; July 2006.
11. Gheorghiade M, Zannad F, Sopko G, et al. Acute heart failure syndromes: current state and framework for future research. *Circulation.* 2005;112:3958-3968.
12. Fonarow GC, Stough WG, Abraham WT, et al. Characteristics, treatments, and outcomes of patients with preserved systolic function hospitalized for heart failure: a report from the OPTIMIZE-HF Registry. *J Am Coll Cardiol.* 2007;50:768-777.
13. Setoguchi S, Stevenson LW, Schneeweiss S. Repeated hospitalizations predict mortality in the community population with heart failure. *Am Heart J.* 2007;154:260-266.
14. Fonarow GC, Abraham WT, Albert NM, et al. Factors identified as precipitating hospital admissions for heart failure and clinical outcomes: findings from OPTIMIZE-HF. *Arch Intern Med.* 2008;168:847-854.
15. Cotter G, Felker GM, Adams KF, et al. The pathophysiology of acute heart failure--is it all about fluid accumulation? *Am Heart J.* 2008;155:9-18.
16. Cotter G, Metra M, Milo-Cotter O, et al. Fluid overload in acute heart failure--re-distribution and other mechanisms beyond fluid accumulation. *Eur J Heart Fail.* 2008;10:165-169.
17. Gheorghiade M, De Luca L, Fonarow GC, et al. Pathophysiologic targets in the early phase of acute heart failure syndromes. *Am J Cardiol.* 2005;96(6A):11G-17G.
18. Metra M, Cotter G, Davison BA, et al. Effect of serelaxin on cardiac, renal, and hepatic biomarkers in the Relaxin in Acute Heart Failure (RELAX-AHF) Development Program: correlation with outcomes. *J Am Coll Cardiol.* 2013;61:196-206.
19. Teerlink JR, Cotter G, Davison BA, et al. Serelaxin, recombinant human relaxin-2, for treatment of acute heart failure (RELAX-AHF): a randomised, placebo-controlled trial. *Lancet.* 2013;381:29-39.
20. Adams KF Jr, Fonarow GC, Emerman CL, et al. Characteristics and outcomes of patients hospitalized for heart failure in the United States: rationale, design, and preliminary observations from the first 100,000 cases in the Acute Decompensated Heart Failure National Registry (ADHERE). *Am Heart J.* 2005;149:209-216.
21. Cleland JG, Swedberg K, Follath F, et al. The EuroHeart Failure survey programme--a survey on the quality of care among patients with heart failure in Europe. Part 1: patient characteristics and diagnosis. *Eur Heart J.* 2003;24:442-463.
22. Nieminen MS, Brutsaert D, Dickstein K, et al. EuroHeart Failure Survey II (EHFS II): a survey on hospitalized acute heart failure patients: description of population. *Eur Heart J.* 2006;27:2725-2736.
23. Collins S, Storrow AB, Kirk JD, et al. Beyond pulmonary edema: diagnostic, risk stratification, and treatment challenges of acute heart failure management in the emergency department. *Ann Emerg Med.* 2008;51:45-57.
24. Gheorghiade M, Vaduganathan M, Ambrosy A, et al. Current management and future directions for the treatment of patients hospitalized for heart failure with low blood pressure. *Heart Fail Rev.* 2013;18:107-122.
25. Pang PS, Cleland JG, Teerlink JR, et al. A proposal to standardize dyspnoea measurement in clinical trials of acute heart failure syndromes: the need for a uniform approach. *Eur Heart J.* 2008;29:816-824.
26. Braunwald E, Bonow RO, Mann DL, et al, eds. *Braunwald's Heart Disease: A Textbook of Cardiovascular Medicine,* 9th ed. 2011; No. 1.
27. Wang CS, FitzGerald JM, Schulzer M, et al. Does this dyspneic patient in the emergency department have congestive heart failure? *JAMA.* 2005;294:1944-1956.
28. Gluecker T, Capasso P, Schnyder P, et al. Clinical and radiologic features of pulmonary edema. *Radiographics.*1999;19:1507-1533.
29. Mahdyoon H, Klein R, Eyler W, et al. Radiographic pulmonary congestion in end-stage congestive heart failure. *Am J Cardiol.* 1989;63:625-627.
30. Okin PM, Devereux RB, Nieminen MS, et al. Electrocardiographic strain pattern and prediction of new-onset congestive heart failure in hypertensive patients: the Losartan Intervention for Endpoint Reduction in Hypertension (LIFE) study. *Circulation.* 2006;113:67-73.

31. Piccini JP, Hernandez AF, Zhao X, et al. Quality of care for atrial fibrillation among patients hospitalized for heart failure. *J Am Coll Cardiol.* 2009;54:1280-1289.
32. Pang PS, Gheorghiade M. Special cases in acute heart failure syndromes: atrial fibrillation and wide complex tachycardia. *Heart Fail Clin.* 2009;5:113-123.
33. Volpicelli G, Elbarbary M, Blaivas M, et al. International evidence-based recommendations for point-of-care lung ultrasound. *Intensive Care Med.* 2012;38:577-591.
34. Gargani L, Frassi F, Soldati G, et al. Ultrasound lung comets for the differential diagnosis of acute cardiogenic dyspnoea: a comparison with natriuretic peptides. *Eur J Heart Fail.* 2008;10:70-77.
35. Secko MA, Lazar JM, Salciccioli LA, Stone MB. Can junior emergency physicians use E-point septal separation to accurately estimate left ventricular function in acutely dyspneic patients? *Acad Emerg Med.* 2011;18:1223-1226.
36. Maisel AS, Krishnaswamy P, Nowak RM, et al. Rapid measurement of B-type natriuretic peptide in the emergency diagnosis of heart failure. *N Engl J Med.* 2002;347:161-167.
37. Maisel A, Mueller C, Adams K Jr, et al. State of the art: using natriuretic peptide levels in clinical practice. *Eur J Heart Fail.* 2008;10:824-839.
38. Pang PS, Jesse R, Collins SP, Maisel A. Patients with acute heart failure in the emergency department: do they all need to be admitted? *J Card Fail.* 2012;18:900-903.
39. Heywood JT, Fonarow GC, Costanzo MR, et al. High prevalence of renal dysfunction and its impact on outcome in 118,465 patients hospitalized with acute decompensated heart failure: a report from the ADHERE database. *J Card Fail.* 2007;13:422-430.
40. Ronco C, Haapio M, House AA, et al. Cardiorenal syndrome. *J Am Coll Cardiol.* 2008;52:1527-1539.
41. Pang PS, Hoffmann U, Shah SJ. Classification of patients with acute heart failure syndromes in the emergency department. *Circ Heart Fail.* 2012;5:2-5.
42. Peacock WF, De Marco T, Fonarow GC, et al. Cardiac troponin and outcome in acute heart failure. *N Engl J Med.* 2008;358:2117-2126.
43. Flaherty JD, Bax JJ, De Luca L, et al. Acute heart failure syndromes in patients with coronary artery disease early assessment and treatment. *J Am Coll Cardiol.* 2009;53:254-263.
44. Flaherty JD, Rossi JS, Fonarow GC, et al. Influence of coronary angiography on the utilization of therapies in patients with acute heart failure syndromes: findings from Organized Program to Initiate Lifesaving Treatment in Hospitalized Patients with Heart Failure (OPTIMIZE-HF). *Am Heart J.* 2009;157:1018-1025.
45. Kociol RD, Pang PS, Gheorghiade M, et al. Troponin elevation in heart failure prevalence, mechanisms, and clinical implications. *J Am Coll Cardiol.* 2010;56:1071-1078.
46. Horwich TB, Patel J, MacLellan WR, Fonarow GC. Cardiac troponin I is associated with impaired hemodynamics, progressive left ventricular dysfunction, and increased mortality rates in advanced heart failure. *Circulation.* 2003;108:833-838.
47. Perna ER, Macin SM, Cimbaro Canella JP, et al. Minor myocardial damage detected by troponin T is a powerful predictor of long-term prognosis in patients with acute decompensated heart failure. *Int J Cardiol.* 2005;99:253-261.
48. Wang NC, Maggioni AP, Konstam MA, et al. Clinical implications of QRS duration in patients hospitalized with worsening heart failure and reduced left ventricular ejection fraction. *JAMA.* 2008;299:2656-2666.
49. Metra M, Nodari S, Parrinello G, et al. Worsening renal function in patients hospitalised for acute heart failure: clinical implications and prognostic significance. *Eur J Heart Fail.* 2008;10:188-195.
50. Smith GL, Lichtman JH, Bracken MB, et al. Renal impairment and outcomes in heart failure: systematic review and meta-analysis. *J Am Coll Cardiol.* 2006;47:1987-1996.
51. Smith GL, Vaccarino V, Kosiborod M, et al. Worsening renal function: what is a clinically meaningful change in creatinine during hospitalization with heart failure? *J Card Fail.* 2003;9:13-25.
52. Gheorghiade M, Abraham WT, Albert NM, et al. Relationship between admission serum sodium concentration and clinical outcomes in patients hospitalized for heart failure: an analysis from the OPTIMIZE-HF registry. *Eur Heart J.* 2007;28:980-988.
53. Gheorghiade M, Filippatos G, De Luca L, Burnett J. Congestion in acute heart failure syndromes: an essential target of evaluation and treatment. *Am J Med.* 2006;119:S3-S10.
54. Lucas C, Johnson W, Hamilton MA, et al. Freedom from congestion predicts good survival despite previous class IV symptoms of heart failure. *Am Heart J.* 2000;140:840-847.
55. Maisel AS, Peacock WF, McMullin N, et al. Timing of immunoreactive B-type natriuretic peptide levels and treatment delay in acute decompensated heart failure: an ADHERE (Acute Decompensated Heart Failure National Registry) analysis. *J Am Coll Cardiol.* 2008;52:534-540.
56. Binanay C, Califf RM, Hasselblad V, et al. Evaluation study of congestive heart failure and pulmonary artery catheterization effectiveness: the ESCAPE trial. *JAMA.* 2005;294:1625-1633.
57. Stevenson LW, Steimle AE, Fonarow G, et al. Improvement in exercise capacity of candidates awaiting heart transplantation. *J Am Coll Cardiol.* 1995;25:163-170.
58. Gheorghiade M, Konstam MA, Burnett JC Jr, et al. Short-term clinical effects of tolvaptan, an oral vasopressin antagonist, in patients hospitalized for heart failure: the EVEREST Clinical Status Trials. *JAMA.* 2007;297:1332-1343.
59. Konstam MA, Gheorghiade M, Burnett JC Jr, et al. Effects of oral tolvaptan in patients hospitalized for worsening heart failure: The EVEREST outcome trial. *JAMA.* 2007;297:1319-1331.
60. Klein L, Massie BM, Leimberger JD, et al. Admission or changes in renal function during hospitalization for worsening heart failure predict postdischarge survival: results from the Outcomes of a Prospective Trial of Intravenous Milrinione for Exacerbation of Chronic Heart Failure (OPTIME-CHF). *Circ Heart Fail.* 2008;1:25-33.
61. Metra M, Davison B, Bettari L, et al. Is worsening renal function an ominous prognostic sign in patients with acute heart failure? The role of congestion and its interaction with renal function. *Circ Heart Fail.* 2012;5:54-62.
62. Peacock W, Emerman C, Costanza M, et al. Acute heart failure mortality is dependent on time to intravenous vasoactive administration [abstract]. *J Card Fail.* 2006;12(6 suppl 1):S117.
63. Vital FM, Saconato H, Ladeira MT, et al. Non-invasive positive pressure ventilation (CPAP or bilevel NPPV) for cardiogenic pulmonary edema. *Cochrane Database Syst Rev.* 2008(3):CD005351.
64. Gray A, Goodacre S, Newby DE, et al. Noninvasive ventilation in acute cardiogenic pulmonary edema. *N Engl J Med.* 2008;359:142-151.
65. McMurray JJ, Adamopoulos S, Anker SD, et al. ESC Guidelines for the diagnosis and treatment of acute and chronic heart failure 2012: The Task Force for the Diagnosis and Treatment of Acute and Chronic Heart Failure 2012 of the European Society of Cardiology. Developed in collaboration with the Heart Failure Association (HFA) of the ESC. *Eur Heart J.* 2012;33:1787-1847.
66. Cotter G, Metzkor E, Kaluski E, et al. Randomised trial of high-dose isosorbide dinitrate plus low-dose furosemide versus high-dose furosemide plus low-dose isosorbide dinitrate in severe pulmonary oedema. *Lancet.* 1998;351:389-393.
67. Levy P, Compton S, Welch R, et al. Treatment of severe decompensated heart failure with high-dose intravenous nitroglycerin: a feasibility and outcome analysis. *Ann Emerg Med.* 2007;50:144-152.
68. Sackner-Bernstein J, Kowalski M, Fox M, Aaronson K. Short-term risk of death after treatment with nesiritide for decompensated heart failure. *JAMA.* 2005;293:1900-1905.
69. Sackner-Bernstein JD, Skopicki HA, Aaronson KD. Risk of worsening renal function with nesiritide in patients with acutely decompensated heart failure. *Circulation.* 2005;111:1487-1491.
70. VMAC Investigators. Intravenous nesiritide vs nitroglycerin for treatment of decompensated congestive heart failure: a randomized controlled trial. *JAMA.* 2002;287:1531-1540.
71. O'Connor CM, Starling RC, Hernandez AF, et al. Effect of nesiritide in patients with acute decompensated heart failure. *N Engl J Med.* 2011;365:32-43.
72. Peacock WF. Initial results from the PROACTION study. *J Emerg Med.* 2006;31:435-436.
73. Konstam MA, Pang PS, Gheorghiade M. Seeking new heights in acute heart failure syndromes: lessons from ASCEND and EVEREST. *Eur Heart J.* 2013;34:1345-1349.
74. Mullens W, Abrahams Z, Francis GS, et al. Sodium nitroprusside for advanced low-output heart failure. *J Am Coll Cardiol.* 2008;52:200-207.
75. Silvers SM, Howell JM, Kosowsky JM, Rokos IC, Jagoda AS, American College of Emergency Physicians. Clinical policy: Critical issues in the evaluation and management of adult patients presenting to the emergency department with acute heart failure syndromes. *Ann Emerg Med.* 2007;49:627-669.
76. Felker GM, Lee KL, Bull DA, et al. Diuretic strategies in patients with acute decompensated heart failure. *N Engl J Med.* 2011;364:797-805.
77. Felker GM, O'Connor CM, Braunwald E, Heart Failure Clinical Research Network I. Loop diuretics in acute decompensated heart failure: necessary? Evil? A necessary evil? *Circ Heart Fail.* 2009;2:56-62.
78. Adams JKF, Fonarow GC, Emerman CL, et al. Characteristics and outcomes of patients hospitalized for heart failure in the United States: rationale, design, and preliminary observations from the first 100,000 cases in the Acute Decompensated Heart Failure National Registry (ADHERE). *Am Heart J.* 2005;149:209-216.
79. Gheorghiade M, Pang PS. Acute heart failure syndromes. *J Am Coll Cardiol.* 2009;53:557-573.
80. Felker GM, O'Connor CM. Inotropic therapy for heart failure: an evidence-based approach. *Am Heart J.* 2001;142:393-401.
81. Bayram M, De Luca L, Massie MB, Gheorghiade M. Reassessment of dobutamine, dopamine, and milrinone in the management of acute heart failure syndromes. *Am J Cardiol.* 2005;96(6A):47G-58G.
82. Aranda JM, Jr., Schofield RS, Pauly DF, et al. Comparison of dobutamine versus milrinone therapy in hospitalized patients awaiting cardiac transplantation: a prospective, randomized trial. *Am Heart J.* 2003;145:324-329.

83. Ungar A, Fumagalli S, Marini M, et al. Renal, but not systemic, hemodynamic effects of dopamine are influenced by the severity of congestive heart failure. *Crit Care Med.* 2004;32:1125-1129.
84. Elkayam U, Ng TM, Hatamizadeh P, et al. Renal vasodilatory action of dopamine in patients with heart failure: magnitude of effect and site of action. *Circulation.* 2008;117:200-205.
85. Giamouzis G, Butler J, Starling RC, et al. Impact of dopamine infusion on renal function in hospitalized heart failure patients: results of the Dopamine in Acute Decompensated Heart Failure (DAD-HF) Trial. *J Card Fail.* 2010;16:922-930.
86. De Backer D, Biston P, Devriendt J, et al. Comparison of dopamine and norepinephrine in the treatment of shock. *N Engl J Med.* 2010;362:779-789.
87. Felker GM, Benza RL, Chandler AB, et al. Heart failure etiology and response to milrinone in decompensated heart failure: results from the OPTIME-CHF study. *J Am Coll Cardiol.* 2003;41:997-1003.
88. Peacock WF, Hollander JE, Diercks DB, et al. Morphine for acute decompensated heart failure: valuable adjunct or a historical remnant? *Acad Emerg Med.* 2005;12(5 suppl 1):97-98.
89. Peacock WF, Hollander JE, Diercks DB, et al. Morphine and outcomes in acute decompensated heart failure: an ADHERE analysis. *Emerg Med J.* 2008;25:205-209.
90. Joynt KE, Jha AK. Thirty-day readmissions--truth and consequences. *N Engl J Med.* 2012;366:1366-1369.
91. Collins SP, Pang PS, Fonarow GC, et al. Is hospital admission for heart failure really necessary? The role of the emergency department and observation unit in preventing hospitalization and rehospitalization. *J Am Coll Cardiol.* 2013;61:121-126.
92. Lee DS, Schull MJ, Alter DA, et al. Early deaths in patients with heart failure discharged from the emergency department: a population-based analysis. *Circ Heart Fail.* 2010;3:228-235.
93. Collins SP, Lindsell CJ, Jenkins CA, et al. Risk stratification in acute heart failure: rationale and design of the STRATIFY and DECIDE studies. *Am Heart J.* 2012;164:825-834.
94. Collins SP, Storrow AB. Acute heart failure risk stratification: can we define low risk? *Heart Fail Clin.* 2009;5:75-83.

CARDIOVASCULAR EMERGENCIES

CHAPTER 8

Bradyarrhythmias

Emily Damuth and Tyler W. Barrett

IN THIS CHAPTER

Recognition of clinically significant bradyarrhythmias

Initial stabilization and management

Pathophysiology

Treatment strategies

Transcutaneous and transvenous pacing

Special causes and their treatment

A resting heart rate of 30 to 40 beats/min might be a goal for emergency physicians devoted to their aerobic health, but that same heart rate in many of our patients can result in significant morbidity and mortality. An inexperienced clinician might underestimate this potentially lethal arrhythmia, thinking that treating bradyarrhythmia in a symptomatic individual is as easy as speeding up the heart rate. Bradyarrhythmias do not have a single cause that can be treated with atropine alone; they arise from a multitude of conduction system abnormalities that require different treatments to restore adequate cardiac output. A physician who neglects to carefully diagnose and treat the underlying cause of the bradyarrhythmia could be the only person in the room whose heart rate increases while the patient decompensates.

Patients with life-threatening bradyarrhythmias often present to the emergency department with ambiguous or vague symptoms such as fatigue or light-headedness. Therefore, it is up to the astute clinician to recognize these subtle presentations and accurately identify the underlying bradyarrhythmia to prevent rapid hemodynamic decompensation.

This chapter provides a framework for recognition of bradyarrhythmias caused by disordered impulse generation (eg, sinus node dysfunction, sinus bradycardia, and exit block) as well as pathologic impulse conduction (atrioventricular [AV] nodal blocks). Emphasis will be placed on differentiating benign bradycardic rhythms from those at risk for progression to cardiogenic shock or arrest.

Initial Stabilization and Management

Although the causes of bradyarrhythmias are innumerable, the initial resuscitation of the patient with symptomatic bradycardia is guided by a single systematic approach. The hallmark of this approach is prioritization of airway and breathing stabilization along with concurrent establishment of large-bore (ie, 14-16 gauge) intravenous access, continuous cardiac monitoring, and placement of defibrillator pads. Once a pulse is confirmed and the patient's circulatory condition permits further assessment, the telemetry monitor and the electrocardiogram (ECG) assume key roles in the rapid diagnosis of bradyarrhythmias.

Initial treatment decisions for patients with bradyarrhythmias are determined by the individual's clinical stability, specifically the presence of hypoperfusion and propensity of the bradyarrhythmia to decompensate to hemodynamic instability. Clinical presentations of bradyarrhythmias vary from an incidental finding in an asymptomatic, trained athlete to cardiovascular collapse in a critically ill patient. In the symptomatic bradycardic patient with syncope, altered mental status, acutely decompensated heart failure, angina, or cardiogenic shock, first-line treatment is rapid intravenous administration of atropine, 0.5 to 1 mg every 3 to 5 minutes to a maximum dose of 3 mg.[1]

Therapeutic vagolysis from atropine administration should be used with caution in the setting of coronary ischemia to avoid increasing myocardial oxygen consumption. In addition, atropine will be ineffective in patients with high-grade AV block at a level below the AV node, as well as in patients who have undergone cardiac transplantation because of surgical cardiac denervation. In these scenarios, pacing and beta-agonists should be used preferentially. Norepinephrine, dopamine, or isoproterenol may be administered as second-line therapy for inotropic or chronotropic effects (Table 8-1). In the bradycardic and hypotensive patient with suspected left ventricular dysfunction, norepinephrine or dopamine would be preferred over isoproterenol to increase inotropy with less vasodilatory effect.

Symptomatic bradyarrhythmias unresponsive to pharmacotherapy require transcutaneous pacing as a bridge to temporary transvenous pacemaker placement. Once a patient's respiratory status and hemodynamic status are stabilized, a complete history, review of current medications, head-to-toe physical examination, and diagnostic studies should be performed to determine the reversibility and proper treatment of the underlying bradyarrhythmia. Time is of the essence in the management of hemodynamically significant bradycardia: the mortality rate reaches 16% in the outpatient setting and 5% in the emergency department.[1] A thorough understanding of normal cardiac conduction is important for the clinician to understand the pathophysiology and appropriate treatment of cardiac conduction disorders.

KEY POINTS

When evaluating the bradycardic patient, quickly assess for signs of hypoperfusion and hemodynamic stability.

Treat the patient's clinical appearance rather than reflexively reacting to the heart rate or ECG rhythm.

Verify the heart rate reported on the cardiac monitor by auscultating with your stethoscope or palpating the carotid pulse.

Important questions to ask:

  Does the examination reveal evidence of hypoperfusion (eg, syncope, altered mental status, angina, decompensated heart failure, or shock)?

  How rapidly is the patient becoming hemodynamically unstable?

  Do I have time to perform and review a 12-lead ECG, or does the patient's airway, breathing, or circulation (ABCs) require immediate intervention?

Normal Cardiac Conduction

The sinuatrial (SA) node serves as the dominant pacemaker during normal conduction, with a discharge rate of 60 to 100 beats/min. The SA node is located at the junction of the right atrium and the superior vena cava and receives blood supply from the SA nodal artery, which arises from the right coronary artery in 60% of the population and the left circumflex artery in the other 40%. The SA nodal impulse depolarizes the atria prior to reaching the AV node, where conduction is delayed to allow atrial contraction and ventricular filling. The long refractory period of the AV node also reduces the rate of ventricular depolarization in supraventricular tachycardia. Conduction can become pathologically prolonged at the level of the AV node, as seen in first-degree AV block, represented by a prolonged PR interval (>200 msec) on a 12-lead ECG. The AV nodal artery supplies the AV node and arises from the right coronary artery in 90% of individuals, with the remaining 10% supplied by the left circumflex artery.[2] The cardiac impulse exits the AV node via the rapidly conducting His-Purkinje system, which depolarizes the ventricular myocardium. In Wenckebach block, conduction delay occurs at the level of the AV node, producing PR prolongation prior to a nonconducted atrial impulse. Mobitz II second-degree AV block, on the other hand, occurs below the AV node and leads to abrupt failure of atrioventricular conduction without preceding PR interval prolongation.

Basic Electrophysiology

The concepts of the action potential might seem relegated to basic science, but they are extremely important when considering the various pharmacologic treatments for bradyarrhythmias For example, consider the bradycardic patient with life-threatening hyperkalemia. Hyperkalemia decreases the difference between myocyte resting potential and threshold potential, making cells more excitable. This occurs because restoration of the cardiac cell resting membrane potential requires potassium efflux and is therefore impaired by hyperkalemia and potentiated by hypocalcemia. Therefore, to treat hyperkalemia-associated bradyarrhythmias, potassium must be pharmacologically

TABLE 8-1.

Vasoactive Medications

Medication	Intropy (beta$_1$)	Chronotropy (beta$_1$)	Vasoconstriction (alpha$_1$)	Vasodilation (beta$_2$)
Dopamine	+++	++	++	+
Isoproterenol	+++	+++	None	+++
Norepinephrine	++	++	+++	None
Epinephrine	+++	+++	+++	++

shifted to the intracellular space and calcium should be administered to restore the cardiac cell's ability to generate an action potential.

Three types of cardiac cells assume distinct roles during electrical excitation. Pacemaker cells exhibit automaticity, meaning they are capable of spontaneous depolarization. His-Purkinje cells rapidly conduct these impulses and have no inherent automaticity. Finally, depolarization of the cardiac myocytes produces mechanical contraction of the atria and ventricles. While the SA and AV nodal pacemaker cells typically initiate depolarization, all of the cardiac cells are capable of assuming this pacemaker cell function. Even cardiac myocytes can display automaticity under pathologic conditions such as ischemia through altered membrane ion channel permeability. The sinus node typically suppresses AV pacemaker generation because the discharge rate exceeds that of the AV node, which in turn fires faster than ventricular myocytes.

An action potential is created when electrical stimulation of cardiac cells alters the resting ionic concentration gradient across the cell membrane. At rest, potassium channels of the cardiac myocyte open while sodium and calcium channels remain closed, allowing the cell interior to generate a negative charge as potassium flows outward down its concentration gradient. This outward positive flow ultimately produces a stable negative resting potential during phase 4 of the action potential. Alteration of this membrane potential triggers a rapid upstroke, or phase 0, of the action potential, as sodium ions move inward and depolarize the myocyte. Repolarization quickly follows in phase 1, where potassium efflux returns the membrane potential to neutral. Phase 2 of the action potential represents further repolarization caused by persistent outward potassium current balanced by inward movement of calcium. During phase 3, potassium efflux surpasses calcium influx, restoring the negative resting membrane potential of phase 4 and terminating repolarization.[3]

Pathologic bradycardia can result from metabolic disturbances or medications capable of altering membrane permeability. For example, quinidine and procainamide can cause pathologic bradycardia through their sodium-channel blocking effects in addition to prolongation of the QT interval. Sodium bicarbonate or magnesium therapy may be given to enhance sodium channel recovery. Similarly, digoxin not only directly suppresses AV nodal conduction but also increases myocardial contractility by inhibiting sodium-potassium pumps, which transiently increases intracellular sodium concentration and calcium influx. Therefore, understanding the physiology of the action potential enhances management of these and other bradyarrhythmias.

Mechanisms of Bradyarrhythmias

Bradyarrhythmias arise when either the generation or conduction of an atrial impulse is disordered.[2] Impaired conduction can occur at the level of the SA node, AV node, or His-Purkinje system. Innervation of the SA and AV nodes is both parasympathetic and sympathetic in origin, so the baseline tone is dictated by the dominant autonomic influence.

Causes of bradyarrhythmias can be broadly categorized as intrinsic or extrinsic (Table 8-2). Intrinsic causes include any primary abnormality of the cardiac conduction system or automaticity and include conditions that infiltrate or disrupt the myocardium such as sarcoidosis and amyloid, myocarditis, and ischemic disease.[1] The most common causes of bradyarrhythmias are extrinsic and include excessive vagal tone, hypoxemia, electrolyte derangement (eg, hyperkalemia, hypokalemia, and hypomagnesemia), and medication side effects or toxicity.[4]

Specific Bradyarrhythmias: Diagnosis and Treatment

Disorders of Impulse Generation

Sinus Node Dysfunction. Sinus node dysfunction (also called sick sinus syndrome) comprises a variety of disorders of impulse formation and conduction in the sinus node and atria, including sinus arrest, sinus exit block, sinus bradycardia, and chronotropic incompetence. Sinus node dysfunction can also be associated with susceptibility to paroxysmal supraventricular tachyarrhythmias, as seen with tachycardia-bradycardia syndrome. Patients with tachycardia-bradycardia syndrome will have episodes of rapid atrial fibrillation, atrial flutter, reentrant supraventricular tachycardia, and junctional tachycardia as well as episodes of bradycardia. The bradycardia is a manifestation of an impaired conduction system. Patients with sinus node

TABLE 8-2.
Causes of Bradycardia

Intrinsic	Extrinsic
Myocardial ischemia	Hypothermia
Infection (viral myocarditis, Lyme disease)	Hypoxia
Inflammatory (collagen vascular disease)	Hypoadrenalism
Idiopathic	Hypothyroidism
Trauma	Hyperkalemia/hypokalemia
Postsurgical	Drugs (antipsychotics, antiarrhythmics)
	Autonomic (vasovagal)

dysfunction may experience bradycardia or prolonged pauses following the pharmacologic or electrical cardioversion of supraventricular tachycardia as a result of the impaired sinus node's failure to recover its normal pacing function. Permanent atrial fibrillation has been shown to cause damage to the SA node and has been associated with progression to symptomatic bradycardia requiring pacemaker placement.[5] Sinus node dysfunction typically occurs in older patients, where SA nodal automaticity is lost secondary to nodal degeneration, fibrosis, infiltration, inflammation, ischemia, or cardiomyopathy.[6] Sinus node dysfunction can also be seen in younger patients with extrinsic influences such as excessive vagal tone, abnormal electrolytes, or medication side effects (eg, toxicity from beta-blockers, calcium channel blockers, clonidine, lithium, digoxin, and amiodarone).

Individuals with sinus node dysfunction have progressive deterioration of sinus node conduction. As a result, they can present to the emergency department with symptoms varying in severity along a spectrum from asymptomatic sinus bradycardia to prolonged sinus arrest requiring emergent pacing. Most patients who experience syncope from sinus bradycardia or pauses are likely to have recurrent symptoms because of the natural history of the disease to progress to node dysfunction.[7] Once hemodynamic stability is achieved, the diagnostic evaluation and treatment should target reversible causes such as electrolyte supplementation, with particular attention to potassium and magnesium. Drug levels (eg, digoxin) should be measured, and antidotes administered for nodal depressant agents, including beta-blockers, calcium channel blockers, lithium, and digoxin. Symptomatic sinus node dysfunction often requires permanent pacing and actually accounts for half of pacemaker implantations in the United States.[8] Therefore, preparation for temporary pacing should be prioritized in conjunction with close hemodynamic monitoring.

KEY POINT

Be wary of elderly patients with bradycardia or sinus pauses after termination of supraventricular tachyarrhythmia. They are at high risk for prolonged sinus arrest.

Sinus Bradycardia. Although classically defined by a heart rate less than 60 beats/min, the presence of symptoms rather than the rate itself determines the pathogenicity of sinus bradycardia. Therapy is reserved for patients with evidence of hypoperfusion, manifested by light-headedness, orthostasis, syncope, altered mental status, focal neurologic deficits, angina, or acutely decompensated heart failure. The causes of bradycardia are innumerable and can be organized as intrinsic or extrinsic in etiology (Table 8-2). Many pathophysiologic states that depress automaticity of the sinus node can be treated by withdrawing the offending agent, administering an antidote, or correcting the underlying cause. For example, severe hypothermia slows impulse conduction through cardiac myocyte potassium channels, which can be reversed with rewarming. Other causes of bradycardia are autonomic, such as the reflex response to hypoxia or increased intracranial pressure.

Atropine is effective in treating hemodynamic compromise if the cause of the instability is rate related. Dopamine or epinephrine infusions can be used as temporizing measures in patients with refractory symptomatic sinus bradycardia while preparation is made for temporary pacing. Consider using norepinephrine infusion for patients requiring adrenergic support in the setting of cardiogenic shock. A subgroup analysis of a large multicenter randomized clinical trial found that the rate of death at 28 days was significantly higher among patients with undifferentiated cardiogenic shock who were treated with dopamine than among those treated with norepinephrine.[9] The trial did not report whether the patients with cardiogenic shock had clinically significant bradycardia or tachycardia.[9] Therefore, dopamine may still be the preferred treatment for patients with cardiogenic shock specifically associated with bradycardia. Permanent pacing is reasonable for symptomatic patients with irreversible causes or symptomatic sinus bradycardia secondary to drug therapy required to manage medical conditions.[7]

Sinus Exit Block. The presentation of sinus exit block can be subtle but nonetheless extremely important to recognize, as it can signify a toxic ingestion or failed conduction from the SA node to the perinodal atrial tissue. In sinus exit block, life-threatening pauses can occur when the conduction of an SA nodal impulse is blocked in the surrounding atria. Similar to blockade at the AV nodal level, sinus exit block is classified into three types. First-degree SA block occurs when initiation of the SA nodal impulse is delayed, which cannot be detected on a surface ECG. In second-degree SA block, both the P wave and associated QRS complex are dropped. Finally, third-degree SA block is characterized by complete absence of P waves, which cannot be distinguished from sinus arrest on a 12-lead ECG.

In severe cases of sinus exit block or sinus arrest, the escape rhythms of ectopic pacemakers might be delayed or inadequate, and the patient presents with clinically significant hypotension. At-risk populations for sinus exit block include elderly patients with sinus node dysfunction; athletes with high vagal tone; patients with inferior myocardial infarction (MI), myocarditis, or vagal stimulation from pain; and those taking beta-blockers, calcium channel blockers, amiodarone, quinidine, or digoxin.

Management begins with recognition of sinus pauses on telemetry or the ECG. The presence of symptomatic pauses longer than 3 seconds or asymptomatic pauses longer than 5 seconds requires treatment.[7] Atropine can augment the SA nodal discharge rate; however, persistent symptomatic pauses necessitate temporary pacing and admission to a critical care unit.[8]

Sinus Arrest. In contrast to sinus exit block, sinus arrest represents failed generation of an SA nodal impulse, rather than blocked conduction to the surrounding atria. Sinus arrest and sinus exit block can both be observed in the setting of toxicity from nodal suppressant agents or as a consequence of ischemia, usually from right coronary artery occlusion. Vagolysis and temporary pacing are reserved for symptomatic sinus pauses. The ECG presented as Figure 8-1 is an example of sinus arrest with no sinus activity (absent P waves and ventricular escape rhythm).

Bradyarrhythmias

> **KEY POINT**
>
> In the patient with prolonged sinus pauses, prepare for temporary pacing immediately by placing defibrillator pads early in the emergency department course. Patients with sinus node failure are likely to progress to hemodynamic instability.

Disorders of Impulse Conduction

Atrioventricular Block. In the normal heart, a physiologic delay in conduction occurs at the AV node, represented by the length of the PR interval, which prevents an uncontrolled ventricular response to supraventricular tachyarrhythmias and allows adequate time for ventricular filling. However, in pathologic AV block, this delay can become prolonged or cause intermittent or even complete failure of AV conduction. AV block is commonly associated with electrolyte abnormalities (ie, hypokalemia and hypomagnesemia); myocardial ischemia or infarction; cardiac surgery; or beta-blocker, calcium channel blocker, amiodarone, or lithium therapy. The 12-lead ECG can help differentiate the location of AV block, which largely determines the clinical significance of the disease. AV block can occur anywhere along the AV nodal complex, including the node itself or the infranodal conduction fibers that make up the bundle of His. Adequate function of the nodal complex depends on adequate right coronary artery perfusion, local parasympathetic tone, and integrity of the conduction fibers.

First-degree AV block is a delay in AV conduction, but all atrial impulses successfully depolarize the ventricle, which is seen as prolongation of the PR interval. Second-degree block at the level of the AV node, typically referred to as Wenckebach, is seen as progressive prolongation of the PR interval prior to total failure of AV node conduction for a single ventricular beat. Following the failed conducted beat, the AV node conduction improves and the PR interval is often normal. This cycle is recurrent, with varying numbers of conducted beats successively lengthening the PR interval prior to the dropped beat.

In contrast to conduction disturbances involving the AV node, diseased infranodal tissues will abruptly fail to conduct, rather showing progressive delay in conduction. The PR interval remains normal for conducted beats. To help identify the location of AV block, examine the regularity of the ventricular response. First- and third-degree AV blocks are regular, and second-degree AV blocks, either nodal or infranodal, are irregular.

It is important to distinguish diseases affecting the AV node from those affecting infranodal tissues because the causes, treatment, and prognosis are very different, as discussed below. Disease in the AV nodal complex can result in either second- or third-degree heart block, but the specific location will determine the likelihood of progression to complete heart block, the reliability of the escape rhythm, and ultimately the need for treatment. Complete AV block resulting from infranodal disease is associated with a distal escape rhythm that is slower (<40 beats/min) and less consistent than block at the level of the AV node.[2]

> **KEY POINTS**
>
> Questions to ask to differentiate the types of AV block:
>
> Is the rhythm regular or irregular?
>
>   Regular (first-degree, fixed second- and third-degree AV block)
>
>   Irregular (second-degree AV block)
>
> Is the QRS complex wide or narrow?

FIGURE 8-1.

Sinus arrest with no sinus activity (absent P waves and ventricular escape rhythm)

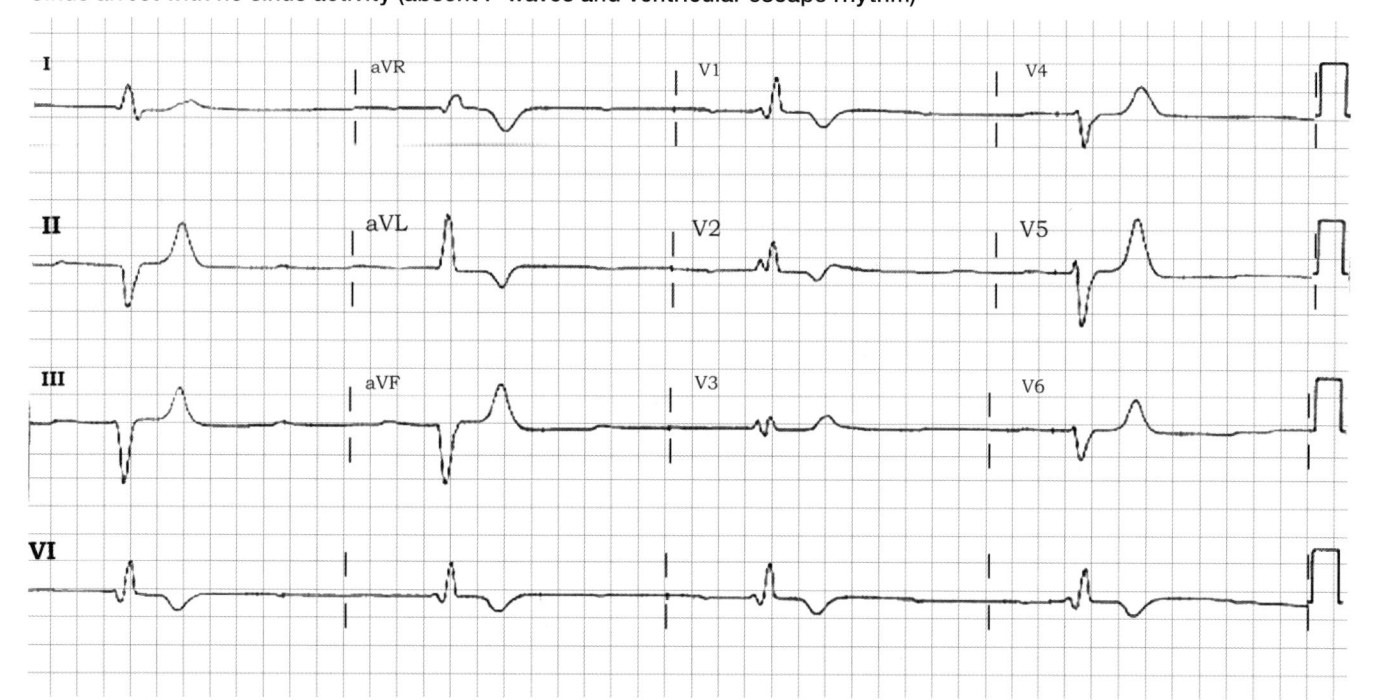

Narrow (first-degree, second-degree Mobitz I, third-degree AV block with junctional escape)

Wide (second-degree Mobitz II AV block, third-degree AV block with ventricular escape)

CASE ONE

A 64-year-old man with a history of hypertension and chronic renal insufficiency is transported to the emergency department via emergency medical services (EMS) following a syncopal event at home. The patient remembers becoming diaphoretic and nauseated about 90 minutes after taking his blood pressure medication. His wife called 911 after finding him unresponsive and bleeding from his scalp. In the emergency department, his blood pressure is 89/47 mm Hg, his heart rate is 69 beats/min, and oxygen saturation is adequate on room air. An ECG is obtained (Figure 8-2).

CASE ONE CONCLUSION

When questioned further about his antihypertensive regimen, the patient admitted that he had not filled the prescription for metoprolol, 100 mg twice daily, that his nephrologist gave him 3 weeks ago. At his primary care appointment the day prior to the emergency department presentation, the patient was persistently hypertensive, so the dosage of metoprolol had been doubled to 200 mg twice daily, because the doctor assumed he was taking the dose prescribed by the nephrologist. The patient then had the new prescription filled and took the higher dose for the first time on the morning of presentation. The patient's emergency department course was uneventful. He was admitted to telemetry for further monitoring after repair of his occipital scalp laceration. His PR interval narrowed gradually throughout the day and, he was discharged home the next day on a reduced dose of beta-blocker.

First-Degree AV Block. First-degree AV block represents an exaggeration of the physiologic delay at the level of the AV node, which allows adequate time for atrial contraction and ventricular filling. This arrhythmia is usually characterized by a regular, narrow rhythm with a constant prolongation of the PR interval greater than 200 msec. First-degree AV block is usually seen as a pharmacologic side effect in patients on beta-blocker, calcium channel blocker, or digoxin therapy but can also be observed in the setting of intrinsic AV nodal disease, inferior MI, myocarditis, or enhanced vagal tone. Because each atrial impulse is still propagated, first-degree AV block is typically considered a benign arrhythmia. Although typically not hemodynamically compromising, first-degree AV block could be a clue to pharmacologic toxicity (eg, involving beta-blockers, amiodarone, or digoxin) or a sign of intrinsic cardiac degeneration or disease.

First-degree AV block can become hemodynamically significant if the PR prolongation becomes severe (>300 msec), which causes the ventricular preload, and ultimately cardiac output, to fall when atrial systole occurs too early during atrial diastole. Therefore, pacing might be required if marked PR prolongation leads to AV dyssynchrony, producing symptoms resembling pacemaker-associated AV dysynchrony.[10]

KEY POINT

Although generally considered benign in the acute setting, first-degree AV block has been reported to double the risk for atrial fibrillation, triple the risk for future pacemaker implantation, and moderately increase the risk of all-cause mortality.[10]

Second-Degree AV Block. In second-degree AV block,

FIGURE 8-2.

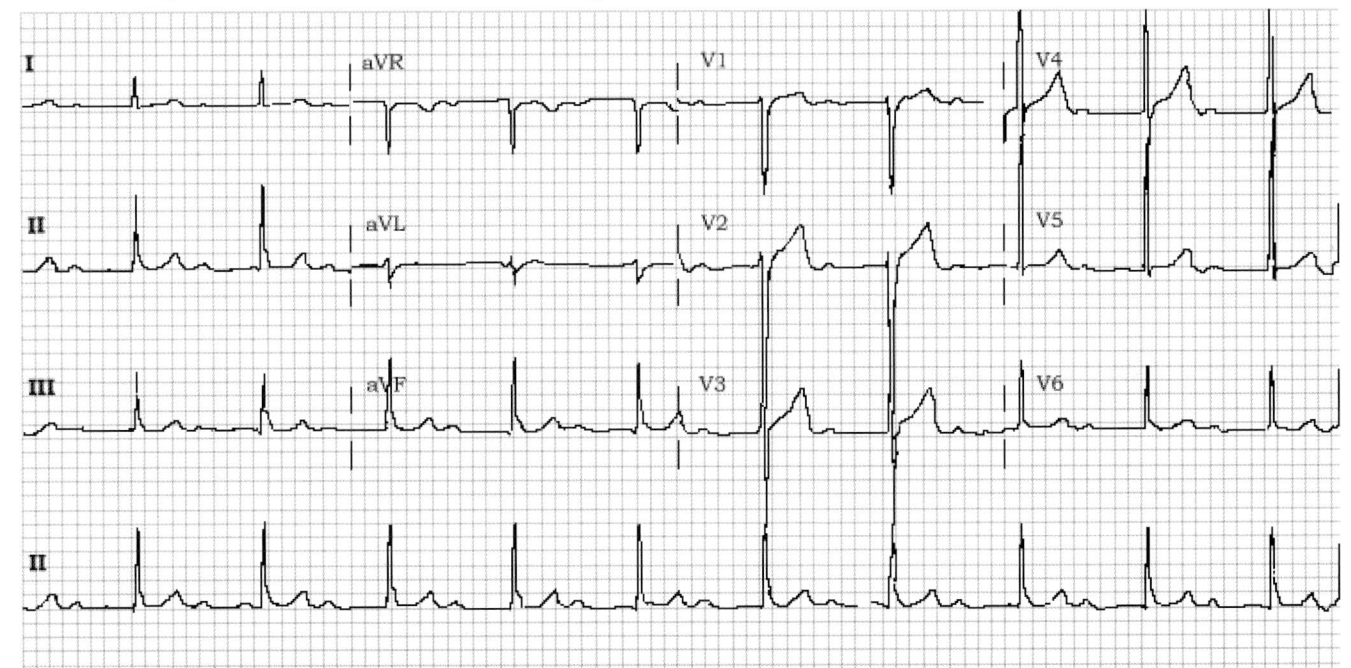

ECG from the patient described in Case One: first-degree AV block

atrial impulses are not consistently conducted to the ventricle, because of disease within the AV node or infranodal tissues. Therefore, a 12-lead ECG demonstrates some P waves that are not followed by a QRS complex. Second-degree AV block is subclassified into two types, which can be differentiated by the constancy of the PR interval and the width of the QRS complex. In Mobitz I second-degree AV block (or Wenckebach), the disease is within the AV node itself, which manifests on the ECG as progressive lengthening of the PR interval. The QRS complex remains narrow because the conduction distal to the AV node is normal. In contrast, Mobitz II AV block is characterized by disease in the conduction tissues distal to the AV node, the His and Purkinje fibers. AV nodal conduction is normal, so the PR interval on the ECG is also normal. The diseased conduction fibers will abruptly fail to conduct a delivered atrial impulse to the ventricle, which is seen as a nonconducted P wave. Because the disease often involves the fibers that constitute the conduction bundles, there is often a co-existing fixed bundle-branch block that produces a widened QRS complex (>120 msec). Intermittent failure of the remaining bundle results in the nonconducted beats. If AV block occurs in a fixed 2:1 interval, the two types of second-degree block cannot be distinguished reliably without an electrophysiology study. However, the width of the QRS complex could help differentiate Mobitz I and II, even in the presence of fixed block.

The location of the block is particularly important, because if the conduction block progresses to third degree, the site of origin of the ventricular escape rhythm (AV node, His bundle, or below the His bundle), rather than the rate itself, determines its stability. The poor automaticity of the His bundle and ventricular tissue makes infranodal escape rhythms generated below or within the His bundle extremely unreliable.

KEY POINT

In general, the more distal the site of block, the slower the escape rhythm. Ventricular pacemakers typically have a rate of 40 beats/min or less, which can lead to insufficient cardiac output and syncope.

CASE TWO

A 38-year-old woman went to a local urgent care center, complaining of subjective fever, productive cough, nasal congestion, and left-sided chest wall pain that she felt only when she coughed or twisted her torso. Several family members had recently had flu-like illnesses. The woman is an avid marathoner and has no chronic medical problems. She has no family history of sudden cardiac death, acute coronary syndrome, or thromboembolic disease. At the urgent care center, a chest radiograph and an ECG were obtained. The radiograph was reported to be normal, leading to the diagnosis of bronchitis and a recommendation for supportive care. However, her ECG (Figure 8-3) was abnormal, so she was instructed to go to the emergency department immediately for evaluation.

CASE TWO CONCLUSION

This patient's ECG shows a sinus rhythm with Mobitz type I (Wenckebach) conduction with a ventricular rate of 63 and no other pathology. This young woman has an incidental finding of Mobitz I without any symptoms. She has not experienced a decrease in exercise tolerance or symptoms likely attributed to an arrhythmia. Her chest wall pain seems most consistent with musculoskeletal pain secondary to coughing. She does not need to be evaluated by a cardiologist in the emergency department and can follow up with her primary care physician for addi-

FIGURE 8-3.

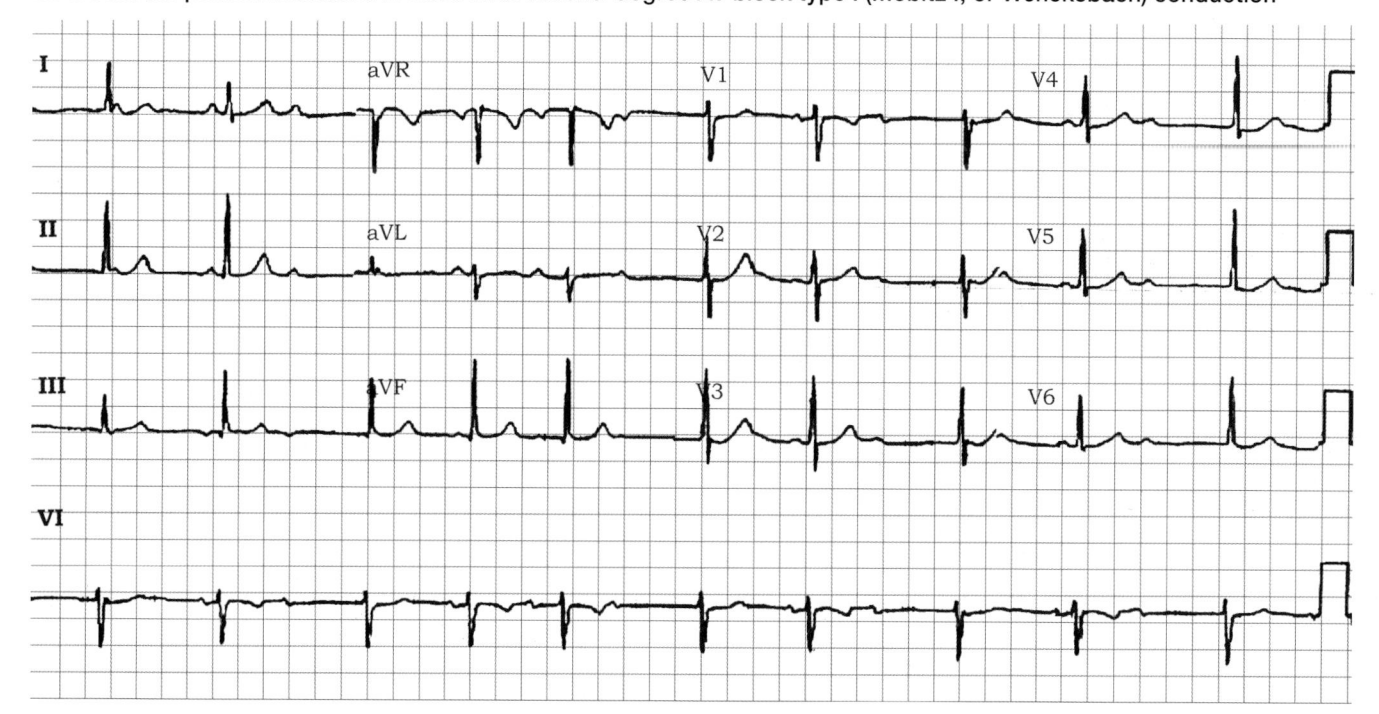

ECG from the patient described in Case Two: second-degree AV block type I (Mobitz I, or Wenckebach) conduction

tional evaluation, which could involve 7-day Holter monitoring and cardiology referral. The patient's arrhythmia is probably secondary to her cardiovascular training as a runner, which produces high vagal tone capable of slowing AV conduction.

The need for pacing in AV block is largely determined by the presence of symptoms in addition to the location of the block. Wenckebach (Mobitz I) AV block is considered a benign arrhythmia because it is usually self-limited and rarely progresses to high-grade AV block. Persistent symptomatic AV block represents an indication for permanent pacemaker placement and temporary pacing in the emergency department.[7]

CASE THREE

A 77-year-old man was visiting a friend in the hospital. When he tried to get up from a chair, he suddenly passed out. He had transient loss of consciousness and a normal blood glucose concentration. He is brought to the emergency department for evaluation. He is alert but responds to questions and verbal commands slowly. He feels nauseated and short of breath but is not experiencing chest pain. He has a history of hypertension and is taking a diuretic and a beta-blocker. He takes no other medications and has not had any recent medication changes. He has not been diagnosed with coronary artery disease. His blood pressure is 88/50 mm Hg and his heart rate is in the 30s. His ECG is shown in Figure 8-4.

CASE THREE CONCLUSION

This patient's ECG showed a sinus rhythm with high-degree Mobitz type II AV block with 3:1 conduction. He had an underlying left bundle-branch block and left atrial abnormality, and his ventricular rate was 32 beats/min. The patient was hypotensive and symptomatic and required emergent treatment, including management of his ABCs and preparation for pacing. Atropine may be considered for this patient and often is given empirically in the prehospital setting; however, his left bundle branch suggests infranodal conduction disease that would not respond to atropine. Atropine can increase the sinus rate and myocardial oxygen requirements in a patient with already impaired perfusion. Transcutaneous pacing would be a preferred option in this patient, since he is at increased risk for progressing to complete heart block. Reversible causes should be evaluated but, given this patient's age and comorbidities, he has significant conduction system disease and will need a permanent pacemaker.

Identification of Mobitz II second-degree block is particularly crucial in the emergency department population, because this bradyarrhythmia can progress suddenly to complete heart block without warning. Therefore, in contrast to Mobitz I AV block, identification of Mobitz II necessitates admission for possible permanent pacemaker placement, even in the absence of symptoms, unless the cause is rapidly reversible.[7] Reversible causes of AV block include electrolyte abnormalities, hypothermia, or AV nodal inflammation after cardiothoracic surgery. When patients present to the emergency department, it is important to recognize high-grade or advanced second-degree AV block, which refers to blockade of two or more consecutive P waves. High-grade second-degree AV block is a variant of Mobitz II with heightened risk of progressing to complete heart block.[11] Additionally, patients with prolonged pauses (>5 seconds) in the presence of atrial fibrillation should also be considered to have advanced AV block.[7]

Third-Degree AV Block or Complete Heart Block. Complete heart block represents complete absence of AV conduction.

FIGURE 8-4.

ECG from the patient described in Case Three: second-degree AV block type II (Mobitz II) conduction with left bundle-branch block

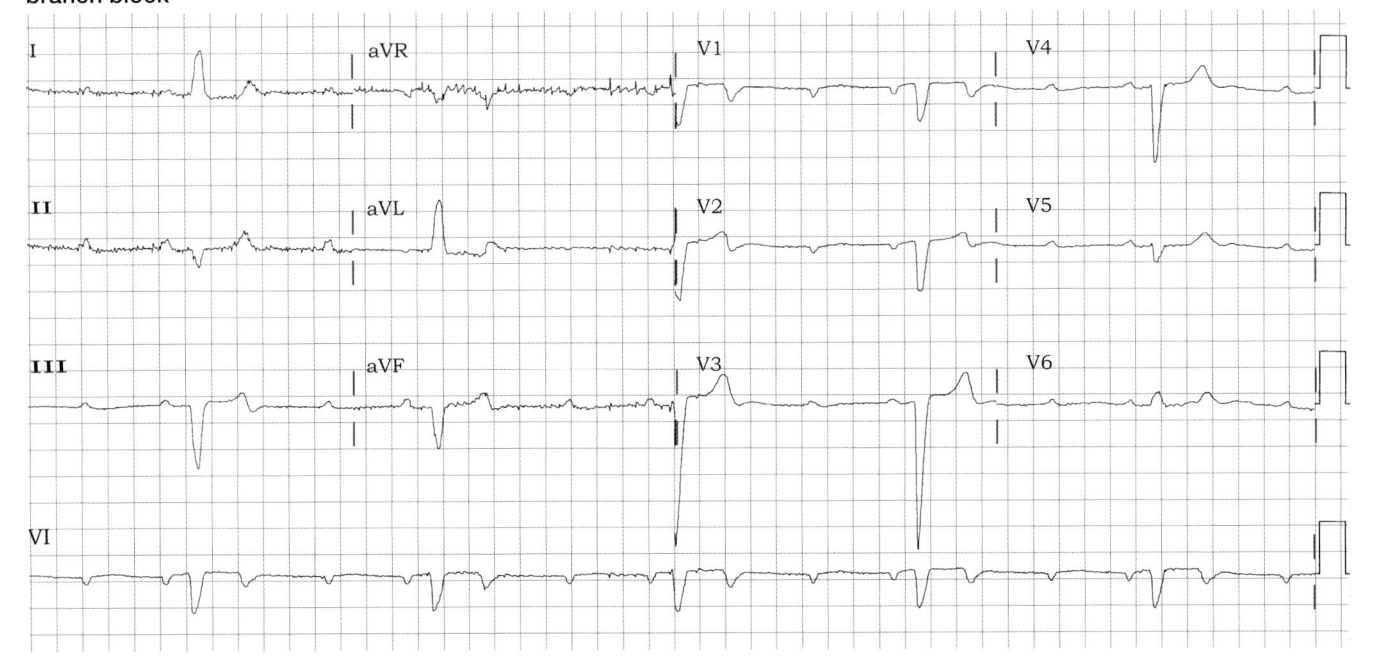

The block can occur in the AV node, in the bundle of His, or in both bundle branches. The atria and ventricles function independently in third-degree AV block: the atrial rate exceeds the ventricular escape rate, indicating AV dissociation.[11] In other words, the P-P interval should be shorter than the R-R interval.

CASE FOUR

An 80-year-old woman is brought to the emergency department following an episode of syncope. She denies head trauma, chest pain, and palpitations. She has a history of hypertension and mild heart failure and takes a beta-blocker and diuretic. She reports feeling increased fatigue over the past week. Immediately prior to the episode, she felt lightheaded and nauseated and was able to guide herself to the floor of her assisted living lunchroom prior to passing out. EMS responded and reported that she had a normal glucose concentration, a blood pressure of 145/90 mm Hg, and a heart rate in the 40s. A 12-lead ECG is obtained (Figure 8-5).

CASE FOUR CONCLUSION

The patient's ECG demonstrated complete heart block. Transcutaneous pacing should be initiated immediately since she has ongoing symptoms. Preparation should be made for transvenous pacemaker insertion with cardiology consultation, which can be performed in the emergency department or the catheterization lab under fluoroscopic guidance, if there is time. Atropine is unlikely to be effective, as the wide QRS complex suggests an infranodal site of blockade. Reversible causes such as medications (eg, the patient's beta-blocker), increased vagal tone, and myocardial ischemia, should be investigated. After insertion of the temporary pacemaker, the patient will need to be closely monitored in a cardiac intensive care unit. If the third-degree heart block does not resolve by withholding beta-blockade, a permanent pacemaker should be placed.

As mentioned previously, the ventricular response in complete heart block is typically regular because of the presence of an escape rhythm. The QRS complex can be narrow or wide, depending on whether the escape rhythm has a junctional (40-60 beats/min) or ventricular (<40 beats/min) origin. Ventricular escape rhythms in complete AV block are slower and less stable and thus should prompt preparation for temporary pacing. Atropine will not be effective in the setting of a wide complex escape rhythm because the location of the blockade is likely infranodal. Dopamine or epinephrine may be used to bridge to pacemaker therapy. Nonrandomized studies show that permanent pacing does improve the survival rate in patients with third-degree AV block.[7]

KEY POINTS

In complete heart block, AV dissociation is demonstrated by an independent atrial rate exceeding the ventricular rate (or P-P interval < R-R interval), with no regular relationship between the P waves and QRS complexes.

Clinical conditions associated with sinus node dysfunction or AV block:

    Inferior or anterior myocardial infarction

    Beta-blocker, calcium channel blocker, amiodarone, lithium, or digoxin therapy

    Myocarditis

    Hyperkalemia

    Hypothermia

    Hypoxemia

    Sleep apnea

FIGURE 8-5.

ECG from the patient described in Case Four: third-degree AV block (complete heart block) with ventricular escape rhythm

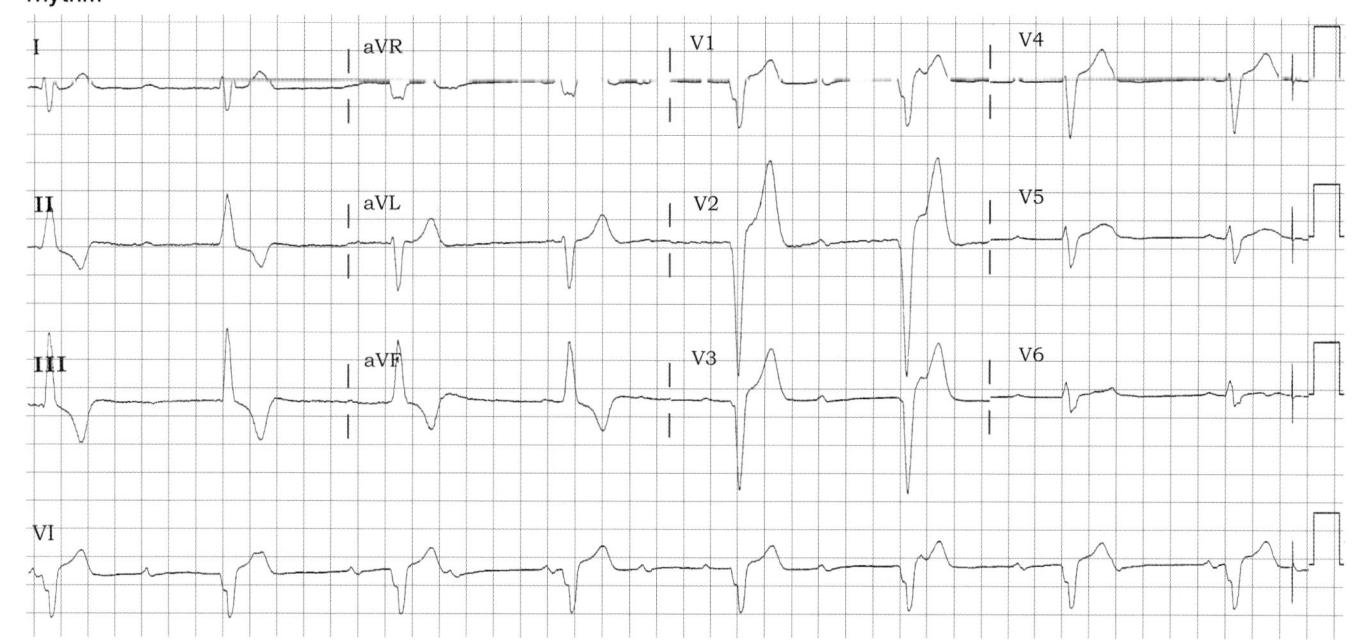

Increased intracranial pressure

Endotracheal suctioning, vomiting, urination, or defecation (enhanced vagal tone)

Bradyarrhythmias Related to Acute Coronary Syndrome

Approximately 25% of acute MIs are complicated by bradyarrhythmias.[12] Sinus node dysfunction and AV block are most commonly seen in patients with inferior MI, as the SA nodal and AV nodal arteries arise from the right coronary artery in most individuals. In fact, sinus bradycardia occurs in 40% to 60% of patients with inferior MI, while AV block occurs in 10% to 25% of cases.[12] AV block during inferior MI usually occurs at the level of the AV node and produces transient first-, second-, or third-degree AV block.

CASE FIVE

While mowing his lawn, a 56-year-old man with known hypertension and diabetes felt the acute onset of substernal chest pressure, nausea, and near syncope. Paramedics found him to be profusely diaphoretic and nauseated. They gave him an aspirin and obtained the 12-lead ECG shown as Figure 8-6, which they transmitted to the receiving hospital.

CASE FIVE CONCLUSION

The prehospital 12-lead ECG clearly shows complete heart block and ST-elevation inferiorly (leads II, III, and aVF) as well as anteriorly (V_1 to V_3). A junctional escape rhythm is present. Given the ongoing myocyte destruction from the presumed occluded right coronary artery and left anterior descending artery, the patient needs urgent revascularization. Regarding the bradyarrhythmia, pacer pads should be placed and pacing should be initiated if the patient becomes symptomatic or hemodynamically unstable. Although AV block is usually a transient complication of impaired perfusion to the AV node from the occluded right coronary artery, heart block associated with anterior infarction tends to be permanent. The patient's junctional escape rhythm could provide compensated cardiac output temporarily, but fluctuations in his heart rate stemming from the impaired conduction can still occur.

AV block secondary to anterior infarction is less common but tends to be permanent. Complete heart block develops in 2.5% of patients with anterior MI compared with 9% of patients with inferior wall MI.[13] However, because the left anterior descending artery supplies the infranodal region, AV block in the setting of anterior wall MI is more likely to be high grade, such as Mobitz II or third-degree with an unstable escape rhythm.[2]

Atropine might be effective in increasing the SA nodal discharge rate and improving conduction in AV block secondary to an inferior MI, but it tends to be ineffective in patients with anterior MI. In addition, atropine should be used with caution during active ischemia to avoid increasing myocardial oxygen demand or precipitating ventricular fibrillation. Keep in mind that hypotension in the setting of acute coronary syndrome can also be caused by ischemic pump failure and might not resolve by simply correcting the bradyarrhythmia. In those cases of ischemic cardiogenic shock, management should focus on revascularization, inotropic therapy (ie, norepinephrine, dobutamine, milrinone), and mechanical support from intra-aortic

FIGURE 8-6.

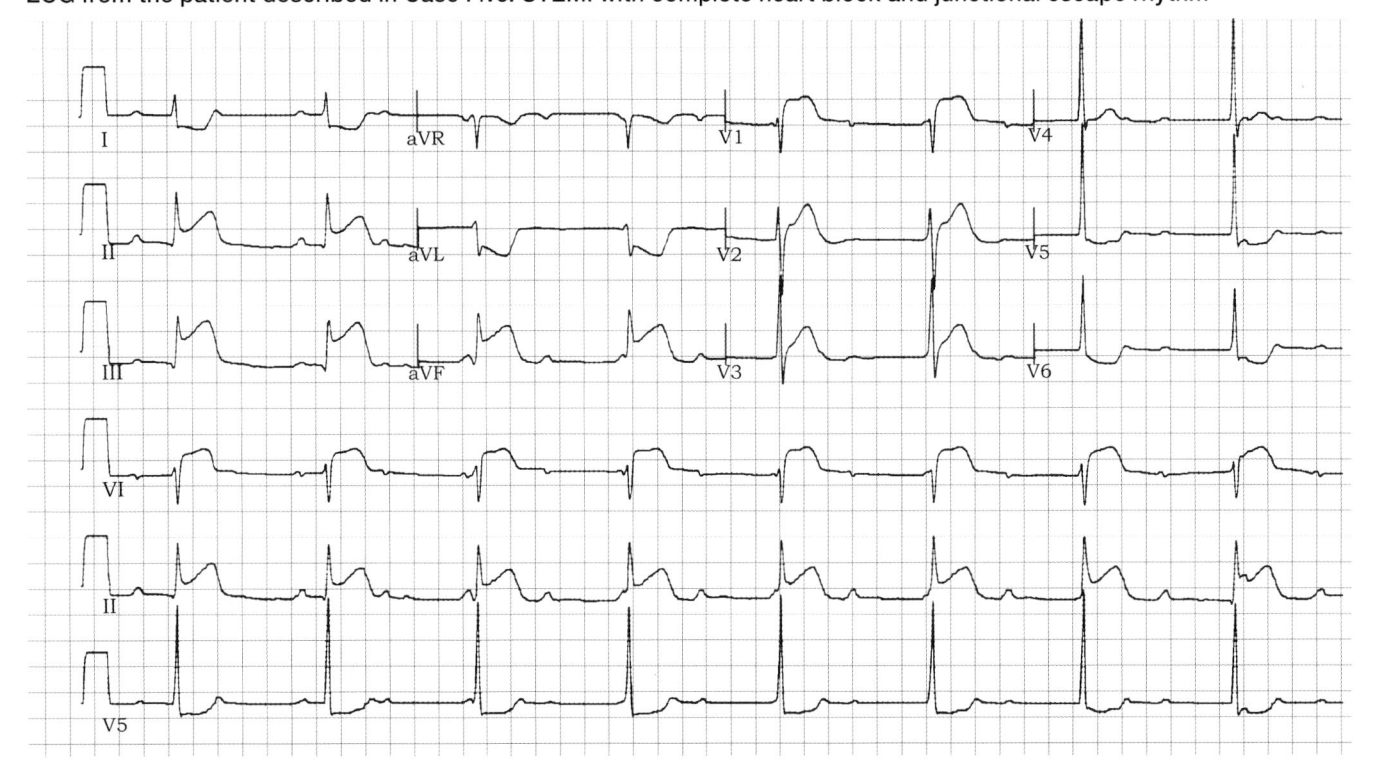

ECG from the patient described in Case Five: STEMI with complete heart block and junctional escape rhythm

balloon pump placement.

Hemodynamically significant bradyarrhythmias in acute coronary syndrome should be treated with temporary cardiac pacing. Bradycardia in the setting of inferior MI is usually transient and likely to need only temporary pacing. AV block in the setting of an anterior MI commonly necessitates permanent pacemaker placement.

KEY POINTS

Conduction disturbances in acute coronary syndrome:
- Inferior myocardial infarction
  - First-, second-, and third-degree AV and SA nodal block
  - Might require temporary pacing, but typically is transient
- Anterior myocardial infarction
  - High-grade second- and third-degree AV block
  - Usually persists, requiring permanent pacing

Common Exogenous Causes of Bradyarrhythmia

Metabolic

Therapeutic hypothermia is now an established therapy used in the emergency department to provide neuroprotection in patients in cardiac arrest, so it is important to understand the effect of cooling on cardiac conduction. At temperatures of 32°C to 34°C, sinus bradycardia and delayed AV or ventricular conduction, manifested by PR and QRS interval prolongation, are commonly observed. In most patients, hypothermia-induced bradyarrhythmias do not become hemodynamically unstable enough to require pacing or medical therapy.[13] Additionally, severe hypothermia from environmental exposure is characteristically associated with Osborne waves, which appear on the ECG as a notch at the end of the QRS interval. Osborne waves are found in nearly 80% of patients with a core temperature below 30°C.[14]

Hypothyroidism is also associated with sinus bradycardia and AV block. The influence of subclinical hypothyroidism (defined by a normal thyroxine level with an elevated thyrotropin level) on cardiac conduction is less well established. However, there have been case reports of patients with subclinical hypothyroidism causing severe bradycardia and transient AV conduction block that were reversed with thyroid hormone supplementation.[15]

Hyperkalemia can produce varying degrees of reversible AV block, including complete heart block. Severely elevated potassium levels can produce a wide QRS rhythm that mandates immediate medical therapy. Even though P waves may not be distinguishable on the 12-lead ECG, this sine wave rhythm does actually originate in the sinus node.

CASE SIX

A 56-year-old man with a history of dilated cardiomyopathy and paroxysmal atrial fibrillation is transported to the emergency department via EMS for weakness. He had been feeling weak for the past day. A friend checked his pulse and found his heart rate to be in the 20s. The patient reports that he had been experiencing vomiting and diarrhea for the past week, with little oral intake. On arrival at the emergency department, his blood pressure is 92/60 mm Hg, with a heart rate of 22 beats/min. His 12-lead ECG is shown in Figure 8-7. His electrolytes were significant for potassium of 6.2, BUN of 56, and creatinine of 3.5.

CASE SIX CONCLUSION

His ECG shows a profound bradycardia, which was interpreted as slow atrial fibrillation and nonspecific inferior T-wave abnormalities. Although the patient's history of atrial fibrillation makes this diagnosis more likely, one should remember that hyperkalemia might result in the disappearance of P waves. The patient was given atropine (a total of 2 mg) by EMS personnel and in the emergency department (a total of 2 mg) for hemodynamic instability. Transcutaneous pacing was initiated in the emergency department as bridge therapy and he was transported emergently to the electrophysiology laboratory for temporary pacing wire placement. The patient was hydrated aggressively for acute renal failure due to volume loss and hyperkalemia. He was treated with intravenous fluids, insulin, glucose, and sodium polystyrene sulfonate (Kayexalate).

Neurologic

Bradyarrhythmias can result from acute intracranial or spinal cord injury. Severe cervical spine injury can disrupt sympathetic innervation of the SA and AV nodes, leading to excessive parasympathetic tone, neurogenic hypotension, and bradycardia. Significantly increased intracranial pressure resulting from traumatic injury, acute stroke, hemorrhage, or mass effect can

FIGURE 8-7.

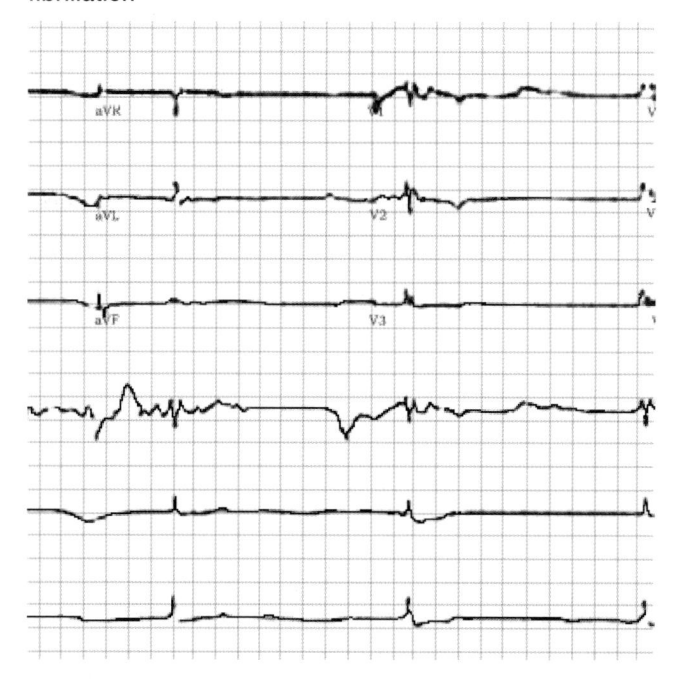

ECG from the patient described in Case Six: slow atrial fibrillation

lead to the Cushing reflex, consisting of hypertension, bradycardia, and irregular respirations, which may be a pre-terminal event.

Toxins/Drugs

The evaluation of the acutely poisoned patient should follow the standard emergency department approach to resuscitation, beginning with stabilization of the airway, breathing, and circulation, in addition to decontamination. Essential history must be obtained from family, witnesses, and emergency medical personnel, including the identity, formulation, and quantity of each substance ingested, to guide antidote and supportive therapy. The possibility of suicide attempt and co-ingestion of additional substances should be entertained. Administration of activated charcoal (1 to 2 g/kg) may be considered for the intubated patient with a protected airway and suspected ingestion time of less than 1 hour prior to presentation.

Overdose of *calcium channel blockers* produces both negative chronotropic and inotropic effects through blockade of voltage-gated calcium channels in cardiac myocytes and conductive tissue.[16] Management of calcium channel blocker toxicity should begin with intravascular volume replacement to counteract toxic vasodilatory effects. Atropine can be effective in treating bradycardia associated with calcium channel blocker poisoning; however, this therapy may be only transiently successful, which should prompt initiation of temporary pacing. Calcium chloride or calcium gluconate therapy is recommended to counteract calcium channel antagonism. A vasopressor such as norepinephrine, epinephrine, dopamine, or phenylephrine is frequently required for hemodynamic support. There is increasing evidence from animal studies to support hyperinsulinemia-euglycemia therapy in calcium channel blocker toxicity.[16] Myocytes need glucose for fuel in states of shock, so it has been hypothesized that hypoinsulinemia perpetuates reduction of vascular tone and inotropy by impeding glucose uptake. Evidence suggests that insulin therapy helps reverse this process.[17] Typical protocols include high-dose insulin infusion (0.5 units/kg/hr) with additional dextrose infusion to target euglycemia.[16]

KEY POINT

Do not rely on calcium administration alone to adequately treat a patient who has intentionally ingested a large volume of a calcium channel blocker. Insulin and glucose should be started early in the symptomatic patient with a calcium channel blocker overdose.

Similarly, *beta-blocker toxicity* causes varying degrees of AV block and intraventricular conduction delay with QRS widening, in addition to reduced inotropy.[18] Glucagon therapy is recommended in patients with beta-blocker toxicity. Glucagon increases automaticity at the SA and AV nodal levels. In addition, it activates adenylate cyclase in the myocardium, which causes chronotropic and inotropic stimulation independent of the antagonized beta-adrenergic receptors.[18] Because of glucagon's short half-life, the initial dose of 50 mcg/kg IV may need to be followed by an infusion.

Lipid emulsion therapy has also been used as a treatment option for refractory cardiovascular collapse secondary to beta-blocker or calcium channel blocker overdose.[19] Published reports demonstrating the effectiveness of this therapy are limited to case reports and series; and lipid emulsion for calcium channel and beta-blocker overdose is not approved by the US Food and Drug Administration. Consultation with the local poison control center and a clinical toxicologist is recommended when considering using lipid emulsion treatment for the critically ill overdose patient.

KEY POINTS

Treatment of an acute intentional beta-blocker drug overdose might require large glucagon doses, which could exhaust a small hospital's inventory. Therefore, it is important to contact the pharmacy early to determine availability. Remember to give an antiemetic, because glucagon can induce vomiting.

Management of cardiac toxidromes:

History is essential.

Identify the specific number and dose of ingested medications.

Consult your local poison control center or toxicologist.

Consider specific antidotes: gastric decontamination if early in presentation, digoxin-specific antibody (cardiac glycosides), calcium (calcium channel blocker), insulin/glucose (calcium channel blocker and beta-blocker), glucagon (beta-blocker).

Conclusion

Management of a patient with a bradyarrhythmia, as with any time-sensitive resuscitation in the emergency department, begins with stabilization of the ABCs. Symptoms of hypoperfusion must be recognized quickly, followed by the rapid administration of atropine or beta-agonist therapy while preparing for possible emergent pacing. After hemodynamic stabilization, 12-lead ECG interpretation is paramount to determine the propensity of the bradyarrhythmia to become unstable or the need for admission for further evaluation or definitive therapy. Each ECG should be examined systematically for rate, regularity, interval prolongation, and ST changes to ensure accurate rhythm identification and avoid overlooking subtle clues as to the cause of the rhythm disturbance.

It is important to consider both intrinsic and extrinsic causes of bradyarrhythmias, so that appropriate treatment is rendered. Acute myocardial ischemia, electrolyte abnormalities, toxic ingestion with nodal depressant agents, neurologic injury, vagal stimulation, hypothermia, and hypothyroidism should all be included in the differential diagnosis and excluded when appropriate.

The emergency physician stands at the front line of distinguishing benign from life-threatening bradyarrhythmias. Proper identification and prompt treatment can save the lives of patients who otherwise would die from complications arising from unrecognized bradyarrhythmias.

Acknowledgments

The authors would like to acknowledge and thank David J. Maron, MD, for his ECG and rhythm strip contributions.

References

1. Sodeck GH, Domanovits H, Meron G, et al. Compromising bradycardia: management in the emergency department. *Resuscitation.* 2007;73:96-102.
2. Kaushik V, Leon AR, Forrester JS, et al. Bradyarrhythmias, temporary and permanent pacing. *Crit Care Med.* 2000;28:N121-N128.
3. Malhotra R, Edelman ER, Lilly LS. Basic cardiac structure and function. In: Lily LS, ed. *Pathophysiology of Heart Disease.* Baltimore, MD: Lippincott Williams & Wilkins; 2003:11-22.
4. Durham D, Worthley LI. Cardiac arrhythmias: diagnosis and management: the bradycardias. *Crit Care Resus.* 2002;4:54-69.
5. Barrett TW, Abraham RL, Jenkins CA, et al. Risk factors for bradycardia requiring pacemaker implantation in patients with atrial fibrillation. *Am J Cardiol.* 2012;110:1315-1321.
6. Dreifus LS, Michelson EL, Kaplinsky E. Bradyarrhythmias: clinical significance and management. *J Am Coll Cardiol.* 1983;1:327-338.
7. Epstein AE, Ellenbogen KA, Freedman RA, et al. 2012 ACCF/AHA/HRS Focused Update Incorporated Into the ACCF/AHA/HRS 2008 Guidelines for Device-Based Therapy of Cardiac Rhythm Abnormalities: a report of the American College of Cardiology/American Heart Association Task Force on Practice Guidelines. *J Am Coll Cardiol.* 2013;61:1-70.
8. Mangrum JM, Dimarco JP. The evaluation and management of bradycardia. *N Engl J Med.* 2000;342:703-709.
9. Debacker D, Biston P, Devriendt J, et al. Comparison of dopamine and norepinephrine in the treatment of shock. *N Engl J Med.* 2010;362:779-789.
10. Cheng S, Keyes MJ, Larson MG, et al. Long-term outcomes in individuals with prolonged PR interval or first-degree atrioventricular block. *JAMA.* 2009;301:2571-2577.
11. Ufberg JW, Clark JS. Bradydysrhythmias and atrioventricular conduction blocks. *Emerg Med Clin North Am.* 2006;24:1-9.
12. Brady WJ, Harrigan RA. Evaluation and management of bradyarrhythmias in the emergency department. *Emerg Med Clin North Am.* 1998;16:364-381.
13. Badhwar N, Kusumoto F, Goldschlager N. Arrhythmias in the coronary care unit. *J Intensive Care Med.* 2012;27:267-289.
14. Sepehrdad R, Paulsen J, Amsterdam EA. The ECG that came in from the cold. *Am J Med.* 2012;125:246-248.
15. Nakayama Y. A case of transient 2:1 atrioventricular block resolved by thyroxine supplementation for subclinical hypothyroidism. *Pacing Clin Electrophysiol.* 2006;29:106-108.
16. Harris NS. Case 24-2006: a 40-year-old woman with hypotension after an overdose of amlodipine. *N Engl J Med.* 2006;355:602-611.
17. Boyer EW, Shannon M. Treatment of calcium channel blocker intoxication with insulin infusion. *N Engl J Med.* 2001;344:1721-1722.
18. Love JN, Enlow B, Klein-Schwartz W, Litovitz TL. Electrocardiographic changes associated with B-blocker toxicity. *Ann Emerg Med.* 2002;40:603-610.
19. Weinberg GL. Lipid emulsion infusion: resuscitation for local anesthetic and other drug overdose. *Anesthesiology.* 2012;117:180-187.

CARDIOVASCULAR EMERGENCIES

CHAPTER 9

Narrow Complex Tachycardia: Diagnosis and Management in the Emergency Department

Amita Sudhir and William J. Brady

IN THIS CHAPTER

Sinus tachycardia

Atrial fibrillation and atrial flutter

Paroxysmal supraventricular tachycardia

Wolff-Parkinson-White syndrome–related narrow complex tachycardia

Multifocal atrial tachycardia

Narrow complex tachycardia (NCT) is a cardiac rhythm with a normal QRS complex duration and a rapid rate. In a very basic sense, NCT is defined as a cardiac rhythm with a QRS complex width of 100 msec or less and a ventricular rate above 100 beats/min. It is not unreasonable to include tachycardias with QRS complex widths of 80 to 100 msec in this definition. As with other electrocardiographic (ECG) diagnoses, the pediatric population has age-appropriate rates and widths for NCT.

These tachycardias arise at or above the level of the atrioventricular (AV) node and span the realm of acute care medicine, with a multitude of arrhythmias, causes, acuity levels, natural histories, management strategies, and outcomes. Prevalences of the various NCT rhythms in the emergency department population are listed in Figure 9-1, and their differential diagnosis is portrayed in Figure 9-2.

These rhythm disturbances span a variety of clinical possibilities, ranging from asymptomatic to very destabilizing. Cardiovascular collapse can be a direct result of the arrhythmia or of the NCT's causative event. For instance, the patient with paroxysmal supraventricular tachycardia (PSVT) can present with significant hypotension, with circulatory shock being a result of the rhythm itself; conversely, a patient with significant hypotension secondary to gastrointestinal hemorrhage can present with sinus tachycardia (ST), with the circulatory shock being a result of the hemorrhage and the rhythm solely a manifestation of hemodynamic compromise. Patients can also present with secondary complications of the NCT such as embolic stroke or peripheral arterial occlusion with atrial fibrillation or atrial flutter.

This chapter focuses on NCT, but it should be noted that any of the rhythm diagnoses discussed here can present as wide complex tachycardia if the patient has aberrant intraventricular conduction such as a fixed or rate-related bundle-branch block. Ventricular preexcitation syndromes with an accessory pathway such as the Wolff-Parkinson-White (WPW) syndrome can also present as supraventricular tachycardia with a widened QRS complex.

KEY POINT

NCTs include a number of arrhythmias, ranging from benign to very destabilizing.

General Approach to the NCT Patient

The patient with NCT should be placed on an ECG monitor; if the situation warrants, a 12-lead ECG should be obtained. Intravenous access should be established. Oxygen administration should be initiated if the peripheral oxygen saturation is

CARDIOVASCULAR EMERGENCIES

less than 94% or if the patient demonstrates respiratory distress. A focused history, including the patient's medical history and medication or recreational drug use, can provide clues to the rhythm diagnosis. The physical examination, again focused on the cardiorespiratory system and the quality of systemic perfusion, is performed while management is initiated. Additional investigations, including laboratory studies and radiographs, may be obtained depending on the presentation. Of course, a single/multilead rhythm strip and a 12-lead ECG provide very important information, leading to rhythm diagnosis in many cases and guiding therapy in most presentations. The following ECG features, discussed in detail for each rhythm in this chapter, should be considered in the analysis: the presence of P waves, P-wave characteristics (morphology, amplitude, number of distinct waves), association of P wave to the QRS complex, ventricular rate, and regularity of the ventricular rate. A diagnostic strategy is presented in Figure 9-3.

KEY POINTS

NCTs occur in all age groups—from neonates to the extreme elderly.

NCTs can result from significant cardiopulmonary illness; they can also be quite innocuous, not indicative of significant underlying pathology.

Management of the various NCTs is based on the rhythm, the patient's presentation, and related clinical issues. The basic therapeutic approach involves consideration of the end-organ impact of the arrhythmia (eg, is cardiogenic shock present?), treatment goals (eg, ventricular rate control and/or rhythm conversion), and management of coexisting pathology. When a tachycardic patient presents to the emergency department with an ECG demonstrating NCT, the initial step should focus on

FIGURE 9-1.

The relative occurrence of NCT in the emergency department population. ST=sinus tachycardia, AFIB=atrial fibrillation, PSVT=paroxysmal supraventricular tachycardia, AFLUT=atrial flutter, MAT=multifocal atrial tachycardia, PAT=paroxysmal atrial tachycardia, AVRT=atrioventricular reciprocating tachycardia (as seen in WPW syndrome).

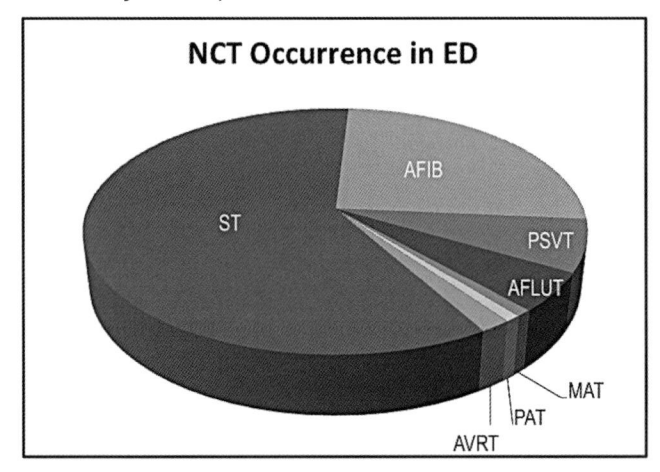

FIGURE 9-2.

Differential considerations of the NCT. A, Sinus tachycardia. B, Atrial fibrillation. C, Atrial flutter. D, Paroxysmal supraventricular tachycardia (AVNRT). E, NCT of WPW syndrome (AVRT; orthodromic tachycardia of WPW). F, Multifocal atrial tachycardia.

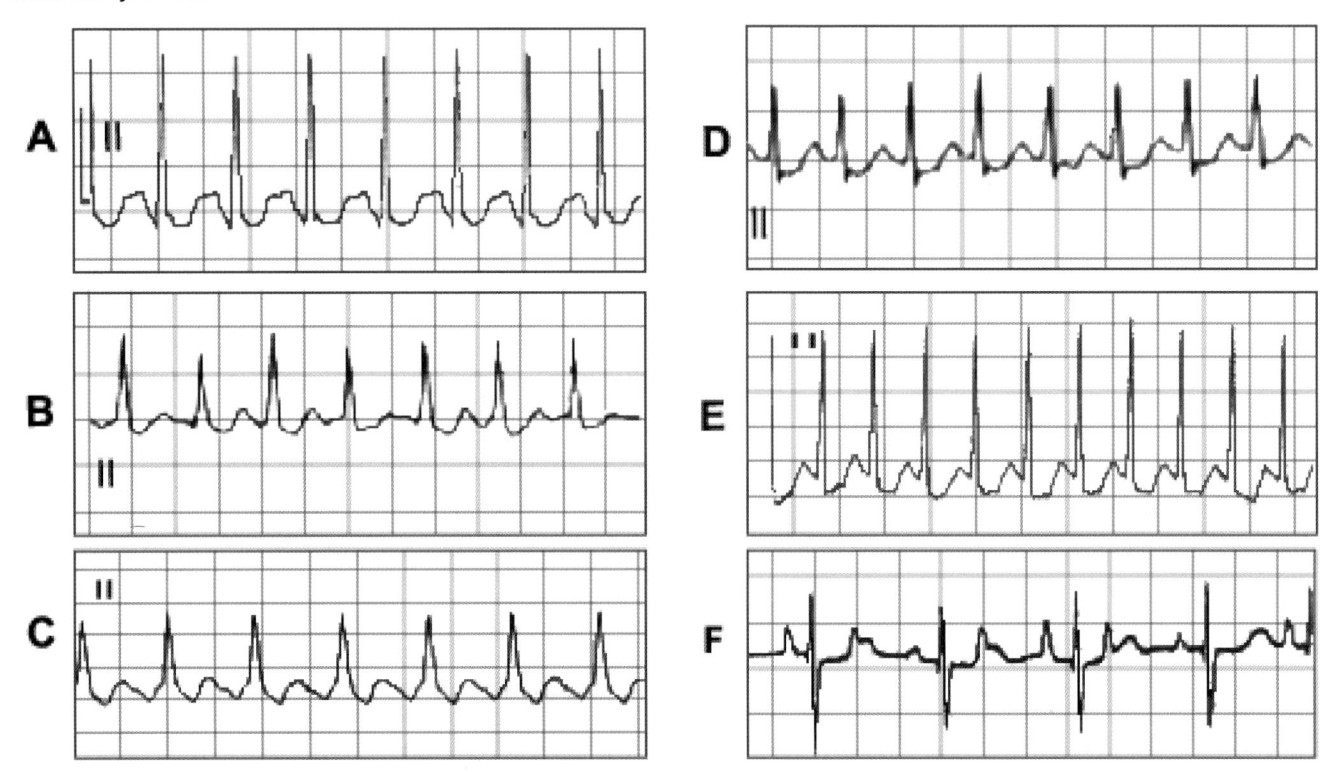

determining the patient's stability. Instability in the setting of NCT suggests the need for urgent intervention. If the patient is deemed to be stable, management is less time sensitive, allowing consideration of therapeutic interventions while the evaluation proceeds. Of course, coexistent issues such as acute heart failure or decompensation of a patient with chronic obstructive pulmonary disease must also be treated.

The various NCTs can be approached with the following therapies: intravenous fluids, supplemental oxygen, vagal maneuvers, adenosine, beta-adrenergic blocking agents, calcium channel blockers, other antiarrhythmic medications, and electrical cardioversion. In most patients, basic supportive therapy involves an intravenous fluid bolus to expand the circulating intravascular volume; such therapy can represent the sole intervention or one component of management. Supplemental oxygen, administered by nasal cannula, facemask, or endotracheal tube, is another important intervention in the patient with NCT. These two interventions are safe for most patients with NCT. Certain NCTs require rhythm-specific therapy (eg, adenosine infusion, diltiazem bolus dosing, or electrical cardioversion), while others need treatment aimed at the underlying cause(s) of the arrhythmia. Determination of patient stability (or lack thereof) will guide early management decisions. Specific management choices are then based on the specific rhythm and the individual patient's presentation. It must be stressed that the list of interventions does not apply to all NCTs; for instance, adenosine would be of no value in a patient with atrial fibrillation with rapid ventricular response, but this drug would be an agent of choice in the management of PSVT.

The general therapeutic approach to the NCT patient is to consider causes of the tachycardia, including hypoxia, fluid deficits or hemorrhage, fever, pain, anxiety, and pharmacologic effects of certain agents. If found, these abnormalities should be addressed. For instance, sinus tachycardia can be precipitated by hypoxia; the simple *administration of oxygen* might correct the problem. In other cases, the NCT is caused by acutely decompensated congestive heart failure with hypoxia; for example, a patient with atrial fibrillation and rapid ventricular response

FIGURE 9-3.

A suggested algorithm for the assessment and diagnosis of NCT in emergency department patients. From: Borloz MP, Mark DG, Pines JM, Brady WJ. ECG differential diagnosis of narrow QRS complex tachycardia: An emergency department-oriented algorithmic approach. *Am J Emerg Med.* 2010;28:379. Copyright 2010. Used with permission from Elsevier.

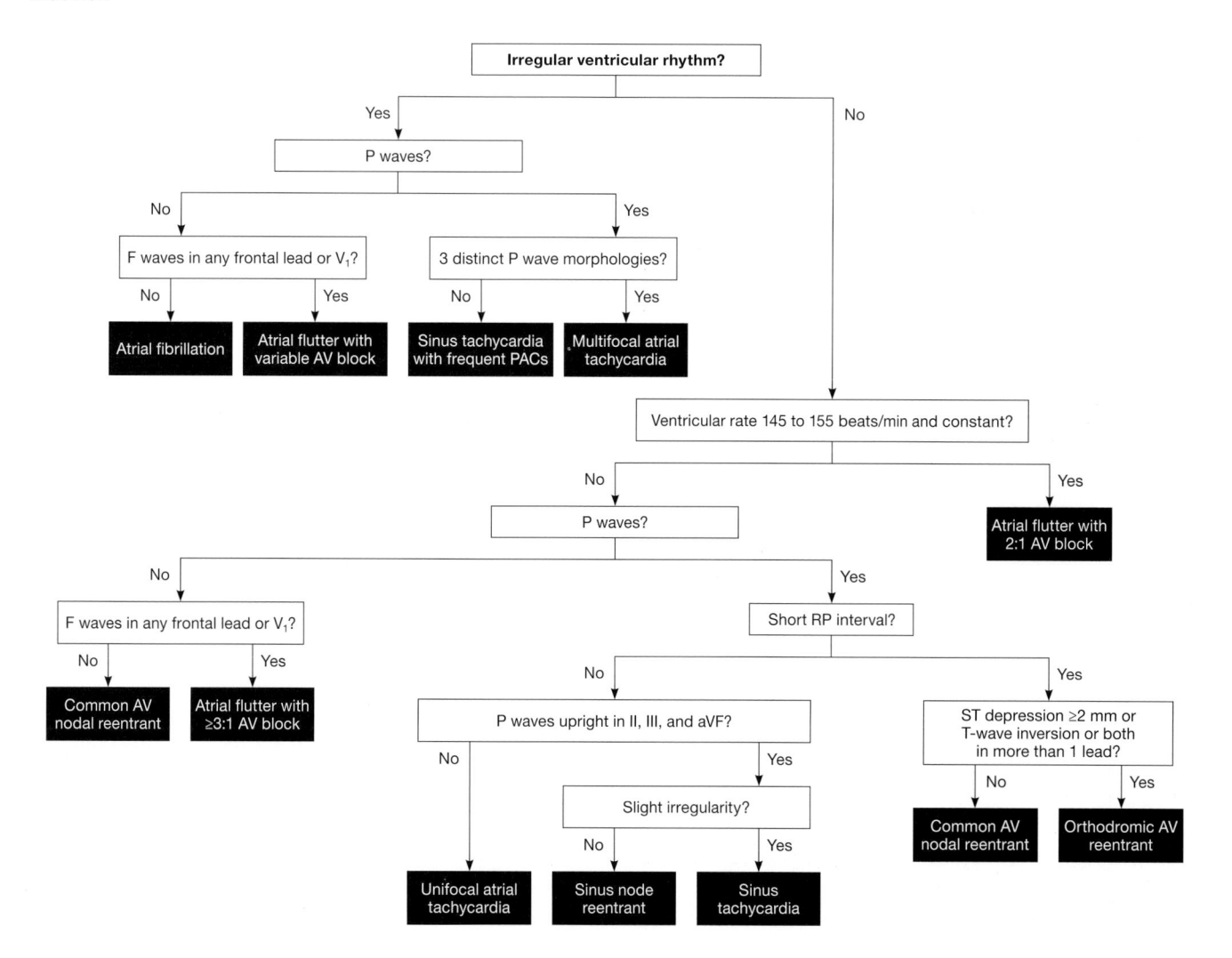

requires oxygen to correct hypoxia resulting from pulmonary edema. In patients without demonstrated oxygen deprivation or respiratory distress, oxygen therapy is usually not required.

Intravenous fluid administration can be of significant value in treating NCT patients who are dehydrated or in circulatory shock. As with oxygen administration, fluid resuscitation becomes the primary therapy in the management of tachycardia in many patients. It is a reasonable early intervention in the tachycardic patient who does not exhibit overt signs of acutely decompensated heart failure with significant pulmonary edema. Sinus tachycardia and atrial fibrillation with rapid ventricular response are excellent examples of NCTs in which intravenous fluid can be a primary intervention. In contrast, patients with PSVT will probably not benefit from intravenous fluid administration, at least as a primary intervention. Generally, normal saline is the fluid of choice. An initial bolus of 0.5 to 1 liter may be given, and then additional fluid may be titrated based on the patient's response. The patient should be assessed for signs of improvement. If the hypovolemia is the result of hemorrhage, administration of blood products may be considered.

An initial therapy, appropriate for only certain NCTs, is the *vagal maneuver*. This intervention can be considered in patients with PSVT, atrial fibrillation, or WPW-related NCT. Vagal maneuvers can be curative if delivered correctly and early in the PSVT patient's clinical course. In fact, if performed early enough, the maneuver converts the rhythm in approximately 20% of such presentations.[1]

Antiarrhythmic agents can be separated into two classes: agents primarily aimed at rate control (the AV node blocking agents, including adenosine, beta-adrenergic blockers, and calcium channel antagonists) and medications focusing on rhythm conversion (amiodarone and procainamide). Of course, there is significant overlap in these two functions with certain medications. *Adenosine* transiently increases potassium efflux and decreases calcium influx into the AV node, profoundly slowing AV conduction and causing momentary ventricular asystole. It is effective in treating only PSVT because it disrupts the reentrant circuit within the AV node. In other rhythm presentations, adenosine produces a momentary block at the AV node, at times revealing important clues regarding the ultimate rhythm diagnosis; for instance, adenosine will reveal obvious flutter waves in the patient with atrial flutter. It should not, however, be used for purely diagnostic purposes but only when the rhythm is reasonably suspicious for PSVT. In this instance, the medication's initial purpose was therapeutic, yet, with a lack of definitive response, diagnostic information can be obtained. Adenosine is a very short-acting agent that profoundly blocks conduction through the AV node. It should be given initially as a rapid 6-mg IV bolus; if this dose is unsuccessful, a 12-mg rapid bolus is given and may be repeated a second time if no response occurs. In certain circumstances of nonresponse to lower doses, a dose of 18 mg IV may be used.[2]

It is important to define a "failure" after administration of adenosine. The serum half-life of the drug is very short; thus, its AV nodal blocking effect is transient and brief. A brief period of AV nodal blockade with near-immediate recurrence of the PSVT is, in fact, not a treatment failure, but a consequence of the medication's duration of effect.[3] In such situations, repeat administration of adenosine at the same dose likely will not be successful. Therefore, a higher dose is needed. Alternatives include the combination of adenosine with another AV nodal blocking agent or another medication. The therapy would include the use of a beta-blocker or a calcium channel blocker, with repeat administration of adenosine.

Many patients with NCT can be treated with an AV nodal blocking agent, with the notable exception of those with sinus tachycardia and most cases of multifocal atrial tachycardia (MAT). In addition to adenosine, other *AV node blocking agents* are available, including beta-adrenergic blockers and calcium channel blockers. These two medication classes may be considered when direct control of the ventricular rate is a desired goal, as in PSVT, atrial fibrillation, atrial flutter, and WPW-related NCT. In general, patients with sinus tachycardia or MAT should not be treated with this approach; rather, the cause should be considered and corrected.

The *beta-adrenergic blocking agents*, or beta-blockers, are an important class of medications in the management of certain NCTs. These medications block beta-receptors, decreasing sympathetic input to the AV node, thereby slowing conduction. Intravenous beta-blockers commonly used for rate control are metoprolol and esmolol. Metoprolol is given as intravenous boluses: 5 mg IV every 5 minutes for a maximum of three doses. Therapeutic end points are satisfactory response, hemodynamic deterioration, or medication maximal dosing. Esmolol, due to its very short duration of action, is administered as a continuous infusion with bolus therapy. The loading dosage for esmolol is 250 to 500 mcg/kg/min administered over 1 minute; an infusion of 50 mcg/kg/min over 4 minutes follows. If therapeutic effects are not observed within 5 minutes, repeat the loading dose up to 4 times as needed, followed by a maintenance infusion at increased dose using increments of 50 mcg/kg/min for 4 minutes at each bolus increase. As the desired blood pressure is approached, reduce the maintenance infusion by 25 to 50 mcg/kg/min or more and titrate to desired effect. Beta-blockers, like the calcium channel blockers, have negative inotropic effects, so the same cautions and contraindications apply.

The *calcium channel antagonists*, or calcium channel blockers, are another important class of medications in the management of NCT. The nondihydropyridine (nonvascular smooth muscle selective) calcium channel blockers—diltiazem and verapamil—block calcium channels in the AV node, thus slowing electrical conduction through it. Because these agents also have negative inotropic effects, they can cause hypotension and exacerbate profound, chronic heart failure. If at all possible, these agents should be avoided in hypotensive patients and in those with significant preexisting heart failure. Diltiazem, administered at a dose of 0.25 mg/kg IV over several minutes, is an appropriate calcium channel blocker for such arrhythmias. If the desired clinical response does not occur, the drug may be repeated at a dose of 0.35 mg/kg IV. Diltiazem can also be infused in continuous fashion for rhythm control at a dose of 10 mg/hr.

Medications with a primary focus of rhythm conversion include amiodarone and procainamide. *Amiodarone* has beta-blocking, calcium channel blocking, and potassium channel blocking effects on the AV node, slowing conduction. Amiodarone is a reasonable choice for the conversion of atrial fibrillation and atrial flutter to sinus rhythm; it can be used as a "back-up" agent for PSVT when other therapies have failed. It can be used in stable patients for chemical cardioversion and in unstable patients as an adjunct to electrical cardioversion. The dosing for amiodarone is 150 mg IV over 10 to 20 minutes; this dose may be repeated once if the clinical response is not satisfactory after 30 to 60 minutes. Caution is advised, because rapid administration can produce hypotension. *Procainamide* is a sodium channel blocker that acts as an antiarrhythmic agent by slowing cardiac conduction. It is an effective agent in stable patients with preserved left ventricular function. It is administered at a dose of 17 mg/kg over 45 minutes to an hour. Alternatively, a more rapid yet observation-intensive mode of administration involves 100- to 200-mg IV boluses given approximately every 5 minutes as tolerated, which allows more expeditious delivery of the drug. Although procainamide is effective, it has two disadvantages: its tendency to produce hypotension and its requirement for slow infusion over 20 to 60 minutes. Rapid infusion can precipitate both hypotension and widening of the QRS complex.

Electrical cardioversion can be considered in certain NCT patients who are unstable because of the arrhythmia or who have not responded to initial pharmacologic measures. The rhythms for which this intervention is most commonly considered are PSVT and atrial fibrillation, but it must be stressed that urgent electrical cardioversion is a rare choice for these rhythms. Atrial flutter rarely requires urgent electrical cardioversion, and sinus tachycardia and MAT are not managed with this approach. The indications for electrical cardioversion in the unstable patient include hypotension and hypoperfusion, altered mentation, acute pulmonary edema, and ischemic chest pain. This definition of instability relies heavily on clinical judgment and the overall appearance of the patient; thus, the bedside clinician is in the best position to determine the need for this intervention. In the stable patient, the need for conversion to sinus rhythm can also be encountered when the patient has not responded to medical therapy (in other words, the rhythm is refractory to medication-based interventions). Atrial fibrillation of new onset can be cardioverted electrically as a first-line treatment, assuming the duration of the arrhythmia is known to be less than 48 hours. This decision, controversial in many ways, is best made in conjunction with cardiology consultation.

Biphasic energy levels range from 25 to 50 joules (J) to maximal energy levels for the particular device (200 to 360 J). In general, PSVT responds to lower energy ranges (50 to 75 J) while atrial fibrillation requires markedly higher settings (starting at 100 J, escalated to the maximum setting). The patient should be sedated for cardioversion if the clinical situation allows. Certain sedation agents can precipitate hypotension and thus should be used with caution, if at all. Synchronized direct-current (DC) cardioversion should be used. Several attempts with increasing energy levels might be needed. Complications of cardioversion, although uncommon, include malig-

FIGURE 9-4.

Sinus tachycardia. The focus for this NCT is in the sinuatrial node. The impulse moves through the atria tissues, arriving at the AV node, and then is transmitted into the ventricle and traverses the intraventricular conduction system.

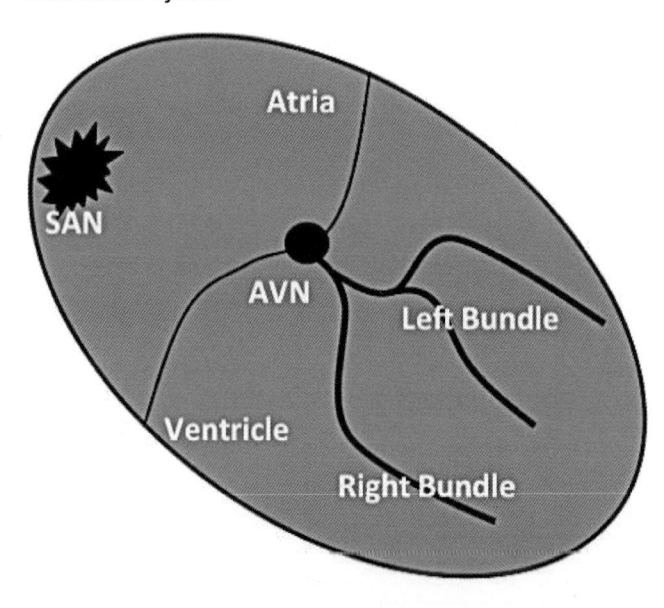

FIGURE 9-5.

Sinus tachycardia in a patient with significant cocaine use

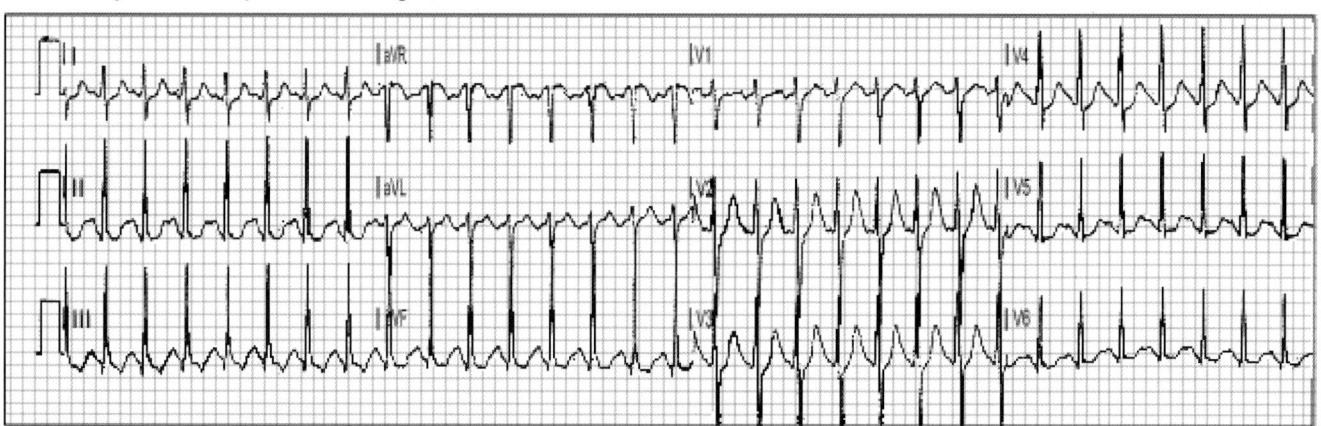

CARDIOVASCULAR EMERGENCIES

nant ventricular arrhythmias, cardiac arrest, and complications from sedation (ie, aspiration). Additionally, the rhythm might not respond (failure to convert).

Caution regarding hemodynamic stability must be exercised here. Not all patients who are unstable and present with one of these arrhythmias require electrical cardioversion. For example, atrial fibrillation can be the primary issue producing hemodynamic compromise. More often, however, it is a manifestation of instability rather than its cause. Thus, electrical cardioversion is not required in all unstable atrial fibrillation presentations.

Narrow Complex Tachycardia Rhythms

Sinus Tachycardia

Sinus tachycardia is the most common NCT encountered in emergency department patients (Figure 9-1) and is found in all segments of this population. It originates from a focus in the sinuatrial (SA) node. Basically, it is sinus rhythm occurring at a rapid rate and should be considered a "reactive" rhythm, occurring in response to a physiologic trigger (Figure 9-4). Generally, sinus tachycardia is a benign rhythm itself and does not cause acute pulmonary edema, hypotension/hypoperfusion, or other end-organ dysfunction. The rate-based definition of sinus tachycardia varies with age, but the etiologic factors are similar in all age groups: hypovolemia resulting from dehydration or blood loss, hypoxia, fever, pain, anxiety, and medication/illicit substance effects. A careful history and examination can identify the underlying cause.

FIGURE 9-6.
Atrial fibrillation with RVR. The foci for this NCT are located in the atria tissues. Multiple atrial foci produce many depolarizations, averaging 600 to 1,200 per minute. These impulses then move through the atria tissues, arriving at the AV node. The AV node allows only a certain number of impulses per unit time to travel through to the ventricles, protecting them from excessively rapid rates. The impulses that are allowed to pass through into the ventricle traverse the intraventricular conduction system.

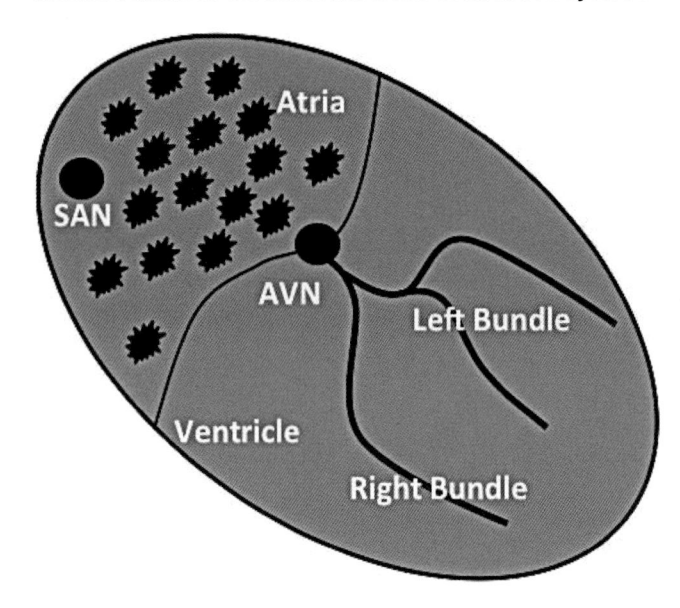

FIGURE 9-7.
Atrial fibrillation with RVR. A, Rhythm strip with chaotic baseline, reflective of the multiple atrial depolarizations. B, 12-lead ECG with atrial fibrillation with RVR; the rate is approximately 170 beats/min, the typical natural history rate for atrial fibrillation.

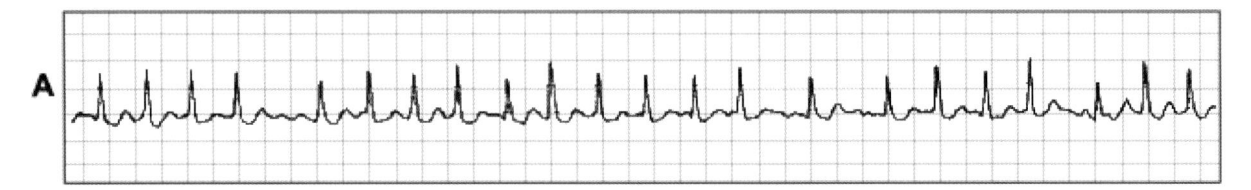

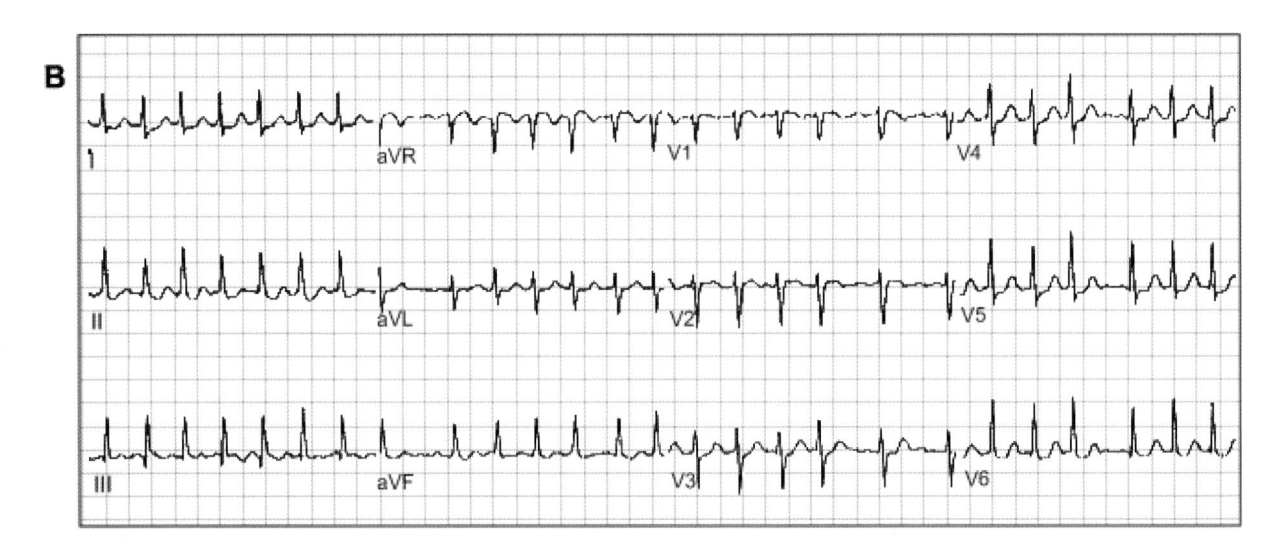

In addition to the physiologic causes of sinus tachycardia is an entity known as the syndrome of inappropriate sinus tachycardia. Individuals with this condition have a high heart rate as well as an exaggerated tachycardic response to exercise. The tachycardia is not a response to a stressor or stimulus. This syndrome is not diagnosed initially in the emergency department. It is best managed by a primary care physician and requires little emergency management besides reassurance, assuming that a physiologic stressor is not detected in the evaluation.

KEY POINT

Sinus tachycardia is a reactive rhythm, occurring in most cases in response to an abnormal physiologic trigger such as hypovolemia, hypoxia, fever, pain, anxiety, or medication/substance effect.

Electrocardiography. Sinus tachycardia (Figure 9-5) is a sinus rhythm with a rate faster than 100 beats/min in adults; infants and children have age-related rates. In addition, a P wave is associated with each QRS complex; the PR and P-P intervals are normal. The P waves are upright, or positive in amplitude, in leads I, II, and III. If the rate is particularly fast (>150 beats/min), the P waves might be "buried" in the QRS complexes, making the rhythm difficult to diagnose. In uncertain cases, the ECG chart speed may be increased, separating the P waves from the QRS complexes and thus facilitating the diagnosis.

Management. The therapeutic approach to sinus tachycardia is based on the underlying cause. Because it is usually a compensatory mechanism resulting from a physiologic stress, the tachycardia should not be addressed directly; rather, the underlying cause should be treated. Intravenous fluid resuscitation is used in patients with hypovolemia and other hypoperfused states. Hypoxia is managed with supplemental oxygen administration and airway support. Febrile patients should be given an antipyretic. Benzodiazepines should be considered in patients whose tachycardia is caused by medication or illicit substance exposure or withdrawal states (assuming treatment is warranted). Pain and anxiety, diagnoses of exclusion as causes of ST, are treated in standard fashion.

AV nodal blocking agents such as beta-blockers and calcium channel blockers have little to no role in the management of sinus tachycardia. A notable exception is aortic dissection and other aortic vascular emergencies, for which a reduction in heart rate is beneficial. Esmolol is the antihypertensive drug of choice in these patients for its negative chronotropic effects. Reducing the heart rate and thus reducing cardiac output is potentially beneficial in preventing further aortic injury.

Disposition. The disposition of patients with sinus tachycardia depends on its cause. The clinician should realize that the presence of tachycardia is a sensitive indicator of risk in patients discharged from the emergency department[4]; patients with a heart rate above 100 beats/min should not be discharged from the emergency department unless a benign explanation for the tachycardia has been documented and/or the abnormal heart rate has been addressed in a satisfactory manner.

Atrial Fibrillation and Atrial Flutter

Atrial fibrillation is the second most common NCT seen in the emergency department (Figure 9-1). Patients can present with a new-onset event or a recurrence; in either case, the rate is frequently rapid and is termed *atrial fibrillation with rapid ventricular response* (RVR). In patients with continuous or intermittent atrial fibrillation, another medical event such as urosepsis or pneumonia can precipitate an exacerbation of the chronic arrhythmia, resulting in atrial fibrillation with RVR. Beyond these typical presentations, a number of other clinical issues can contribute to the development of atrial fibrillation with RVR; for instance, patients can present with paroxysmal atrial fibrillation associated with hyperthyroidism, resulting from hypokalemia and/or hypomagnesemia, or following excessive ethanol intoxication (the holiday heart syndrome).[5]

KEY POINT

Atrial fibrillation, atrial flutter, and multifocal atrial tachycardia most often occur in patients with significant underlying cardiopulmonary disease.

The mechanism of atrial fibrillation appears to be the production of multiple depolarizations by microreentrant wavelets in the atria. The rate of atrial depolarization is extremely rapid—600 to 1,200 per minute (Figure 9-6). Paroxysms of atrial fibrillation can be triggered by alterations in autonomic tone and/or ectopic foci, which are frequently located in or around the pulmonary veins.[6,7] From a macroscopic pathologic perspective, a common theme found in most patients with atrial fibrillation is dilation and/or stiffening of the atrial structures, resulting from years of chronic cardiovascular illness (eg, poorly treated hypertension, ischemic heart disease, valvular heart disease). Patients do not tolerate atrial fibrillation with RVR hemodynamically for a number of reasons, including the excessively rapid ventricular rate and the loss of the "atrial kick," the atrial contraction component of ventricular filling. These patients are at risk of thromboembolism leading to stroke and other peripheral ischemic presentations.

Atrial fibrillation with RVR is also seen in patients with WPW syndrome; in fact, this form of atrial fibrillation is the second most frequently encountered rhythm disturbance seen in association with the syndrome, occurring in 20% to 25% of patients with symptomatic arrhythmia. This form of atrial fibrillation (discussed in Chapter 10) actually presents with a very rapid, irregular rhythm and widened, bizarre appearing QRS complexes.

Electrocardiography of atrial fibrillation. Atrial fibrillation presents with a characteristic ECG appearance (Figure 9-7). The cardiac rhythm is irregular with no pattern to the irregularity (an irregularly irregular rhythm). P waves are absent, reflecting the electrical chaos in the atrial tissues, with depolarization occurring at rate of 600 to 1,200 per minute; the baseline can be isoelectric and flat or chaotic with fibrillatory waves of varying morphology (Figure 9-7A). The ventricular rate varies, but most often a ventricular response of approximately 170 beats/min is seen. This rate represents the "naturally occurring" (ie, not altered by other disease state or medications) rate of atrial fibrillation (Figure 9-7B). The irregularity of the rhythm, particularly in situations involving RVR, can be difficult to detect with the naked eye; ECG calipers or another measuring method might be required to recognize the irregularity. The QRS complex is narrow in most presentations. Preexisting bundle-branch block or rate-related bundle dysfunction can produce a widened QRS complex, producing the irregular wide complex tachycardia.

It has been suggested that the amplitude of the fibrillatory waves can suggest the underlying cause of atrial fibrillation. Fine fibrillatory waves (<0.5 mm in amplitude) are associated with ischemic heart disease, while coarse waves (>0.5 mm in amplitude) signify left atrial enlargement likely related to chronic hypertension and valvular disease.

Atrial flutter shares many issues with atrial fibrillation; in fact, atrial flutter is frequently confused clinically with "coarse" atrial fibrillation. Atrial fibrillation is quite common, but atrial flutter occurs much less often (Figure 9-1). Atrial flutter most commonly results from a macroreentrant circuit within the right atrium. Causes of atrial flutter are similar to those of atrial fibrillation. From the hemodynamic perspective, patients tend to tolerate atrial flutter better than atrial fibrillation. Atrial flutter results from a single atrial focus (Figure 9-8), so the atrial kick remains intact. The rapid ventricular rate, however, can produce decompensation. Lastly, thromboembolism occurs in the atrial flutter patient at a rate similar to that among patients with atrial fibrillation.

Electrocardiography of atrial flutter. The ECG diagnosis of atrial flutter is more challenging (Figure 9-9) than the diagnosis of atrial fibrillation. Atrial flutter can be regular or irregular (Figures 9-9 and 9-10). Identifiable P waves are present. They are seen with a single morphology and appear as downward deflections, called flutter waves, which resemble a saw blade and have a sawtooth appearance (Figures 9-9B and 9-9C). These waves are best seen in leads, II, III, aVF, and V$_1$. In atrial flutter, they are frequently inverted in leads I, II, and/or III, which is a major point of distinction from sinus tachycardia (Figure 9-9B). Both rhythms are NCTs, yet the P waves are upright in all three limb leads with ST. Most commonly, the atrial rate is regular, usually at 300 beats/min, with a range from 250 to 350 beats/min. Less commonly, atrial rates vary from 340 to 430 beats/min.

Although 1:1 atrioventricular conduction is possible, some form of AV block is usually present, which directly affects the ventricular rate. Most often, a 1:2 conduction pattern is seen, with two atrial depolarizations for every one ventricular depolarization; this magnitude of the block produces a ventricular rate around 150 beats/min (Figure 9-9). A 3:1 conduction pattern, or AV block, results in a ventricular rate of 100 beats/min. Although the degree of AV block is often fixed, it can also be variable, yielding an irregular ventricular response (Figure 9-10).

A NCT that is regular, at a rate of approximately 150 beats/min, strongly suggests atrial flutter with 2:1 conduction. This is the "naturally occurring" rate for atrial flutter, which is unaffected by other disease states or medications (Figure 9-9B). As with atrial fibrillation, the QRS complex is narrow. Preexisting bundle-branch block or rate-related bundle dysfunction can widen the QRS complex, producing a wide complex tachycardia.

Management. The vast majority of atrial fibrillation and atrial flutter emergency department presentations are related to rapid ventricular rates; thus, management largely focuses on the patient with atrial fibrillation or atrial flutter complicated by RVR. New-onset atrial fibrillation typically presents with RVR; "exacerbations" of preexisting arrhythmia similarly can present with rapid rates. In either case, the management of both atrial fibrillation and atrial flutter focuses on three basic goals: identification and treatment of rhythm-related instability, ventricular rate control aimed at reduction of rapid response, and rhythm termination with conversion to sinus rhythm. As noted above, atrial fibrillation can be destabilizing, requiring urgent intervention, while atrial flutter much less often presents with significant hemodynamic compromise.

In patients with new-onset arrhythmia with RVR who are profoundly unstable, primarily due to the rapid rhythm, urgent electrical cardioversion is the most appropriate therapy. This scenario is uncommon and can be difficult to recognize. More often, atrial fibrillation and atrial flutter with RVR present less dramatically. In fact, the issue of hemodynamic instability is not a "yes or no" phenomenon. Rather, stability must be considered along a clinical spectrum, with consideration of the exacerbating factors and their impact on hemodynamic status. Furthermore, most patients with RVR likely are experiencing tachycardia due to a secondary event such as hypovolemia, fever, hypoxia, or pain. For instance, the patient with a history of atrial fibrillation can present with gastrointestinal bleeding and hypovolemia; a tachycardic response is appropriate for this

FIGURE 9-8.

Atrial flutter. The focus for this NCT is in the atria; note that, in contrast to atrial fibrillation, atrial flutter has one focus. The impulse then moves through the atria tissues, arriving at the AV node. The impulse then is transmitted into the ventricle and traverses the intraventricular conduction system.

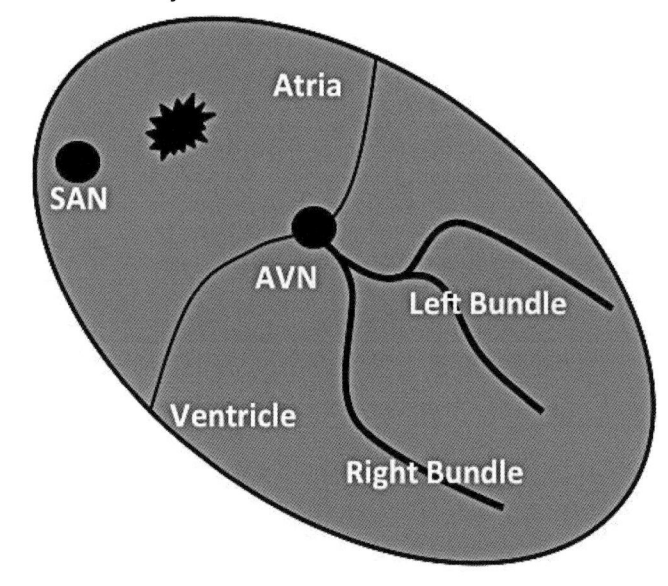

Narrow Complex Tachycardia

patient's hemorrhage-related hypovolemia. Similar statements can be made regarding dehydration and absolute hypovolemia; sepsis with elevated temperature, relative hypovolemia, and inefficient perfusion; and trauma with hemorrhagic shock.

The most appropriate management of patients experiencing RVR focuses on the underlying issue responsible for the tachycardic response. Infusion of intravenous normal saline and/or blood products, as appropriate for the clinical situation, can markedly reduce the response. Correction of hypoxia, reduction of fever, and pain management, in the appropriate patient, will

FIGURE 9-9.

Atrial flutter with a ventricular rate of 150 beats/min. A, Rhythm strip demonstrating atrial flutter. The arrow indicates flutter waves. B, 12-lead ECG with NCT at a rate of 150 beats/min, the natural history rate for atrial flutter. The P waves are not upright in leads I, II, and III. The combination of a regular rhythm with rate of 150 beats/min and inverted P waves in the limb leads suggests atrial flutter. C, Atrial flutter (150 beats/min) with flutter waves (arrows) in leads II and III in three patients.

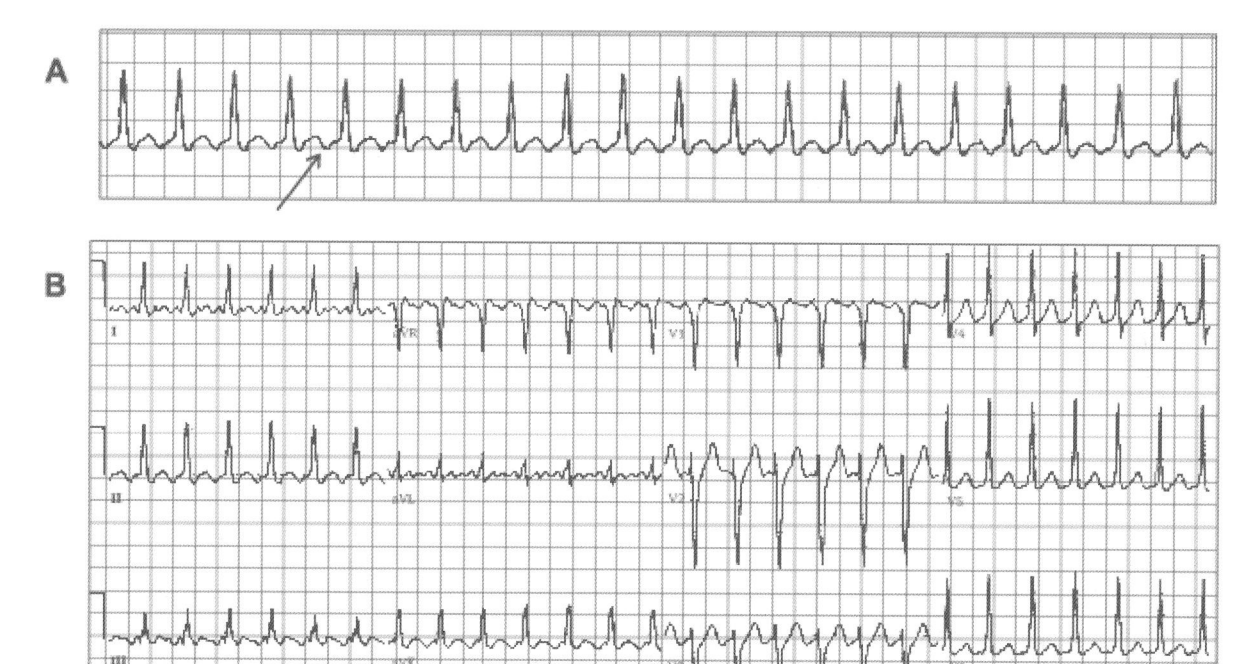

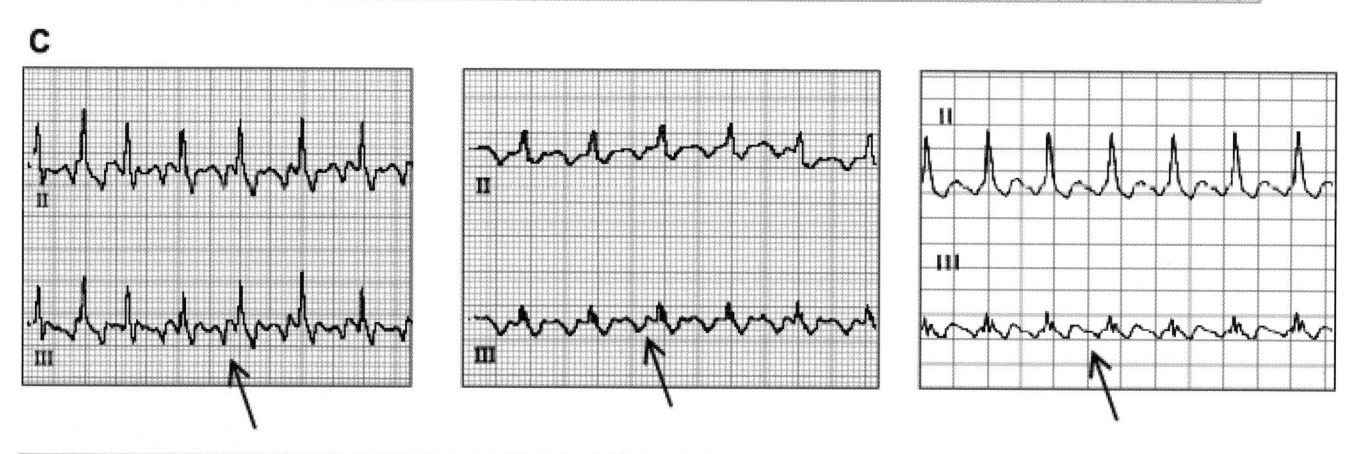

FIGURE 9-10.

Atrial flutter with variable conduction (ie, variable block)

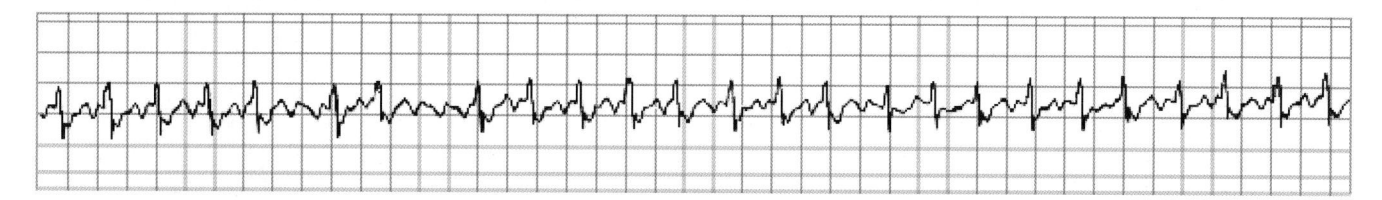

CARDIOVASCULAR EMERGENCIES

FIGURE 9-11.

PSVT. In most instances of PSVT, the focus is located in the AV node, but, in a minority of PSVT patients, the focus is in the atrial tissues. A, The impulse originates in the AV node. The impulse then is transmitted into the ventricle and traverses the intraventricular conduction system. B, The impulse originates from a focus in the atria. It travels through atrial tissues to the AV node, is transmitted into the ventricle, and traverses the intraventricular conduction system.

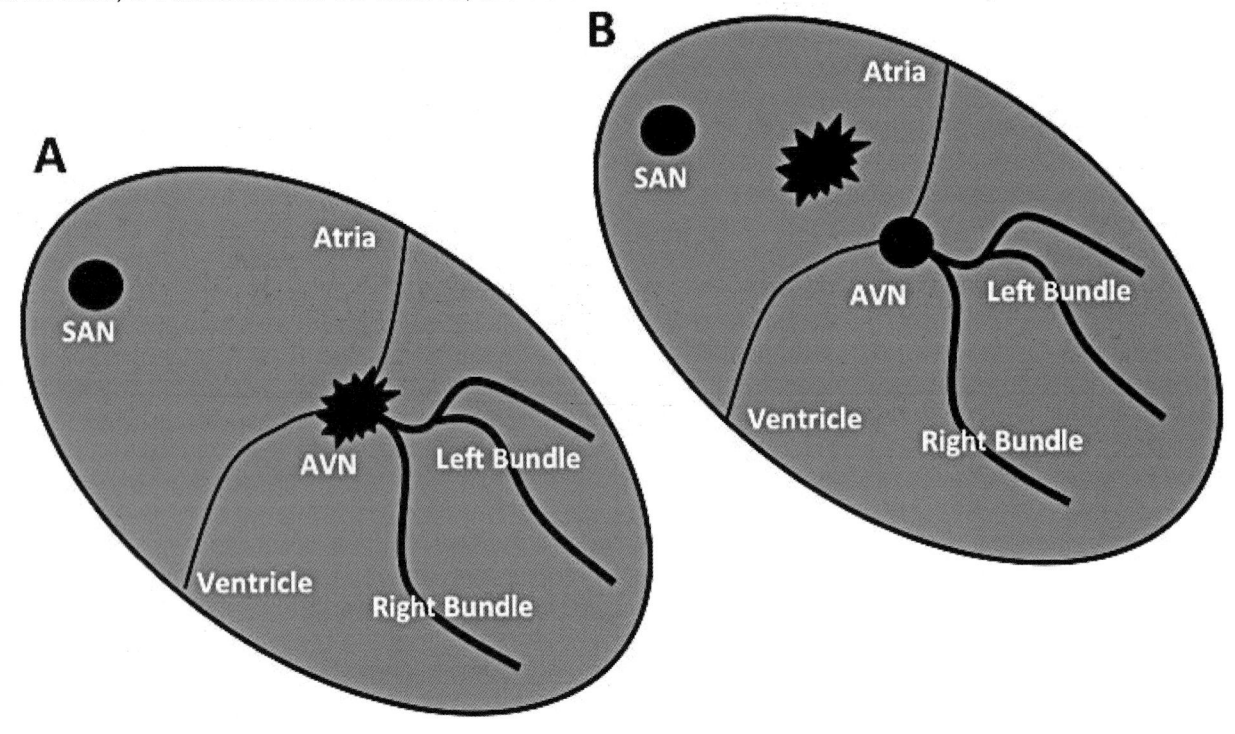

FIGURE 9-12.

PSVT, also known as AV nodal reciprocating tachycardia. A, PSVT with large, prominent QRS complexes. B, PSVT with small, less prominent QRS complexes. C, PSVT with retrograde P waves (arrow). D, PSVT after electrical cardioversion to sinus tachycardia. The arrowheads indicate the monitor-defibrillator is set on synchronized cardioversion.

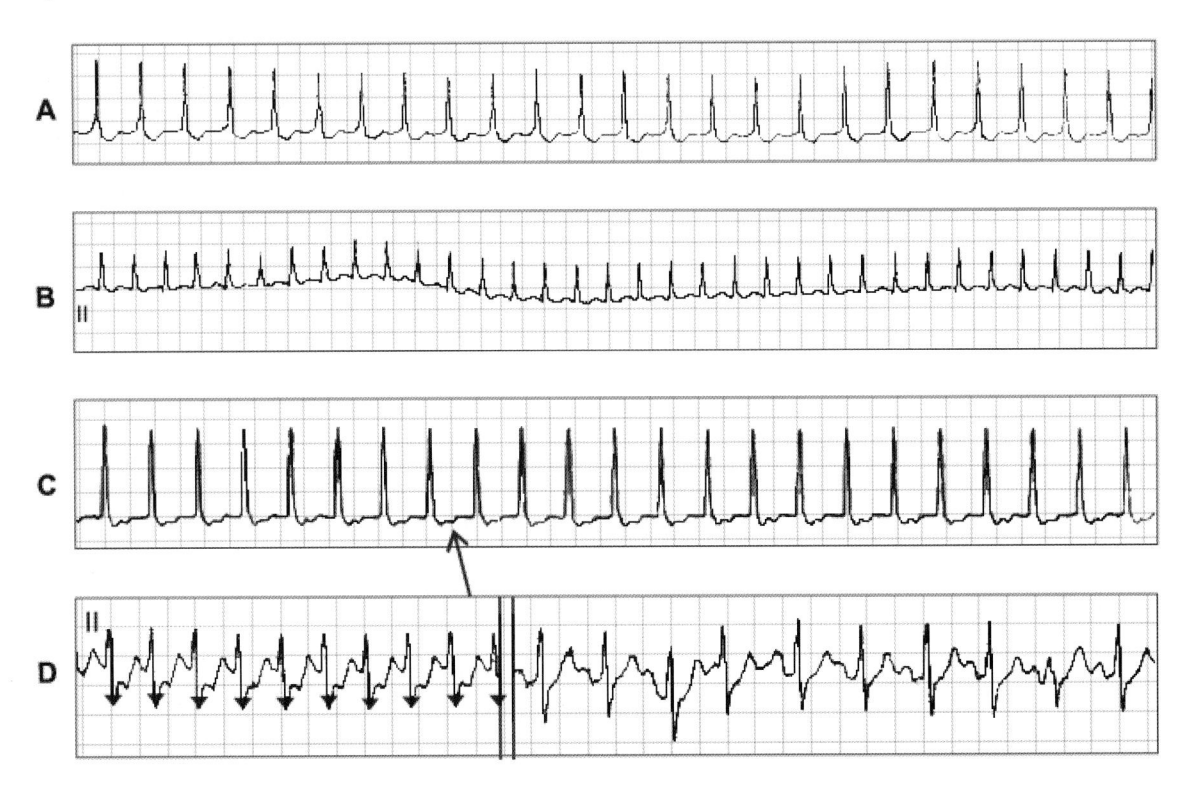

also lower the ventricular rate. Attempts at electrical cardioversion in these patients can be problematic and are ill advised.

Electrical cardioversion can be appropriate for the patient with RVR and hemodynamic instability thought to be caused primarily by the rapid rate. Biphasic energy levels should start at 75 to 100 J, with escalation as appropriate depending on the patient's response. Sedation-assisted electrical cardioversion is most appropriate, but the administration of sedatives to a hypotensive patient can be problematic. The bedside clinical assessment will guide such choices. Appropriate agents include etomidate, ketamine, propofol, and midazolam; fentanyl can be added for pain management at the clinician's discretion.

Once instability has been considered and addressed appropriately, the next task involves reducing the ventricular rate; in fact, ventricular rate control is the primary task of the emergency clinician in the vast majority of patient contacts. Ventricular rate control can be accomplished via two strategies: intravascular volume expansion with normal saline, as discussed above, or the use of AV node blocking agents, essentially "gaining control of the AV node." Intravenous calcium channel blockers or beta-adrenergic blockers are the most appropriate agents. Diltiazem is an excellent choice in this setting and can be used safely in patients with mild to moderate chronic left ventricular dysfunction. Metoprolol is another reasonable choice. Esmolol, using standard bolus and infusion, can be used if the patient's hemodynamic status is tenuous. The drug's relatively short serum half-life allows more of a "turn-on/turn-off" capability if the patient's condition deteriorates.

Interestingly, amiodarone can be employed in this rate-control strategy because of its beta-blocking and calcium channel

FIGURE 9-13.

PSVT (AV nodal reciprocating tachycardia) in a young woman

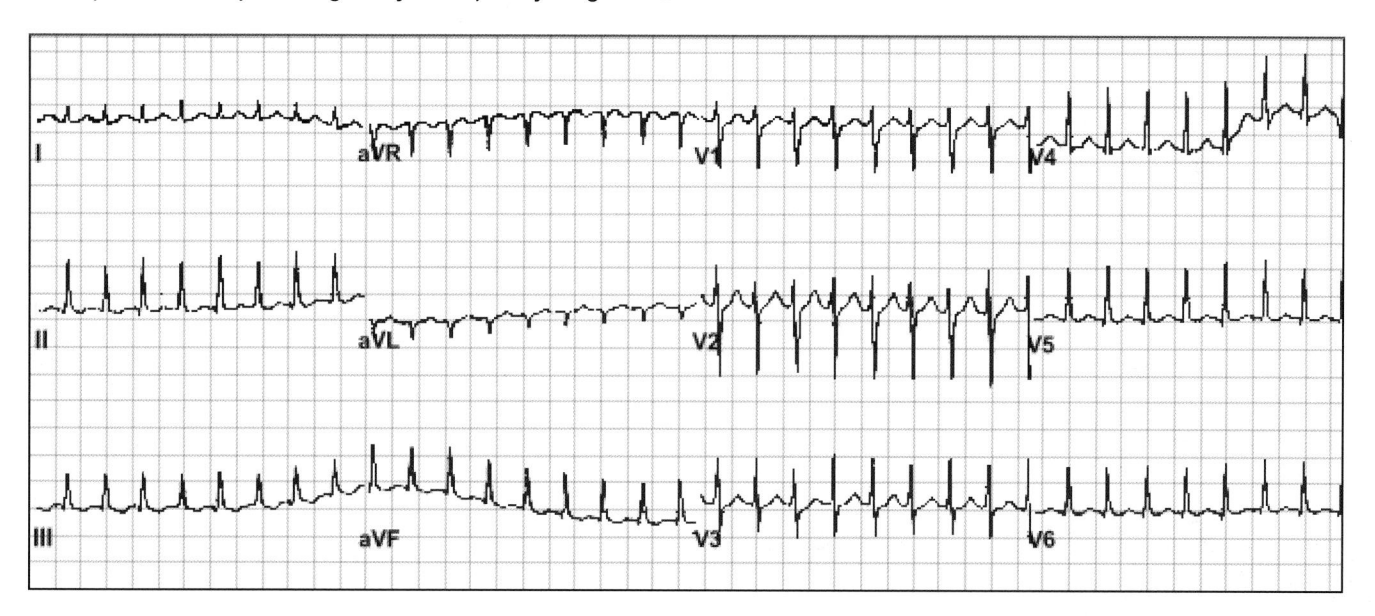

FIGURE 9-14.

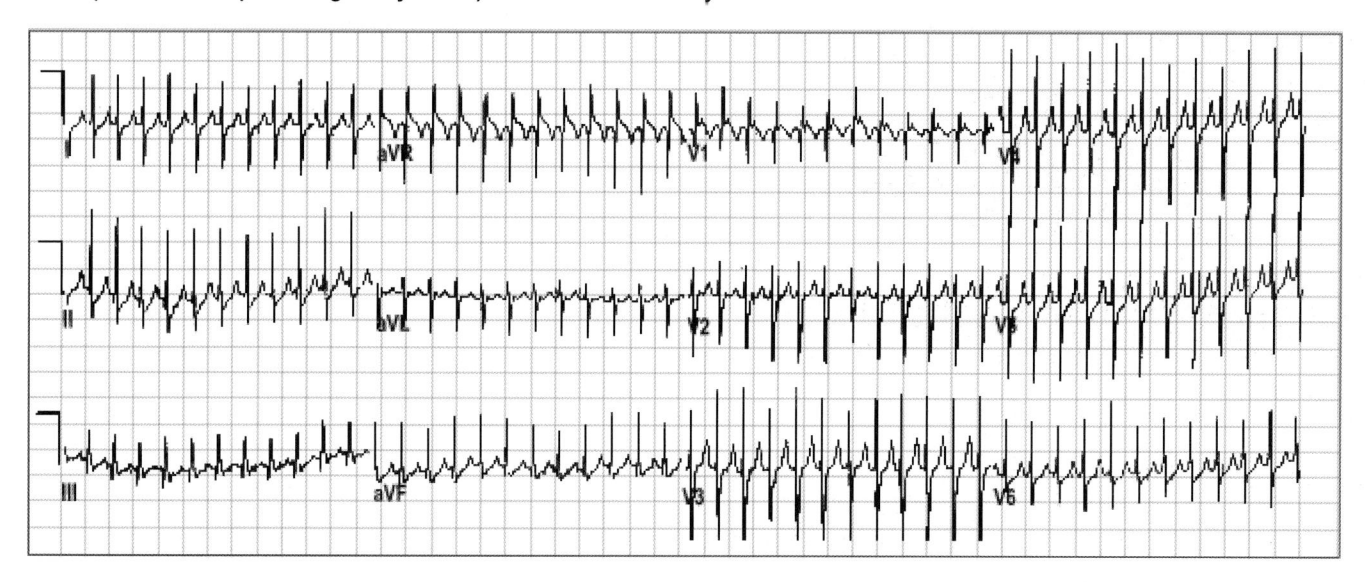

PSVT (AV nodal reciprocating tachycardia) in a 9-month-old boy

blocking abilities. Adequate rate control should be a primary issue for the emergency physician to address in atrial fibrillation scenarios. Lastly, the unstable patient may be treated urgently with rate control rather than electrical cardioversion initially.

Rate control by itself significantly reduces related symptoms. The continued presence of atrial fibrillation either at a controlled rate or with continued tachycardia, however, can still produce unwanted clinical manifestations. Recall that an organized atrial contraction, the atrial kick, contributes to left ventricular filling. The loss of atrial contraction's ventricular filling can continue to produce unpleasant manifestations despite adequate rate control. Therefore, the final consideration focuses on rhythm conversion from atrial fibrillation to sinus rhythm. This conversion is quite difficult to attain, and the practice is controversial.

Rhythm conversion can be accomplished using medications or electrical therapy. The parenteral medications that may be administered include procainamide, amiodarone, and ibutilide. Electrical therapy is performed in similar fashion to the description for the unstable patient. In either choice of management strategy, the patient should be electively converted only if the duration of the arrhythmia is known to be less than 2 days. Beyond this 48-hour period, significant clot formation is possible within the left-sided cardiac chambers. Conversion with clot in the left heart can result in embolism, leading to stroke or peripheral ischemia syndromes.

Numerous studies suggest that a significant portion of patients with new-onset atrial fibrillation spontaneously convert to sinus rhythm within 24 hours after onset and evaluation, assuming rate control is achieved and disruptions in the "internal milieu" are corrected.[8-11] This very high rate of "spontaneous" conversion, coupled with the results of numerous atrial fibrillation trials demonstrating that rate control is similar to rhythm control, argues in favor of an initial rate-focused strategy.[10,11] For instance, the AFFIRM and RACE trials demon-

FIGURE 9-15.

PSVT (AV nodal reciprocating tachycardia) with retrograde P waves (arrows)

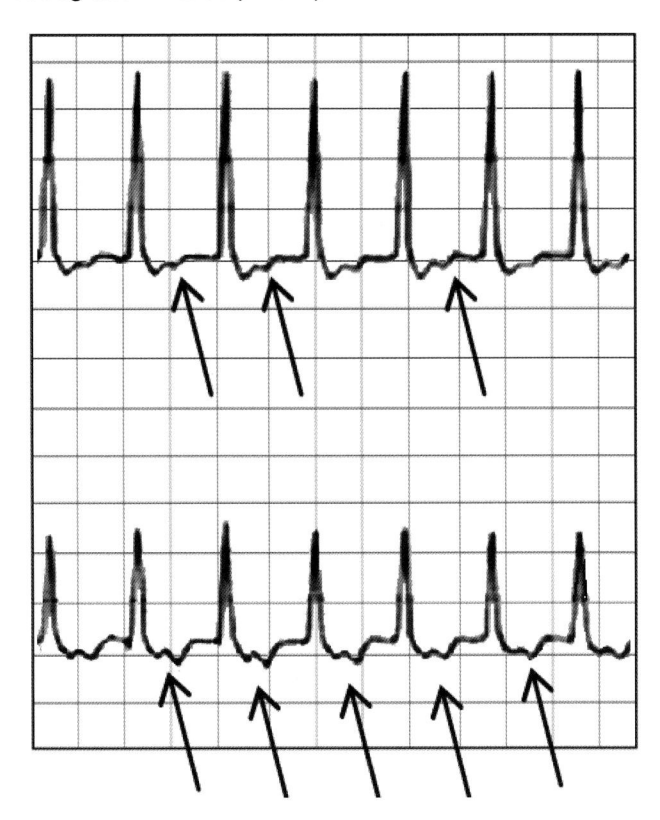

FIGURE 9-16.

PSVT (AV nodal reciprocating tachycardia) with rate-related ST-segment depression (arrows) in leads V_4, V_5, and V_6 in a 29-year-old woman. Coronary ischemia was not noted in the evaluation, during the arrhythmias, or after conversion to sinus rhythm.

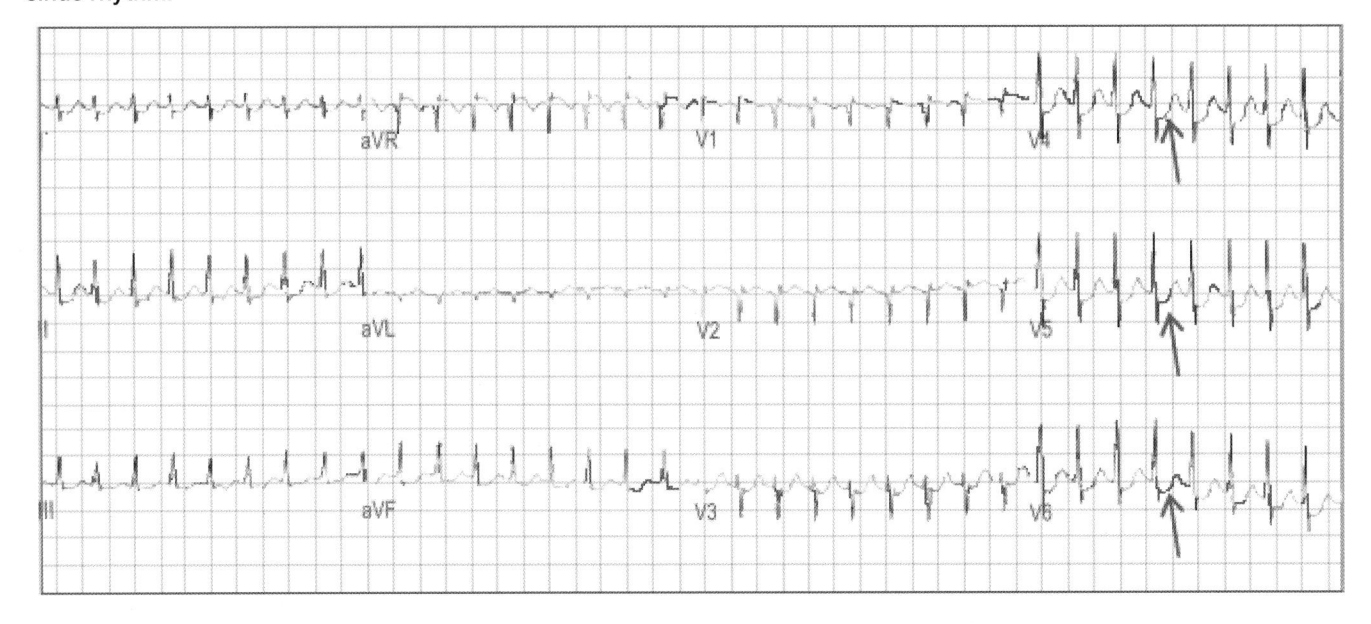

strated no significant difference in quality-of-life issues, control of symptoms, and the occurrence of adverse events between the rate- and rhythm-control groups.[10,11] Therefore, a patient with new-onset atrial fibrillation who is stable may certainly be managed with rate control alone, as an inpatient or outpatient, depending on other clinical variables.

The rhythm-conversion perspective, however, notes that earlier attempts at cardioversion are more likely to be successful in both the short and long term. There is no easy answer to this rhythm conversion question. Consultation with a cardiologist can be pursued to determine the need for non-urgent electrical cardioversion.

Disposition. Disposition decisions for the atrial fibrillation/atrial flutter patient are based on several issues, including the overall clinical situation, the response to emergency department treatment of the arrhythmia, the management strategies that are selected, and the patient's history of the rhythm disorder (ie, new onset versus recurrence). The patient with acute decompensation of the cardiopulmonary systems complicated by atrial fibrillation or atrial flutter with RVR likely requires admission to the hospital for management of the various issues. Prompt conversion to normal sinus rhythm without recurrence can allow discharge from the emergency department, but this scenario is not often encountered in these patients. Of course, if the arrhythmia recurs or management of the initial rhythm is difficult, admission is a likely course of action. The management strategy chosen for a particular patient can affect care; for instance, electrical cardioversion in the appropriate patient likely will require observation in a short-stay or equivalent unit. Finally, patients with new-onset atrial fibrillation or atrial flutter can be admitted to the hospital for further management and evaluation of the rhythm disorder and related causes. In select patients with appropriate and timely outpatient resources, discharge to home with followup may be considered, assuming all other clinical variables are non-issues.

Paroxysmal Supraventricular Tachycardia

PSVT is the third most common NCT in the emergency department population, following sinus tachycardia and atrial fibrillation (Figure 9-1).[1] This tachycardia most frequently results from an abnormal focus located within the AV node. In 80% to 90% of cases, the focus is found in the AV node (Figure 9-11A); in the remainder of cases, it is located in the atrial tissues (Figure 9-11B). PSVT is seen in all age groups, from the young infant to the extremely elderly. It is seen frequently in younger patients, particularly women. Ultimately benign in most cases, PSVT can cause significant cardiovascular instability. Despite the presentation, PSVT presents in the absence of known cardiovascular disease for most patients. The rare patient presents with PSVT as a manifestation of an underlying issue and thus requires management of the arrhythmias and the causative problem.[1] In fact, the rhythm can largely be considered a nuisance—a cardiovascular hiccup—and not a threat to life.

Patients present with a range of symptoms and signs. Palpitations, chest pain, pounding sensations in the neck and chest, dyspnea, dizziness, and syncope are common complaints expressed by patients with PSVT. Interestingly, the vast majority report a sensation of "pounding in the neck," which results from concomitant atrial and ventricular contraction, elevated right atrial pressures, and flow reversal from the right atrium to the systemic venous system. In fact, the absence of this symptom is a strong negative predictor of PSVT in the NCT patient.[12] The examination might reveal only a regularly occurring tachycardia; in other instances, hypotension, other signs of hypoperfusion (eg, altered mentation), and pulmonary edema can be seen.

KEY POINT

Paroxysmal supraventricular tachycardia, although potentially destabilizing in its presentation, is usually a benign rhythm.

Approximately 80% to 90% of patients with PSVT demonstrate an arrhythmia focus in the AV node; in the remaining patients, the PSVT has an atrial focus (Figure 9-11). Two to three percent of PSVT-appearing arrhythmias are, in fact, WPW-related NCT, the narrow complex atrioventricular reciprocating tachycardia (AVRT).

Electrocardiography. From the ECG perspective (Figures 9-12, 9-13, and 9-14), PSVT is a narrow QRS complex tachycardia. The QRS complex is of normal width, usually less than 80 msec in duration; on occasion, it is minimally widened, with a width of no more than 100 msec. PSVT is rapid and regular. In the adult patient, the rate is usually 170 to 180 beats/min but can range from as low as 130 to as high as 260. In children, the rate can approach 240 to 260 beats/min, particularly in infants (Figure 9-14).

P waves are usually not seen. Since atrial and ventricular depolarizations usually occur almost simultaneously, the P waves are frequently buried in the QRS complex and are totally obscured; in fact, in 80% of PSVT cases, the P wave is not observed on the ECG. In a minority of presentations, a retrograde P wave is noted (Figures 9-9C and 9-15), indicating conduction from, rather than to, the AV node. The AV nodal impulse moves in retrograde fashion back into the atria. The retrograde P wave can be found either before, during, or after the QRS complex; frequently, it is inverted in the limb leads. If the P wave occurs before the QRS complex, no measurable PR interval is noted. If the P wave occurs after the QRS complex, it can distort the terminal portion of the QRS complex, producing a "pseudo" S wave in the inferior leads and a "pseudo" R wave in V_1.

Finally, ST-segment depression is noted at times in this NCT, particularly in leads V_4, V_5, and V_6 (Figure 9-16). This ST-segment deviation is likely a result of the rate (ie, rate-related ST-segment depression). When this ECG finding is observed, additional evaluation and management of an acute coronary event are not required unless other clinical data suggest the need for them.

Management. In most instances, PSVT is managed appropriately and easily, with favorable patient outcome. Since the vast majority of PSVT cases result from a problem in the AV node, it is not surprising that vagal maneuvers, adenosine, and other AV nodal blocking agents are successful in rhythm management and ultimate conversion. Vagal maneuvers are success-

CARDIOVASCULAR EMERGENCIES

ful in 20% of patients, particularly if used early in the rhythm's course. If vagal maneuvers are unsuccessful, intravenous adenosine is most often curative. It is the uncommon patient who requires a beta-blocker or calcium channel blocker. In such cases, the patient has not responded to intravenous adenosine, likely because of its ultra-short serum half-life. The use of an agent with a longer serum half-life can assist in the conversion to sinus rhythm; this therapy can be used in full dose or partial dose combined with repeat adenosine administration. In patients with recalcitrant PSVT or unstable presentations, electrical cardioversion may be employed. In the very uncommon case of the patient with an active, inciting cardiovascular event, the cause of the PSVT is managed in standard fashion, appropriate for the particular event.

Disposition. Prompt conversion to normal sinus rhythm without recurrence can allow discharge from the emergency department. In general, patients with PSVT can be discharged safely, assuming their postconversion course is unremarkable. The vast majority of PSVT patients do not experience significant, additional pathophysiologic events; thus, "treat what you see" is the appropriate mindset for PSVT in the emergency department.[1] Of course, admission is a likely course of action if the arrhythmia recurs, management of the initial rhythm is difficult, or an active event is occurring.

Wolff-Parkinson-White Syndrome

The WPW syndrome, a ventricular preexcitation disorder, allows an anomalous connection between the atria and ventricles, providing the substrate for supraventricular arrhythmia. The actual incidence of symptomatic arrhythmia seen in patients with the classic WPW ECG triad (shortened PR interval, delta wave, and minimally widened QRS complex) is unknown. The most frequently encountered rhythm disturbance seen in patients with this syndrome is NCT, encountered in 90% of those with a symptomatic arrhythmia.

WPW NCT is also known as AV reentrant, or reciprocating, tachycardia (AVRT) because of the associated conduction pattern (Figure 9-17): the atrial impulse travels anterograde through the AV node, with ventricular activation occurring through the

FIGURE 9-17.

AVRT in the WPW syndrome. The focus for this NCT is located in the supraventricular tissues, originating with a premature beat. The impulse then moves from atrial tissues to ventricular tissues via the AV node. In a large reentry loop, the impulse moves in retrograde fashion from the ventricular tissues to atrial tissues via the accessory pathway. This reentry loop perpetuates itself, producing the regular NCT. As the reentry phenomenon continues, the impulses traverse the intraventricular conduction system.

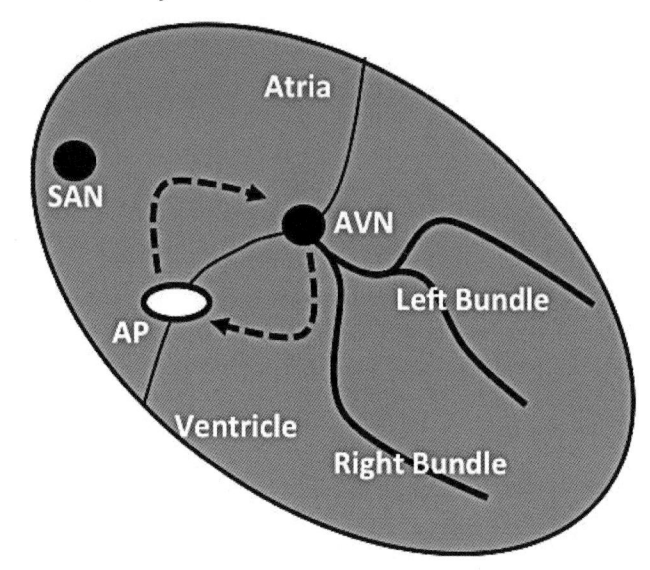

FIGURE 9-18.

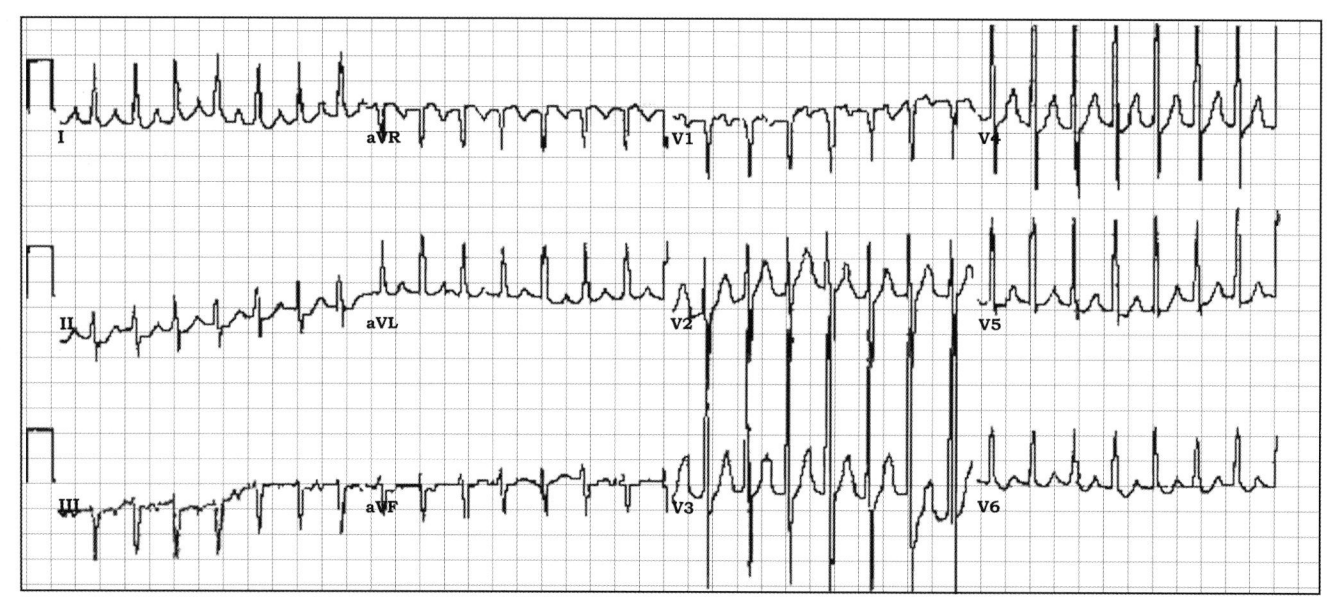

AVRT with a regularly occurring narrow QRS complex and a ventricular rate of approximately 175 beats/min in the WPW syndrome

normal conduction system. The impulse then returns to the atria in retrograde fashion via the accessory pathway, the anomalous connection between the atria and ventricles. This type of conduction in WPW syndrome is called *orthodromic*, indicating an anterograde direction of impulse movement through the AV node. Thus, this rhythm is best described as orthodromic AVRT.

Typical PSVT, the NCT not associated with WPW syndrome, is known as AV nodal reentrant tachycardia (AVNRT). The inclusion of the "N" in this descriptor highlights the involvement of the AV node as the focus of the reentry loop compared with WPW AVRT, in which the reentry loop involves the AV node, the accessory pathway, and the atrial and ventricular tissues.

Electrocardiography. The ECG features of orthodromic AVRT are shown in Figures 9-18 and 9-19: a narrow QRS complex, without a delta wave (since the ventricles are being activated through the normal conduction pathway), with ventricular rates ranging from 160 to 220 beats/min in the adult (Figure 9-18) and 180 to 260 beats/min in a child (Figure 9-19). The QRS complex is, of course, narrow with a width less than 80 to 100 msec in duration and occurs in a very rapid, regular fashion. In most instances, P waves are not noted (occasionally, a P wave is seen immediately before or after the QRS complex, representing retrograde atrial activation [the retrograde P wave]). This form of WPW NCT resembles "typical" PSVT in many ways, and they can be extremely difficult to differentiate (Figure 9-20).

Management. The initial treatment of orthodromic AVRT focuses on two issues: the patient's stability on presentation and an awareness of the arrhythmia's properties aimed at an interruption of the reentrant circuit. As in the therapeutic approach to any tachyarrhythmia, electrical cardioversion should be applied to all patients with hemodynamic instability, manifested by altered systemic perfusion, mental status changes, ischemic chest pain, or dyspnea caused by acute pulmonary edema.

In the hemodynamically stable patient, the first therapeutic intervention should be with vagal maneuvers (carotid sinus massage, Valsalva, and ice water face immersion), which can temporarily block conduction through the AV node. Vagal maneuvers are more likely to be successful in the termination of the arrhythmia when applied soon after initiation of the tachycardia, since sympathetic tone tends to increase as the duration of the tachycardia lengthens. If vagal maneuvers fail, the next therapeutic step is the use of medications that prolong the refractory period of the AV node. In the orthodromic AVRT (ie, the narrow complex variety of arrhythmia), the use of AV node blocking agents is both correct and appropriate. This choice of intervention is markedly different than for the other two symptomatic arrhythmias of WPW syndrome—wide QRS complex AVRT and preexcited atrial fibrillation with wide QRS complex. In these two WPW rhythm presentations, AV node blocking agents are contraindicated.

The first choice of AV nodal blockade is adenosine, a very short-acting agent that blocks the AV node and interrupts the reentrant circuit. Adenosine is generally a safe choice with an excellent record of successful arrhythmia termination. If adenosine fails, additional treatment of the orthodromic tachycardia can be provided with several AV node blocking medications, including calcium channel antagonists and beta-adrenergic blocking agents such as intravenous diltiazem, metoprolol, or esmolol. Additionally, procainamide is effective by producing block in the accessory conduction pathway. A note of caution, however, is advised in this situation: procainamide is slower to

FIGURE 9-19.

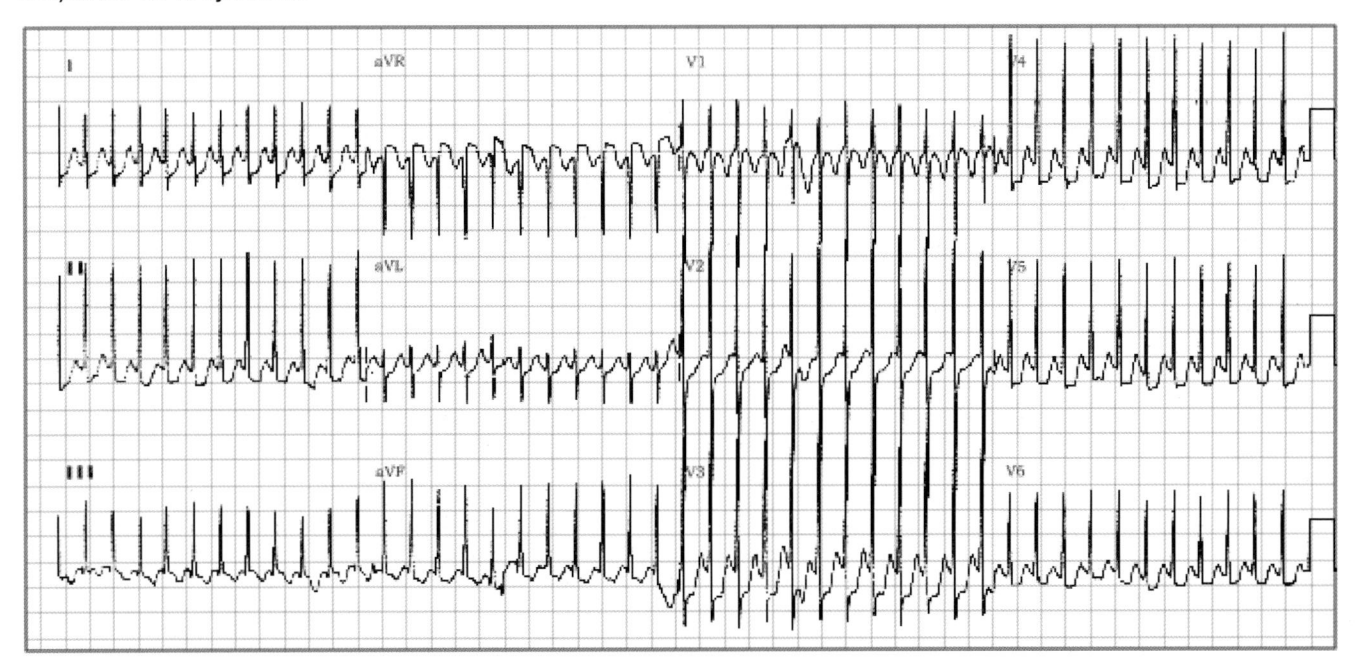

AVRT with a regularly occurring narrow QRS complex and an extremely rapid ventricular rate (approximately 260 beats/min) in the WPW syndrome

act than the calcium channel antagonists and beta-adrenergic blocking agents with respect to arrhythmia termination.

KEY POINT

AVRT, the most common arrhythmia of the WPW syndrome, is an NCT that is similar in appearance to PSVT. This NCT can be treated with AV nodal blocking agents, again similar to PSVT.

Disposition. Prompt conversion to normal sinus rhythm without recurrence can allow discharge from the emergency department. If this course of management is chosen, prompt cardiology followup is needed. Alternatively, admission to the hospital with consideration for electrophysiologic study and potential cardiac ablation is also appropriate. If the arrhythmia recurs or management of the initial rhythm is difficult, admission is a likely course of action.

Multifocal Atrial Tachycardia

MAT, an uncommon form of NCT, is classified as a subtype of atrial tachycardia. Other terms used to describe this NCT are *chaotic atrial tachycardia* and *chaotic atrial rhythm*, reflecting the lack of understanding of the arrhythmia's pathophysiology. Thus, it is understandable that multiple names have been used to describe this arrhythmia; the most appropriate term remains *multifocal atrial tachycardia*. The prevalence of MAT is quite low, ranging from 0.05% to 0.35%; furthermore, considering the range of NCTs seen in the emergency department, MAT represents less than 3% of all such cases. It is usually seen in older patients with acute exacerbations of chronic pulmonary or cardiopulmonary disease. It has also been described postoperatively and in conditions involving hypoxia, as in pneumonia, pulmonary embolism, and acute pulmonary edema. For instance, a recent review of inpatients with MAT revealed that their typical age was 70. Their mortality rate during hospitalization was almost 50%, probably related to age and comorbidities rather than to MAT itself.[13]

The pathophysiology of MAT is uncertain. In fact, the mechanism responsible for its development is not specifically known but likely involves abnormal automaticity or triggered activity. Reentry phenomenon is not involved. Regardless of the mechanism of the arrhythmia, multiple different foci are noted in the atria, discharging at random. The impulses are conducted to the ventricle, producing an irregular ventricular rhythm (Figure 9-21). Electrolyte abnormalities, including hypomagnesemia and hypokalemia, probably contribute to its genesis. This observation is based on the fact that replacement therapy can convert MAT to sinus rhythm.[14] Of course, acute exacerbations of chronic obstructive pulmonary disease and other cardiopulmonary illnesses with hypoxia are seen in association with MAT. Management of these underlying conditions with resolution of the hypoxia is also associated with MAT conversion to sinus rhythm.

Electrocardiography. The ECG definition of MAT includes a consideration of the P waves, QRS complexes, rate, and regularity (Figure 9-22). Three distinct P waves are observed in any single ECG lead; they are usually best seen in leads II, III, aVF, and V_1. Interestingly, certain authorities require that the three P waves must be separate and distinct from the sinus rhythm-produced P waves, thus requiring three non-sinus P

FIGURE 9-20.

A comparison of AVNRT (ie, PSVT) (A) with AVRT of WPW syndrome (B)

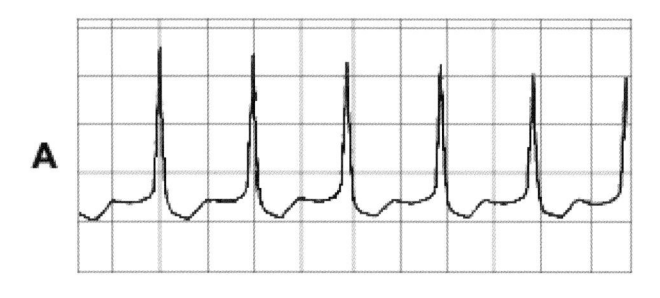

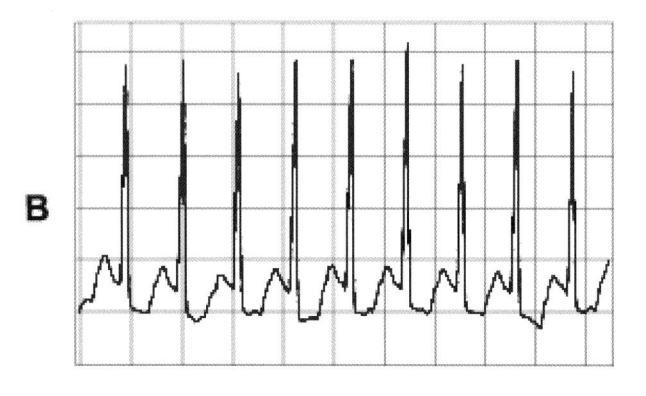

FIGURE 9-21.

MAT. The foci for this NCT are found in the atria; note that several different foci are active in MAT. The impulse, regardless of its atrial source, moves through the atrial tissues, arriving at the AV node. The impulse then is transmitted into the ventricle and traverses the intraventricular conduction system.

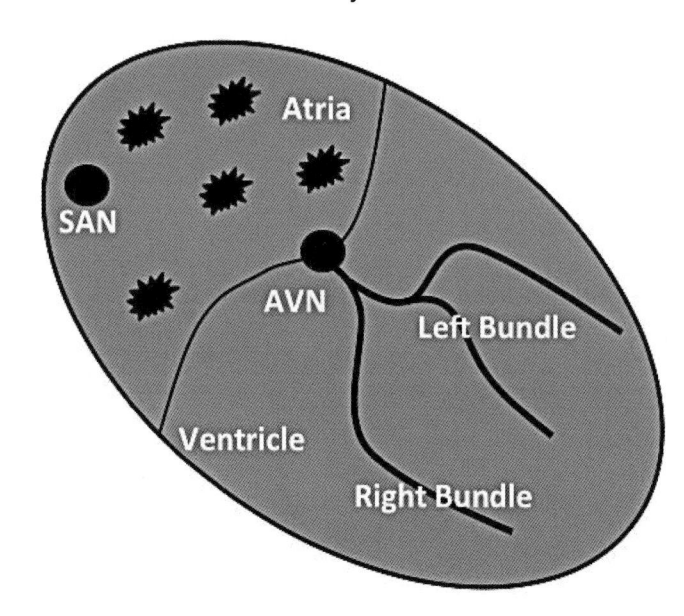

waves for the diagnosis.

The isoelectric baseline should be flat between P-QRS-T cycles, an important feature that distinguishes MAT from atrial fibrillation with its chaotic baseline. The QRS complexes are irregular without apparent pattern to the irregularity. The QRS complex is usually narrow unless preexisting bundle-branch, rate-related aberrant intraventricular conduction, or a preexisting accessory pathway is present. The P-P, PR, and R-R intervals are all irregular. Particularly rapid forms of MAT are difficult to identify and distinguish from atrial fibrillation with the irregularly irregular rhythm (Figure 9-23). The treatment approaches to MAT and atrial fibrillation are quite different; thus, it is vital to look for and identify the different P waves with a flat isoelectric baseline.

Management. The initial management of MAT focuses on treatment of the underlying cause: the use of bronchodilators with intravenous steroids for chronic obstructive pulmonary disease exacerbations, nitrates and positive-pressure external ventilation for pulmonary edema, intravenous fluids with oxygen and antibiotics for pneumonia. This approach most often involves correcting hypoxia, improving oxygenation, addressing electrolyte and acid-base abnormalities, and withdrawing inciting medications. In addition, intravenous fluid should be used if significant hypovolemia is suspected. On occasion, ventricular rate control may be used with calcium channel blockade. MAT is not amenable to electrical cardioversion; thus, hypotension in the setting of rapid MAT is not managed with electrical cardioversion but rather with correction of the underlying issue(s).[13]

KEY POINT

Management goals in the patient with MAT most often include treatment of the underlying, exacerbating events such as chronic obstructive pulmonary disease or pneumonia. In rare cases, direct rate control may be used if other methods are not effective.

Disposition. Admission decisions for patients experiencing MAT are driven almost entirely by the underlying cause of the arrhythmia.

FIGURE 9-22.

MAT. Note the rapid, irregular rhythm with at least three P-wave morphologies in a single ECG lead.

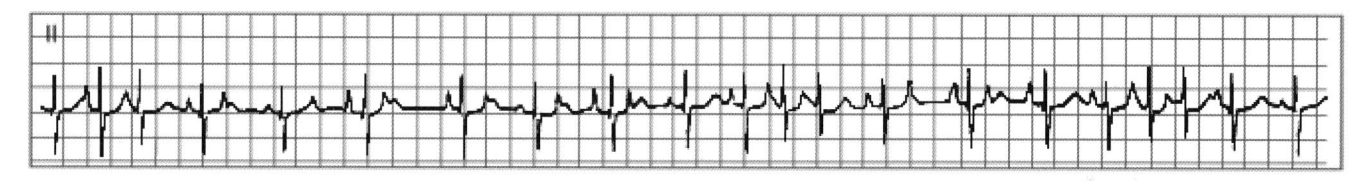

FIGURE 9-23.

Comparison of atrial fibrillation with MAT. Both rhythms are irregular without apparent regularity to the pattern. A, Atrial fibrillation with no identifiable P waves. B, MAT with distinct, identifiable P waves of multiple morphology.

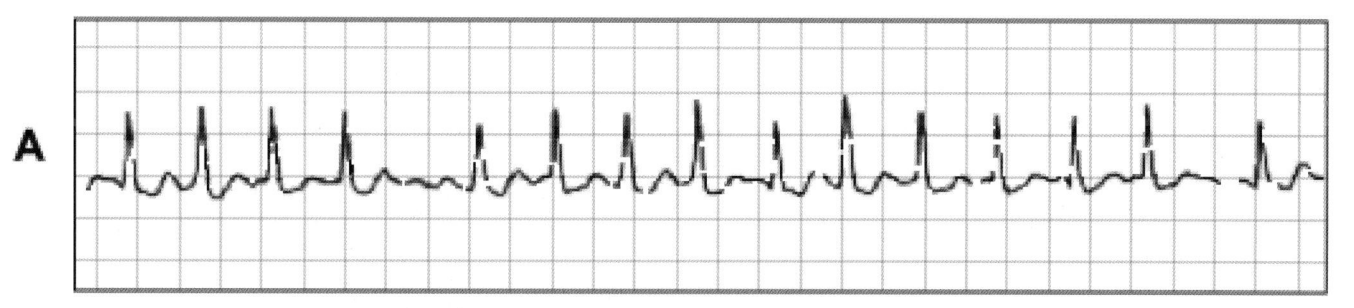

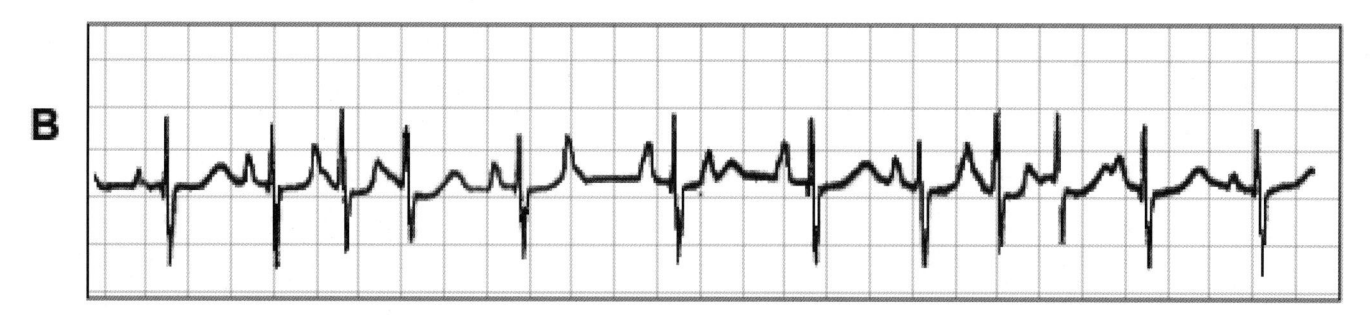

References

1. Luber S, Brady WJ, Joyce T, Perron AD. Paroxysmal supraventricular tachycardia: Outcome after emergency department care. *Am J Emerg Med.* 2001;19:40-42.
2. Monteleone P, Sochor MS, Brady WJ: Deadly dysrhythmias. In Winters M, DeBlieux P, Marcolini E, et al (eds). *Emergency Department Resuscitation of the Critically Ill.* Dallas, Texas: American College of Emergency Physicians; 2011.
3. Brady WJ, DeBehnke DJ, Wickman LL, Lindbeck G. Treatment of out-of-hospital supraventricular tachycardia: adenosine vs. verapamil. *Acad Emerg Med.* 1996;3:574-585.
4. Slkar DP, Crandall CS, Loeliger E, et al. Unanticipated death after discharge home from the emergency department. *Ann Emerg Med.* 2007;49:735-745.
5. Crozier I, Melton I, Pearson S. Management of atrial fibrillation in the emergency department. *Int Med J.* 2003;33:182-185.
6. Bettoni M, Zimmerman M. Autonomic tone variations before the onset of paroxysmal atrial fibrillation. *Circulation.* 2002;105:2753-2759.
7. Haïssaguerre M, Jaïs P, Shah DC, et al. Spontaneous initiation of atrial fibrillation by ectopic beats originating in the pulmonary veins. *N Engl J Med.* 1998;339:659-666.
8. Ergene U, Ergene O, Fowler J, et al. Must antidysrhythmic agents be given to all patients with new-onset atrial fibrillation? *Am J Emerg Med.* 1999;17:659-662.
9. Digitalis in Acute Atrial Fibrillation (DAAF) Trial Group. Intravenous digoxin in acute atrial fibrillation: results of a randomized, placebo-controlled multicentre trial in 239 patients. *Eur Heart J.* 1997;18:649-654.
10. Olshansky B, Rosenfeld LE, Warner AL, et al. The atrial fibrillation follow-up investigation of rhythm management (AFFIRM) study. *J Am Coll Cardiol.* 2004;43:1209-1210.
11. Hagens VE, Van Gelder IC, Crijins HJ, et al. The RACE study in perspective: rate control versus electrical cardioversion of persistent atrial fibrillation. The RACE study. *Cardiac Electrophys Rev.* 2003;7:118-121.
12. Gürsoy S, Steurer G, Brugada J, et al. Brief report: the hemodynamic mechanism of pounding in the neck in atrioventricular nodal reentrant tachycardia. *N Engl J Med.* 1992;327:772-774.
13. McCord J, Borzak S. Multifocal atrial tachycardia. *Chest.* 1998;113:203-209.
14. Iseri LT, Fairshter RD, Hardemann JL, et al. Magnesium and potassium therapy in multifocal atrial tachycardia. *Am Heart J.* 1985;110:789-794.

CHAPTER 10

Wide Complex Tachycardia

Keith A. Marill and David F.M. Brown

IN THIS CHAPTER

Differential diagnosis

Supraventricular tachycardia

Ventricular tachycardia

Polymorphic ventricular tachycardia

Diagnosis

Supraventricular tachycardia versus ventricular tachycardia

Treatment

Prognosis and disposition

Wide complex tachycardia (WCT) generally refers to a rapid heart rhythm (>100 beats/min in adults) and a wide morphology QRS complex observed on the electrocardiogram (ECG) (>120 msec). Heart rate is normally determined by the sinus node, which is the fastest intrinsic pacemaker in the heart. Tachycardia occurs when the intrinsic sinus rate is accelerated or other cardiac tissue with pacemaker activity supersedes the sinus rate. Heart rate varies with age, so the threshold of 100 beats/min is most appropriate in adults, and a higher age-related threshold may be considered in children. The QRS complex represents the ECG signature of the electrical depolarization or activation of the ventricles. Normally, ventricular activation is tightly synchronized because of rapid simultaneous conduction of the electrical depolarization signal to both the left and right ventricular endocardium from the atrioventricular (AV) node by the His-Purkinje fibers. If the Purkinje fibers are damaged, or excitation of the ventricles occurs via an alternate mechanism, then normal synchronization might be lost. The duration between initial and final activation of the ventricles will be increased and the QRS complex widened.

Patients with WCT most commonly present with complaints of palpitations, chest discomfort, shortness of breath, or syncope. They may be normotensive or hypotensive. Advanced age, underlying heart disease, and faster heart rate are associated with greater danger and instability.

The differential diagnosis of WCT is broad and the morbidity rate, mortality rate, and therapeutic implications vary widely. In addition to multiple intrinsic cardiologic diseases, a variety of pathologic conditions extrinsic to the heart can exert multiple local effects leading to WCT (Table 10-1). These extrinsic pathologic conditions include metabolic derangements, particularly those leading to hyperkalemia, toxicologic insults such as those causing myocardial sodium channel blockade that slows the depolarization process, and inappropriate extrinsic pacing by an implanted or external pacemaker device. Regarding intrinsic cardiologic disease, WCT is often classified based on whether the tachycardic pacemaker or pacemaker circuit involves tissue superior to the ventricles (supraventricular tachycardia [SVT]) or is located solely within the ventricular mass (ventricular tachycardia [VT]).

Differential Diagnosis

The most important metabolic derangement associated with WCT is advanced hyperkalemia. The rapid movement of potassium across the myocardial cell membrane via dedicated potassium channels is most prominently responsible for repolarization of the myocardium during the transition from systole to diastole. This ventricular repolarization corresponds to the

T-wave deflection on the ECG. Thus, hyperkalemia is initially evidenced by prominent peaked T-wave morphology. If the serum potassium level continues to rise, myocardial function becomes profoundly poisoned. This leads directly to compromised cardiac output, tachycardia, and a wide, rounded QRS morphology. Severe hyperkalemia can lead to progressive ventricular instability, fibrillation, and death if not promptly reversed.

The conditions most commonly associated with severe hyperkalemia in the emergency setting are chronic renal insufficiency or failure, sometimes associated with chronic hemodialysis. Renal function can deteriorate for many reasons, often with associated oliguria or anuria and fluid overload manifested by dyspnea, pulmonary rales, and peripheral edema on examination. An interruption in routine hemodialysis, which could be related to altered mental function, psychiatric illness, noncompliance, or another event, can lead to hyperkalemia in patients with known renal failure for whom hemodialysis has been prescribed.

Decreased sodium channel function is the most common end point in patients with toxicologic causes of WCT. The QRS complex is the electrical manifestation of ventricular depolarization, which is caused by the movement of sodium ions across the myocardial cell membrane into the cell through specific intracellular sodium channels. Any pharmaceutical agent or poison that interferes with myocardial sodium channel function can slow the depolarization process and widen the QRS complex. Classically, the most important and effective agents are the antiarrhythmics in the Vaughn Williams Ia classification, including procainamide and quinidine. Other important agents include the cyclic antidepressants, which poison the sodium channel when ingested in overdose, the class Ic antiarrhythmics (eg, flecainide and propafenone), diphenhydramine, carbamazepine, cocaine, and phenothiazines. In overdose, these agents can also cause tachycardia. Tachycardia can be multifactorial because of the decreased efficiency of systolic contraction and reduced cardiac output, as well as a prominent anticholinergic effect for the Ia antiarrhythmics, cyclic antidepressants, diphenhydramine, and phenothiazines.

By virtue of localized endocardial pacing that does not use the His-Purkinje fiber system, endocardial ventricular pacing almost always causes a wide QRS complex. An accelerated pacing rate can be a response to a number of conditions, depending on the pacing system and programming. A dual-lead system could sense a sinus or supraventricular tachycardia and pace the ventricles rapidly. Pacemaker-mediated tachycardia can also occur with dual-chamber pacemakers. A premature ventricular contraction initiates a reentrant loop of excitation, with retrograde conduction from the ventricles to the atria, and the pacemaker provides the antegrade limb, with atrial sensing and ventricular excitation.

TABLE 10-1.

Differentiating SVT from VT: Characteristics Suggestive of VT

History
Prior diagnosis of VT (prior SVT suggests SVT)
Prior myocardial infarction
Age over 35 years
Male sex
Prior diagnosis of WPW syndrome suggests SVT
Physical examination
Evidence of AV dissociation (variable first heart sound or abnormal jugular venous pulsation)
Cardiovascular stability is *not* predictive
ECG
Heart rate is not predictive
Frontal QRS axis 180 to 270 degrees
QRS interval larger than 140 msec for RBBB pattern or larger than 160 msec for LBBB pattern, or RS interval greater than 100 msec
Positive or negative concordance across the precordial leads
Wide QRS morphology grossly different from QRS morphology in sinus rhythm
Evidence of atrioventricular dissociation (fusion and capture beats)
Diagnostic interventions
No response to AV nodal blockade (ie, Valsalva maneuver, adenosine)

> **KEY POINT**
>
> Consider hyperkalemia, agents that block sodium channel function, and rapid paced rhythms in the differential for any WCT.

Supraventricular Tachycardia

SVT manifests with a wide QRS complex via three primary mechanisms. First, any supraventricular rhythm can have an associated wide QRS complex if there is aberrant conduction in the His-Purkinje system. Aberrant conduction to the ventricles means that one or two of the three limbs of the Purkinje system demonstrate abnormally slow or absent conduction and thus synchronized activation of the ventricles is lost. The result is a wide QRS complex (Figure 10-1). The QRS morphology can demonstrate a right or left bundle-branch block (RBBB, LBBB) depending on the Purkinje bundle(s) affected. Aberrancy can be permanent because of damage to a Purkinje bundle (eg, RBBB or LBBB) or temporary. Sometimes, abnormal Purkinje conduction occurs only at high heart rates because the specialized conduction tissue has had insufficient time to repolarize and is still refractory. This situation is called *rate-related bundle-branch block*. Aberrant conduction can also occur as a result of therapy that causes sodium channel blockade such as administration of class Ia and Ic antiarrhythmics (Figure 10-2).

Second, an accessory tract connection might be present between the atria and ventricles, separate and apart from the AV node. When conduction occurs from the atria to the ventricles via an accessory tract, it is called *antegrade*. When conduction occurs in the reverse direction—from the ventricles to the atria—it is called *retrograde*. In the presence of an accessory tract, any atrial rhythm such as sinus or atrial fibrillation can conduct in an antegrade fashion through the accessory tract to the ventricles. This pathway of conduction generally does not connect with or use the His-Purkinje system and thus does not lead to synchronized ventricular excitation. Ventricular activation via an accessory tract is more akin to a premature ventricular contraction, in which the ventricles are initially activated at the site of the accessory tract connection and the wave of depolarization spreads from that point across the ventricular myocardium. The process can be thought of as a three-dimensional version of the waves that emanate from a stone thrown into a still pond. The resulting ventricular depolarization process is slow and manifests with a wide QRS complex.

When an accessory tract provides antegrade conduction in sinus rhythm, the normal delay in conduction through the AV node is bypassed, and there is relatively early excitation, or preexcitation, of the ventricles. This is manifested by a shortened PR interval on the ECG and an abnormal slurred upstroke to the QRS complex in addition to a widened QRS. These are the characteristics of the Wolff-Parkinson-White (WPW) syndrome. The WPW syndrome is defined by the presence of an accessory pathway that demonstrates antegrade conduction in sinus rhythm. Patients with WPW syndrome are thus prone to all of the arrhythmias associated with accessory tract conduction described in this section. An accessory tract that does not conduct in an antegrade fashion during sinus rhythm but is able to conduct during and facilitate arrhythmias is called a *concealed accessory tract*.

Third, a reentrant or circus rhythm uses both the AV node and an accessory pathway or, more rarely, two accessory pathways. Reentrant conduction means there is a circular pattern of depolarization that is continuous and sufficiently rapid to supersede the sinus node as the pacemaker of the heart. If the pattern of depolarization descends down the AV node and retrograde up the accessory tract, then it is termed *orthodromic*. This is the most common pattern. In the presence of orthodromic reentry, the QRS complex is narrow if His-Purkinje conduction is normal but wide if His-Purkinje conduction is aberrant.

Alternatively, depolarization can occur antegrade down the accessory tract and retrograde back up the AV node. This less common pattern is called *antidromic conduction*. The QRS complex will necessarily be wide in the setting of antidromic conduction because activation of the ventricles does not occur via the His-Purkinje system but rather as described above for accessory tract conduction.

It is useful to distinguish irregular from regular WCT. Irregular means the time interval between beats varies. A rhythm is regularly irregular if the variation in time between beats occurs in a regular recurring pattern. Among the SVT causes of WCT, the ventricular response to atrial fibrillation generally remains irregular whether conduction occurs through the AV node or an accessory tract. For rapid WCT with rates in the neighborhood of 200 beats/min or above, an irregular rhythm as well as variable QRS complexes are important clues suggestive of underlying atrial fibrillation and WPW syndrome with accessory tract conduction (Figure 10-3). Reentrant rhythms generally produce a regular WCT because of their recurrent and regular pattern of excitation. Atrial flutter is most commonly produced by a reentrant circuit in the right atrium, and thus the ventricular response is regular or perhaps regularly irregular due to second-degree heart block.

> **KEY POINTS**
>
> SVT manifests with a wide QRS complex if there is:
>
> Aberrant conduction in the His-Purkinje system (ie, right or left bundle block) which can be baseline or rate related,
>
> Conduction from the atria to the ventricles via an accessory tract,
>
> A reentrant or circus rhythm that uses both an accessory pathway and the AV node or, more rarely, two accessory pathways.

Ventricular Tachycardia

VT occurs when a native ventricular rhythm that does not involve the AV node or supraventricular tissue occurs at a rate that supersedes the sinus and other supraventricular pacemakers. VT generally demonstrates a wide QRS complex because it does not use the His-Purkinje system in a coordinated fashion for ventricular activation. VT is most commonly caused by a reentrant circuit of depolarization within the ventricular myo-

CARDIOVASCULAR EMERGENCIES

FIGURE 10-1.
A, Regular WCT with a normal axis and a rate of approximately 150 beats/min. Note the multiple regular deflections in the inferior leads, suggestive of atrial flutter at 300 beats/min with 2:1 block and aberrant conduction. B, The diagnosis is proved, with increased AV nodal blockade to 3:1 conduction exposing saw-tooth atrial deflections (see lead V_4).

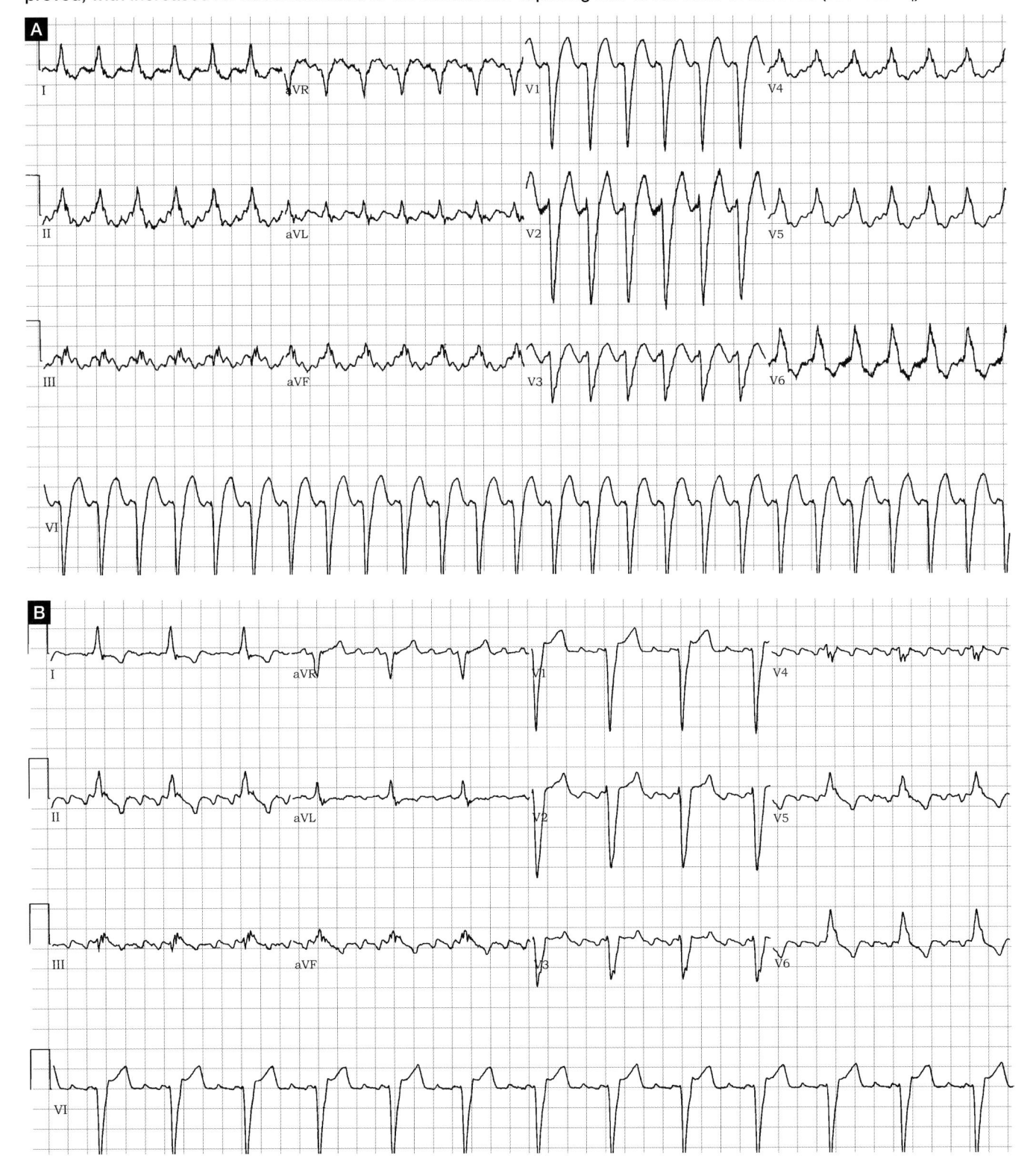

Wide Complex Tachycardia

FIGURE 10-2.

A 72-year-old woman who has a history of atrial fibrillation following a pulmonary vein isolation procedure and is taking the class Ic antiarrhythmic dofetilide presents with palpitations. Her heart rate is approximately 150 beats/min and the QRS duration is 128 msec (A). The morphology spontaneously converted from wide (A) to narrow (B), then the ventricular response was controlled with calcium channel blockade, with resulting 2:1 conduction (C). Dofetilide treatment likely contributed to the presenting wide QRS complex morphology. Note the negative precordial concordance with WCT (although the rhythm proved to be supraventricular).

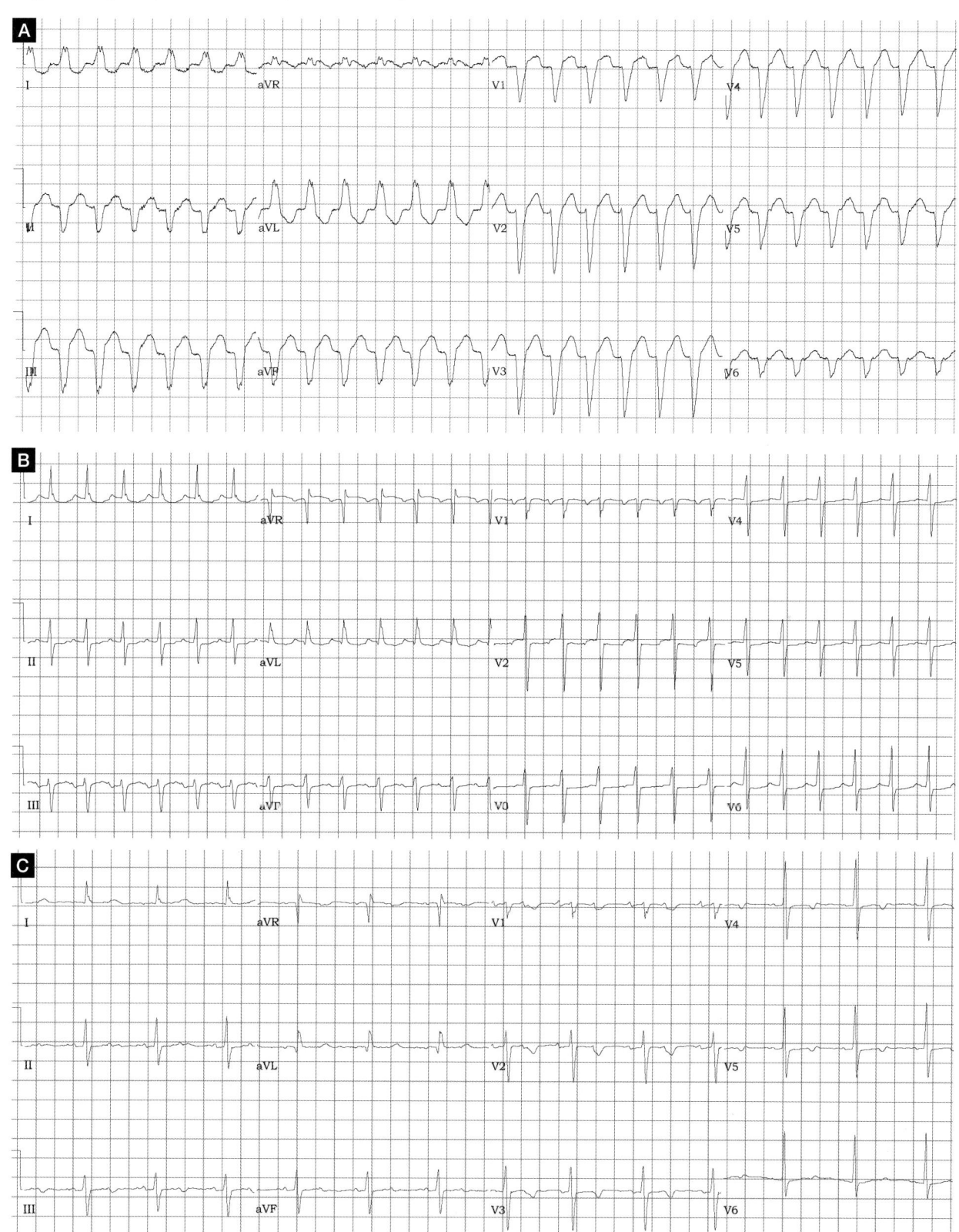

cardium. Often this is caused by the presence of a scar from a previous myocardial infarction (MI). The scar tissue provides an electrically silent island that the reentrant wave can circle. The surrounding heterogeneous peri-infarct tissue and fibrosis provide the substrate for a slower conducting limb of the reentrant circuit, which gives the remaining tissue time to depolarize before the wave of excitation returns. The rhythm is most commonly regular with a uniform QRS morphology, called *monomorphic*.

A variety of other structural heart diseases can cause reentrant VT. Myocardial scar resulting from prior repair of congenital heart disease can lead to VT such as right ventricular outflow tract VT associated with repair of tetralogy of Fallot. Congestive heart failure is associated with an increased rate of VT. Dilated nonischemic cardiomyopathy is associated with a particular type called *bundle-branch reentrant VT*. Hypertrophic cardiomyopathy and arrhythmogenic right ventricular dysplasia can be associated with diffuse scarring and myofibril disarray, which promote reentry.

Another mechanism responsible for VT is enhanced automaticity resulting from a steepening of the phase 4 slope of depolarization in the myocardial action potential cycle. This could occur for a variety of reasons, including an intrinsic abnormality in ion channel function, enhanced responsiveness to or excessive sympathetic tone, or medication or drug toxicity. Digoxin overdose, a classic cause of enhanced automaticity, often results in bidirectional VT, which is a specific morphologic type of VT with QRS morphology that alternates every other beat. Other agents that can cause VT in overdose are sympathomimetics such as amphetamines and cocaine, theophylline, and thyroid hormone. Enhanced automaticity can be exacerbated by metabolic abnormalities such as hypokalemia and hypoxia.

VT can be triggered by delayed afterdepolarizations. Delayed after-depolarizations are oscillatory changes in cell membrane voltage that occur after completion of myocardial repolarization. They can occur in the setting of exercise or increased sympathetic tone, and the resulting VT often initiates in the right ventricular outflow tract. They can also be induced in congestive heart failure and initiate VT.

Atrial activity might or might not be associated with ventricular activity during VT.[1] Half of patients with VT have a dissociation of atrial and ventricular activity; a separate slower supraventricular pacemaker depolarizes the atria. One-third of patients with VT have 1:1 retrograde conduction from the ventricles backward up the AV node to the atria. The remainder demonstrate a variety of retrograde conduction with second-degree block such as 2:1 or Wenckebach (Figure 10-4).

Polymorphic Ventricular Tachycardia

VT with varying QRS morphology is called *polymorphic*. The duration of the QT interval in the native rhythm that precedes polymorphic VT is an important factor in classifying this condition. Polymorphic VT in association with a normal QT interval is most commonly associated with ischemic heart disease and acute myocardial ischemia. The morphology varies from irregularly changing amplitude and shape to a more orga-

FIGURE 10-3.

Atrial fibrillation with wide QRS complexes: is this aberrancy or conduction via bypass tract? High rate (shortest R-R interval is about 200 msec) and high beat-to-beat QRS variability (seen in lead V$_2$) favor the diagnosis of bypass tract conduction (WPW syndrome). The risk of sudden death is inversely associated with the length of the shortest R-R interval, with 240 msec (6 small boxes) suggesting higher risk.

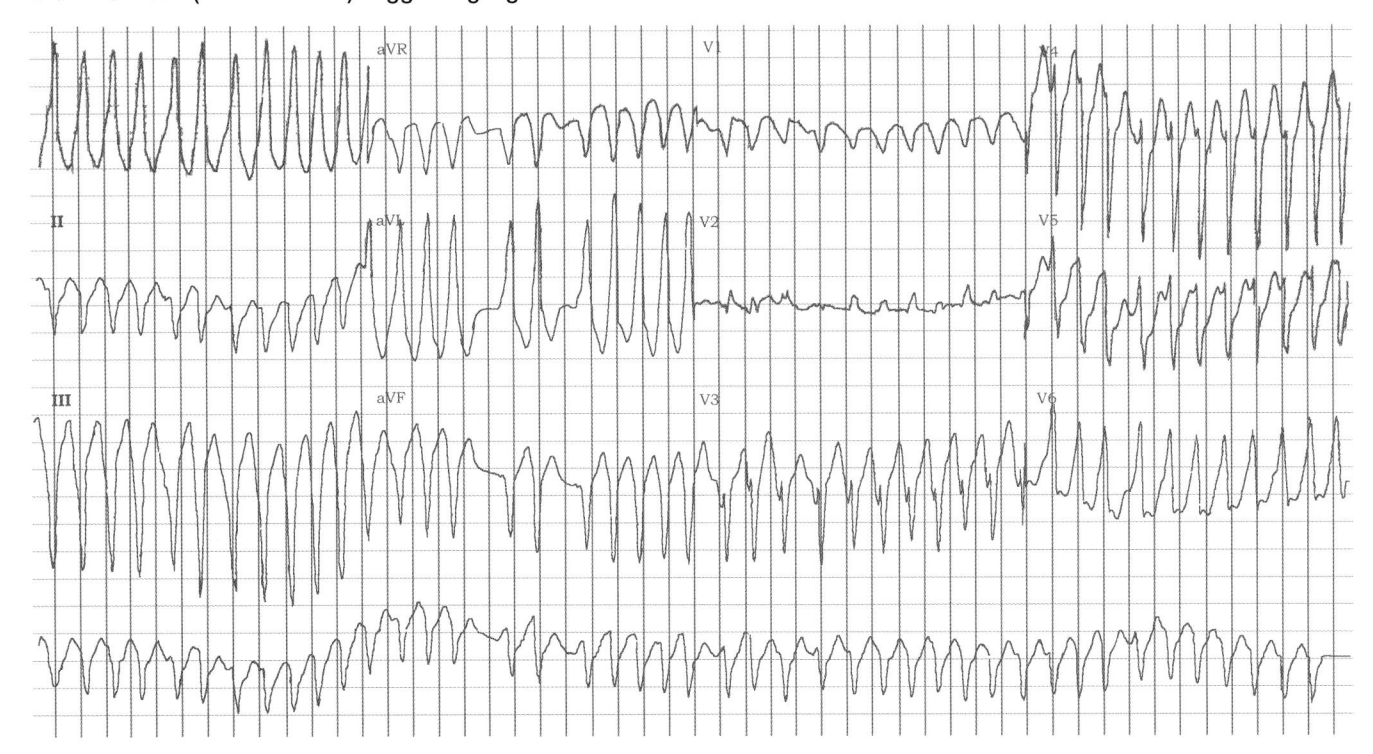

FIGURE 10-4.

A 52-year-old woman with a history of MI presented with relatively narrow tachycardia. Ventricular deflections march through regularly, whereas a regularly irregular pattern of P waves is noted (see V_1 rhythm strip). The ventricles are conducting in a retrograde direction to the atria with a lengthening conduction interval (arrows) and ultimately dropped P wave. This retrograde V-to-A Wenckebach conduction confirms the diagnosis of VT. The short arrows indicate the initial retrograde VA conduction, the medium-length arrows indicate the following longer retrograde VA conduction, and the longest arrows indicate absence or dropped conduction before the cycle repeats.

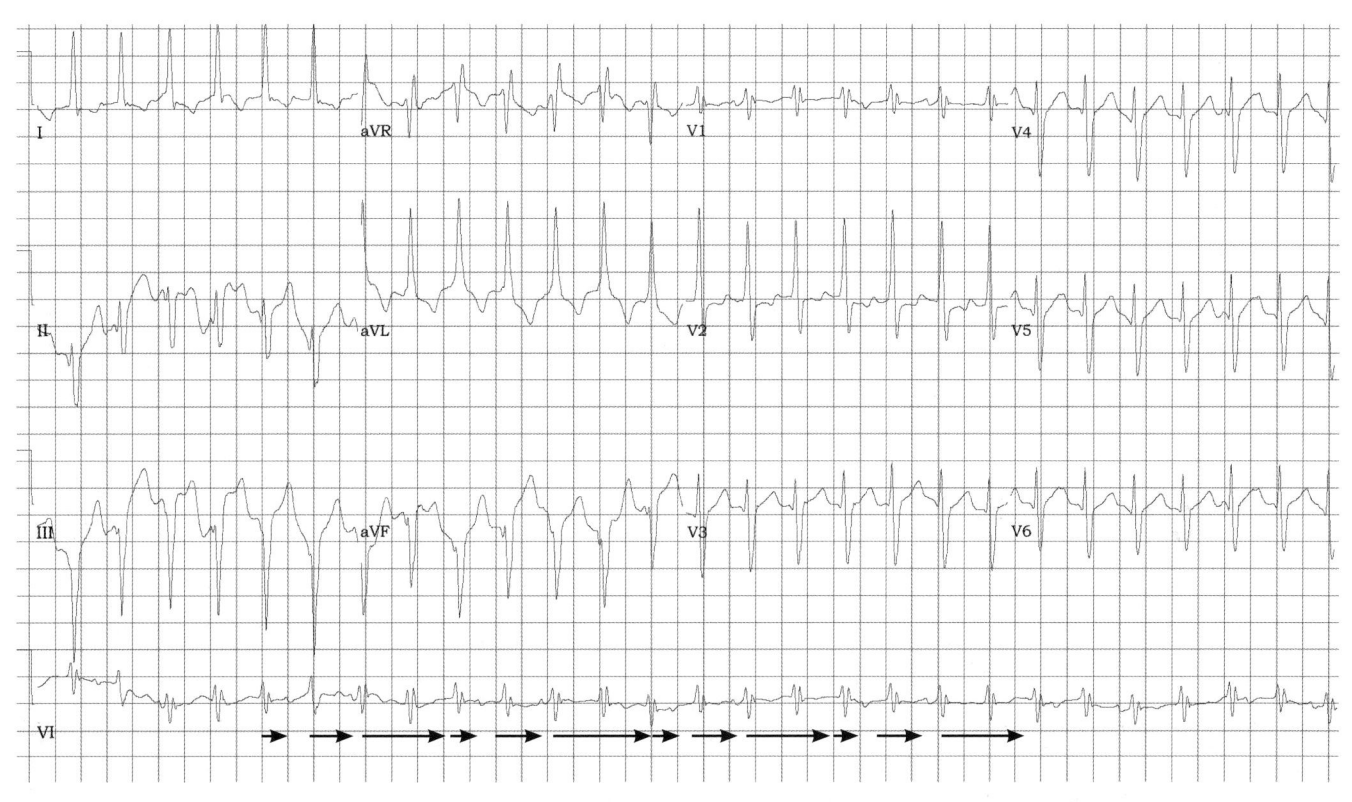

FIGURE 10-5.

A 57-year-old man who has a history of nonischemic cardiomyopathy, has had cardioverter-defibrillator implantation, is now taking amiodarone, and has a long QT interval (QTc 511 msec) experiences an initial PVC that causes a long R-R interval (left arrow). Then a second PVC follows a short R-R interval and occurs within the T wave of the preceding beat, leading to TdP. The second PVC occurs during the relative refractory period of the myocardium. Episodes were recurrent and refractory despite maximal medical therapy and pacing at increased heart rate and resolved only after sedation with mechanical ventilation.

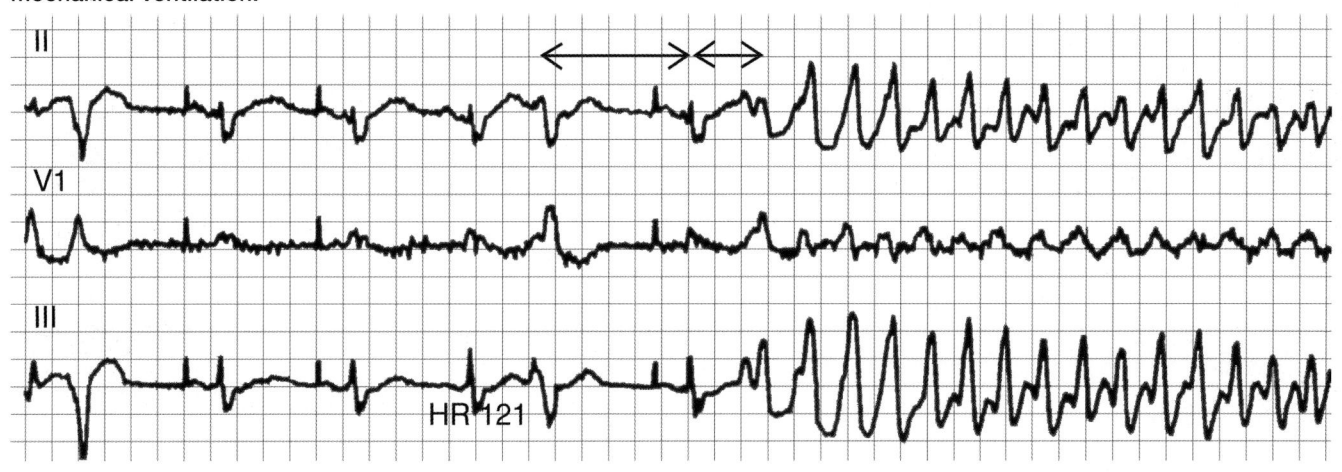

nized sinusoidal pattern.

Torsade de pointes (TdP) is a particularly important type of polymorphic VT, defined by a sinusoidal-appearing undulation of the QRS amplitude, a prolonged QT interval, and a long-short sequence of R-R interval duration on onset[2] (Figure 10-5). TdP is an unstable rhythm that can spontaneously terminate back to sinus rhythm or degenerate to ventricular fibrillation (VF) and sudden death.

A long QT interval, which by definition is necessary to initiate TdP, might be congenital, stemming from defects in the cardiac ion channel conducting or support proteins. QT prolongation can be caused by a decrease in function of the myocardial repolarizing potassium channels or, alternatively, an increase or persistence in conduction of the depolarizing sodium or excitatory calcium channels. A long QT interval can also be acquired as a result of metabolic abnormalities such as hypokalemia, hypomagnesemia, acidosis, or ischemia or of therapeutic or toxic medication affects from the class Ia, Ic, and III antiarrhythmics as well as many other agents. The medication effects can be complex and interact such that some medicines directly affect myocardial channel function while others simply alter the metabolism of the offending agents. The concept of repolarization reserve has been developed to suggest that each individual can withstand a certain degree of QT prolongation without subsequent TdP, and this reserve might be related to a number of congenital and acquired factors, including progressive cardiac disease and failure.[3]

Although Brugada syndrome is not associated with QT-interval prolongation, it is thought to be caused by a variety of genetic defects that decrease sodium channel function.[4] The result can be polymorphic VT, VF, or sudden cardiac death. Brugada syndrome is diagnosed based on the ECG characteristics of a pattern of RBBB and an elevation of more than 2 mm at the J point, with a slowly descending ST segment in conjunction with flat or negative T waves in the right precordial leads V_1, V_2, or V_3 (Figure 10-6). In addition, the patient or a family member would have a history of syncope, inducible polymorphic ventricular tachycardia or ventricular fibrillation, or sudden death from cardiac causes but no obvious structural cause of sudden death.[4-6] The significance of the Brugada pattern on the ECG without personal or family risk factors for sudden death is uncertain.

Brugada syndrome seems to be most prevalent in Southeast Asian populations. It is responsible for some cases of the nocturnal sudden death described as "laitai" (death during sleep) in Thailand, "bangungut" (to rise and moan during sleep and then die) in the Philippines, and "pokkuri" (unexpected sudden death from cardiac causes at night) in Japan.[7] The clinical manifestations are nine times as common among men as among women, often first occurring in the third or fourth decade of life and in patients at rest or during sleep.

KEY POINTS

VT with varying QRS morphology is called *polymorphic*.

TdP is defined by a sinusoidal-appearing undulation of the QRS amplitude, a prolonged QT interval, and a long-short sequence of R-R interval duration on onset.

Causes of polymorphic VT include metabolic abnormalities, ischemia, therapeutic or toxic medication effects, and genetic conduction defects such as Brugada syndrome.

Making the Diagnosis

As is typical throughout emergency medicine, a careful history of illness is critical to making the correct diagnosis when a patient comes to an emergency department with WCT. A history of renal disease, the use of renal-toxic medicines, or an acute decrease in urine output should all raise concern for the possibility of hyperkalemia. A serum potassium measurement can usually be obtained rapidly with a blood gas measurement. Hyperkalemia is associated with a characteristic progression of ECG changes, beginning with tall, sharp peaking of the T waves and leading to eventual wide, rounded tachycardic QRS complexes. It is often difficult to discern whether the pacemaker is from the sinus node or if VT has developed, but the primary treatment remains emergent lowering of the serum potassium concentration.

A history of medication overdose, evidence of psychiatric ill-

FIGURE 10-6.

A 34-year-old man with no relevant medical history was found unresponsive at night with VF arrest. The baseline ECG shows the characteristic incomplete RBBB pattern and ST elevations in V_1 and V_2, indicative of Brugada syndrome.

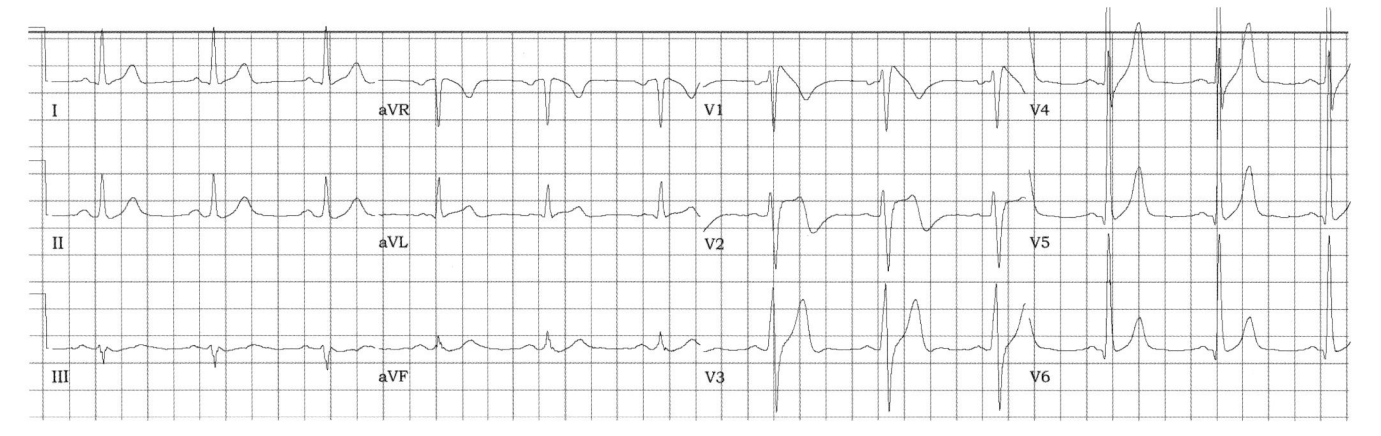

ness or acute behavioral disturbance, or altered mental status should all raise suspicion for cyclic antidepressant or antipsychotic overdose in the setting of WCT. The emergency physician should seek collateral history from emergency medical service personnel, friends, or family members and medication history from any available records to assess for this concern. A toxicologic screen will ultimately be valuable, but it is generally not available in a timely manner to guide initial therapeutic decisions. The emergency physician often needs to assume overdose and treat this worst case scenario pending further available information.

Similar to many disease processes, toxicity from cyclic antidepressants and other agents that hinder fast sodium channel conduction does not seem to affect the depolarization kinetics of the bundle branches and myocardium in a perfectly homogeneous manner. As a result, the ECG might demonstrate relatively specific suggestive characteristics. First, because these medicines have anticholinergic characteristics, ventricular tachyarrhythmias are almost always preceded by sinus tachycardia. There is also relative delay in depolarization of the right side of the heart, which is manifested by a widened QRS complex and right-axis deviation of the terminal 30 msec of the QRS complex. Thus, there is a prominent R wave in lead aVR and an S wave in leads I and aVL. A widened QRS interval and right-axis deviation of the terminal 30 msec are both more pronounced and more persistent in cyclic antidepressant overdose patients who develop ventricular arrhythmias and seizures.[8]

Supraventricular versus Ventricular Tachycardia

The distinction between SVT and VT in patients with *regular* WCT has important therapeutic and prognostic implications. The history, physical examination, and ECG can all provide useful clues, although it is often difficult to make a definitive diagnosis in the emergency department (Table 10-2). It is useful to consider the odds of VT versus SVT and, by applying Bayesian theory, to assess the likelihood ratios for individual tests or characteristics that can be used to adjust the odds. In general, for adults presenting to an emergency department with stable WCT, the pretest odds of VT versus SVT are about 3:1 (75% patients with VT).[9]

The most important factor suggestive of VT is a history of MI, with a positive likelihood ratio of 13.[10] If the pretest odds of VT are 3:1, then without any other information, the post-test odds of VT for a patient with a history of MI can be calculated as 3 × 13 = 39, or 39:1. This corresponds to a 39 ÷ (39+1) × 100 = 97.5% chance of VT. Other characteristics associated with an increased likelihood of prior MI or cardiomyopathy such as male sex, age over 35 years, history of coronary artery bypass graft, and ejection fraction less than 35% are also associated with an increased likelihood of VT.[11] Being younger than 35 years of age could increase the odds of SVT by a factor of 6.

The degree of cardiovascular stability should not be used to distinguish between SVT and VT. Patients with VT can walk into an emergency department. In theory, a number of physical examination characteristics can be used to distinguish these two mechanisms of WCT. AV dissociation occurs when VT is present and the atria are depolarized separately and intrinsically at a slower rate without retrograde ventriculoatrial (VA) conduction. Variation in the first heart sound or jugular venous pulsation can result from AV dissociation.[12] In practice, these examination findings usually cannot be identified with sufficient certainty to make a definitive diagnosis of VT in the emergency department.

ECG characteristics that can be useful in distinguishing SVT from VT include QRS duration, frontal plane QRS axis, QRS concordance across the precordial leads, QRS morphology, and AV dissociation, including the presence of capture or fusion beats. Heart rate has not proved to be a useful differentiator.[1] With the advent of implantable cardioverter-defibrillators and programming to terminate VT above rates of 180 to 200 beats/min with antitachycardia pacing algorithms, it can be theorized that the average heart rate of patients presenting to the emergency department with VT would decrease since more rapid VT should have been automatically terminated in the field. However, the heart rate of patients experiencing VT presenting to the emergency department has not decreased substantially.[11] Although heart rate is not a good differentiator of underlying diagnoses, it is a critical factor in determining cardiovascular stability. Patients with extremely elevated heart rates for age, regardless of underlying mechanism, require expeditious attention and termination of the WCT to avoid life-threatening decompensation.

The dominant pacemaker in VT emanates from within the ventricular myocardium and most commonly does not use the His-Purkinje system to facilitate conduction. As a result, the duration of the QRS interval is usually markedly prolonged and the axis of depolarization can be highly abnormal both in the frontal plane and across the precordium. This is generally not the case for SVT with aberrant conduction, where the His-Purkinje system remains at least partly functional and used. However, for SVT with conduction through a peripherally located accessory tract, the ventricles can also be activated, with an unusual and asymmetric wave of depolarization across the ventricular myocardium. Thus, none of the predictive morphologic QRS characteristics is truly diagnostic.

The QRS duration tends to be longer in VT. A duration of more than 160 msec increases the odds of VT by a factor of 4.6 and is relatively specific but insensitive.[13,14] Brugada and colleagues[15] developed an algorithm to differentiate SVT from VT. The second node in the algorithm denotes an RS interval larger than 100 msec in the precordial leads as 98% specific for VT. The RS interval is measured from the onset of the R wave to the nadir of the S wave. However, all measurements of depolarization duration can be confounded by concurrent therapy that affects fast sodium channel function, particularly class I antiarrhythmics.

A bizarre QRS axis in the frontal plane between 180 and 270 degrees could be highly specific for VT, but recent data suggest this finding is only moderately predictive.[13,14] Concordance can be thought of as an extreme axis across the precordial leads. Positive concordance means all of the QRS complexes across the precordial leads have a primarily positive deflection, and negative concordance means they are all primarily negative.

These correspond to ventricular depolarization emanating from the back or front of the heart, respectively. While only demonstrating approximately 10% sensitivity, positive and negative concordance are more than 90% specific and approximately 85% specific, respectively, for VT[13] (Figure 10-7). Brugada and colleagues utilized the absence of an RS complex throughout the precordial leads, which is also a reflection of a highly abnormal precordial axis, as the first node in their diagnostic algorithm.[15] Specifically, to be positive, this criterion means an RS complex with positive followed by negative deflection is not present in any of the precordial leads.

The presence of RBBB versus LBBB is not predictive of SVT versus VT. Multiple researchers have attempted to identify more subtle morphologies within the bundle-branch block categories that could be predictive.[1,15] While variable scientific success has been met, the rules developed are often complex and subtle and have had limited clinical impact and utility in the emergency department.[16,17] WCT with a bundle-branch block pattern similar to that observed in sinus rhythm suggests but does not prove SVT.[18] An interesting alternative approach that demonstrated 90% sensitivity and 67% to 85% specificity for VT is to assume a diagnosis of VT unless the QRS morphology is consistent with a typical RBBB or LBBB.[19]

As discussed above, AV dissociation is present in approximately 50% of patients with VT. Thus, if the clinician could always identify AV dissociation if it is present, then the maximal sensitivity of AV dissociation for VT would be 50%. AV dissociation can be identified by P waves that occur on a regular basis, but not at the same rate or with the same interval with respect to QRS complexes. The key to identifying AV dissociation is "marching out" these P waves in the midst of WCT (Figure 10-8). AV dissociation is also suggested by fusion and capture beats. Fusion beats are QRS deflections caused, in part, by ongoing VT but are also, in part, activated by a supraventricular excitation that arrives almost simultaneously. Capture beats are QRS deflections that are entirely activated by supraventricular excitation via the His-Purkinje system and occur just before an expected beat within ongoing VT (Figure 10-9). In practice, AV dissociation can be identified only approximately half of the time when present; so its sensitivity and specificity are approximately 25% and more than 95%, respectively.

SVT with a reentrant circuit that involves the AV node can terminate in response to increased vagal tone and AV block, and SVT that is conducted to the ventricles via the AV node

TABLE 10-2.

Wide Complex Tachycardia: Differential Diagnosis

Extrinsic factors
Hyperkalemia
Sodium channel blocking toxicity
Inappropriate electrical pacing
Other toxicities contributing to VT (see below)
Intrinsic factors
SVT
Aberrant conduction (persistent or rate related)
Accessory tract conduction
Antidromic reentrant circuit
Antegrade accessory conduction of tachycardic atrial rhythms (such as atrial fibrillation, atrial flutter, atrial tachycardia, sinus tachycardia)
VT
Monomorphic
– Reentrant VT (due to scarring from previous MI or repair of congenital heart disease, congestive cardiomyopathy, hypertrophic cardiomyopathy, arrhythmogenic right ventricular dysplasia)
– Enhanced automaticity (caused by genetic abnormalities, toxicity, or exercise)
– Triggered (ie, due to delayed afterdepolarizations such as those that occur with right ventricular outflow tract VT)
Polymorphic
– Associated with normal QT interval (ischemic)
– Associated with long QT interval (called torsade de pointes), caused by genetic abnormalities, metabolic derangement, or toxicity
– Brugada syndrome

may demonstrate temporarily decreased conduction in response to vagal stimulation. Increased vagal tone would be unlikely to alter VT. Vagal maneuvers such as carotid massage after ruling out carotid bruit or the Valsalva maneuver might terminate SVT or block AV conduction and thus suggest or diagnose the presence of SVT. Adenosine infusion can have a comparable effect and is useful for diagnosing WCT of uncertain origin.[11,20,21] If the WCT is irregular, suggesting atrial fibrillation, or if there is reason to suspect atrial flutter with WPW syndrome and accessory tract conduction, then adenosine is contraindicated because it can enhance accessory tract conduction and further increase the heart rate.[22]

KEY POINTS

For adults presenting to an emergency department with stable WCT, the historical pretest odds of VT versus SVT are about 3:1 (75% chance).

The most important factor suggestive of VT is a history of MI, with a positive likelihood ratio of 13.

ECG evidence of AV dissociation is highly specific for VT.

The degree of cardiovascular stability should not be used to distinguish between SVT and VT.

Treatment

Treatment of WCT is highly dependent on the suspected underlying cause (Figure 10-10). When hyperkalemia or toxicity or overdose with a cyclic antidepressant or another medication is diagnosed, it should be treated appropriately with standard regimens.

When pacemaker-associated tachycardia is suspected, the emergency physician should first make a diligent attempt to confirm the diagnosis and rule out other causes of appropriate tachycardic pacemaker function. If pacemaker-associated tachycardia remains the most likely diagnosis, then it can be terminated by resetting the pacemaker to an asynchronous non-sensing paced mode. This can be accomplished by application of an appropriate magnet to the chest; the result is ventricular pacing at a rate determined by the manufacturer.

If the WCT mechanism is likely SVT and the patient is stable, then intravenous administration of adenosine is often a reasonable first therapeutic intervention. The major exception is when the presence of an accessory tract and antegrade conduction of atrial flutter or fibrillation with a rapid and wide ventricular response are suspected. In this case, adenosine is contraindicated because it can enhance accessory tract conduction. Reentrant atrioventricular tachycardia that uses the AV node for one limb and an accessory tract for the other limb of the circuit would be likely to terminate with adenosine treatment. However, it can be difficult to distinguish this rhythm from atrial flutter with antegrade accessory tract conduction. For this reason, it might be safest to avoid adenosine whenever an

FIGURE 10-7.

A 58-year-old man with a history of nonischemic cardiomyopathy who had undergone cardioverter-defibrillator implantation and was now taking metoprolol, amiodarone, and mexiletine presented with recurrent implanted cardioverter-defibrillator shocks. In his ECG, the upward rightward axis, markedly wide QRS complex, negative precordial concordance, and AV dissociation (vertical markings are provided below the rhythm strip) are all consistent with VT. Lidocaine infusion was initiated but stopped when the patient experienced a seizure. His condition improved after administration of increased doses of his oral regimen.

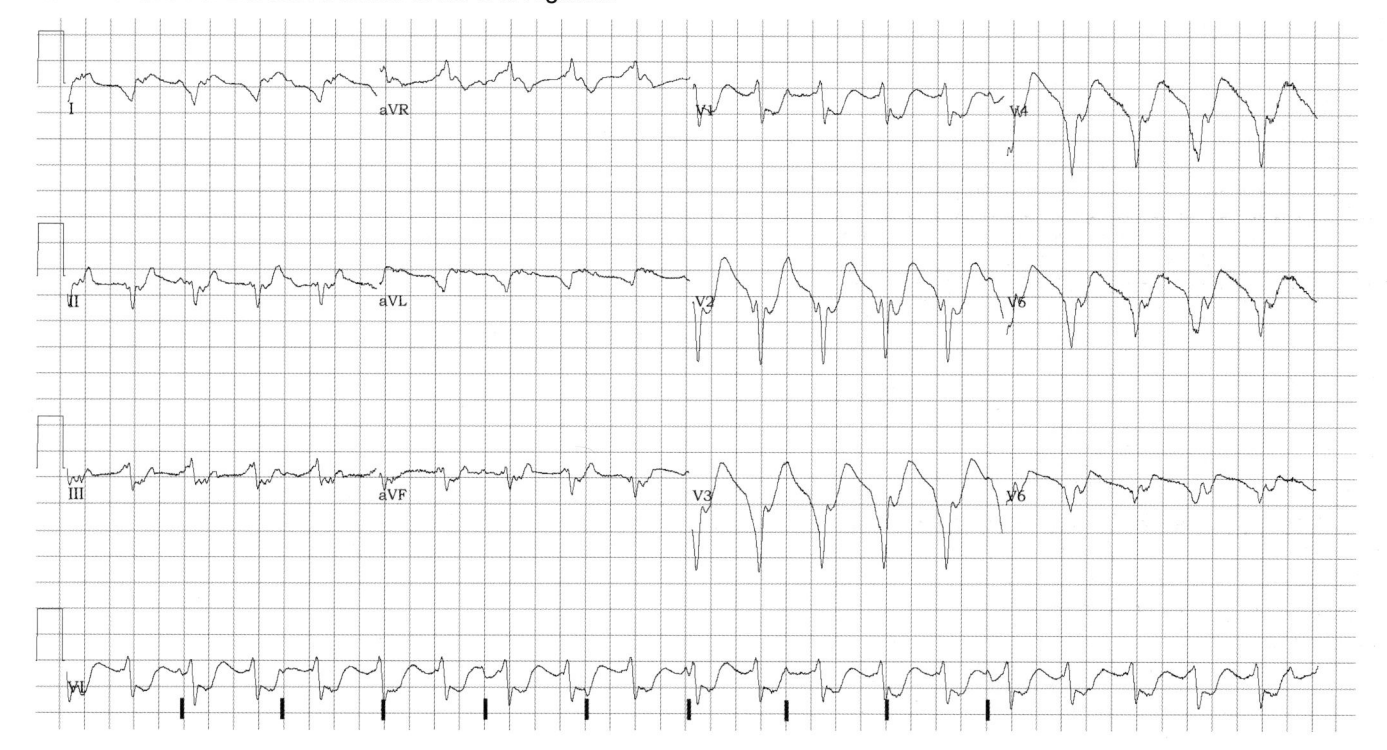

accessory tract is known to be present. Similarly, other agents that decrease AV nodal conduction such as calcium channel and beta-adrenergic blockers can also enhance accessory tract conduction and should be avoided in patients with WCT.

For SVT in the presence of a known accessory tract, intravenous administration of procainamide is most commonly recommended to terminate WCT. Procainamide generally slows conduction and prolongs the refractory period of the accessory tract tissue.[23,24] It may terminate a reentrant SVT and terminate or decrease the ventricular response to atrial fibrillation and flutter with accessory tract conduction. Intravenous administration of amiodarone has also been recommended for such patients but the evidence for its benefit in the emergency department setting is limited. Furthermore, the initial effect of amiodarone infusion is AV nodal blockade. This raises similar theoretic concern for increased conduction down an accessory pathway as for other AV nodal blocking agents, discussed above.[25]

If the ventricular rate is highly accelerated or myocardial

FIGURE 10-8.

A 52-year-old woman with a history of bipolar illness and myocardial infarction came to the emergency department for help with depression. During the assessment, incidental tachycardia was noted. It was not responsive to adenosine or amiodarone, so the patient was electrically cardioverted. Her ECG shows a relatively narrow QRS complex (125 msec) and no right upward axis or concordance. However, it demonstrated clear AV dissociation (note the vertical markers at the P waves) consistent with VT.

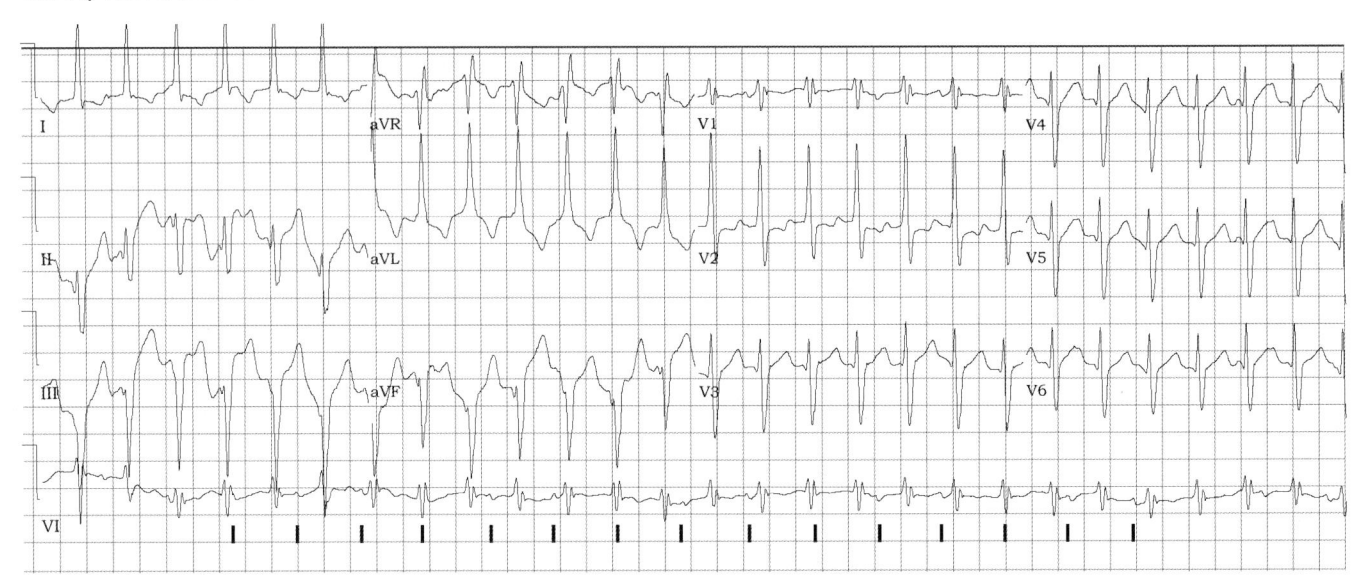

FIGURE 10-9.

A 57-year-old man without a history of heart disease presented to the emergency department after experiencing dyspnea on exertion with chest tightness and palpitations during the past month. His ECG demonstrates WCT with occasional narrow capture beats, suggesting VT. Capture beats occur because supraventricular activity "captures" the ventricle prior to the VT beat. His VT was terminated successfully with procainamide. The patient had extensive coronary artery disease and underwent four-vessel coronary artery bypass grafting.

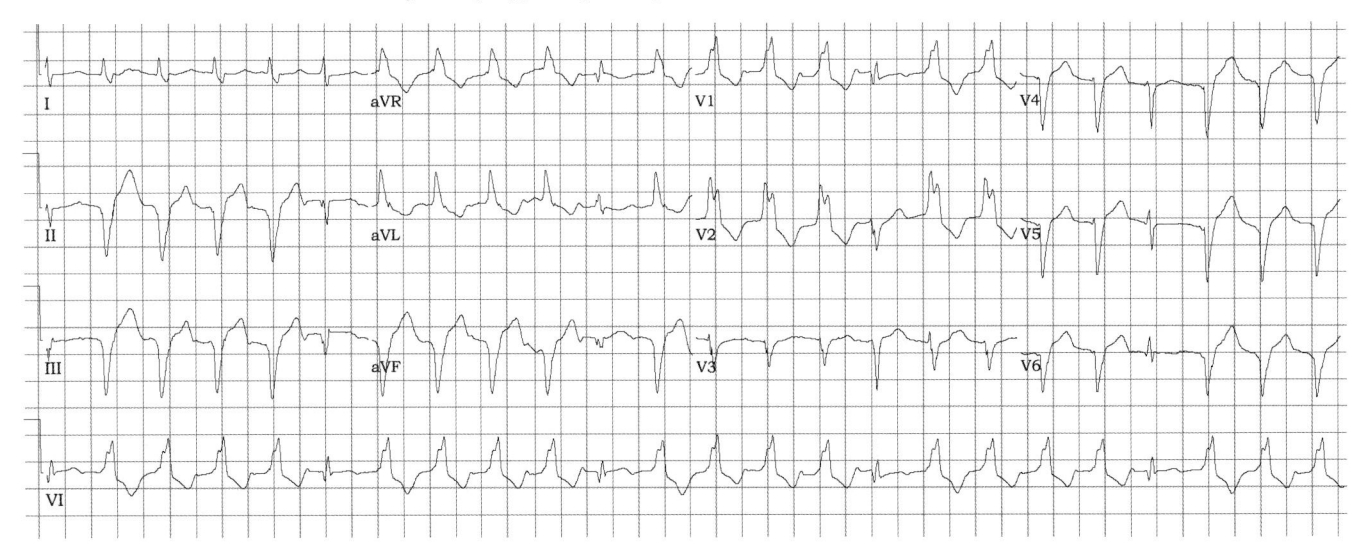

function is severely compromised, then SVT may be unstable, with symptoms of chest pain, shortness of breath, lightheadedness, or frank syncope. Synchronized direct current cardioversion, with sedation if possible, might be the safest therapeutic course. Synchronization of the shock with the ongoing SVT decreases the likelihood of inadvertent stimulation on the upstroke of the T wave ("R on T") and resulting VF. Although direct current cardioversion will not alter sinus tachycardia, it will terminate other SVTs approximately 90% of the time, and adverse effects beyond the initial discomfort are rare.

Stable VT has also been treated with a variety of medicines. The most effective antiarrhythmics to terminate sustained monomorphic VT are intravenous procainamide and racemic sotalol.[26,27] The relevant mechanism of action for both agents is likely delaying repolarization and increasing the QT interval and refractory period duration. A prolonged myocardial refractory period disrupts the circuit of reentrant depolarization in the ventricular myocardium. Unfortunately, procainamide predictably causes a decrease in blood pressure, and intravenous sotalol, which remains unavailable in the United States, rarely causes TdP. Neither lidocaine nor amiodarone causes a rapid increase in refractory period duration after acute intravenous administration.[28] Both agents are relatively safe but poorly effective for terminating VT.[29] However, amiodarone may be more effective at both terminating and preventing VT over the ensuing hours after administration.[30]

A few uncommon types of VT, including right ventricular outflow tract VT, are particularly sensitive to adenosine and verapamil.[31] However, the intravenous administration of verapamil has been associated with precipitous cardiovascular collapse in patients with VT and in infants with SVT.[32,33] Given the rarity of these VT mechanisms and the difficulty of making a definitive diagnosis in the emergency department, it is wisest for emergency physicians to avoid the use of verapamil for WCT, unless the patient has a clearly defined history of a particular sensitive VT and safe previous treatment. Adenosine is unlikely to benefit most patients with VT and should be avoided when VT is strongly suspected.

The recommended treatment for pulseless VT is defibrillation, and the safest and most effective treatment for stable or unstable VT is direct current cardioversion. The success rate for VT termination is above 90%. However, when VT is recurrent, suppressive medical therapy must be considered. The best medicine for this indication is uncertain, but beta-adrenergic blockers (eg, metoprolol) as well as amiodarone, lidocaine, and procainamide have been used.[34]

The treatment of polymorphic VT in the setting of a normal QT interval most commonly centers on the treatment of coronary ischemia and revascularization.[35] Beta-blockade, lidocaine, or amiodarone can also be helpful to suppress recurrent VT.

TdP is generally unstable with inadequate perfusion and should be cardioverted immediately. Intravenous magnesium, usually administered as an initial dose of 2 grams magnesium sulfate, has also been used to terminate TdP and prevent recurrence.[36] Because the QT interval is rate dependent and longer with lower heart rates, TdP is promoted in the setting of bradycardia. Interventions that accelerate the heart rate and prevent TdP include electrical pacing, preferably transvenous, or, if transcutaneous, with appropriate sedation for discomfort, and

FIGURE 10-10.

Algorithm for treatment of wide complex tachycardia

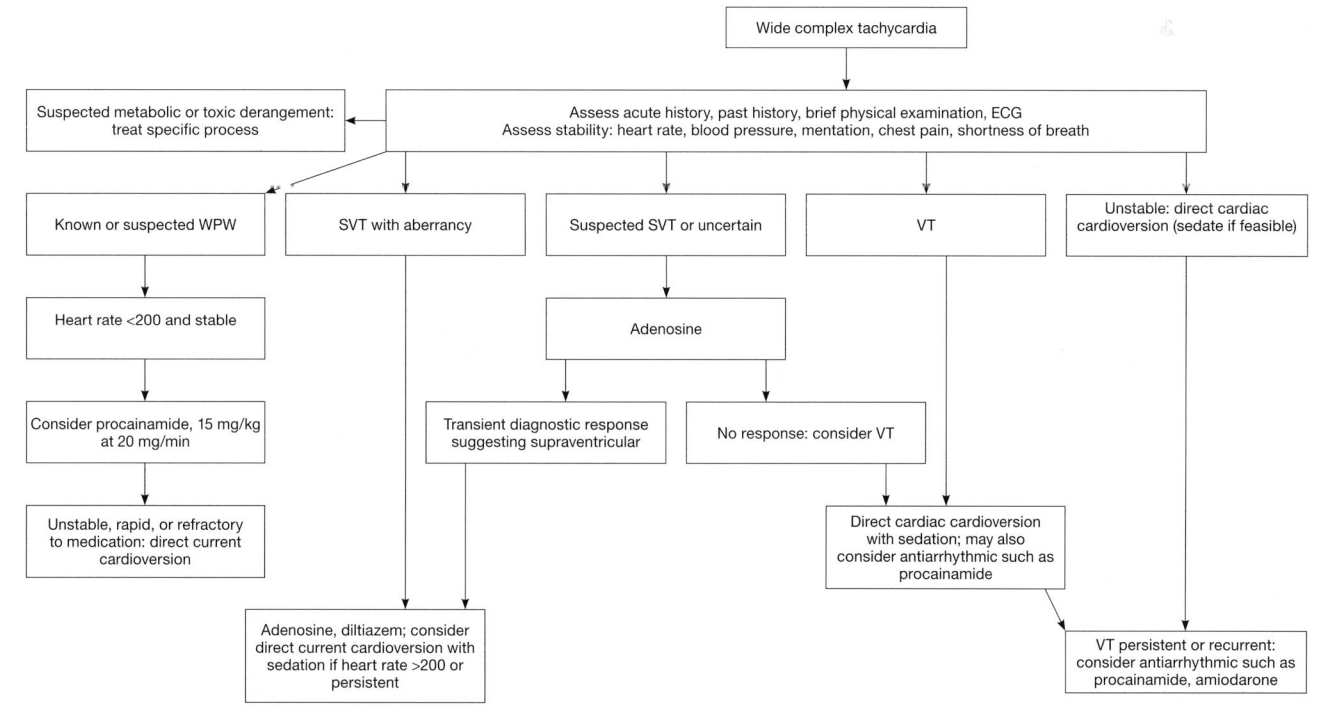

Note: All direct cardiac cardioversion should be synchronized, if possible.

infusion of an adrenergic stimulant such as isoproterenol. Class I and III antiarrhythmic agents are generally contraindicated because they can further prolong the QT interval and increase QT dispersion. Patients with congenital long-QT syndrome generally require cardioverter-defibrillator implantation.

The best treatment for VT/VF in association with Brugada syndrome is cardioversion or defibrillation. The best emergent treatment to prevent recurrent VT/VF for these patients is uncertain. Because the mechanism is thought to most commonly be deficient sodium channel function, the class Ia sodium channel blocking antiarrhythmic agent procainamide has been used to unmask the ECG phenotype and should be avoided therapeutically. Paradoxically, quinidine, another class Ia agent that also blocks the transient outward current, has shown some therapeutic benefit.[37] Ultimately, implanted cardioverter-defibrillator placement is the mainstay of long-term treatment.

KEY POINTS

If the WCT mechanism is likely SVT and the patient is stable, then intravenous administration of adenosine is often a reasonable first therapeutic intervention. However, adenosine should be avoided when an accessory tract is known or suspected to be present.

Calcium channel and beta-adrenergic blockers should be avoided unless the patient has a clearly defined history of a particular sensitive VT and safe previous treatment.

For stable SVT in the presence of a known accessory tract, intravenous administration of procainamide is most commonly recommended to terminate WCT.

For unstable SVT, synchronized direct current cardioversion, with sedation if possible, is the safest therapeutic course. The most effective antiarrhythmic to terminate sustained monomorphic VT is intravenous procainamide (intravenous racemic sotalol, which is also highly effective, is unavailable in the United States).

The recommended treatment for pulseless VT is defibrillation, and the safest and most effective treatment for stable or unstable VT is direct current cardioversion.

VT/VF in association with congenital disorders such as Brugada syndrome or congenital long-QT syndrome generally require cardioverter-defibrillator implantation.

TdP with inadequate perfusion should be cardioverted immediately. Intravenous magnesium and interventions that accelerate the heart rate may terminate TdP and prevent recurrence in the acute setting.

Prognosis and Disposition

The prognosis and disposition of patients with WCT depend on the underlying nature and severity of cardiac disease as well as the rhythm mechanism. Severe metabolic and toxicologic conditions causing WCT generally require both emergent treatment to terminate WCT and definitive therapy and hospital admission. WCT associated with implanted cardiac devices requires electrophysiologist interrogation and adjustment of the device's programming or other definitive therapy.

If the mechanism of WCT is known to be SVT based on acute findings or the patient's history, and the tachyarrhythmia is hemodynamically well tolerated, then discharge with close clinic followup after a period of emergency department observation after termination of the WCT is reasonable. If the patient is older or has compromised cardiac function or if the WCT is not hemodynamically well tolerated, then a more conservative approach with admission to an observation unit or the hospital is likely warranted. Marked rapid ventricular response to SVT, as observed with atrial flutter or fibrillation with antegrade accessory tract conduction, likely warrants hospital admission and evaluation by an electrophysiologist.

Many SVT rhythms are amenable to medical or definitive catheter ablation therapy. Atrial flutter and fibrillation also warrant consideration of anticoagulant therapy.

VT is most commonly associated with ischemic or advanced heart disease and generally portends a worse prognosis than SVT. If the WCT mechanism is uncertain, then it is safest to presume the presence of VT and treat accordingly. Patients with VT generally require hospital admission for further care. Without an obvious reversible cause, patients with VT are at risk for recurrence and decompensation to VF and sudden cardiac death. Consequently, patients, particularly those with a compromised ejection fraction of less than 35%, may be treated with an implanted cardioverter-defibrillator. The device is designed to prevent sudden cardiac death, but it cannot prevent the inexorable advancement of heart failure often observed in these patients. In fact, increased frequency of implanted cardioverter-defibrillator activation is associated with a worse prognosis.[38] Nevertheless, the incidence of VT seems to have decreased along with improvements in the care of patients with acute MI over the past few decades. The treatment options available for the treatment of VT, including catheter ablation and device therapy, have also taken remarkable steps forward and we anticipate that improvements will continue to emerge in the future.

References

1. Wellens HJ, Bar FW, Lie KI. The value of the electrocardiogram in the differential diagnosis of a tachycardia with a widened QRS complex. *Am J Med*. 1978;64:27-33.
2. Kay GN, Plumb VJ, Arciniegas JG, et al. Torsade de pointes: the long-short initiating sequence and other clinical features: observations in 32 patients. *J Am Coll Cardiol*. 1983;2:806-817.
3. Roden DM. Taking the idio out of idiosyncratic—predicting torsades de pointes. *Pacing Clin Electrophysiol*. 1998;21:1029-1034.
4. Benito B, Brugada R, Brugada J, et al. Brugada syndrome. *Prog Cardiovasc Dis*. 2008;51:1-22.
5. Antzelevitch C, Brugada P, Borggrefe M, et al. Brugada syndrome: report of the Second Consensus Conference. *Heart Rhythm*. 2005;2:429-440 [erratum, *Heart Rhythm*. 2005;2:905].
6. Brugada P, Brugada R, Brugada J. Should patients with an asymptomatic Brugada electrocardiogram undergo pharmacological and electrophysiological testing? *Circulation*. 2005;112:279-292.
7. Parrish RG, Tucker M, Ing R, et al. Sudden unexplained death syndrome in Southeast Asian refugees: a review of CDC surveillance. *MMWR CDC Surveill Summ*. 1987;36(SS-1):43SS-53SS.
8. Liebelt EL, Ulrich A, Francis PD, Woolf A. Serial electrocardiogram changes in acute tricyclic antidepressant overdoses. *Crit Care Med*. 1997;25:1721-1726.
9. Wrenn K. Management strategies in wide QRS complex tachycardia. *Am J Emerg Med*. 1991;9:592-597.
10. Baerman JM, Morady F, DiCarlo LA, Buitleir MD. Differentiation of ventricular tachycardia from supraventricular tachycardia with aberration: value of the clinical history. *Ann Emerg Med*. 1987;16:40-43.
11. Marill KA, Wolfram S, deSouza IS, et al. Adenosine for wide-complex tachycardia: efficacy and safety. *Crit Care Med*. 2009;37:2512-2518.

12. Garratt CJ, Griffith MJ, Young G, et al. Value of physical signs in the diagnosis of ventricular tachycardia. *Circulation.* 1994;90:3103-3107.
13. Akhtar M, Shenasa M, Jazayeri M, et al. Wide QRS complex tachycardia. *Ann Intern Med.*1988;109:905-912.
14. Marill KA. Diagnostic testing and the average absolute likelihood ratio: application to diagnosing wide QRS complex tachycardia and other emergency department diseases. *Am J Emerg Med.* 2012;30:1895-1906.
15. Brugada P, Brugada J, Mont L, et al. A new approach to the differential diagnosis of a regular tachycardia with a wide QRS complex. *Circulation.* 1991;83:1649-1659.
16. Wellens HJ. Ventricular tachycardia: diagnosis of broad QRS complex tachycardia. *Heart.* 2001;86:579-585.
17. Goldberger ZD, Rho RW, Page RL. Approach to the diagnosis and initial management of the stable adult patient with a wide complex tachycardia. *Am J Cardiol.* 2008;101:1456-1466.
18. Halperin BD, Kron J, Cutler JE, et al. Misdiagnosing ventricular tachycardia in patients with underlying conduction disease and similar sinus and tachycardia morphologies. *West J Med.* 1990;152:677-682.
19. Griffith MJ, Garratt CJ, Mounsey P, Camm AJ. Ventricular tachycardia as default diagnosis in broad complex tachycardia. *Lancet.* 1994;343:386-388.
20. Griffith MJ, Linker NJ, Ward DE, et al. Adenosine in the diagnosis of broad complex tachycardia. *Lancet.* 1988;1:672-675.
21. Rankin AC, Oldroyd KG, Chong E, et al. Value and limitations of adenosine in the diagnosis and treatment of narrow and broad complex tachycardias. *Br Heart J.* 1989;62:195-203.
22. Brodsky MA, Allen BJ, Grimes JA, Gold C. Enhanced atrioventricular conduction during atrial flutter after intravenous adenosine (letter). *N Engl J Med.* 1994;330:288-289.
23. Sellers TD, Compabell RWF, Bashore TM, et al. Effects of procainamide and quinidine sulfate in the Wolff-Parkinson-White syndrome. *Circulation.* 1977;55:15-22.
24. Boahene KA, Klein GJ, Yee, R, et al. Termination of acute atrial fibrillation in the Wolff-Parkinson-White syndrome by procainamide and propafenone: importance of atrial fibrillatory cycle length. *J Am Coll Cardiol.* 1990;16:1408-1414.
25. Tijunelis MA, Herbert ME. Myth: Intravenous amiodarone is safe in patients with atrial fibrillation and Wolff-Parkinson-White syndrome in the emergency department. *CJEM.* 2005;7:262-265.
26. Gorgels AP, van den Dool A, Hofs A, et al. Comparison of procainamide and lidocaine in terminating sustained monomorphic ventricular tachycardia. *Am J Cardiol.*1996;78:43-46.
27. Ho DS, Zecchin RP, Richards DA, et al. Double-blind trial of lignocaine versus sotalol for acute termination of spontaneous sustained ventricular tachycardia. *Lancet.* 1994;344:18-23.
28. Morady F, Dicarlo LA, Krol RB, et al: Acute and chronic effects of amiodarone on ventricular refractoriness, intraventricular conduction and ventricular tachycardia induction. *J Am Coll Cardiol.* 1986;7:148-157.
29. Marill KA, deSouza IS, Nishijima DK, et al. Amiodarone is poorly effective for the acute termination of ventricular tachycardia. *Ann Emerg Med.* 2006;47:217-224.
30. Scheinman MM, Levine JH, Cannom DS, et al. Dose-ranging study of intravenous amiodarone in patients with life-threatening ventricular tachyarrhythmias. *Circulation.* 1995;92:3264-3272.
31. Lerman BB, Belardinelli L, West GA, et al. Adenosine-sensitive ventricular tachycardia: evidence suggesting cyclic AMP-mediated triggered activity. *Circulation.* 1986;74:270-280.
32. Rankin AC, Rae AP, Cobbe SM. Misuse of intravenous verapamil in patients with ventricular tachycardia. *Lancet.* 1987;2(8557):472-474.
33. Buxton AE, Marchlinski FE, Doherty JU, et al. Hazards of intravenous verapamil for sustained ventricular tachycardia. *Am J Cardiol.* 1987;59:1107-1110.
34. Credner SC, Klingenheben T, Mauss O, et al. Electrical storm in patients with transvenous implantable cardioverter-defibrillators: incidence, management and prognostic implications. *J Am Coll Cardiol.* 1998;32:1909-1915.
35. Wolfe CL, Nibley C, Bhandari A, et al. Polymorphous ventricular tachycardia associated with acute myocardial infarction. *Circulation.* 1991;84:1543-1551.
36. Tzivoni D, Banai S, Schuger C, et al. Treatment of torsade de pointes with magnesium sulfate. *Circulation.* 1988;77:392-397.
37. Belhassen B, Glick A, Viskin S. Efficacy of quinidine in high-risk patients with Brugada syndrome. *Circulation.* 2004;110:1731-1737.
38. Moss AJ, Schuger C, Beck CA, et al. Reduction in inappropriate therapy and mortality through ICD programming. *N Engl J Med.* 2012;367:2275-2283.

CARDIOVASCULAR EMERGENCIES

CHAPTER 11

Syncope

James V. Quinn

IN THIS CHAPTER

Pathophysiology

Causes of syncope

Initial evaluation with consideration of diagnostic testing

Risk stratification tools and their limitations

Emergency department disposition

Syncope is a symptom complex comprising a brief loss of consciousness associated with an inability to maintain postural tone that resolves spontaneously without medical intervention. Most patients return to their baseline neurologic function. Near-syncope, a premonition of syncope without loss of consciousness, shares the same basic pathophysiologic process as syncope and the same risks.[1]

One in four people will experience an episode of syncope during his or her lifetime. Syncope accounts for 1% to 2% of emergency department visits each year and up to 6% of hospital admissions, resulting in more than $2.4 billion in hospital admission costs annually in the United States.[2-5]

Pathophysiology

A reduction of cerebral perfusion by 35%, or complete disruption for 5 to 10 seconds, will cause most people to lose consciousness or develop symptoms. Usually, an inciting event causes a drop in cardiac output, which decreases oxygen and substrate delivery to the brain.[6] Less commonly, vasospasm or other alterations in flow reduce central nervous system blood flow. After syncope, most patients are in a horizontal position, thereby decreasing the required perfusing pressure to retain consciousness. The change in position in combination with either the response of autonomic autoregulatory centers or reversion to a perfusing cardiac rhythm will result in spontaneous return of consciousness without any permanent change in neurologic function.

KEY POINTS

Syncope is common, and significant health care resources are expended in its evaluation and management.

Syncope is usually a benign symptom but occasionally is life threatening.

Despite the inciting condition, all forms of syncope have a common pathophysiologic mechanism.

Causes of Syncope

The causes of syncope are numerous, from common benign disorders to less common life-threatening processes (Table 11-1), and can be divided into specific categories, as follows: cardiac, reflex mediated, neurologic, and unknown. Each category carries its own prognostic implications. In the Framingham Heart Study, 7,814 patients were followed for 17 years, and 822 reported syncope over that time. People with documented heart disease and syncope had twice the death rate of those without syncope, and those with syncope with a neurologic cause were 50% more likely to die. Those with an unknown cause also had a significantly increased risk of death of 30%, whereas those with neurally mediated or vasovagal syncope had a lower risk of death than the study's general population cohort.[7] These findings indicate that diagnosis of syncope in the emergency department can be helpful in classifying patients and can be used as part of the risk-stratification process. Some studies have reported that the cause of syncope remains unknown after emergency department evaluation in as many as 60% of patients.[8,9] Other investigators, however, have shown that with a more careful history and aggressive approach the rate of those with an unclear cause for their syncope after emergency department evaluation can be reduced to 20%.[10,11]

Cardiac Syncope

Syncope of cardiac origin is associated with the greatest risk of death over a lifetime and is a harbinger of sudden death.[7,12] The risk of sudden cardiac death is what inhibits most emergency physicians from discharging patients with syncope of unknown cause. Sudden death is almost always caused by an arrhythmia, and the incidence is increased in patients with structural heart disease,[13] for whom the 6-month incidence of death is reported to be as high as 10%.[14]

Syncope from arrhythmias is typically sudden and not associated with prodromal symptoms. A variety of arrhythmias can cause syncope; nonperfusing ventricular tachycardia and ventricular fibrillation leading to asystole are lethal and cause the greatest concern.[15] Less lethal bradyarrhythmias and tachyarrhythmias can also lead to transient cerebral hypoperfusion; however, there is no absolute high or low heart rate that will produce a loss of consciousness. Both the autonomic nervous system's ability to compensate for a decrease in cardiac output and the degree of cerebrovascular atherosclerotic disease have a role in whether certain arrhythmias become symptomatic.[16,17] A bradyarrhythmia in the setting of normal blood pressure is more likely to be an incidental finding on an electrocardiogram (ECG) rather than the actual cause of syncope, although it should prompt further investigation.[18]

Arrhythmias can occur in people with structurally normal hearts but with genetic conditions such as Brugada syndrome or long or short QT syndromes[19] and in those with catecholamine-associated polymorphic ventricular tachycardia. Ar-

TABLE 11-1.

Causes of Syncope

Cardiac	Myxoma
Arrhythmias	Pericardial disease
Atrial fibrillation or flutter	Pulmonary embolism
Bradyarrhythmias	Pulmonary hypertension
Short or long QT interval	Tricuspid stenosis
Pacemaker malfunction	Other valvular heart disease
Second- or third-degree heart block	**Reflex Mediated**
Sinus node disease	Breath holding
Stokes-Adams attack	Carotid sinus syndrome
Supraventricular tachycardia	Orthostatic hypotension
Tachyarrhythmias	Situational
Torsade de pointes	Cough
Ventricular tachycardia	Defecation
Structural disease	Micturition
Aortic dissection	Neuralgia
Aortic stenosis	Swallow
Cardiomyopathy	Vasovagal
Congenital heart disease	**Neurologic**
Mitral stenosis	Migraine
Myocardial infarction	Subclavian steal
Myocardial ischemia	Transient ischemic attacks

rhythmias associated with electrolyte disorders (eg, hyperkalemia and hypomagnesemia [torsade de pointes]) or drug-related disorders (eg, tricyclic antidepressant overdose)[12,20] can be fatal. In people with structural heart disease, arrhythmias can be caused by underlying damage in the conduction system of the heart[21] and therefore can often be predicted by a patient's history or careful ECG analysis.[22] Structural heart disease can also cause syncope because it hampers the heart's ability to increase cardiac output[13,23] in response to physical exertion and to vasodilation from medication or heat. Normally, cardiac output increases to compensate for a decrease in systemic vascular resistance in order to maintain arterial perfusion; but when cardiac output is fixed because of structural abnormality, compensation is limited, leading to a decrease in arterial perfusion.

Syncope related to structural heart disease has several classic presentations. Valvular heart disease such as aortic stenosis should be excluded as a cause of syncope in the elderly.[24] The classic presentation is chest pain, dyspnea on exertion, and syncope. Hypertrophic cardiomyopathy, characterized by asymmetric left ventricular hypertrophy leading to obstruction, should be suspected in young patients who faint while exercising. Patients with acute pulmonary embolism can have pulmonary outflow obstruction, which can present as syncope.[25] Cardiomyopathy is the most common form of structural heart disease that decreases cardiac output, possibly leading to syncope.[23,26,27]

Vasovagal Syncope

Vasovagal syncope, often referred to as reflex-mediated or neurally mediated syncope, is usually benign and recurrent.[28] This type of syncope is associated with inappropriate vasodilation, bradycardia, or both. It is the result of inappropriate vagal tone, either directly or as an excessive response to increased sympathetic stimulation.[29,30]

Vasovagal syncope is often associated with a sensation of increased warmth and can be accompanied by preceding lightheadedness (prodrome) with sweating and nausea. A slow, progressive onset with the associated prodrome usually suggests vasovagal syncope. It can occur after exposure to an unexpected or unpleasant sight, sound, or smell; fear; severe pain; emotional distress; surgical instrumentation; coughing; defecation; or micturition. Therefore, it is often referred to as situational syncope. It can also occur in association with prolonged standing or kneeling in a crowded or warm environment, when the vagus nerve can become stimulated, resulting in reflex bradycardia and vasodilation. Upright tilt-table testing can be used to diagnose vasovagal syncope.[6,31]

Carotid sinus hypersensitivity, characterized by bradycardia or hypotension, is another type of reflex-mediated syncope. The carotid body contains pressure-sensitive receptors that can generate two autonomic responses. Most common is an abnormal vagal response, leading to bradycardia and asystole lasting more than 3 seconds. Less common is a vasodepressor response that decreases blood pressure more than 50 mm Hg without a significant change in heart rate.[32]

Neurologic Syncope

Neurologic disorders are rarely the primary cause of syncope, but they must be considered in any patient with syncope and signs or symptoms of central nervous system pathology. Non-neurologic syncope is, by definition, transient in nature and results in a return to baseline neurologic function. Patients with loss of consciousness followed by persistent neurologic deficits or altered mental status are not experiencing true syncope.

Brainstem ischemia can cause sudden brief episodes of loss of consciousness. These episodes are typically associated with other symptoms and physical findings of posterior circulation ischemia such as diplopia, vertigo, or nausea and involve the reticular activating system in the brain stem.

Subclavian steal is a rare cause of brainstem ischemia,[33] characterized by an abnormal narrowing of the subclavian artery proximal to the origin of the vertebral artery. With exercise of the ipsilateral arm, blood is shunted or "stolen" from the vertebral-basilar system to the subclavian artery supplying the arm muscles. Anatomically, it is more common on the left. Physical examination might reveal decreased pulse volume and diminished blood pressure in the affected arm. Other causes of brainstem ischemia include vertebral-basilar atherosclerotic disease and basilar artery migraines.

Subarachnoid hemorrhage is a potentially devastating disease process that can cause syncope, but it is usually accompanied by other signs and symptoms such as headache, focal neurologic deficits, or persistent altered mental status. The frequency with which spontaneous subarachnoid hemorrhage causes syncope is not really known. Traumatic subarachnoid hemorrhage from a head injury is more common and is the result of the syncope, not the cause.[34]

Seizure can be confused with syncope (Table 11-2).[35-37] During an episode of syncope, people often exhibit brief tonic-clonic movements. Confusion (a postictal state) after "syncope" lasting more than 15 minutes and associated with tongue biting, incontinence, or an epileptic aura suggests a seizure diagnosis. *Most people who have a seizure have a history of it. New-onset seizure in adults is unusual and usually occurs in people who have experienced neurologic injury.*

Most cases of syncope stemming from neurologic causes are easily recognized. Routine neurodiagnostic testing of syncope patients is not recommended unless the episode is associated with neurologic symptoms or significant head trauma.

Other Causes of Syncope

Syncope can also be caused by orthostasis and medication.[38] Medications can cause orthostasis or arrhythmias, which can affect the young and old.[39,40]

As one ages, the adrenergic receptor responsiveness of both the heart and the peripheral blood vessels gradually decreases. This decreased adrenergic responsiveness contributes to the diminished chronotropic response seen after orthostatic stresses in the elderly. Furthermore, elderly patients with structural heart disease have trouble increasing cardiac output to accommodate postural changes, which can be exacerbated by dehydration and some medications. When assessing an elderly patient, cardiac causes should be reasonably excluded before focusing on orthostasis as the cause of syncope. Positive orthostatic changes have been documented in up to 40% of asymptomatic patients over the age of 70 years and in about a quarter of those younger than 60.[40,41] For consideration of orthostasis as a reason for syncope, patients should have symptoms associated with a drop in systolic pressure of more than 20 mm Hg and/or an absolute value below 90 mm Hg.[41,42]

KEY POINTS

Syncope stemming from cardiac disorders and resulting in sudden death from arrhythmia causes the greatest concern.

Syncope with a neurologic basis is rare.

Vasovagal or situational syncope is almost always benign but can be difficult to diagnose with certainty.

Patients with unclear causes of syncope should be stratified according to risk.

Patient Evaluation

Emergency department evaluation of the patient with syncope should have the goal of making a specific diagnosis and guiding disposition based on the risk associated with that diagnosis. When the cause of syncope is unknown, risk stratification is the most practical approach. Risk stratification is based on a careful history, a thorough physical examination, and ECG interpretation. Other testing should be guided by the findings of these core components.

History

A clinical history should be obtained from the patient and any witness of the event. Emphasis should be placed on the symptoms or occurrences preceding the loss of consciousness, the characteristics of the loss of consciousness, and the symptoms after regaining consciousness. The history should include position, environmental stimuli, and the involvement of strenuous activity. All warning symptoms should be documented as part of the search for prodromal symptoms or situations consistent with vasovagal or situational syncope. Neurologic symptoms such as headache, vertigo, or focal weakness and cardiac symptoms such as chest pain or palpitations should be elicited, as should the duration of loss of consciousness and any resuscitative efforts such as chest compressions.

Symptoms associated with syncope that should raise concern include chest pain (acute myocardial infarction, aortic dissection, pulmonary embolism, aortic stenosis), palpitations (arrhythmia), shortness of breath (pulmonary embolism), headache (subarachnoid hemorrhage), and abdominal/back pain (leaking abdominal aortic aneurysm, ruptured ectopic pregnancy). A sudden event and events associated with exertion should increase suspicion of a cardiac arrhythmia or structural cardiopulmonary disease.

Concurrent illness or substance use should be documented. The patient's medical history should include questions regarding underlying structural heart disease, including congenital heart disease, valvular heart disease, coronary artery disease, and cardiomyopathy. It should also include details about previous cardiopulmonary events, including myocardial infarction, pulmonary embolism, ventricular arrhythmias, and heart failure.

The patient's use of medications should be recorded, including over-the-counter medications such as laxatives and herbal supplements. Patients who are dieting aggressively to lose weight might have an electrolyte disturbance or could be taking amphetamine-like medications. A family history is important in regard to arrhythmias, sudden cardiac death, and other cardiac risks. Special attention should be given to patients presenting after single-car motor vehicle crashes (many of them have a history of driving off the road).

Seizure is the most common event mistaken as syncope. Mild, brief, tonic-clonic activity ("convulsive syncope") can accompany syncope of any cause. The patient's history is very important in differentiating syncope from seizure.[43] A classic aura or postictal confusion and muscle pain indicate seizure, whereas characteristic prodromal symptoms of nausea and diaphoresis suggest reflex-mediated (vasovagal) syncope. Witnessed head

TABLE 11-2.

Differentiating Seizure from Syncope

	Syncope	Seizure
Movement characteristics	Light shaking	Generalized, violent tonic-clonic movement
Duration of movements	Brief, resolves without intervention, not recurrent	Longer than 15 seconds, can recur
Postictal period	Brief, often less than a few minutes before spontaneous return to baseline	Depends on duration of seizure, but often more than 15 minutes, with gradual clearing of confusion before return to baseline; can be accompanied by physical achiness
Prodrome	Can have vagal symptoms of warmth, diaphoresis, nausea	Can have aura of visual or olfactory stimuli and posturing
Incontinence/tongue biting	Unusual	Occasional
Laboratory abnormalities	B-type natriuretic peptide levels can increase over time in arrhythmogenic syncope	Creatine phosphokinase and lactate levels might be elevated after prolonged seizure

turning or unusual posture during the event is consistent with seizure. A prolonged postictal phase is characteristic of seizure. Prolonged delays in returning to baseline function in a patient with syncope and normal blood pressure or glucose would be highly atypical of vasovagal syncope. Urinary incontinence is not useful in the distinction. Tongue biting is specific for seizure but has poor sensitivity.[44]

Physical Examination

Evidence of trauma without defensive injuries to the hands or knees should raise suspicion of a sudden event, but patients with noncardiac syncope are also just as likely to suffer significant facial and head trauma. The physical examination should focus on the cardiovascular and neurologic systems. The strength of pulses in the extremities should be compared, left versus right; asymmetry should increase suspicion of aortic dissection or subclavian steal. The presence of orthostatic hypotension and its symptoms should be sought. To appropriately evaluate orthostasis, the patient should lie supine for 5 minutes and then rise to a standing position. After standing, blood pressure measurements should be taken two to three times over the next few minutes. A decrease in systolic blood pressure of more than 20 mm Hg, especially if the pressure is less than 90 mm Hg, or the precipitation of symptoms is considered positive for orthostasis. Cardiac examination might reveal the murmurs of hypertrophic cardiomyopathy or aortic stenosis. The neurologic examination could uncover findings of focal neurologic disease or evidence of autonomic instability (eg, peripheral neuropathy). Rectal examination should be considered to evaluate for gastrointestinal bleeding.

Electrocardiogram

A 12-lead ECG should almost always be obtained. Even though the ECG leads to a diagnosis in only a small number of patients, it is simple, inexpensive, and important in risk stratification.[45] The ECG should be evaluated for evidence of cardiopulmonary disease, acute ischemia, arrhythmia, heart block, and prolonged QT interval. Because the normal QT interval will vary based on rate, a corrected QT (QTc) interval is often calculated by the ECG computer using the Bazett formula [$QTc = QT/\sqrt{(RR)}$]. A prolonged QTc interval (Figure 11-1) has a variable definition, but the literature defines it as an interval larger than 470 msec, with intervals larger than 500 msec being most associated with ventricular arrhythmias (eg, torsade de pointes).[22,46,47] Potential causes of a prolonged QTc include hypokalemia, hypomagnesemia, hypocalcemia, Type IA medications, hypothermia, elevated intracranial pressure, and congenital prolonged QT syndrome. Many of these causes of prolonged QTc are reversible in the emergency department, and patients should therefore be evaluated for these causes and treated accordingly.

The ECG should also be scrutinized for evidence of ventricular pre-excitation, the most common form of which is Wolff-Parkinson-White (WPW) syndrome. Patients with WPW syndrome are at risk for extreme tachyarrhythmias, the most deadly type being atrial fibrillation. Patients with WPW syndrome who present with syncope should be monitored and admitted for ablation of the accessory pathway. WPW syndrome is discussed in further detail in Chapters 9 and 10.

Less common causes of syncope that should be identified on the ECG include Brugada syndrome and hypertrophic cardiomyopathy. Brugada syndrome is presumed to be caused by a sodium channelopathy that predisposes patients to develop sudden episodes of polymorphic tachycardia. The tachycardia may abort spontaneously, in which case patients present complaining of syncope, or the tachycardia may degenerate into ventricular fibrillation and produce sudden death. These patients have structurally normal hearts, and therefore the only method of confirming the diagnosis is via electrophysiologic studies. Patients presenting with syncope who demonstrate "classic" ECG findings of Brugada syndrome (Figure 11-2) should be promptly referred to an electrophysiologist for definitive testing and placement of an internal cardioverter-defibrillator. Medical therapies have not been found to be effective.

Hypertrophic cardiomyopathy is a common cause of sudden death in otherwise healthy teens and young adults. The condition is most common in males and often occurs during exertion. These patients have underlying hypertrophy of the interventricular septum that produces obstruction to ventricular outflow, leading to ventricular arrhythmias. Patients typically present with atypical chest pain, near-syncope, syncope, or sudden death. The ECG almost always demonstrates large-amplitude QRS complexes suggesting left or biventricular hypertrophy, and frequently there are also deep narrow Q waves in the inferior or lateral leads (Figure 11-3). When the diagnosis is suspected, a Doppler echocardiogram should be obtained for definitive diagnosis. Patients should be started on beta-blockers, counseled to avoid exertion, and referred to cardiology for chronic management.

In general, any new ECG changes, particularly any non-sinus rhythms noted during emergency department monitoring, are important. Recent studies have shown that any left bundle conduction abnormalities, old or new, should generate particular concern in patients with acute syncope. While in the emergency department, patients should be monitored for abnormal rhythms to reasonably exclude a cardiac cause of the syncope.[48]

Other Testing

Laboratory testing should be directed by findings in the history and physical examination. A complete blood count is generally indicated, especially in patients suspected of being anemic. A female of reproductive age should have a urine pregnancy test. Electrolyte abnormalities and creatine phosphokinase elevation might implicate seizures as a cause of syncope. The B-type natriuretic peptide (BNP) or pro-BNP level appears to be associated with risk of serious cardiovascular outcome and death. Reed and colleagues found that a BNP level higher than 300 pg/mL in the setting of syncope suggests risk of serious outcome.[49] However, the value of a single BNP measurement has been questioned with regard to the timing of the draw in relation to the event. Serial samples might be of more value.[50]

It is unclear whether BNP adds any value over a history of heart failure or structural disease.[51,52] An echocardiogram allows evaluation for structural heart disease; this procedure may

CARDIOVASCULAR EMERGENCIES

FIGURE 11-1.

Prolonged QTc. The QTc interval here is 653 msec. This was caused by severe hypocalcemia, and once the calcium level was corrected, the QTc normalized.

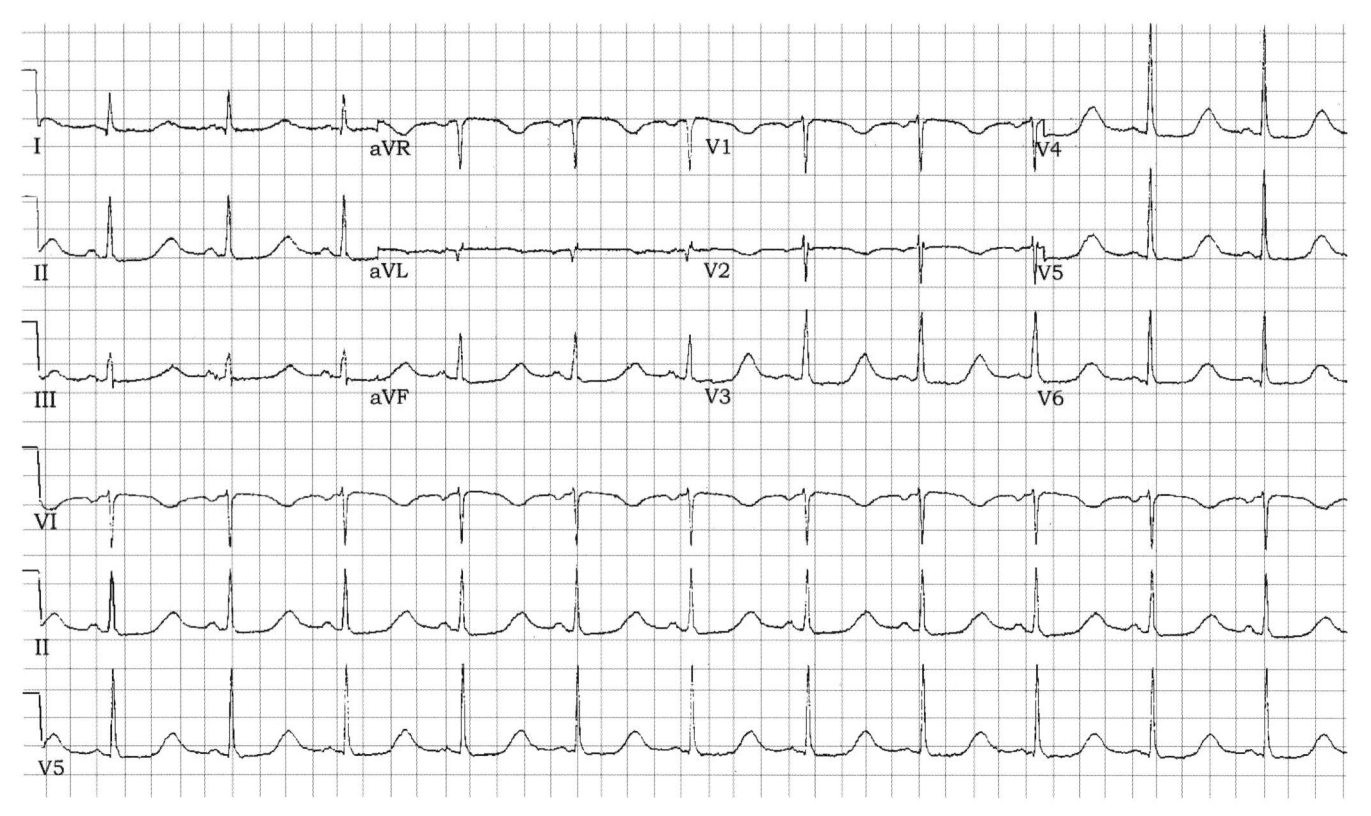

FIGURE 11-2.

The Brugada Syndrome. The ECG demonstrates a classic Brugada syndrome appearance: incomplete or complete right bundle-branch block appearance in leads V_1 through V_2 (sometimes extending to lead V_3) and associated ST-segment elevation leading to inverted T waves.

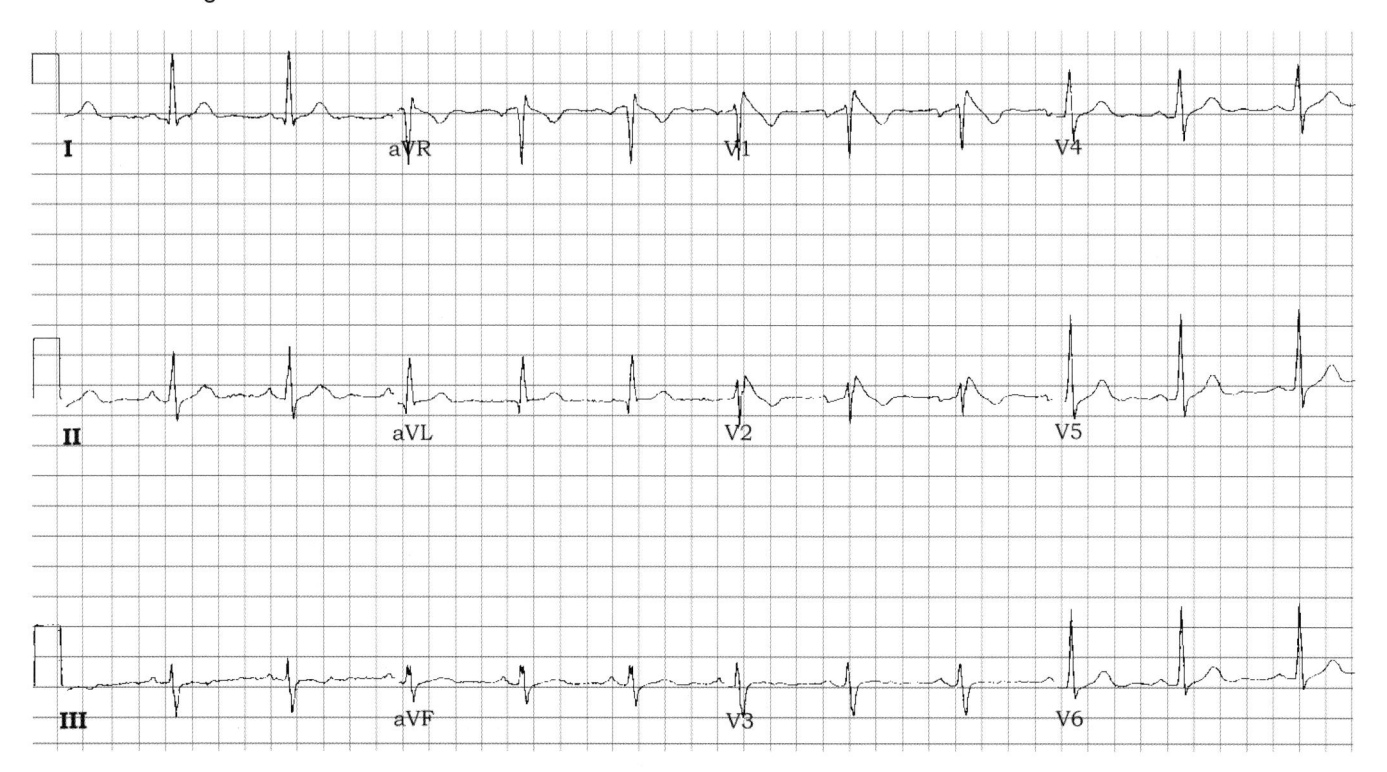

be done based on risk. Routine echocardiography has not been shown to be useful or practical in the emergency department evaluation of syncope.[53]

Neurologic Testing

When the history or physical examination does not suggest a neurologic cause for syncope, the clinical yield of routine computed tomography (CT), electroencephalography, or lumbar puncture is very low. A head CT scan or magnetic resonance imaging scan is not warranted in asymptomatic patients who have experienced an isolated event, have no neurologic symptoms, and have no significant head trauma.[54,55]

KEY POINTS

A careful history and physical examination can help delineate the cause of syncope.

An ECG and monitoring in the emergency department are almost always warranted.

The use of other imaging and testing should be guided by the findings on history and physical examination.

Disposition and Followup

Diagnosis Established

Patients with syncope of cardiac or neurologic origin should be admitted. Patients with vasovagal, orthostatic, and medication-related syncope have no increased risk of cardiovascular morbidity or mortality and do not need to be hospitalized if the precipitating factor has been addressed.

Unexplained Syncope

Even after extensive evaluation, many patients are diagnosed with syncope of unknown cause. Those left with an unknown cause can be further risk stratified to allow safe and efficient disposition from the emergency department.[10,11]

Several studies have assessed risk stratification variables to identify patients at risk of both short-term and 1-year morbidity and mortality. Martin and associates studied consecutive emergency department patients with syncope to identify predictors of arrhythmia and death at 1 year.[56] Significant risk factors were a history of arrhythmia, an abnormal ECG, a history of heart failure, and age above 45 years. Quinn and colleagues assessed adverse outcomes at 7 and 30 days in their derivation and validation of the San Francisco Syncope Rule.[3,57] The significant predictors of adverse events that they identified are listed in Table 11-3. Inconsistencies in attempts to validate the San Francisco Syncope Rule have been related primarily to inconsistencies in the definition of syncope and the application of the predictor variables.[58] The Osservatorio Epidemiologico sulla Sincope nel Lazio study group developed a risk score based on predictors of death at 1 year, which they found to be an abnormal ECG, a history of cardiovascular disease (including heart failure), age above 65 years, and syncope without prodrome.[59] Sarasin and colleagues developed a prediction score for subsequent arrhythmia in patients with unexplained syncope after a standard emergency department evaluation.[60] They found the significant

FIGURE 11-3.

Hypertrophic cardiomyopathy. The ECG demonstrates large amplitude QRS complexes and deep narrow Q waves in the lateral leads I and aVL. Q waves may be present in leads V_5 through V_6 as well, or they may be limited to the inferior leads. These Q waves are characteristically narrow, unlike infarction-related Q waves, which are typically at least 40 msec wide.

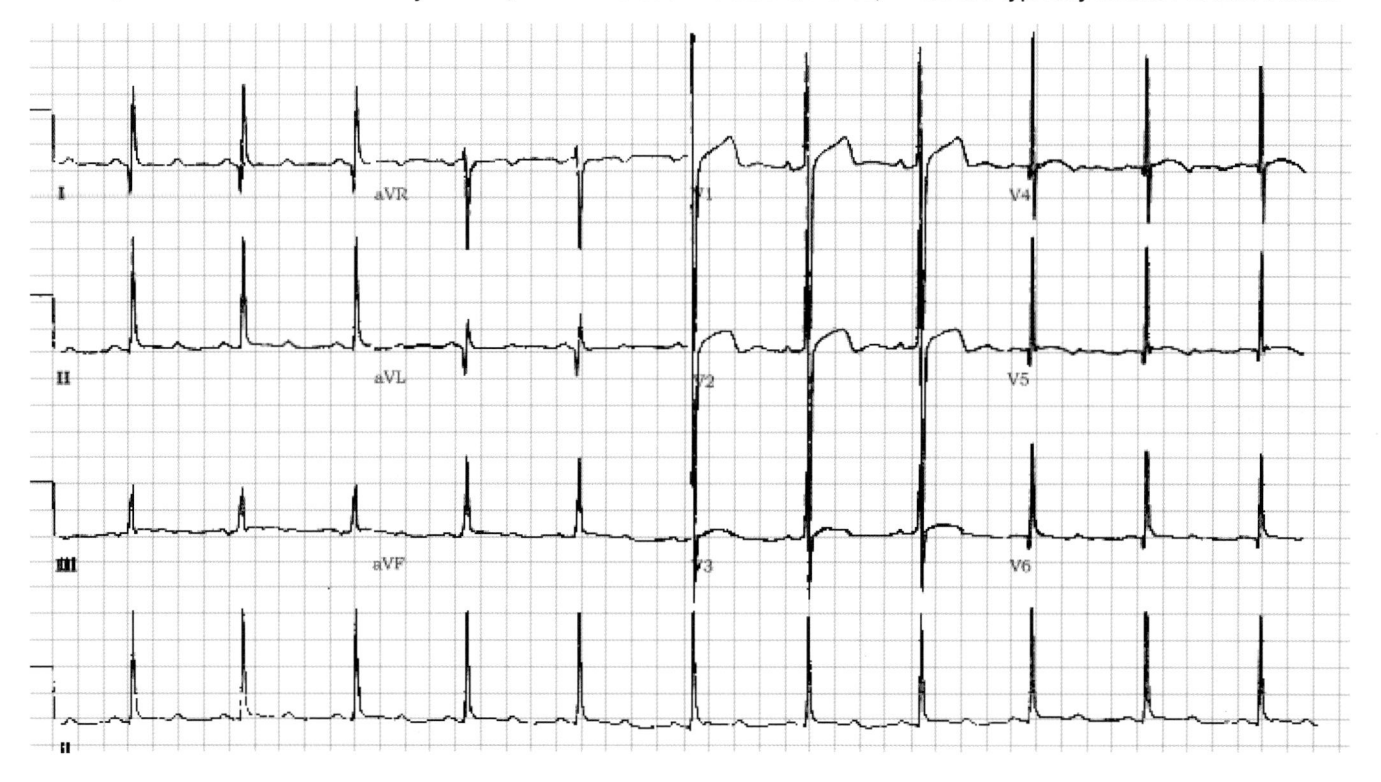

variables to be an abnormal ECG, a history of heart failure, and age above 65 years.

Using the risk factors identified in these studies can help clinicians determine patients' risk and appropriate disposition. Although the validation studies have limitations, they did yield the consistent conclusions that an abnormal ECG or rhythm on monitoring and a history of heart disease (particularly structural heart disease especially characterized by a history of heart failure) are clear risk factors.

KEY POINTS

Patients with abnormal ECGs, non-sinus rhythms, and structural heart disease are at high risk for serious outcomes following syncope.

General risk is increased with advanced age.

Low-risk patients who are asymptomatic and appear to be well may be considered for discharge.

Inpatient Evaluation

The value and cost effectiveness of admission and testing in the inpatient setting have been questioned.[61,62] With the exception of patients with acute life-threatening diagnoses (eg, stroke, aortic dissection), the goal of the inpatient evaluation is focused on identifying underlying heart disease and detecting life-threatening arrhythmias. All admitted patients require

TABLE 11-3.
Predictors of Adverse Events in the San Francisco Syncope Rule[3,57]

History of heart failure
Abnormal ECG
Rhythm other than sinus (eg, during monitoring or on repeated ECGs)
Conduction delays
New changes as minimal as first-degree atrioventricular block
Morphologic changes to the QRS complex or ST segment not evident on previous tracings
Hematocrit less than 30
Shortness of breath
Systolic blood pressure less than 90 mm Hg in the emergency department

FIGURE 11-4.
Emergency department disposition of adult patients with syncope[71]

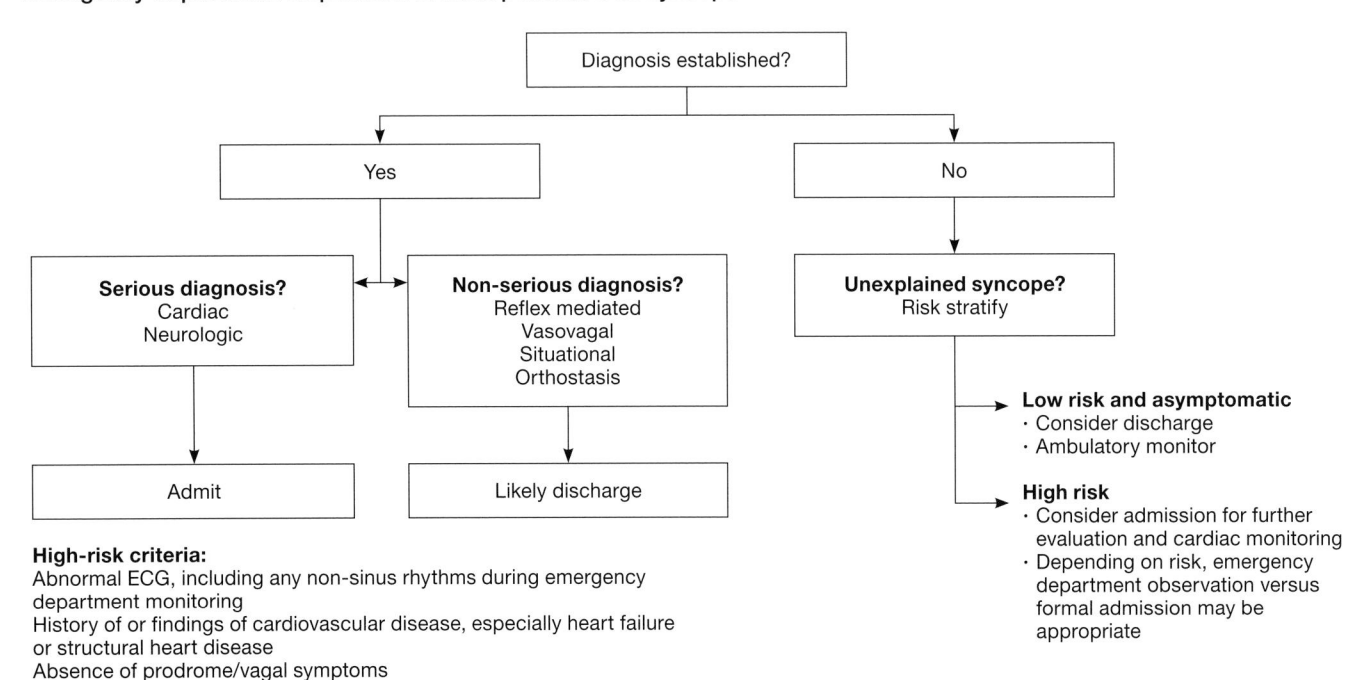

Diagnosis established?
- Yes
  - Serious diagnosis? (Cardiac, Neurologic) → Admit
  - Non-serious diagnosis? (Reflex mediated, Vasovagal, Situational, Orthostasis) → Likely discharge
- No
  - Unexplained syncope? Risk stratify
    - Low risk and asymptomatic
      - Consider discharge
      - Ambulatory monitor
    - High risk
      - Consider admission for further evaluation and cardiac monitoring
      - Depending on risk, emergency department observation versus formal admission may be appropriate

High-risk criteria:
Abnormal ECG, including any non-sinus rhythms during emergency department monitoring
History of or findings of cardiovascular disease, especially heart failure or structural heart disease
Absence of prodrome/vagal symptoms
Persistent low blood pressure (SBP <90 mm Hg)
Family history of sudden cardiac death (especially in young individuals)
Advanced age

continuous ECG monitoring. Arrhythmia as the cause of syncope is confirmed in patients with recurrent symptoms during a monitored arrhythmia and excluded in patients with recurrent symptoms during sinus rhythm. High-risk patients should be admitted and monitored as inpatients. If the initial monitoring period does not reveal any abnormalities, monitoring in the outpatient setting for prolonged periods of time has the best diagnostic yield.[63-65] An echocardiogram should be performed on patients with known or suspected heart disease to evaluate for valvular disorders and cardiomyopathies in order to determine overall cardiac function. Echocardiographic abnormalities are usually clinically apparent and will seldom be found in patients with a normal cardiac examination and ECG.[53] Stress testing is useful to identify exercise-induced arrhythmias or ischemia or to reproduce exertional syncope once hypertrophic cardiomyopathy has been excluded by echocardiography. Electrophysiology testing is typically reserved for patients with documented arrhythmia, preexcitation syndromes, or underlying heart disease.[15]

Outpatient Evaluation

Patients appropriate for outpatient syncope evaluation (the most cost-effective approach) are those thought to be at low risk for serious cardiac arrhythmias.[66] Long-term monitoring, which includes ambulatory or event monitors, is useful to further evaluate potential arrhythmias. The duration of monitoring is debatable, but monitors are now more portable and can be worn for longer periods,[65] which allows for detection of more abnormalities and increases diagnostic yield.[67,68]

Tilt-table testing is also suggested for patients with recurrent, unexplained syncope.[29,31] Tilt-testing is designed to identify reflex-mediated syncope by rapidly moving the patient from a supine position on the tilt table to an upright position of 60° for 45 minutes. A positive end point is reached if syncope, hypotension, or the patient's typical symptoms are reproduced. Repeat testing with isoproterenol or sublingual nitroglycerin is performed if the initial evaluation is negative.[16]

KEY POINTS

Cardiac monitoring in the inpatient or outpatient setting has the greatest value in identifying arrhythmias.

Prolonged monitoring improves diagnostic yield.

Practice Guidelines

Various specialty guidelines contain recommendations for evaluation and disposition based on risk factors.[69,70] The disposition of emergency department patients based on guidelines promulgated by the American College of Emergency Physicians is summarized in Figure 11-4.[71]

References

1. Grossman SA, Babineau M, Burke L, et al. Do outcomes of near syncope parallel syncope? *Am J Emerg Med*. 2011;30:203-206.
2. Blanc JJ, L'Her C, Touiza A, et al. Prospective evaluation and outcome of patients admitted for syncope over a 1 year period. *Eur Heart J*. 2002;23:815-820.
3. Quinn JV, Stiell IG, McDermott DA, et al. Derivation of the San Francisco Syncope Rule to predict patients with short-term serious outcomes. *Ann Emerg Med*. 2004;43:224-232.
4. Numeroso F, Mossini G, Spaggiari E, et al. Syncope in the emergency department of a large northern Italian hospital: incidence, efficacy of a short-stay observation ward and validation of the OESIL risk score. *Emerg Med J*. 2010;27:653-658.
5. Sun BC, Emond JA, Camargo CA Jr. Direct medical costs of syncope-related hospitalizations in the United States. *Am J Cardiol*. 2005;95:668-671.
6. Ammirati F, Colivicchi F, Di Battista G, et al. Variable cerebral dysfunction during tilt induced vasovagal syncope. *Pacing Clin Electrophysiol*. 1998;21(11 Pt 2):2420-2425.
7. Soteriades ES, Evans JC, Larson MG, et al. Incidence and prognosis of syncope. *N Engl J Med*. 2002;347:878-885.
8. Hori S. Diagnosis of patients with syncope in emergency medicine. *Keio J Med*. 1994;43:185-191.
9. Gilman JK. Syncope in the emergency department: a cardiologist's perspective. *Emerg Med Clin North Am*. 1995;13:955-971.
10. Alboni P, Brignole M, Menozzi C, et al. Diagnostic value of history in patients with syncope with or without heart disease. *J Am Coll Cardiol*. 2001;37:1921-1928.
11. Kapoor WN. A standardized sequential clinical examination identified probable causes of syncope in 69% of patients. *ACP J Club*. 2002;136:77.
12. Juang JM, Huang SK. Brugada syndrome—an under-recognized electrical disease in patients with sudden cardiac death. *Cardiology*. 2004;101:157-169.
13. Efthimiadis GK, Parcharidou DG, Giannakoulas G, et al. Left ventricular outflow tract obstruction as a risk factor for sudden cardiac death in hypertrophic cardiomyopathy. *Am J Cardiol*. 2009;104:695-699.
14. Kapoor WN. Syncope. *N Engl J Med*. 2000;343:1856-1862.
15. Chen LY, Jahangir A, Decker WW, et al. Score indices for predicting electrophysiologic outcomes in patients with unexplained syncope. *J Interv Card Electrophysiol*. 2005;14:99-105.
16. Brembilla-Perrot B, Muhanna I, Marcon O, et al. Increased sensitivity of electrophysiological study by isoproterenol infusion in unexplained syncope. *Int J Cardiol*. 2006;106:82-87.
17. Brembilla-Perrot B, Beurrier D, de la Chaise AT, et al. Significance and prevalence of inducible atrial tachyarrhythmias in patients undergoing electrophysiologic study for presyncope or syncope. *Int J Cardiol*. 1966;53:61-69.
18. Diaz-Castro O, Puchol A, Almendral J, et al. Predictors of in-hospital ventricular fibrillation or torsades de pointes in patients with acute symptomatic bradycardia. *J Electrocardiol*. 2004;37:55-60.
19. Liu JF, Jons C, Moss AJ, et al. Risk factors for recurrent syncope and subsequent fatal or near-fatal events in children and adolescents with long QT Syndrome. *J Am Coll Cardiol*. 2011;57:941-950.
20. Mok NS, Chan NY. Brugada syndrome presenting with sustained monomorphic ventricular tachycardia. *Int J Cardiol*. 2004;97:307-309.
21. Middlekauff HR, Stevenson WG, Saxon LA. Prognosis after syncope: impact of left ventricular function. *Am Heart J*. 1993;125:121-127.
22. Aggarwal A, Sherazi S, Levitan B, et al. Corrected QT interval as a predictor of mortality in elderly patients with syncope. *Cardiol J*. 2011;18:395-400.
23. Middlekauff HR, Stevenson WG, Stevenson LW, et al. Syncope in advanced heart failure: high risk of sudden death regardless of origin of syncope. *J Am Coll Cardiol*. 1993;21:110-116.
24. Kapoor WN. Evaluation and outcome of patients with syncope. *Medicine*. 1990;69:160-175.
25. Wolfe TR, Allen TL. Syncope as an emergency department presentation of pulmonary embolism. *J Emerg Med*. 1998;16:27-31.
26. Olshansky B, Poole JE, Johnson G, et al. Syncope predicts the outcome of cardiomyopathy patients: analysis of the SCD-HeFT study. *J Am Coll Cardiol*. 2008;51:1277-1282.
27. Padhi PK, Patel DK, Mohanty PK, et al. Factors predicting morbidity and mortality in idiopathic dilated cardiomyopathy—an inhospital survey. *J Assoc Physicians India*. 2006;54:587-588.
28. Sumner GL, Rose MS, Koshman ML, et al. Recent history of vasovagal syncope in a young, referral-based population is a stronger predictor of recurrent syncope than lifetime syncope burden. *J Cardiovasc Electrophysiol*. 2010;21:1375-1380.
29. Boehm KE, Morris EJ, Kip KT, et al. Diagnosis and management of neurally mediated syncope and related conditions in adolescents. *J Adolesc Health*. 2001;28:2-9.
30. Grubb BP, Jorge Sdo C. A review of the classification, diagnosis, and management of autonomic dysfunction syndromes associated with orthostatic intolerance. *Arq Bras Cardiol*. 2000;74:537-552.
31. de Castro RR, da Nobrega AC. Elderly patients with unexplained syncope: what should be considered a positive tilt test response? *Auton Neurosci*. 2006;126-127:169-173.
32. Coplan NL. Carotid sinus hypersensitivity and syncope: cause/effect or true/true/unrelated. *Arch Intern Med*. 2006;166:491-492.
33. Brignole M, Alboni P, Benditt D, et al. Guidelines on management (diagnosis and treatment) of syncope. *Eur Heart J*. 2001;22:1256-1306.

34. Frontera JA, Parra A, Shimbo D, et al. Cardiac arrhythmias after subarachnoid hemorrhage: risk factors and impact on outcome. *Cerebrovasc Dis.* 2008;26:71-78.
35. Abubakr A, Wambacq I. The diagnostic value of EEGs in patients with syncope. *Epilepsy Behav.* 2005;6:433-434.
36. Ammirati F, Colivicchi F, Di Battista G, et al. Electroencephalographic correlates of vasovagal syncope induced by head-up tilt testing. *Stroke.* 1998;29:2347-2351.
37. Libman MD, Potvin L, Coupal L, et al. Seizure vs. syncope: measuring serum creatine kinase in the emergency department. *J Gen Intern Med.* 1991;6:408-412.
38. Hanlon JT, Linzer M, MacMillan JP, et al. Syncope and presyncope associated with probable adverse drug reactions. *Arch Intern Med.* 1990;150:2309-2312.
39. Walker BD, Krahn AD, Klein GJ, et al. Drug induced QT prolongation: lessons from congenital and acquired long QT syndromes. *Curr Drug Targets Cardiovasc Haematol Dis.* 2003;3:327-335.
40. Mussi C, Ungar A, Salvioli G, et al. Orthostatic hypotension as cause of syncope in patients older than 65 years admitted to emergency departments for transient loss of consciousness. *J Gerontol A Biol Sci Med Sci.* 2009;64:801-806.
41. Atkins D, Hanusa B, Sefcik T, et al. Syncope and orthostatic hypotension. *Am J Med.* 1991;91:179-185.
42. Sarasin FP, Louis-Simonet M, Carballo D, et al. Prevalence of orthostatic hypotension among patients presenting with syncope in the ED. *Am J Emerg Med.* 2002;20:497-501.
43. Sheldon R, Rose S, Ritchie D, et al. Historical criteria that distinguish syncope from seizures. *J Am Coll Cardiol.* 2002;40:142-148.
44. Brigo F, Nardone R, Bongiovanni LG. Value of tongue biting in differential diagnosis between epileptic seizures and syncope. *Seizure.* 2012;21:568-572.
45. Cerrone M, Priori SG. Routine electrocardiogram and medical history in syncope: a simple approach can identify most high-risk patients. *Europace.* 2009;11:1411-1412.
46. Liu JF, Jons C, Moss AJ, et al. Risk factors for recurrent syncope and subsequent fatal or near-fatal events in children and adolescents with long QT Syndrome. *J Am Coll Cardiol.* 2011;57:941-950.
47. Jimenez-Candil J, Diego M, Cruz Gonzalez I, et al. Relationship between the QTc interval at hospital admission and the severity of the underlying ischaemia in low and intermediate risk people studied for acute chest pain. *Int J Cardiol.* 2008;126:84-91.
48. Quinn J, McDermott D. Electrocardiogram findings in emergency department patients with syncope. *Acad Emerg Med.* 2011;18:714-718.
49. Reed MJ, Newby DE, Coull AJ, et al. The ROSE (risk stratification of syncope in the emergency department) study. *J Am Coll Cardiol.* 2010;55:713-717.
50. Costantino G, Solbiati M, Casazza G, et al. Usefulness of N-terminal pro-B-type natriuretic peptide increase as a marker for cardiac arrhythmia in patients with syncope. *Am J Cardiol.* 2014;113(1):98-102.
51. Reed MJ, Newby DE, Coull AJ, et al. Role of brain natriuretic peptide (BNP) in risk stratification of adult syncope. *Emerg Med J.* 2007;24:769-773.
52. Costantino G, Solbiati M, Pisano G, et al. NT-pro-BNP for differential diagnosis in patients with syncope. *Int J Cardiol.* 2009;137:298-299.
53. Sarasin FP, Junod AF, Carballo D, et al. Role of echocardiography in the evaluation of syncope: a prospective study. *Heart.* 2002;88:363-367.
54. Grossman SA, Fischer C, Bar JL, et al. The yield of head CT in syncope: a pilot study. *Intern Emerg Med.* 2007;2:46-49.
55. Narayanan V, Keniston A, Albert RK. Utility of emergency cranial computed tomography in patients without trauma. *Acad Emerg Med.* 2012;19:E1055-E1060.
56. Martin TP, Hanusa BH, Kapoor WN. Risk stratification of patients with syncope. *Ann Emerg Med.* 1997;29:459-466.
57. Quinn J, McDermott D, Stiell I, et al. Prospective validation of the San Francisco Syncope Rule to predict patients with serious outcomes. *Ann Emerg Med.* 2006;47:448-454.
58. Saccilotto RT, Nickel CH, Bucher HC, et al. San Francisco Syncope Rule to predict short-term serious outcomes: a systematic review. *CMAJ.* 2011;183:E1116-E1126.
59. Colivicchi F, Ammirati F, Melina D, et al. Development and prospective validation of a risk stratification system for patients with syncope in the emergency department: the OESIL risk score. *Eur Heart J.* 2003;24:811-819.
60. Sarasin FP, Hanusa BH, Perneger T, et al. A risk score to predict arrhythmias in patients with unexplained syncope. *Acad Emerg Med.* 2003;10:1312-1317.
61. Tattersall LC, Reed MJ. The inpatient management of syncope. *Emerg Med J.* 2010;27:870-872.
62. Mendu ML, McAvay G, Lampert R, et al. Yield of diagnostic tests in evaluating syncopal episodes in older patients. *Arch Intern Med.* 2009;169:1299-1305.
63. Benezet-Mazuecos J, Ibanez B, Rubio JM, et al. Utility of in-hospital cardiac remote telemetry in patients with unexplained syncope. *Europace.* 2007;9:1196-1201.
64. Sarasin FP, Carballo D, Slama S, et al. Usefulness of 24-h Holter monitoring in patients with unexplained syncope and a high likelihood of arrhythmias. *Int J Cardiol.* 2005;101:203-207.
65. Assar MD, Krahn AD, Klein GJ, et al. Optimal duration of monitoring in patients with unexplained syncope. *Am J Cardiol.* 2003;92:1231-1233.
66. Krahn AD, Klein GJ, Yee R, et al. Cost implications of testing strategy in patients with syncope: randomized assessment of syncope trial. *J Am Coll Cardiol.* 2003;42:495-501.
67. Krahn AD, Klein GJ, Yee R, et al. Use of an extended monitoring strategy in patients with problematic syncope. Reveal Investigators. *Circulation.* 1999;99:406-410.
68. Bass EB, Curtiss EI, Arena VC, et al. The duration of Holter monitoring in patients with syncope. Is 24 hours enough? *Arch Intern Med.* 1990;150:1073-1078.
69. Cooper PN, Westby M, Pitcher DW, et al. Synopsis of the National Institute for Health and Clinical Excellence Guideline for management of transient loss of consciousness. *Ann Intern Med.* 2011;155:543-549.
70. Moya A, Sutton R, Ammirati F, et al. Guidelines for the diagnosis and management of syncope (version 2009). *Eur Heart J.* 2009;30:2631-2671.
71. Huff JS, Decker WW, Quinn JV, et al. Clinical policy: critical issues in the evaluation and management of adult patients presenting to the emergency department with syncope. *Ann Emerg Med.* 2007;49:431-444.

CHAPTER 12

Modern Management of Cardiac Arrest

Joshua C. Reynolds

IN THIS CHAPTER

Circulatory support

Defibrillation

Airway

Oxygenation

Ventilation

Pharmacotherapy

Devices

Regionalization of care

A universal termination-of-resuscitation rule

Novel future directions

Out-of-hospital cardiac arrest (OHCA) is a profound clinical and public health challenge, both in the United States and across the globe. The incidence of OHCA is highest in Australia (113 per year per 100,000 population), followed by North America (94 per year per 100,000 population), Europe (86 per year per 100,000 population), and Asia (55 per year per 100,000 population).[1] Cardiovascular disease is the most common cause of OHCA, and death from cardiovascular disease accounts for one third of annual deaths in the United States.[2] The incidence of OHCA from a presumed cardiac cause is highest in North America (55 per year per 100,000 population), followed by Australia (44 per year per 100,000 population), Europe (35 per year per 100,000 population), and Asia (32 per year per 100,000 population).[1] OHCA is more likely to have a cardiac cause in patients older than 35 years and a noncardiac cause in patients younger than 35.[3] In fact, 83% of cardiac arrests occurring in patients under 19 years are noncardiac in origin.[4] Health care providers are notoriously inaccurate in identifying the cause of OHCA, often underestimating noncardiac origins.[5,6]

Outcomes from OHCA vary markedly by region, as documented by a 10-site North American resuscitation research consortium with a total catchment population of 21.4 million.[7] Among cardiac arrest victims treated by emergency medical services (EMS) personnel, the median survival rate to hospital discharge was 8.4% (interquartile range: 5.4%-10.4%) with survival rates ranging from 3% to 16.3% across the country. The survival rate was markedly higher in patients with ventricular fibrillation as the initial rhythm. In this subpopulation, the median survival rate to hospital discharge was 22% (interquartile range: 15%-24.4%), with survival rates ranging from 7.7% to 39.9% across the same geographic locales.

General Management Considerations

Cardiac arrest is a dynamic disease. Few clinical presentations strain the multitasking and leadership abilities of emergency physicians more. However, astute clinicians must realize that they are orchestrating only one portion of a larger series of events, each of which directly affects patient outcome. Prehospital and emergency department resuscitation to achieve return of spontaneous circulation (ROSC) is only one small piece of the puzzle. Layperson recognition of cardiac arrest, activation of the EMS system, and provision of bystander cardiopulmonary resuscitation (CPR) are equally important. Likewise, the critical care, inpatient, and rehabilitation phases play crucial roles in attaining neurologically favorable survival. This larger view of cardiac arrest care is embodied in the success of bundled postresuscitation care packages that boost rates of neurologically favorable survival among patients who attain ROSC.[8]

Circulatory Support

Pulse Checks

It is increasingly clear that both lay rescuers and health care providers have difficulty performing accurate pulse checks.[9-17] When assessing an unresponsive patient, health care providers tend to be more accurate in recognizing cardiac arrest when they assess breathing and heart rate sequentially rather than simultaneously.[18] The initial assessment of an unresponsive patient can be confounded by agonal respirations, which are common after cardiac arrest.[19-22] The presence of agonal respirations should not preclude initiating CPR.

Chest Compressions

The recommended depth for chest compressions is at least 2 inches for adults. This recommendation comes from several "before-and-after" studies of EMS systems that implemented new regional protocols.[23,24] A compression depth of at least 2 inches improved defibrillation success and ROSC compared with historical controls. No human trial has directly compared these depths, so there is insufficient evidence to recommend an upper limit on chest compression depth.

Allowing complete chest recoil is recommended to maximize the hemodynamic effects of CPR. Animal data suggest improved mean arterial pressure, coronary perfusion pressure, cardiac output, and myocardial blood flow with complete recoil.[25,26] No studies have been performed in humans to specifically compare complete and incomplete chest recoil during CPR.

The recommended rate of chest compressions is at least 100 compressions per minute. One study of inhospital cardiac arrests demonstrated an association between chest compression rates above 80 per minute and ROSC.[27] There is no known association between chest compression rate and survival.[28]

A related metric for CPR is chest compression fraction—larger fractions correlate with higher rates of survival to hospital discharge. Chest compression fraction is the proportion of total resuscitation time during which chest compressions are provided. In one study, the highest rate of survival to hospital discharge was achieved with a chest compression fraction greater than 0.60.[28] This fraction corresponded to chest compression rates of 100 to 127 per minute. To maximize chest compression fraction, interruptions in chest compressions must be minimized, especially those for ventilations, pulse checks, rhythm analysis, defibrillation, and postdefibrillation assessment. These tasks are addressed in turn throughout this chapter.

New monitor/defibrillator technologies include computerized algorithms that remove chest compression artifact from the electrocardiogram (ECG) during CPR (Figure 12-1). The filtered signal reveals the underlying rhythm. In simulated models of human ECG recordings with CPR artifact, ECG processing afforded 90% to 98% sensitivity and 80% to 89% specificity in identifying a shockable rhythm during ongoing chest compressions.[29-34]

The recommended compression-to-ventilation ratio for health care providers is 30:2. This ratio represents a compromise between maintaining a pressure gradient with continuous chest compressions and oxygenation/ventilation. The recommended ratio of 30:2 started with the 2005 update of guidelines from the International Liaison Committee on Resuscitation. Since then, evidence regarding improved outcomes with this ratio has been mixed. Two studies demonstrated an increased survival rate with a ratio of 30:2 compared with historical controls using 15:2,[35,36] while others failed to show the same benefit.[37,38]

There is a quality gap between recommended CPR parameters and actual performance. Despite recommendations, CPR performed by health care providers is frequently too slow and too shallow, with incomplete recoil.[39-43] Real-time feedback devices are readily available for CPR performance. These devices typically consist of an accelerometer that is placed between the rescuer's hands and the victim's anterior chest wall. They display real-time data on rate, depth, recoil, and chest compression fraction. These devices improve CPR quality, but, unfortunately, this strategy has not translated into improved survival rates.[23,24,44-50]

The association between chest compression fraction and sur-

FIGURE 12-1.

ECG signal filtering during chest compressions

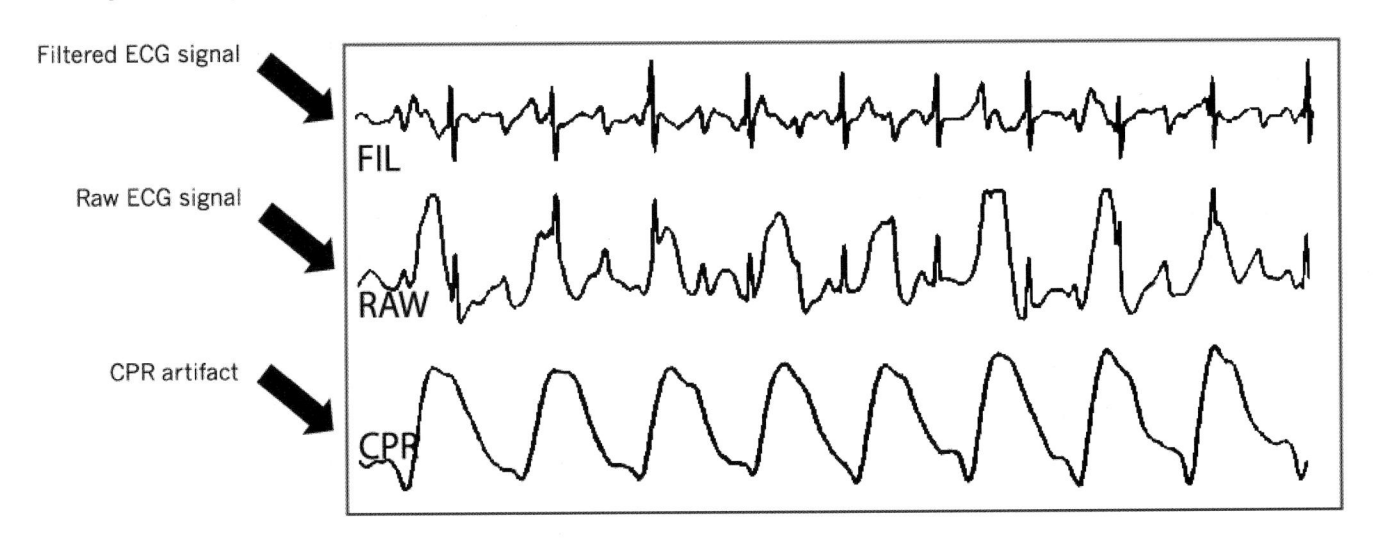

vival to hospital discharge begs the question: What if CPR consisted only of chest compressions? The concept of continuous chest compressions (also called *chest-compression-only CPR* or *hands-only CPR*) has been evaluated for lay rescuers as a means of reducing the barriers associated with initiating bystander CPR. Continuous chest compressions provided by lay rescuers result in improved survival compared with no bystander CPR.[51-58] However, the evidence is mixed for the use of this technique by EMS personnel. Some studies have suggested that continuous chest compressions are better than traditional CPR,[59-62] while others find no benefit.[63-65] A multicenter, randomized clinical trial is being conducted to compare the two techniques.[66]

KEY POINTS

Assess patients thought to be in cardiac arrest for a pulse and abnormal breathing. Agonal respirations should not preclude initiating CPR.

Perform high-quality, minimally interrupted chest compressions with a depth of 2 inches or more, at a rate of 100 or more compressions per minute, allowing full chest recoil.

Accelerometer-based, real-time feedback devices improve CPR quality.

There is insufficient evidence to support the routine use of continuous chest compressions, but this technique may be considered in special circumstances. A clinical trial has been launched to compare CPR techniques.

Defibrillation

Defibrillator Type and Energy Selection

Several types of defibrillators are commercially available. Each of them has proprietary energy waveforms (eg, biphasic truncated exponential, pulsed biphasic, rectilinear biphasic, damped sinusoid monophasic, and monophasic truncated exponential). Biphasic defibrillators are more prevalent than monophasic defibrillators because they are more successful at terminating ventricular fibrillation (VF).[67-73] However, a randomized controlled trial showed no difference in survival between defibrillator types.[74] Emergency physicians should be familiar with the defibrillator types used at their institutions and the manufacturer's recommendations for energy selection. The recommended energy for biphasic defibrillation is typically 150 to 200 joules.[75,76] If in doubt regarding the energy recommended for a particular device, use the device-specific maximal energy for patients in cardiac arrest with either pulseless ventricular tachycardia or VF.

Defibrillation Timing

The optimal timing of defibrillation is a contested issue. One proposed benefit of CPR is reperfusion of myocardial tissue, which washes out inflammatory mediators and restores high-energy phosphate substrates. CPR is thought to prime the myocardium to receive a rescue shock. However, in two randomized controlled trials, 1.5 to 3 minutes of CPR before the first defibrillation attempt did not improve survival, even after stratification by EMS response interval.[42,77] In contrast, a third randomized controlled trial found a benefit of CPR before defibrillation when the EMS response interval was more than 4 or 5 minutes.[78]

VF waveform analysis can be used to guide the optimal timing of defibrillation. Various waveform parameters, for example, slope, frequency, amplitude, and longitudinal similarity, have been used to quantify the VF waveform. The VF waveform correlates with coronary perfusion pressure[79] and myocardial ATP concentration.[80] Many retrospective studies confirmed the feasibility of predicting defibrillation success with quantitative waveform analysis[81-103]; however, no prospective studies have been performed to evaluate the impact on patient outcomes.

Stacked shocks (successive defibrillations without resuming CPR) have no demonstrable survival benefit[104] and unnecessarily interrupt chest compressions; therefore, this approach to cardiac resuscitation should not be used.

Perishock Pauses in Chest Compressions

The perishock pause interval is the break in chest compressions before (preshock pause) and after (postshock pause) a defibrillation. Adjusting for typical prognostic variables, patients who receive preshock pauses longer than 20 seconds are half as likely to survive to hospital discharge as those for whom the preshock pause is less than 10 seconds. Interestingly, postshock pauses do not have the same association. Overall, every 5-second increase in the perishock pause interval (up to 50 seconds) is associated with a 14% reduction in survival to hospital discharge.[105]

One technique used to minimize the preshock pause in chest compressions is charging the defibrillator during chest compressions. Care providers tend to instinctively cease chest compressions while the defibrillator is charging. This interruption is unnecessary, provided there is adequate communication between the person performing chest compressions, the person operating the defibrillator, and the team leader. A second technique is "hands-on defibrillation," which Lloyd and associates tested in a feasibility study.[106] In their study design, mock rescuers wearing polyethylene gloves compressed the chests of patients undergoing elective (external) biphasic cardioversion. Compressing with 20 pounds of downward force, rescuers were exposed to low levels of leakage current that was both imperceptible and below the recommended safety standards for leakage current. This feasibility study was performed under specific circumstances, and further evaluation is needed before the technique can be extrapolated to other conditions. (The author and the associate editor of this chapter can personally attest to safely performing chest compressions while wearing polyethylene gloves during external defibrillation with a biphasic defibrillator.)

Palpable pulses are typically absent immediately after defibrillation.[107,108] Furthermore, health care providers have difficulty correctly identifying central pulses as an indication to stop CPR.[14] Increasing the number of interruptions during CPR reduces the rates of ROSC and survival.[109] In a study of witnessed, VF OHCA, immediate resumption of CPR after defibrillation was associated with an improved survival rate.[35,110]

KEY POINTS

Know the defibrillator model used in your institution as well as the manufacturer's recommended energy selection.

For witnessed arrests leaving a shockable rhythm, it is reasonable to defibrillate before starting CPR. For unwitnessed arrests leaving a shockable rhythm, it is reasonable to perform CPR before defibrillating.

Minimize the perishock pause interval by continuing chest compressions while the defibrillator is charging, delivering a single shock, and immediately resuming chest compressions. Do not delay CPR for rhythm analysis or a pulse check.

Hands-on defibrillation appears to be safe under specific conditions.

Airway

Adjuncts

The airway adjuncts used most commonly by health care providers are oropharyngeal and nasopharyngeal tubes. They have a long history of use in a variety of clinical scenarios, but their use during human CPR has not been studied. Two case reports have documented the inadvertent intracranial insertion of a nasopharyngeal airway in patients with basilar skull fractures.[111,112]

Cricoid Pressure

The original intent of applying cricoid pressure was to reduce gastric inflation during ventilation with a bag valve mask. The studies that demonstrated this effect applied much higher tidal volumes than those currently recommended.[113,114] More recent data have shown that cricoid pressure hampers the placement of both supraglottic and endotracheal airways. In addition, it impairs laryngeal mask airway placement and subsequent ventilation.[115-122] And it affects tracheal intubation in several ways, as follows: by increasing time to intubation, by decreasing success rates, and by diminishing the laryngoscopic view.[115-130] Cricoid pressure should not be performed routinely during airway management in cardiac arrest.

Advanced Airways

Prehospital advanced airway management is a controversial topic that is beyond the scope of this chapter. The rate of adverse events during intubation attempts becomes unacceptably high if prehospital care providers do not receive active, continued training and skills maintenance.[131-136] The same can likely be said for all types of health care providers. Whether in the prehospital setting or in the emergency department, prolonged attempts at advanced airway management unnecessarily interrupt chest compressions, especially when acceptable alternatives are available.

Evidence is mixed regarding the optimal timing of advanced airway management during cardiac arrest resuscitation. Analysis of a large inhospital cardiac arrest registry (25,000 patients) found that earlier airway management (within 5 minutes) was associated with improved 24-hour survival.[137] In OHCA, intubations performed within 12 minutes into the resuscitation were associated with improved survival, compared with intubations performed after 13 minutes.[138] A bundled care package of delayed intubation, passive oxygen delivery via nonrebreathing mask during CPR, and minimally interrupted chest compressions improved the rate of neurologically intact survival to hospital discharge among adults who experienced witnessed OHCA and then had a shockable rhythm.[59]

Supraglottic airways represent an acceptable alternative to endotracheal intubation during cardiac arrest resuscitation. Ventilation through a variety of supraglottic devices results in arterial blood gas values similar to those that can be achieved with traditional bag-valve-mask ventilation.[139-140] Additionally, ventilation through a laryngeal mask airway results in less regurgitation (3.5%) than ventilation with a bag valve mask (12.4%).[141] Supraglottic airways perform as well as, or better than, endotracheal intubation in terms of insertion success rates, time to insertion, and ventilation parameters.[142-150] Supraglottic airways are also excellent rescue devices for difficult/failed intubations in cardiac arrest.[143,144,148,151-156] Data are mixed regarding the outcomes of cardiac arrest patients when supraglottic airway devices are used. One retrospective study that compared endotracheal intubation to the use of an esophageal tracheal Combitube found no differences in rates of ROSC or survival.[149] Another found that patients ventilated with a laryngeal mask airway had a higher rate of ROSC than a control group that underwent endotracheal intubation.[151]

Confirmation of the correct placement of an airway device is a crucial step in airway management. The best available standard is continuous waveform capnography, which has 100% sensitivity and 100% specificity in cardiac arrest.[157,158] If this option is not available, then the combination of a colorimetric end-tidal carbon dioxide (CO_2) detector and clinical assessment is an acceptable alternative.

KEY POINTS

It is reasonable to place an oropharyngeal or a nasopharyngeal airway in a patient being ventilated with a bag valve mask. Do not use a nasopharyngeal airway in patients with suspected basilar skull fracture.

Cricoid pressure impairs supraglottic and endotracheal airway insertion and is not recommended.

Evidence is insufficient regarding the optimal timing of advanced airway management. The timing depends on the circumstances of the cardiac arrest, local guidelines, and the rescuer's level of training.

Supraglottic airways are a reasonable alternative to endotracheal intubation during cardiac arrest resuscitation. They are also an excellent back-up rescue airway.

Continuous waveform capnography is the best available standard for confirmation of correct airway placement. The use of a colorimetric detector in conjunction with clinical assessment is an acceptable alternative.

Oxygenation

The current convention is to oxygenate with 100% fraction

of inspired oxygen (FIO_2) during CPR. No studies have compared the use of 100% FIO_2 with titrated FIO_2 during CPR for adults in cardiac arrest. Animal data suggest that 100% FIO_2 results in worse neurologic outcomes compared with 21% FIO_2.

Passive oxygenation during chest compressions is a technique proposed to minimize interruptions. It is predicated on cycles of successive chest wall compression and recoil, which generate passive airflow while applying high-flow oxygen via nonrebreathing mask. If the tidal volumes generated are greater than the dead space, oxygenated air is moved into the lungs. If the tidal volumes generated are insufficient to overcome the dead space, the turbulent mixing of air can still result in molecular diffusion and subsequent gas exchange, similar to high-frequency oscillatory ventilation. In two human studies, passive oxygen delivery through a Boussignac tube at 15 liters/min with ongoing chest compressions generated gas exchange and hemodynamics that were at least equal to if not better than those achieved with standard positive-pressure oxygenation through an endotracheal tube; no difference in clinical outcome was noted.[63,64] However, a simplified cardiac arrest protocol consisting of passive oxygenation via nonrebreathing mask and continuous chest compressions resulted in improved rates of neurologically intact survival to hospital discharge in adults who experienced witnessed cardiac arrest and had a subsequent shockable initial rhythm.[61,62] A multicenter, randomized clinical trial is currently underway to evaluate this technique.[66]

KEY POINTS

There is a knowledge gap about the best FIO_2 to employ during cardiac arrest resuscitation. In the absence of contradictory data, 100% FIO_2 remains the current recommendation.

There is insufficient evidence to support the routine use of passive oxygenation. This technique may be considered in special circumstances. A clinical trial is underway to answer this question.

Ventilation

The only human data on ventilation parameters during CPR are about respiratory rate. No reports have addressed minute ventilation or peak inspiratory pressure. The ventilatory rate is frequently too high during cardiac arrest resuscitation, and the use of real-time CPR feedback devices results in delivered ventilation rates closer to those recommended in the guidelines.[48] Animal data suggest that hyperventilation is associated with diminished hemodynamics and survival,[159] but there is no human evidence that avoiding hyperventilation improves the rate of ROSC or survival.

End-tidal CO_2 monitoring represents one of the few modes of physiologic feedback available during resuscitation. Increases in end-tidal CO_2 typically herald ROSC.[160,161] Additionally, end-tidal CO_2 values higher than 10 mm Hg during CPR are associated with ROSC,[162] while values below 10 mm Hg during CPR are associated with nonsurvival.[163-168] End-tidal CO_2 has not been evaluated specifically as a tool to guide resuscitation interventions in real time.

KEY POINTS

There is a knowledge gap about the best ventilation parameters during cardiac arrest resuscitation. Based on animal data, hyperventilation should be avoided.

End-tidal CO_2 values below 10 mm Hg are associated with low probability of survival, but data are insufficient for the creation of specific prognostic cut-offs at different time intervals.

End-tidal CO_2 monitoring can provide feedback about resuscitation effectiveness.

Pharmacotherapy

Clinical trials of resuscitation drugs have demonstrated, at best, short-term outcome improvements (eg, rate of ROSC). No trial of any medication employed during resuscitation has demonstrated improved rates of survival to hospital discharge. A three-arm randomized trial that compared 1) intravenous access and resuscitation drugs (epinephrine, amiodarone, atropine, and vasopressin), 2) no intravenous access or resuscitation drugs, and 3) placebo in adults who experienced OHCA found no difference in the rate of survival to hospital discharge or neurologic outcome between the three arms.[169] This trial was conducted before the advent of specialized postresuscitation care, so it might be necessary to reevaluate resuscitation drugs in this setting.

No direct human evidence is available to define the optimal timing of drug delivery during cardiac arrest resuscitation. Subgroup analyses of clinical trials suggest a decrease in the survival rate for every minute drug delivery is delayed after collapse,[170,171] but this is probably biased by the simultaneous delay of prehospital care. Animal data suggest that time to drug administration is an independent predictor of ROSC.[172]

Vasopressors

The scientific community has finally achieved clinical equipoise about epinephrine in cardiac arrest.[173] There has never been a placebo-controlled study that attributed an increased rate of survival to hospital discharge to epinephrine. Furthermore, the largest study to date, involving a Japanese cohort of more than 400,000 prospectively matched patients, demonstrated that prehospital administration of epinephrine increased ROSC but decreased survival and 1-month functional outcomes.[174] A rigorous, prospective, randomized, placebo-controlled trial is needed to evaluate the effectiveness of this medication. Vasopressin offers no survival advantage over epinephrine.[175-177] Epinephrine plus vasopressin offers no survival advantage over epinephrine alone.[178,179]

Atropine

At best, atropine offers no survival benefit for patients in cardiac arrest.[180-182] At worst, it is associated with diminished survival.[183-185]

Antiarrhythmics (Amiodarone, Lidocaine, Procainamide)

Amiodarone is superior to lidocaine for treating refractory

shock or recurrent ventricular tachycardia/VF,[170,171] and procainamide is associated with short-term survival in VF.[182] However, no antiarrhythmic has ever demonstrated an improved rate of survival to hospital discharge. A multicenter, randomized clinical trial is currently underway to address this question.[186]

Intravenous Fluids

No human studies have compared resuscitation with intravenous fluids to resuscitation without intravenous fluids during cardiac arrest.[187] Animal data suggest a decrease in coronary perfusion pressure with intravenous fluid administration during CPR.[188-190] Hypertonic intravenous fluids have been investigated preliminarily: one small, randomized controlled trial found no benefit of hypertonic intravenous fluids over isotonic intravenous fluids during cardiac arrest resuscitation.[191] Additionally, two studies found no improvement in ROSC using ice-cold intravenous fluids compared with room temperature intravenous fluids during CPR.[192,193]

Specific Causes (Case-by-Case Basis)

There is no evidence that the routine use of buffers (eg, sodium bicarbonate) improves outcome from cardiac arrest.[194-197] In fact, buffering agents might worsen outcome.[185,198-200]

Three randomized controlled trials of routine calcium administration during cardiac arrest showed no survival benefit.[201-203] Two additional studies associated routine calcium administration with worsened survival rate to hospital discharge.[185,204] Calcium should still be considered for specific causes of cardiac arrest (eg, hypocalcemia, hypermagnesemia, calcium channel blocker overdose, and wide QRS complexes).

Four randomized controlled trials of routine magnesium administration during VF cardiac arrest showed no survival benefit over placebo.[205-208] Magnesium should still be considered for specific causes of cardiac arrest (eg, torsade de pointes).

No short-term or long-term benefit is gained from the routine administration of fibrinolytics during cardiac arrest resuscitation.[209,210] However, the risk of intracranial hemorrhage is increased.[210] Fibrinolytics should still be considered for specific causes of cardiac arrest (eg, myocardial infarction, pulmonary embolism).

KEY POINTS

Resuscitation drugs need to be reevaluated in the context of modern, postresuscitation care.

The routine use of vasopressors might improve the rate of ROSC, but there is no evidence they improve survival rates or neurologic outcome. In fact, they might worsen long-term outcomes.

Antiarrhythmics might have short-term benefit but have never been associated with survival or neurologic outcome. A clinical trial is underway to answer this question.

Sodium bicarbonate does not improve outcomes; in fact, it could be harmful.

Calcium, magnesium, and fibrinolytics should be considered only for specific causes of cardiac arrest.

Devices

Mechanical chest compression devices might have a role in the future of cardiac arrest resuscitation, but evidence remains insufficient to support or refute the routine use of a mechanical device as opposed to traditional human CPR.[211] Many types of devices have been developed, as follows: active compression-decompression devices, load-distributing band devices, piston devices, and Lund University Cardiac Arrest System (LUCAS) devices. A number of case reports and case series have described the deployment of mechanical CPR devices as a bridge to therapy during CT scan, percutaneous coronary intervention, and cannulation for extracorporeal membrane oxygenation (ECMO).

The impedance threshold device was designed to decrease intrathoracic pressure, thereby improving venous return to the heart and subsequent cardiac output during CPR. It operates via a one-way valve that selectively impedes passive air entry during the decompression phase of CPR. Four randomized controlled trials failed to show a benefit in the rate of survival to hospital discharge or neurologic outcome.[212-215]

KEY POINTS

Mechanical CPR might have a role as a bridge to therapy or alternative reperfusion strategies.

The impedance threshold device offers no demonstrable benefit in neurologically favorable survival from cardiac arrest.

Regionalization of Care

Regionalized systems of care that coordinate prehospital care systems with receiving centers have been established for the time-efficient management of trauma, ST-elevation myocardial infarction, and acute stroke. Several case-control studies have highlighted the effectiveness of bundled postresuscitation care, demonstrating improved outcomes compared with historical controls.[8,216-220] Many medical care providers in outlying community hospitals treat post–cardiac arrest patients infrequently, because of the low rates of resuscitation associated with bystander and prehospital care. Regionalized cardiac arrest centers increase referral volumes and thereby care providers' experience.[221] The positive correlation between greater provider experience (or procedural volume) for complex diagnoses (or procedures) and better patient outcome has been well documented.[222]

Evidence continues to accumulate regarding improved outcomes when cardiac arrest patients are treated at regionalized centers (Table 12-1). Wnent and associates,[223] in an urban setting in Germany, described the influence of the prehospital emergency physician's choice of admitting hospital on patient outcome after cardiac arrest. A total of 434 patients were admitted to hospitals in this study: 39% to centers with the ability to perform percutaneous coronary intervention (PCI) and 61% to hospitals without PCI capabilities. Adjusting for confounders, patients who were transported to a PCI center were more than three times as likely to survive with favorable neurologic outcome. Cha and colleagues[224] studied the records of more than 27,000 Korean patients who were transported to a hospital with CPR in progress. Even with longer transport intervals, patients who were transported to high-volume centers were more likely to survive to hospital discharge compared with those taken to low-volume centers.

One of the common barriers to implementation of regionalized cardiac arrest care is patient transport. Bypassing a local hospital to transport a cardiac arrest patient to a more distant resuscitation center is a controversial topic. However, two recent studies demonstrated that prehospital transport time does not independently affect patient outcome after cardiac arrest.[225,226] This conclusion suggests that a modest increase in the transport interval could benefit patients because of the higher level of care available at the specialty center.

Interfacility transfer for postresuscitation care is a related issue. Critically ill, recently resuscitated cardiac arrest patients are inherently at risk for deterioration en route. Hartke and associates[227] evaluated the records of 248 resuscitated patients who had been transported to tertiary care facilities. With a median transport time of 63 minutes (interquartile range: 51-81 minutes), they found that re-arrest was uncommon (6%) and that critical events (hypotension or hypoxia) affected 23% of patients during transport. Most critical events occurred within the first hour of transport, and 27% occurred at the referring facility prior to departure. Patients on vasopressors were most likely to suffer critical events. The authors weighed the risk of transport against the overall survival rate of 53% and the 29% survival rate of patients who experienced a critical event. They proposed that resuscitated patients referred to a regional center from outlying facilities derive benefit from transport to a cardiac arrest center, with an acceptable risk of decompensation en route.

A Universal Termination-of-Resuscitation Rule

In an attempt to establish universally applicable prehospital termination of resuscitation rules, Morrison and coworkers[228] prospectively validated an established set of termination-of-resuscitation rules for basic life support providers (Table 12-2) in a cohort of 2,145 OHCA patients. These rules demonstrated 100% specificity for recommending transport of potential survivors and a positive predictive value of 100% for death. The predicted transport rate was 46%.

A universal set of termination-of-resuscitation rules could minimize practice variation among physicians providing online medical control. It could also improve resource utilization and EMS safety by reducing the number of patients transported to the hospital. However, reducing the number of patients transported may impede the development of new strategies and techniques for patients currently deemed "un-resuscitatable." Universal termination-of-resuscitation rules open the possibility for rare, but occasional, premature termination of resuscitation.

TABLE 12-1.

Proposed Clinical Services for Regionalized Cardiac Arrest Centers

Neurologic services
Induced hypothermia
Continuous electroencephalographic monitoring
Seizure management
Neurology consultation
Neurosurgical consultation
Cerebral imaging (computed tomography, magnetic resonance imaging, perfusion studies)
Neurophysiologic testing (evoked potentials)
Prognostication services
Critical care services
Ventilator management
Glucose control
Goal-directed hemodynamic management
Cardiovascular services
Cardiac catheterization/PCI
Coronary artery bypass grafting
Intraaortic balloon pump
Cardiovascular mechanical support devices
ECMO
Transplant surgery consultation
Electrophysiology consultation
Internal cardioverter-defibrillator placement
Other services
Physical medicine and rehabilitation consultation
Physical and occupational therapy
Social work
Organ donation
Outpatient physical and occupational therapy
Outpatient neurological rehabilitation
Outpatient psychological services

TABLE 12-2.

Validated Rules for Prehospital Termination of Resuscitation

1. No return of spontaneous circulation prior to transport
2. No shock administered
3. Arrest not witnessed by EMS personnel

Novel Future Directions

A modern view of cardiac arrest resuscitation must look to novel resuscitation paradigms. Examples include "crowdsourcing" first responders, mapping the locations of public automatic external defibrillators (AED) with mobile media, and extracorporeal life support (ECLS).

Dispatching Lay Rescuers via SMS Mobile Phone Messages

Crowdsourcing is the process of outsourcing tasks to a distributed group of people. Scholten and associates[229] described a prehospital dispatch system in the Netherlands, which uses SMS alerts (ie, text messages) to crowdsource lay rescuers to suspected cardiac arrest victims while simultaneously dispatching traditional EMS providers. To create this system, 2,168 lay rescuers enlisted and provided their home and work addresses. Based on these addresses, lay rescuers who lived or worked in a victim's vicinity were notified via SMS alert to proceed to the location of a suspected OHCA and begin CPR. Additional lay rescuers close to a public AED were notified via SMS alert to obtain the device and proceed to the patient's location. Over a 3-month period, this system was activated for 52 patients with suspected cardiac arrest. More than 3,000 individual SMS alerts were sent to 2,287 laypersons, and action was taken based on 579 alerts. Aid was provided for 47 patients. Laypersons started early CPR, performed early defibrillation, assisted EMS personnel, or took care of family members. Laypersons arrived before EMS personnel in 21 cases (45%), started CPR and/or performed defibrillation for 18 patients (38%), and assisted EMS personnel in 9 cases (19%).

Geographic Mapping of AEDs

The untrained public can use AEDs effectively. The location of many of the 1 million AEDs sold in the United States over the past 20 years is unknown; there is no central registry of AED locations. AED registration is the responsibility of the device owner, and the requirements for registration differ by region. Bystanders might pass public AEDs during their daily activities but then not remember the AED location when it is needed, or they might be completely unaware that an AED is nearby. Merchant and associates[230] described an endeavor to create a central registry of public AEDs in Philadelphia. Through a public contest, participants took pictures of AEDs with their mobile phones and submitted them to a central repository. A total of 1,429 public AEDs were catalogued over 8 weeks by 313 teams and individuals. This central repository could be distributed in the form of a mobile phone application or other social media platform with a built-in mapping function.

FIGURE 12-2.

Summary of data supporting/refuting interventions during cardiac arrest resuscitation

Unknown
- Monitoring ventilation parameters
- Optimal F_{IO_2} during CPR
- Hands-on defibrillation

Detrimental Interventions
- Cricoid pressure
- "Stacked" defibrillations
- Perishock pauses in CPR
- Prolonged advanced airway management that interrupts CPR

Beneficial Interventions
- Minimally interrupted, high-quality chest compressions
- Airway confirmation with continuous waveform capnometry
- Maximizing chest compression fraction
- Compression-only CPR for lay rescuers

Unclear (likely detrimental)
- Epinephrine
- Vasopressin
- Atropine
- Routine calcium
- Routine sodium bicarbonate
- Routine fibrinolytics

Unclear (likely beneficial)
- Oro- and naso-pharyngeal airways
- Filtered ECG signals
- Biphasic defibrillators
- Continuous chest compressions with passive oxygenation
- Supraglottic airways
- Real-time CPR feedback devices
- Timing defibrillation with ventricular fibrillation waveform measures

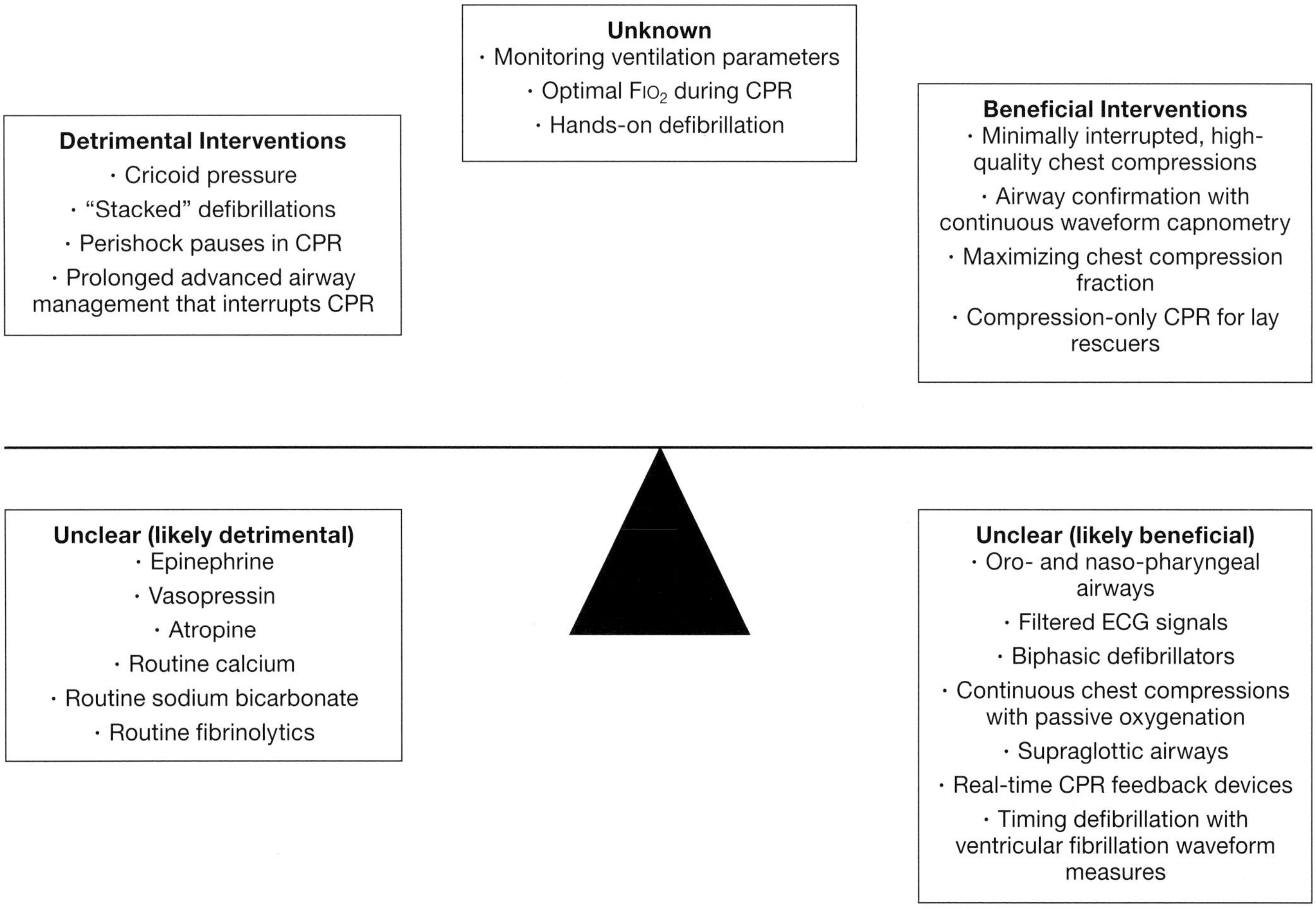

Extracorporeal Life Support

ECLS, the incorporation of ECMO into cardiac arrest resuscitation, is a resource-intensive therapy that has been deployed successfully overseas to boost the rate of neurologically favorable survival in select candidates who experienced OHCA. Japan has one of the most sophisticated ECLS systems.[231] Eligible patients have to satisfy the following criteria: age 18 to 74 years, bystander-witnessed cardiac arrest, presumed cardiac cause of arrest, less than 15-minute estimated interval from collapse until EMS arrival, shockable rhythm, and persistent cardiac arrest on arrival to the hospital. Eligible patients are cannulated percutaneously for ECMO in the emergency department, with CPR in progress. Once ECMO is initiated, patients are cooled rapidly with the ECMO circuit while receiving urgent coronary angiography, PCI if indicated, and intra-aortic balloon pumping. There is a clear, step-wise relationship between outcome and quartiles of the collapse-to-ECMO and ECMO-to-34°C intervals. The optimal cut-off in the Japanese ECLS system is 55.5 minutes for the collapse-to-ECMO interval and 21.5 minutes for the ECMO-to-34°C interval. Survival with favorable neurologic outcome is more than 50% when the ECMO-to-34°C interval is less than 21.5 minutes, regardless of the collapse-to-ECMO interval. A cumulative review of the Japanese ECLS literature indicated that 1,282 patients who experienced OHCA between 1983 and 2008 received ECLS.[232] Among the 516 cases with available outcome data, 27% survived to hospital discharge. Approximately half of the survivors had mild or no neurologic disability. A randomized comparison of ECLS and traditional resuscitation is being performed in Prague, Czech Republic.[233]

ECLS for OHCA has been slow to catch on the United States, but programs are commencing in some cities. In the emergency-physician-led ECLS program in San Diego, California, for example, patients must satisfy the following criteria to be eligible for the intervention: any CPR initiated within 10 minutes after arrest, initial rhythm other than asystole, less than 10-minute EMS transport time, less than 60 minutes total time in cardiac arrest, and lack of preexisting severe neurologic disease.[234] A tiered, three-stage pathway is used for ECLS implementation, with opportunity to exit the pathway at each stage. Over a 1-year period, 18 patients met inclusion criteria, and ECLS was initiated successfully in 8 of them. Five (63%) survived to hospital discharge with a good neurologic outcome.

Conclusion

Prehospital and emergency department resuscitation to achieve ROSC are only two links in a long chain of survival. Local and regional systems of care must optimize both the preceding and succeeding links to improve outcomes from cardiac arrest (Figure 12-2).

Minimally interrupted, high-quality chest compressions are the cornerstone of cardiac arrest resuscitation. However, CPR is not a destination therapy; it is a temporizing bridge to allow the identification and correction of underlying pathology.

Continuing chest compressions while the defibrillator is charging minimizes unnecessary interruptions. Continuation of chest compressions during defibrillation is feasible under specific circumstances.

The role of advanced airways remains controversial in cardiac arrest resuscitation. Supraglottic airways are an acceptable alternative to traditional endotracheal intubation.

No resuscitation drug has ever demonstrated improved survival to hospital discharge or neurologic outcome.

There is clinical equipoise for epinephrine in cardiac arrest. A rigorous, prospective, randomized, placebo-controlled trial is needed.

Modern management of cardiac arrest should occur in a regionalized cardiac arrest center.

We could be reaching the limit of refining traditional CPR. New resuscitation paradigms are needed to achieve more than modest improvements in patient outcome.

References

1. Sayre MR, Koster RW, Botha M, et al. Part 5: Adult basic life support: 2010 International Consensus on Cardiopulmonary Resuscitation and Emergency Cardiovascular Care Science With Treatment Recommendations. *Circulation.* 2010;122(16 suppl 2):S298-S324.
2. Writing Group Members, Roger VL, Go AS, Lloyd-Jones DM, et al. Heart disease and stroke statistics – 2012 update: a report from the American Heart Association. *Circulation.* 2012;125:e2-e220.
3. Herlitz J, Svensson L, Engdahl J, et al. Characteristics of cardiac arrest and resuscitation by age group: An analysis from the Swedish cardiac arrest registry. *Am J Emerg Med.* 2007;25:1025-1031.
4. Ong ME, Stiell I, Osmond MH, et al. Etiology of pediatric out-of-hospital cardiac arrest by coroner's diagnosis. *Resuscitation.* 2006;68:335-342.
5. Kuisma M, Alaspaa A. Out-of-hospital cardiac arrests of non-cardiac origin: Epidemiology and outcome. *Eur Heart J.* 1997;18:1122-1128.
6. Kurkciyan I, Meron G, Behringer W, et al. Accuracy and impact of presumed cause in patients with cardiac arrest. *Circulation.* 1998;98:766-771.
7. Nichol G, Thomas E, Callaway CW, et al. Regional variation in out-of-hospital cardiac arrest incidence and outcome. *JAMA.* 2008;300:1423-1431.
8. Sunde K, Pytte M, Jacobsen D, et al. Implementation of a standardised treatment protocol for post resuscitation care after out-of-hospital cardiac arrest. *Resuscitation.* 2007;73:29-39.
9. Bahr J, Klingler H, Panzer W, et al. Skills of lay people in checking the carotid pulse. *Resuscitation.* 1997;35:23-26.
10. Brennan RT, Braslow A. Skill mastery in public CPR classes. *Am J Emerg Med.* 1998;16:653-657.
11. Chamberlain D, Smith A, Woollard M, et al. Trials of teaching methods in basic life support (3): Comparison of simulated CPR performance after first training and at 6 months, with a note on the value of re-training. *Resuscitation.* 2002;53:179-187.
12. Eberle B, Dick WF, Schneider T, et al. Checking the carotid pulse check: Diagnostic accuracy of first responders in patients with and without a pulse. *Resuscitation.* 1996;33:107-116.
13. Lapostolle F, Le Toumelin P, Agostinucci JM, et al. Basic cardiac life support providers checking the carotid pulse: performance, degree of conviction, and influencing factors. *Acad Emerg Med.* 2004;11:878-880.
14. Liberman M, Lavoie A, Mulder D, Sampalis J. Cardiopulmonary resuscitation: errors made by pre-hospital emergency medical personnel. *Resuscitation.* 1999;42:47-55.
15. Moule P. Checking the carotid pulse: diagnostic accuracy in students of the healthcare professions. *Resuscitation.* 2000;44:195-201.
16. Nyman J, Sihvonen M. Cardiopulmonary resuscitation skills in nurses and nursing students. *Resuscitation.* 2000;47:179-184.
17. Tibballs J, Russell P. Reliability of pulse palpation by healthcare per- sonnel to diagnose paediatric cardiac arrest. *Resuscitation.* 2009;80:61-64.
18. Albarran JW, Moule P, Gilchrist M, Soar J. Comparison of sequential and simultaneous breathing and pulse check by healthcare professionals during simulated scenarios. *Resuscitation.* 2006;68:243-249.
19. Bang A, Herlitz J, Martinell S. Interaction between emergency medical dispatcher and caller in suspected out-of-hospital cardiac arrest calls with focus on agonal breathing: a review of 100 tape recordings of true cardiac arrest cases. *Resuscitation.* 2003;56:25-34.
20. Bohm K, Rosenqvist M, Hollenberg J, et al. Dispatcher-assisted telephone-guided cardiopulmonary resuscitation: An underused lifesaving system. *Eur J Emerg Med.* 2007;14:256-259.

21. Bobrow BJ, Zuercher M, Ewy GA, et al. Gasping during cardiac arrest in humans is frequent and associated with improved survival. *Circulation*. 2008;118:2550-2554.

22. Vaillancourt C, Verma A, Trickett J, et al. Evaluating the effectiveness of dispatch-assisted cardiopulmonary resuscitation instructions. *Acad Emerg Med*. 2007;14:877-883.

23. Kramer-Johansen J, Myklebust H, Wik L, et al. Quality of out-of-hospital cardiopulmonary resuscitation with real time automated feedback: a prospective interventional study. *Resuscitation*. 2006;71:283-292.

24. Edelson DP, Litzinger B, Arora V, et al. Improving in-hospital cardiac arrest process and outcomes with performance debriefing. *Arch Intern Med*. 2008;168:1063-1069.

25. Yannopoulos D, McKnite S, Aufderheide TP, et al. Effects of incomplete chest wall decompression during cardiopulmonary resuscitation on coronary and cerebral perfusion pressures in a porcine model of cardiac arrest. *Resuscitation*. 2005;64:363-372.

26. Zuercher M, Hilwig RW, Ranger-Moore J, et al. Leaning during chest compressions impairs cardiac output and left ventricular myocardial blood flow in piglet cardiac arrest. *Crit Care Med*. 2010;38:1141-1146.

27. Abella BS, Sandbo N, Vassilatos P, et al. Chest compression rates during cardiopulmonary resuscitation are suboptimal: a prospective study during in-hospital cardiac arrest. *Circulation*. 2005;111:428-434.

28. Christenson J, Andrusiek D, Everson-Stewart S, et al. Chest compression fraction determines survival in patients with out-of-hospital ventricular fibrillation. *Circulation*. 2009;120:1241-1247.

29. Eilevstjonn J, Eftestol T, Aase SO, et al. Feasibility of shock advice analysis during CPR through removal of CPR artefacts from the human ECG. *Resuscitation*. 2004;61:131-141.

30. Aramendi E, de Gauna SR, Irusta U, et al. Detection of ventricular fibrillation in the presence of cardiopulmonary resuscitation artefacts. *Resuscitation*. 2007;72:115-123.

31. Li Y, Bisera J, Tang W, Weil MH. Automated detection of ventricular fibrillation to guide cardiopulmonary resuscitation. *Crit Pathw Cardiol*. 2007;6:131-134.

32. Li Y, Bisera J, Geheb F, et al. Identifying potentially shockable rhythms without interrupting cardiopulmonary resuscitation. *Crit Care Med*. 2008;36:198-203.

33. Ruiz de Gauna S, Ruiz J, Irusta U, et al. A method to remove CPR artefacts from human ECG using only the recorded ECG. *Resuscitation*. 2008;76:271-278.

34. Irusta U, Ruiz J, de Gauna SR, et al. A least mean-square filter for the estimation of the cardiopulmonary resuscitation artifact based on the frequency of the compressions. *IEEE Trans Biomed Eng*. 2009;56:1052-1062.

35. Steinmetz J, Barnung S, Nielsen SL, et al. Improved survival after an out-of-hospital cardiac arrest using new guidelines. *Acta Anaesthesiol Scand*. 2008;52:908-913.

36. Sayre MR, Cantrell SA, White LJ, et al. Impact of the 2005 American Heart Association cardiopulmonary resuscitation and emergency cardiovascular care guidelines on out-of-hospital cardiac arrest survival. *Prehosp Emerg Care*. 2009;13:469-477.

37. Hostler D, Rittenberger JC, Roth R, et al. Increased chest compression to ventilation ratio improves delivery of CPR. *Resuscitation*. 2007;74:446-452.

38. Baker PW, Conway J, Cotton C, et al. Defibrillation or cardiopulmonary resuscitation first for patients with out-of-hospital cardiac arrests found by paramedics to be in ventricular fibrillation? A randomised control trial. *Resuscitation*. 2008;79:424-431.

39. Abella BS, Alvarado JP, Myklebust H, et al. Quality of cardiopulmonary resuscitation during in-hospital cardiac arrest. *JAMA*. 2005;293:305-310.

40. Wik L, Kramer-Johansen J, Myklebust H, et al. Quality of cardiopulmonary resuscitation during out-of-hospital cardiac arrest. *JAMA*. 2005;293:299-304.

41. Aufderheide TP, Pirrallo RG, Yannopoulos D, et al. Incomplete chest wall decompression: a clinical evaluation of CPR performance by EMS personnel and assessment of alternative manual chest compression-decompression techniques. *Resuscitation*. 2005;64:353-362.

42. Van Hoeyweghen RJ, Bossaert LL, Mullie A, et al. Quality and efficiency of bystander CPR. Belgian Cerebral Resuscitation Study Group. *Resuscitation*. 1993;26:47-52.

43. Valenzuela TD, Kern KB, Clark LL, et al. Interruptions of chest compressions during emergency medical systems resuscitation. *Circulation*. 2005;112:1259-1265.

44. Niles D, Nysaether J, Sutton R, et al. Leaning is common during in-hospital pediatric CPR, and decreased with automated corrective feedback. *Resuscitation*. 2009;80:553-557.

45. Chiang WC, Chen WJ, Chen SY, et al. Better adherence to the guidelines during cardiopulmonary resuscitation through the provision of audio-prompts. *Resuscitation*. 2005;64:297-301.

46. Kern KB, Sanders AB, Raife J, et al. A study of chest compression rates during cardiopulmonary resuscitation in humans: the importance of rate-directed chest compressions. *Arch Intern Med*. 1992;152:145-149.

47. Berg RA, Sanders AB, Milander M, et al. Efficacy of audio-prompted rate guidance in improving resuscitator performance of cardiopulmonary resuscitation on children. *Acad Emerg Med*. 1994;1:35-40.

48. Abella BS, Edelson DP, Kim S, et al. CPR quality improvement during in-hospital cardiac arrest using a real-time audiovisual feedback system. *Resuscitation*. 2007;73:54-61.

49. Fletcher D, Galloway R, Chamberlain D, et al. Basics in advanced life support: a role for download audit and metronomes. *Resuscitation*. 2008;78:127-134.

50. Gruben KG, Romlein J, Halperin HR, Tsitlik JE. System for mechanical measurements during cardiopulmonary resuscitation in humans. *IEEE Trans Biomed Eng*. 1990;37:204-210.

51. Hallstrom A, Cobb L, Johnson E, Copass M. Cardiopulmonary resuscitation by chest compression alone or with mouth-to-mouth ventilation. *N Engl J Med*. 2000;342:1546-1553.

52. Iwami T, Kawamura T, Hiraide A, et al. Effectiveness of bystander-initiated cardiac-only resuscitation for patients with out-of-hospital cardiac arrest. *Circulation*. 2007;116:2900-2907.

53. Ong ME, Ng FS, Anushia P, et al. Comparison of chest compression only and standard cardiopulmonary resuscitation for out-of-hospital cardiac arrest in Singapore. *Resuscitation*. 2008;78:119-126.

54. Wik L, Steen PA, Bircher NG. Quality of bystander cardiopulmonary resuscitation influences outcome after prehospital cardiac arrest. *Resuscitation*. 1994;28:195-203.

55. Bohm K, Rosenqvist M, Herlitz J, et al. Survival is similar after standard treatment and chest compression only in out-of-hospital bystander cardiopulmonary resuscitation. *Circulation*. 2007;116:2908-2912.

56. SOS-KANTO Study Group. Cardiopulmonary resuscitation by bystanders with chest compression only (SOS-KANTO): an observational study. *Lancet*. 2007;369:920-926.

57. Waalewijn RA, Tijssen JG, Koster RW. Bystander initiated actions in out-of-hospital cardiopulmonary resuscitation: results from the Amsterdam Resuscitation Study (ARRESUST). *Resuscitation*. 2001;50:273-279.

58. Olasveengen TM, Wik L, Steen PA. Standard basic life support vs. continuous chest compressions only in out-of-hospital cardiac arrest. *Acta Anaesthesiol Scand*. 2008;52:914-919.

59. Bobrow BJ, Ewy GA, Clark L, et al. Passive oxygen insufflation is superior to bag-valve-mask ventilation for witnessed ventricular fibrillation out-of-hospital cardiac arrest. *Ann Emerg Med*. 2009;54:656-662.

60. Bobrow BJ, Clark LL, Ewy GA, et al. Minimally interrupted cardiac resuscitation by emergency medical services for out-of-hospital cardiac arrest. *JAMA*. 2008;299:1158-1165.

61. Kellum MJ, Kennedy KW, Barney R, et al. Cardiocerebral resuscitation improves neurologically intact survival of patients with out-of-hospital cardiac arrest. *Ann Emerg Med*. 2008;52:244-252.

62. Kellum MJ, Kennedy KW, Ewy GA. Cardiocerebral resuscitation improves survival of patients with out-of-hospital cardiac arrest. *Am J Med*. 2006;119:335-340.

63. Bertrand C, Hemery F, Carli P, et al. Constant flow insufflation of oxygen as the sole mode of ventilation during out-of-hospital cardiac arrest. *Intensive Care Med*. 2006;32:843-851.

64. Saissy JM, Boussignac G, Cheptel E, et al. Efficacy of continuous insufflation of oxygen combined with active cardiac compression-decompression during out-of-hospital cardiorespiratory arrest. *Anesthesiology*. 2000;92:1523-1530.

65. Krischer JP, Fine EG, Weisfeldt ML, et al. Comparison of prehospital conventional and simultaneous compression-ventilation cardiopulmonary resuscitation. *Crit Care Med*. 1989;17:1263-1269.

66. ClinicalTrials.gov. A service of the US National Institutes of Health. Registry and results database of publicly and privately supported clinical studies of human participants conducted around the world. Available at: http://www.clinicaltrials.gov. Accessed March 10, 2014.

67. Morrison LJ, Dorian P, Long J, et al. Out-of-hospital cardiac arrest rectilinear biphasic to monophasic damped sine defibrillation waveforms with advanced life support intervention trial (ORBIT). *Resuscitation*. 2005;66:149-157.

68. Schneider T, Martens PR, Paschen H, et al. Multicenter, randomized, controlled trial of 150-J biphasic shocks compared with 200- to 360-J monophasic shocks in the resuscitation of out-of-hospital cardiac arrest victims. *Circulation*. 2000;102:1780-1787.

69. van Alem AP, Chapman FW, Lank P, et al. A prospective, randomised and blinded comparison of first shock success of monophasic and biphasic waveforms in out-of-hospital cardiac arrest. *Resuscitation*. 2003;58:17-24.

70. Carpenter J, Rea TD, Murray JA, et al. Defibrillation waveform and post-shock rhythm in out-of-hospital ventricular fibrillation cardiac arrest. *Resuscitation*. 2003;59:189-196.

71. Freeman K, Hendey GW, Shalit M, Stroh G. Biphasic defibrillation does not improve outcomes compared to monophasic defibrillation in out-of-hospital cardiac arrest. *Prehosp Emerg Care*. 2008;12:152-156.

72. Gliner BE, White RD. Electrocardiographic evaluation of defibrillation shocks delivered to out-of-hospital sudden cardiac arrest patients. *Resuscitation*. 1999;41:133-144.

73. Hess EP, Atkinson EJ, White RD. Increased prevalence of sustained return of spontaneous circulation following transition to biphasic waveform defibrillation. *Resuscitation*. 2008;77:39-45.

74. Kudenchuk PJ, Cobb LA, Copass MK, et al. Transthoracic incremental monophasic versus biphasic defibrillation by emergency responders (TIMBER): a randomized comparison of monophasic with biphasic waveform ascending energy defibrillation for the resuscitation of out-of-hospital cardiac arrest due to ventricular fibrillation. *Circulation.* 2006;114:2010-2018.
75. Stiell IG, Walker RG, Nesbitt LP, et al. BIPHASIC Trial: a randomized comparison of fixed lower versus escalating higher energy levels for defibrillation in out-of-hospital cardiac arrest. *Circulation.* 2007;115:1511-1517.
76. Walsh SJ, McClelland AJ, Owens CG, et al. Efficacy of distinct energy delivery protocols comparing two biphasic defibrillators for cardiac arrest. *Am J Cardiol.* 2004;94:378-380.
77. Jacobs IG, Finn JC, Oxer HF, Jelinek GA. CPR before defibrillation in out-of-hospital cardiac arrest: a randomized trial. *Emerg Med Australas.* 2005;17:39-45.
78. Wik L, Hansen TB, Fylling F, et al. Delaying defibrillation to give basic cardiopulmonary resuscitation to patients with out-of-hospital ventricular fibrillation: a randomized trial. *JAMA.* 2003;289:1389-1395.
79. Reynolds JC, Salcido DD, Menegazzi JJ. Correlation between coronary perfusion pressure and quantitative ECG waveform measures during resuscitation of prolonged ventricular fibrillation. *Resuscitation.* 2012;83:1497-1502.
80. Salcido DD, Menegazzi JJ, Suffoletto BP, et al. Association of intramyocardial high energy phosphate concentrations with quantitative measures of the ventricular fibrillation electrocardiogram waveform. *Resuscitation.* 2009;80:946-950.
81. Weaver WD, Cobb LA, Dennis D, et al. Amplitude of ventricular fibrillation waveform and outcome after cardiac arrest. *Ann Intern Med.* 1985;102:53-55.
82. Yang Z, Lu W, Harrison RG, et al. A probabilistic neural network as the predictive classifier of out-of-hospital defibrillation outcomes. *Resuscitation.* 2005;64:31-36.
83. Box MS, Watson JN, Addison PS, et al. Shock outcome prediction before and after CPR: a comparative study of manual and automated active compression-decompression CPR. *Resuscitation.* 2008;78:265-274.
84. Brown CG, Dzwonczyk R, Martin DR. Physiologic measurement of the ventricular fibrillation ECG signal: estimating the duration of ventricular fibrillation. *Ann Emerg Med.* 1993;22:70-74.
85. Callaway CW, Sherman LD, Mosesso VN Jr, et al. Scaling exponent predicts defibrillation success for out-of-hospital ventricular fibrillation cardiac arrest. *Circulation.* 2001;103:1656-1661.
86. Eftestol T, Sunde K, Aase SO, et al. Predicting outcome of defibrillation by spectral characterization and nonparametric classification of ventricular fibrillation in patients with out-of-hospital cardiac arrest. *Circulation.* 2000;102:1523-1529.
87. Eftestol T, Wik L, Sunde K, et al. Effects of cardiopulmonary resuscitation on predictors of ventricular fibrillation defibrillation success during out-of-hospital cardiac arrest. *Circulation.* 2004;110:10-15.
88. Eftestol T, Losert H, Kramer-Johansen J, et al. Independent evaluation of a defibrillation outcome predictor for out-of-hospital cardiac arrested patients. *Resuscitation.* 2005;67:55-61.
89. Gundersen K, Kvaloy JT, Kramer-Johansen J, et al. Identifying approaches to improve the accuracy of shock outcome prediction for out-of-hospital cardiac arrest. *Resuscitation.* 2008;76:279-284.
90. Gundersen K, Kvaloy JT, Kramer-Johansen J, et al. Using within-patient correlation to improve the accuracy of shock outcome prediction for cardiac arrest. *Resuscitation.* 2008;78:46-51.
91. Gundersen K, Kvaloy JT, Kramer-Johansen J, et al. Development of the probability of return of spontaneous circulation in intervals without chest compressions during out-of-hospital cardiac arrest: an observational study. *BMC Med.* 2009;7:6.
92. Gundersen K, Nysaether J, Kvaloy JT, et al. Chest compression quality variables influencing the temporal development of ROSC-predictors calculated from the ECG during VF. *Resuscitation.* 2009;80:177-182.
93. Jekova I, Mougeolle F, Valance A. Defibrillation shock success estimation by a set of six parameters derived from the electrocardiogram. *Physiol Meas.* 2004;25:1179-1188.
94. Li Y, Ristagno G, Bisera J, et al. Electrocardiogram waveforms for monitoring effectiveness of chest compression during cardiopulmonary resuscitation. *Crit Care Med.* 2008;36:211-215.
95. Neurauter A, Eftestol T, Kramer-Johansen J, et al. Prediction of countershock success using single features from multiple ventricular fibrillation frequency bands and feature combinations using neural networks. *Resuscitation.* 2007;73:253-263.
96. Olasveengen TM, Eftestol T, Gundersen K, et al. Acute ischemic heart disease alters ventricular fibrillation waveform characteristics in out-of hospital cardiac arrest. *Resuscitation.* 2009;80:412-417.
97. Ristagno G, Gullo A, Berlot G, et al. Prediction of successful defibrillation in human victims of out-of-hospital cardiac arrest: a retrospective electrocardiographic analysis. *Anaesth Intensive Care.* 2008;36:46-50.
98. Russell ME, Friedman MI, Mascioli SR, et al. Off-label use: an industry perspective on expanding use beyond approved indications. *J Interv Cardiol.* 2006;19:432-438.
99. Snyder DE, White RD, Jorgenson DB. Outcome prediction for guidance of initial resuscitation protocol: shock first or CPR first. *Resuscitation.* 2007;72:45-51.
100. Watson JN, Uchaipichat N, Addison PS, et al. Improved prediction of defibrillation success for out-of-hospital VF cardiac arrest using wavelet transform methods. *Resuscitation.* 2004;63:269-275.
101. Watson JN, Addison PS, Clegg GR, et al. Practical issues in the evaluation of methods for the prediction of shock outcome success in out-of-hospital cardiac arrest patients. *Resuscitation.* 2006;68:51-59.
102. Jagric T, Marhl M, Stajer D, et al. Irregularity test for very short electrocardiogram (ECG) signals as a method for predicting a successful defibrillation in patients with ventricular fibrillation. *Transl Res.* 2007;149:145-151.
103. Strohmenger HU, Lindner KH, Brown CG. Analysis of the ventricular fibrillation ECG signal amplitude and frequency parameters as predictors of countershock success in humans. *Chest.* 1997;111:584-589.
104. Jost D, Degrange H, Verret C, et al. DEFI 2005: a randomized controlled trial of the effect of automated external defibrillator cardiopulmonary resuscitation protocol on outcome from out-of-hospital cardiac arrest. *Circulation.* 2010;121:1614-1622.
105. Cheskes S, Schmicker RH, Christenson J, et al. Perishock pause: an independent predictor of survival from out-of-hospital shockable cardiac arrest. *Circulation.* 2011;124:58-66.
106. Lloyd MS, Heeke B, Walter PF, et al. Hands-on defibrillation: an analysis of electrical current flow through rescuers in direct contact with patients during biphasic external defibrillation. *Circulation.* 2008;117:2510-2514.
107. van Alem AP, Sanou BT, Koster RW. Interruption of cardiopulmonary resuscitation with the use of the automated external defibrillator in out-of-hospital cardiac arrest. *Ann Emerg Med.* 2003;42:449-457.
108. Rea TD, Shah S, Kudenchuk PJ, et al. Automated external defibrillators: To what extent does the algorithm delay CPR? *Ann Emerg Med.* 2005;46:132-141.
109. Eftestol T, Sunde K, Steen PA. Effects of interrupting precordial compressions on the calculated probability of defibrillation success during out-of-hospital cardiac arrest. *Circulation.* 2002;105:2270-2273.
110. Rea TD, Helbock M, Perry S, et al. Increasing use of cardiopulmonary resuscitation during out-of-hospital ventricular fibrillation arrest: survival implications of guideline changes. *Circulation.* 2006;114:2760-2765.
111. Schade K, Borzotta A, Michaels A. Intracranial malposition of nasopharyngeal airway. *J Trauma.* 2000;49:967-968.
112. Muzzi DA, Losasso TJ, Cucchiara RF. Complication from a nasopharyngeal airway in a patient with a basilar skull fracture. *Anesthesiology.* 1991;74:366-368.
113. Petito SP, Russell WJ. The prevention of gastric inflation: a neglected benefit of cricoid pressure. *Anaesth Intensive Care.* 1988;16:139-43.
114. Lawes EG, Campbell I, Mercer D. Inflation pressure, gastric insufflation and rapid sequence induction. *Br J Anaesth.* 1987;59:315-318.
115. Asai T, Barclay K, Power I, Vaughan RS. Cricoid pressure impedes placement of the laryngeal mask airway and subsequent tracheal intubation through the mask. *Br J Anaesth.* 1994;72:47-51.
116. Asai T, Barclay K, Power I, Vaughan RS. Cricoid pressure impedes placement of the laryngeal mask airway. *Br J Anaesth.* 1995;74:521-525.
117. Ansermino JM, Blogg CE. Cricoid pressure may prevent insertion of the laryngeal mask airway. *Br J Anaesth.* 1992;69:465-467.
118. Aoyama K, Takenaka I, Sata T, Shigematsu A. Cricoid pressure impedes positioning and ventilation through the laryngeal mask airway. *Can J Anaesth.* 1996;43:1035-1040.
119. Brimacombe J, White A, Berry A. Effect of cricoid pressure on ease of insertion of the laryngeal mask airway. *Br J Anaesth.* 1993;71:800-802.
120. Gabbott DA, Sasada MP. Laryngeal mask airway insertion using cricoid pressure and manual in-line neck stabilisation. *Anaesthesia.* 1995;50:674-676.
121. Xue FS, Mao P, Li CW, et al. Influence of pressure on cricoid on insertion Pro-Seal laryngeal mask airway and ventilation function [in Chinese]. *Zhongguo Wei Zhong Bing Ji Jiu Yi Xue.* 2007;19:532-535.
122. Li CW, Xue FS, Xu YC, et al. Cricoid pressure impedes insertion of, and ventilation through, the ProSeal laryngeal mask airway in anesthetized, paralyzed patients. *Anesth Analg.* 2007;104:1195-1198.
123. McNelis U, Syndercombe A, Harper I, et al. The effect of cricoid pressure on intubation facilitated by the gum elastic bougie. *Anaesthesia.* 2007;62:456-459.
124. Harry RM, Nolan JP. The use of cricoid pressure with the intubating laryngeal mask. *Anaesthesia.* 1999;54:656-659.
125. Noguchi T, Koga K, Shiga Y, Shigematsu A. The gum elastic bougie eases tracheal intubation while applying cricoid pressure compared to a stylet. *Can J Anaesth.* 2003;50:712-717.
126. Asai T, Murao K, Shingu K. Cricoid pressure applied after placement of laryngeal mask impedes subsequent fibreoptic tracheal intubation through mask. *Br J Anaesth.* 2000;85:256-261.
127. Snider DD, Clarke D, Finucane BT. The "BURP" maneuver worsens the glottic view when applied in combination with cricoid pressure. *Can J Anaesth.* 2005;52:100-104.

128. Smith CE, Boyer D. Cricoid pressure decreases ease of tracheal intubation using fibreoptic laryngoscopy (WuScope System). *Can J Anaesth.* 2002;49:614-619.
129. Heath ML, Allagain J. Intubation through the laryngeal mask: a technique for unexpected difficult intubation. *Anaesthesia.* 1991;46:545-548.
130. Levitan RM, Kinkle WC, Levin WJ, et al. Laryngeal view during laryngoscopy: a randomized trial comparing cricoid pressure, backward-upward-rightward pressure, and bimanual laryngoscopy. *Ann Emerg Med.* 2006;47:548-555.
131. Bradley JS, Billows GL, Olinger ML, et al. Prehospital oral endotracheal intubation by rural basic emergency medical technicians. *Ann Emerg Med.* 1998;32:26-32.
132. Sayre MR, Sakles JC, Mistler AF, et al. Field trial of endotracheal intubation by basic EMTs. *Ann Emerg Med.* 1998;31:228-233.
133. Katz SH, Falk JL. Misplaced endotracheal tubes by paramedics in an urban emergency medical services system. *Ann Emerg Med.* 2001;37:32-37.
134. Jones JH, Murphy MP, Dickson RL, et al. Emergency physician-verified out-of-hospital intubation: miss rates by paramedics. *Acad Emerg Med.* 2004;11:707-709.
135. Wirtz DD, Ortiz C, Newman DH, Zhitomirsky I. Unrecognized misplacement of endotracheal tubes by ground prehospital providers. *Prehosp Emerg Care.* 2007;11:213-218.
136. Timmermann A, Russo SG, Eich C, et al. The out-of-hospital esophageal and endobronchial intubations performed by emergency physicians. *Anesth Analg.* 2007;104:619-623.
137. Wong ML, Carey S, Mader TJ, et al. Time to invasive airway placement and resuscitation outcomes after inhospital cardiopulmonary arrest. *Resuscitation.* 2010;81:182-186.
138. Shy BD, Rea TD, Becker LJ, et al. Time to intubation and survival in prehospital cardiac arrest. *Prehosp Emerg Care.* 2004;8:394-399.
139. Rumball CJ, MacDonald D. The PTL, Combitube, laryngeal mask, and oral airway: a randomized prehospital comparative study of ventilatory device effectiveness and cost-effectiveness in 470 cases of cardiorespiratory arrest. *Prehosp Emerg Care.* 1997;1:1-10.
140. SOS-KANTO Study Group. Comparison of arterial blood gases of laryngeal mask airway and bag-valve-mask ventilation in out-of-hospital cardiac arrests. *Circ J.* 2009;73:490-496.
141. Stone BJ, Chantler PJ, Baskett PJ. The incidence of regurgitation during cardiopulmonary resuscitation: a comparison between the bag valve mask and laryngeal mask airway. *Resuscitation.* 1998;38:3-6.
142. Frass M, Frenzer R, Rauscha F, et al. Ventilation with the esophageal tracheal Combitube in cardiopulmonary resuscitation: promptness and effectiveness. *Chest.* 1988;93:781-784.
143. Atherton GL, Johnson JC. Ability of paramedics to use the Combitube in prehospital cardiac arrest. *Ann Emerg Med.* 1993;22:1263-1268.
144. Rabitsch W, Schellongowski P, Staudinger T, et al. Comparison of a conventional tracheal airway with the Combitube in an urban emergency medical services system run by physicians. *Resuscitation.* 2003;57:27-32.
145. Rumball C, Macdonald D, Barber P, et al. Endotracheal intubation and esophageal tracheal Combitube insertion by regular ambulance attendants: a comparative trial. *Prehosp Emerg Care.* 2004;8:15-22.
146. Samarkandi AH, Seraj MA, el Dawlatly A, et al. The role of laryngeal mask airway in cardiopulmonary resuscitation. *Resuscitation.* 1994;28:103-106.
147. Staudinger T, Brugger S, Watschinger B, et al. Emergency intubation with the Combitube: comparison with the endotracheal airway. *Ann Emerg Med.* 1993;22:1573-1575.
148. Staudinger T, Brugger S, Roggla M, et al. Comparison of the Combitube with the endotracheal tube in cardiopulmonary resuscitation in the prehospital phase [in German]. *Wien Klin Wochenschr.* 1994;106:412-415.
149. Cady CE, Weaver MD, Pirrallo RG, et al. Effect of emergency medical technician-placed Combitubes on outcomes after out-of-hospital cardiopulmonary arrest. *Prehosp Emerg Care.* 2009;13:495-499.
150. Verghese C, Prior-Willeard PF, Baskett PJ. Immediate management of the airway during cardiopulmonary resuscitation in a hospital without a resident anaesthesiologist. *Eur J Emerg Med.* 1994;1:123-125.
151. Deakin CD, Peters R, Tomlinson P, et al. Securing the pre-hospital airway: a comparison of laryngeal mask insertion and endotracheal intubation by UK paramedics. *Emerg Med J.* 2005;22:64-67.
152. Calkins TR, Miller K, Langdorf MI. Success and complication rates with prehospital placement of an esophageal-tracheal combitube as a rescue airway. *Prehosp Disaster Med.* 2006;21:97-100.
153. Guyette FX, Wang H, Cole JS. King airway use by air medical providers. *Prehosp Emerg Care.* 2007;11:473-476.
154. Tentillier E, Heydenreich C, Cros AM, et al. Use of the intubating laryngeal mask airway in emergency pre-hospital difficult intubation. *Resuscitation.* 2008;77:30-34.
155. Timmermann A, Russo SG, Rosenblatt WH, et al. Intubating laryngeal mask airway for difficult out-of-hospital airway management: a prospective evaluation. *Br J Anaesth.* 2007;99:286-291.
156. Martin SE, Ochsner MG, Jarman RH, et al. Use of the laryngeal mask airway in air transport when intubation fails. *J Trauma.* 1999;47:352-357.
157. Grmec S. Comparison of three different methods to confirm tracheal tube placement in emergency intubation. *Intensive Care Med.* 2002;28:701-704.
158. Silvestri S, Ralls GA, Krauss B, et al. The effectiveness of out-of-hospital use of continuous end-tidal carbon dioxide monitoring on the rate of unrecognized misplaced intubation within a regional emergency medical services system. *Ann Emerg Med.* 2005;45:497-503.
159. Aufderheide TP, Sigurdsson G, Pirrallo RG, et al. Hyperventilation-induced hypotension during cardiopulmonary resuscitation. *Circulation.* 2004;109:1960-1965.
160. Bhende MS, Thompson AE. Evaluation of an end-tidal CO_2 detector during pediatric cardiopulmonary resuscitation. *Pediatrics.* 1995;95:395-399.
161. Sehra R, Underwood K, Checchia P. End tidal CO_2 is a quantitative measure of cardiac arrest. *Pacing Clin Electrophysiol.* 2003;26(part 2):515-517.
162. Grmec S, Kupnik D. Does the Mainz Emergency Evaluation Scoring (MEES) in combination with capnometry (MEESc) help in the prognosis of outcome from cardiopulmonary resuscitation in a pre-hospital setting? *Resuscitation.* 2003;58:89-96.
163. Grmec S, Klemen P. Does the end-tidal carbon dioxide (ETCO2) concentration have prognostic value during out-of-hospital cardiac arrest? *Eur J Emerg Med.* 2001;8:263-269.
164. Kolar M, Krizmaric M, Klemen P, et al. Partial pressure of end-tidal carbon dioxide successful predicts cardiopulmonary resuscitation in the field: a prospective observational study. *Crit Care.* 2008;12:R115.
165. Levine RL, Wayne MA, Miller CC. End-tidal carbon dioxide and outcome of out-of-hospital cardiac arrest. *N Engl J Med.* 1997;337:301-306.
166. Wayne MA, Levine RL, Miller CC. Use of end-tidal carbon dioxide to predict outcome in prehospital cardiac arrest. *Ann Emerg Med.* 1995;25:762-767.
167. Ahrens T, Schallom L, Bettorf K, et al. End-tidal carbon dioxide measurements as a prognostic indicator of outcome in cardiac arrest. *Am J Crit Care.* 2001;10:391-398.
168. Sanders AB, Kern KB, Otto CW, et al. End-tidal carbon dioxide monitoring during cardiopulmonary resuscitation: a prognostic indicator for survival. *JAMA.* 1989;262:1347-1351.
169. Olasveengen TM, Sunde K, Brunborg C, et al. Intravenous drug administration during out-of-hospital cardiac arrest: a randomized trial. *JAMA.* 2009;302:2222-2229.
170. Dorian P, Cass D, Schwartz B, et al. Amiodarone as compared with lidocaine for shock-resistant ventricular fibrillation. *N Engl J Med.* 2002;346:884-890.
171. Kudenchuk PJ, Cobb LA, Copass MK, et al. Amiodarone for resuscitation after out-of-hospital cardiac arrest due to ventricular fibrillation. *N Engl J Med.* 1999;341:871-878.
172. Rittenberger JC, Menegazzi JJ, Callaway CW. Association of delay to first intervention with return of spontaneous circulation in a swine model of cardiac arrest. *Resuscitation.* 2007;73:154-160.
173. Callaway CW. Questioning the use of epinephrine to treat cardiac arrest. *JAMA.* 2012;307:1198-1200.
174. Hagihara A, Hasegawa M, Abe T, et al. Prehospital epinephrine use and survival among patients with out-of-hospital cardiac arrest. *JAMA.* 2012;307:1161-1168.
175. Wenzel V, Krismer AC, Arntz HR, et al. A comparison of vasopressin and epinephrine for out-of-hospital cardiopulmonary resuscitation. *N Engl J Med.* 2004;350:105-113.
176. Stiell IG, Hebert PC, Wells GA, et al. Vasopressin versus epinephrine for inhospital cardiac arrest: a randomised controlled trial. *Lancet.* 2001;358:105-109.
177. Aung K, Htay T. Vasopressin for cardiac arrest: a systematic review and meta-analysis. *Arch Intern Med.* 2005;165:17-24.
178. Callaway CW, Hostler D, Doshi AA, et al. Usefulness of vasopressin administered with epinephrine during out-of-hospital cardiac arrest. *Am J Cardiol.* 2006;98:1316-1321.
179. Gueugniaud PY, David JS, Chanzy E, et al. Vasopressin and epinephrine vs. epinephrine alone in cardiopulmonary resuscitation. *N Engl J Med.* 2008;359:21-30.
180. Coon GA, Clinton JE, Ruiz E. Use of atropine for brady-asystolic prehospital cardiac arrest. *Ann Emerg Med.* 1981;10:462-467.
181. Tortolani AJ, Risucci DA, Powell SR, et al. In-hospital cardiopulmonary resuscitation during asystole: therapeutic factors associated with 24-hour survival. *Chest.* 1989;96:622-626.
182. Stiell IG, Wells GA, Hebert PC, et al. Association of drug therapy with survival in cardiac arrest: limited role of advanced cardiac life support drugs. *Acad Emerg Med.* 1995;2:264-273.
183. Engdahl J, Bang A, Lindqvist J, et al. Can we define patients with no and those with some chance of survival when found in asystole out of hospital? *Am J Cardiol.* 2000;86:610-614.
184. Engdahl J, Bang A, Lindqvist J, et al. Factors affecting short- and long-term prognosis among 1069 patients with out-of-hospital cardiac arrest and pulseless electrical activity. *Resuscitation.* 2001;51:17-25.

185. van Walraven C, Stiell IG, Wells GA, et al; the OTAC Study Group. Do advanced cardiac life support drugs increase resuscitation rates from in-hospital cardiac arrest? *Ann Emerg Med*. 1998;32:544-553.
186. Amiodarone, lidocaine or neither for out-of-hospital cardiac arrest due to ventricular fibrillation or tachycardia (ALPS). Available at: http://www.ClinicalTrials.gov. Accessed March 10, 2014.
187. Morrison LJ, Deakin CD, Morley PT, et al. Part 8: Advanced life support: 2010 International Consensus on Cardiopulmonary Resuscitation and Emergency Cardiovascular Care Science With Treatment Recommendations. *Circulation*. 2010;122(16 suppl 2):S345-S421.
188. Ditchey RV, Lindenfeld J. Potential adverse effects of volume loading on perfusion of vital organs during closed-chest resuscitation. *Circulation*. 1984;69:181-189.
189. Voorhees WD, Ralston SH, Kougias C, Schmitz PM. Fluid loading with whole blood or Ringer's lactate solution during CPR in dogs. *Resuscitation*. 1987;15:113-123.
190. Gentile NT, Martin GB, Appleton TJ, et al. Effects of arterial and venous volume infusion on coronary perfusion pressures during canine CPR. *Resuscitation*. 1991;22:55-63.
191. Bender R, Breil M, Heister U, et al. Hypertonic saline during CPR: feasibility and safety of a new protocol of fluid management during resuscitation. *Resuscitation*. 2007;72:74-81.
192. Bruel C, Parienti JJ, Marie W, et al. Mild hypothermia during advanced life support: a preliminary study in out-of-hospital cardiac arrest. *Crit Care*. 2008;12:R31.
193. Kamarainen A, Virkkunen I, Tenhunen J, et al. Prehospital induction of therapeutic hypothermia during CPR: a pilot study. *Resuscitation*. 2008;76:360–363.
194. Dybvik T, Strand T, Steen PA. Buffer therapy during out-of-hospital cardiopulmonary resuscitation. *Resuscitation*. 1995;29:89-95.
195. Vukmir RB, Katz L. Sodium bicarbonate improves outcome in prolonged prehospital cardiac arrest. *Am J Emerg Med*. 2006;24:156-161.
196. Aufderheide TP, Martin DR, Olson DW, et al. Prehospital bicarbonate use in cardiac arrest: a 3-year experience. *Am J Emerg Med*. 1992;10:4-7.
197. Suljaga-Pechtel K, Goldberg E, Strickon P, et al. Cardiopulmonary resuscitation in a hospitalized population: prospective study of factors associated with outcome. *Resuscitation*. 1984;12:77-95.
198. Skovron ML, Goldberg E, Suljaga-Petchel K. Factors predicting survival for six months after cardiopulmonary resuscitation: multivariate analysis of a prospective study. *Mt Sinai J Med*. 1985;52:271-275.
199. Delooz H, Lewi PJ. Are inter-center differences in EMS-management and sodium-bicarbonate administration important for the outcome of CPR? The Cerebral Resuscitation Study Group. *Resuscitation*. 1989;17(suppl):S199-S206.
200. Roberts D, Landolfo K, Light R, Dobson K. Early predictors of mortality for hospitalized patients suffering cardiopulmonary arrest. *Chest*. 1990;97:413-419.
201. Stueven HA, Thompson BM, Aprahamian C, Tonsfeldt DJ. Calcium chloride: reassessment of use in asystole. *Ann Emerg Med*. 1984;13(part 2):820-822.
202. Stueven HA, Thompson B, Aprahamian C, et al. The effectiveness of calcium chloride in refractory electromechanical dissociation. *Ann Emerg Med*. 1985;14:626-629.
203. Stueven HA, Thompson B, Aprahamian C, et al. Lack of effectiveness of calcium chloride in refractory asystole. *Ann Emerg Med*. 1985;14:630-632.
204. Stueven H, Thompson BM, Aprahamian C, et al. Use of calcium in prehospital cardiac arrest. *Ann Emerg Med*. 1983;12:136-139.
205. Allegra J, Lavery R, Cody R, et al. Magnesium sulfate in the treatment of refractory ventricular fibrillation in the prehospital setting. *Resuscitation*. 2001;49:245-249.
206. Thel MC, Armstrong AL, McNulty SE, et al; Duke Internal Medicine Housestaff. Randomised trial of magnesium in in-hospital cardiac arrest. *Lancet*. 1997;350:1272-1276.
207. Fatovich DM, Prentice DA, Dobb GJ. Magnesium in cardiac arrest (the MAGIC trial). *Resuscitation*. 1997;35:237-241.
208. Hassan TB, Jagger C, Barnett DB. A randomised trial to investigate the efficacy of magnesium sulphate for refractory ventricular fibrillation. *Emerg Med J*. 2002;19:57-62.
209. Abu-Laban RB, Christenson JM, Innes GD, et al. Tissue plasminogen activator in cardiac arrest with pulseless electrical activity. *N Engl J Med*. 2002;346:1522-1528.
210. Bottiger BW, Arntz HR, Chamberlain DA, et al. Thrombolysis during resuscitation for out-of-hospital cardiac arrest. *N Engl J Med*. 2008;359:2651-2662.
211. Shuster M, Lim SH, Deakin CD, et al. Part 7: CPR techniques and devices: 2010 International Consensus on Cardiopulmonary Resuscitation and Emergency Cardiovascular Care Science with Treatment Recommendations. *Circulation*. 2010;122(16 suppl 2):S338-S344.
212. Plaisance P, Lurie KG, Vicaut E, et al. Evaluation of an impedance threshold device in patients receiving active compression-decompression cardiopulmonary resuscitation for out of hospital cardiac arrest. *Resuscitation*. 2004;61:265-271.
213. Plaisance P, Lurie KG, Payen D. Inspiratory impedance during active compression-decompression cardiopulmonary resuscitation: A randomized evaluation in patients in cardiac arrest. *Circulation*. 2000;101:989-994.
214. Aufderheide TP, Pirrallo RG, Provo TA, et al. Clinical evaluation of an inspiratory impedance threshold device during standard cardiopulmonary resuscitation in patients with out-of-hospital cardiac arrest. *Crit Care Med*. 2005;33:734-740.
215. Wolcke BB, Mauer DK, Schoefmann MF, et al. Comparison of standard cardiopulmonary resuscitation versus the combination of active compression-decompression cardiopulmonary resuscitation and an inspiratory impedance threshold device for out-of-hospital cardiac arrest. *Circulation*. 2003;108:2201-2205.
216. Knafelj R, Radsel P, Ploj T, et al. Primary percutaneous coronary intervention and mild induced hypothermia in comatose survivors of ventricular fibrillation with ST-elevation acute myocardial infarction. *Resuscitation*. 2007;74:227-234.
217. Wolfrum S, Pierau C, Radke PW, et al. Mild therapeutic hypothermia in patients after out-of-hospital cardiac arrest due to acute ST-segment elevation myocardial infarction undergoing immediate percutaneous coronary intervention. *Crit Care Med*. 2008;36:1780-1786.
218. Oddo M, Schaller MD, Feihl F, et al. From evidence to clinical practice: effective implementation of therapeutic hypothermia to improve patient outcome after cardiac arrest. *Crit Care Med*. 2006;34:1865-1873.
219. Rittenberger JC, Guyette FX, Tisherman SA, et al. Outcomes of a hospital-wide plan to improve care of comatose survivors of cardiac arrest. *Resuscitation*. 2008;79:198-204.
220. Gaieski DF, Band RA, Abella BS, et al. Early goal-directed hemodynamic optimization combined with therapeutic hypothermia in comatose survivors of out-of-hospital cardiac arrest. *Resuscitation*. 2009;80:418-424.
221. Donnino MW, Rittenberger JC, Gaieski D, et al. The development and implementation of cardiac arrest centers. *Resuscitation*. 2011;82:974-978.
222. Birkmeyer JD, Stukel TA, Siewers AE, et al. Surgeon volume and operative mortality in the United States. *N Engl J Med*. 2003;349:2117-2127.
223. Wnent J, Seewald S, Heringlake M, et al. Choice of hospital after out-of-hospital cardiac arrest—a decision with far-reaching consequences: a study in a large German city. *Crit Care*. 2012;16(5):R164. [Epub ahead of print].
224. Cha WC, Lee SC, Shin SD, et al. Regionalisation of out-of-hospital cardiac arrest care for patients without prehospital return of spontaneous circulation. *Resuscitation*. 2012;83:1338-1342.
225. Spaite DW, Bobrow BJ, Vadeboncoeur TF, et al. The impact of prehospital transport interval on survival in out-of-hospital cardiac arrest: implications for regionalization of postresuscitation care. *Resuscitation*. 2008;79:61-66.
226. Spaite DW, Stiell IG, Bobrow BJ, et al. Effect of transport interval on out-of-hospital cardiac arrest survival in the OPALS study: implications for triaging patients to specialized cardiac arrest centers. *Ann Emerg Med*. 2009;54:256-257.
227. Hartke A, Mumma BE, Rittenberger JC, et al. Incidence of re-arrest and critical events during prolonged transport of post-cardiac arrest patients. *Resuscitation*. 2010;81:938-942.
228. Morrison LJ, Verbeek PR, Zhan C, et al. Validation of a universal prehospital termination of resuscitation clinical prediction rule for advanced and basic life support providers. *Resuscitation*. 2009;80:324-328.
229. Scholten AC, van Manen JG, van der Worp WE, et al. Early cardiopulmonary resuscitation and use of Automated External Defibrillators by laypersons in out-of-hospital cardiac arrest using an SMS alert service. *Resuscitation*. 2011;82:1273-1278.
230. Merchant RM, Asch DA, Hershey JC, et al. A crowdsourcing, mobile media, challenge to locate automated external defibrillators. *Circulation*. 2012;126:A57.
231. Nagao K, Kikushima K, Watanabe K, et al. Early induction of hypothermia during cardiac arrest improves neurological outcomes in patients with out-of-hospital cardiac arrest who undergo emergency cardiopulmonary bypass and percutaneous coronary intervention. *Circ J*. 2010;74:77-85.
232. Morimura N, Sakamoto T, Nagao K, et al. Extracorporeal cardiopulmonary resuscitation for out-of-hospital cardiac arrest: s review of the Japanese literature. *Resuscitation*. 2011;82:10-14.
233. Belohlavek J, Kucera K, Jarkovsky J, et al. Hyperinvasive approach to out-of hospital cardiac arrest using mechanical chest compression device, prehospital intraarrest cooling, extracorporeal life support and early invasive assessment compared to standard of care: a randomized parallel groups comparative study proposal. "Prague OHCA study". *J Transl Med*. 2012;10:163.
234. Bellezzo JM, Shinar Z, Davis DP, et al. Emergency physician-initiated extracorporeal cardiopulmonary resuscitation. *Resuscitation*. 2012;83:966-970.

CARDIOVASCULAR EMERGENCIES

CHAPTER 13

Post–Cardiac Arrest Syndrome

Gail Delfin and Benjamin S. Abella

IN THIS CHAPTER

Pathophysiology

Clinical features

Initial evaluation and treatment

Special considerations

Regionalization of post–cardiac arrest care

Practice guidelines

The rate of survival to discharge after cardiac arrest remains less than 20% in most hospitals and communities.[1] As many as 50% of survivors suffer a range of persistent disabilities as a result of the event and subsequent reperfusion injury processes.[1] It is important that emergency physicians are well prepared to address the goals of immediate post–cardiac arrest therapy: to optimize systemic perfusion, to encourage metabolic homeostasis, and to support organ system function to maximize the potential for neurologic recovery.[2] The purpose of this chapter is to describe the post–cardiac arrest syndrome (PCAS) and its implications for clinical care. Emphasis will be placed on the management of patients undergoing targeted temperature management (TTM), a form of whole-body cooling employed after resuscitation from cardiac arrest (also known as therapeutic hypothermia). This relatively new and evolving therapy represents the cornerstone of postresuscitation care and is becoming more prevalent in emergency department practice.

Pathophysiology

Based on the pathophysiology of ischemia-reperfusion injury, PCAS is triggered by the abrupt return of spontaneous circulation (ROSC) after the complete loss of blood flow during the arrest. Representing an overlapping set of injury processes, the clinical manifestations of PCAS include cerebral edema, myocardial dysfunction, and systemic inflammatory response with associated hypotension and shock state.[3] These phenomena can be compounded by the persistent pathology that caused the original arrest event (such as untreated myocardial ischemia or pulmonary embolism).

On a cellular level, PCAS is characterized by aberrant mitochondrial function and activation of programmed cell death pathways through various mechanisms, including the release of cytochrome C and disruption of oxidative phosphorylation.[4,5] At the humoral level, reperfusion triggers immune activation pathways, escalating levels of cytokines such as interleukin-6 and tumor necrosis factor alpha.[6] Anomalous neutrophil and coagulation activation occur, similar to the inflammatory changes and cellular activation observed in sepsis. Additionally, oxygen free radicals such as superoxide and hydrogen peroxide are generated during PCAS, leading to tissue injury in the brain and vascular endothelium[7] (Figure 13-1).

Clinical Features

The cellular and vascular insults associated with PCAS become manifest within minutes to hours following cardiac arrest and ROSC. Cerebral edema with a concomitant increase in intracranial pressure can develop soon after ROSC; herniation is a possible consequence of this swelling, often causing death within the first 72 hours after resuscitation.[8] Myocardial stunning is evident on echocardiography as global hypokinesis and a markedly reduced ejection fraction. Stunning can persist for 48 to 72 hours and often requires inotropic/vasopressor support.[9,10] Fortunately, this myocardial depression often fully reverses as the post–cardiac arrest course progresses. Inflammation can precipitate vascular leak, intravascular fluid loss, and a subsequent drop in the systemic vascular resistance, resulting in marked hypotension and organ hypoperfusion. Bacteremia and infectious complications can become evident in the days following resuscitation from cardiac arrest because of bacterial translocation from the gastrointestinal tract, as demonstrated in animal models.[11] Acute kidney injury is associated with PCAS, especially in the presence of postresuscitation cardiogenic shock.[12,13] Tubular cell injury from ATP depletion and apoptotic cellular death has been documented in laboratory models.[14] Recent evidence suggests that, in post–cardiac arrest patients with cardiogenic shock treated with TTM, aggressive volume administration during the first 6 hours following ROSC correlates with significant reduction in kidney injury.[15]

Relative adrenal insufficiency is prevalent following resuscitation from cardiac arrest[16,17] and can contribute to vasopressor-dependent shock. Although the incidence of adrenal insufficiency can be high following cardiac arrest, it is infrequently considered and deserves further investigation to determine whether treatment with corticosteroids will improve outcomes.[18]

Initial Evaluation and Treatment

Cardiovascular instability and neurologic injury are the major causes of death during hospitalization after cardiac arrest.[19] Post–cardiac arrest care is highly time sensitive and includes management of patients across a wide spectrum of illness—from the patient who is awake and hemodynamically stable to the unstable, comatose patient who requires treatment for persistent and significant post–cardiac arrest pathophysiology. Assessment and treatment of dysfunction in multiple organ systems simultaneously is often required.

After ROSC and the establishment of a secure airway, oxygenation and ventilation should be optimized. Although 100% oxygen is usually delivered during resuscitation, to prevent oxygen toxicity, current international resuscitation guidelines recommend prompt titration of oxygen to lower fraction of inspired oxygen (F_{IO_2}) levels to maintain arterial pulse oximetry above 94%. This concept is still under active investigation and not yet well established by prospective clinical studies.[3] Resuscitation guidelines also recommend the avoidance of hyperventilation, which can adversely affect cardiac output and cerebral blood flow. A goal arterial partial pressure of carbon dioxide ($Paco_2$) of 40 to 45 mm Hg is advised.[2]

KEY POINT

During post–cardiac arrest care, promptly titrate oxygen delivery to maintain the pulse oximetry reading above 94%. Ventilate to a $Paco_2$ of 40 to 45 mm Hg.

Hypotension is frequently present in the resuscitated cardiac arrest patient. Some investigations have suggested the possible benefit of utilizing an algorithmic approach to early goal-directed hemodynamic optimization.[20] Although early goal-directed therapy has been employed in the treatment of sepsis,[21] no randomized controlled trials have been performed to demonstrate the benefit in PCAS. Based on the limited available evidence, the following hemodynamic goals are recommended: mean arterial pressure, above 65 mm Hg; central venous pressure (CVP), 8 to 12 mm Hg; central venous oxygen saturation ($Scvo_2$), above 70%; urine output, more than 0.5 mL/kg/hr; and a normal or decreasing serum lactate level over the first 24 hours of care.[3] Although the serum lactate concentration can be quite high immediately following resuscitation, it is of little prognostic value; lactate clearance over the first 12 to 24 hours is the more important parameter with regard to subsequent clinical course.[22]

If hemodynamic goals are not achieved despite aggressive fluid resuscitation, vasoactive agents might be required. Bedside echocardiography and central venous pressure measurements might be helpful to guide therapy. Inotropes and/or vasopressors could be required. No specific vasoactive agent or combination has been shown to be superior in treating cardiovascular dysfunction after cardiac arrest, although laboratory studies

FIGURE 13-1.

Ischemia-reperfusion injury and elements of the PCAS. TTM attenuates the inflammatory and cellular processes that lead to clinical injury.

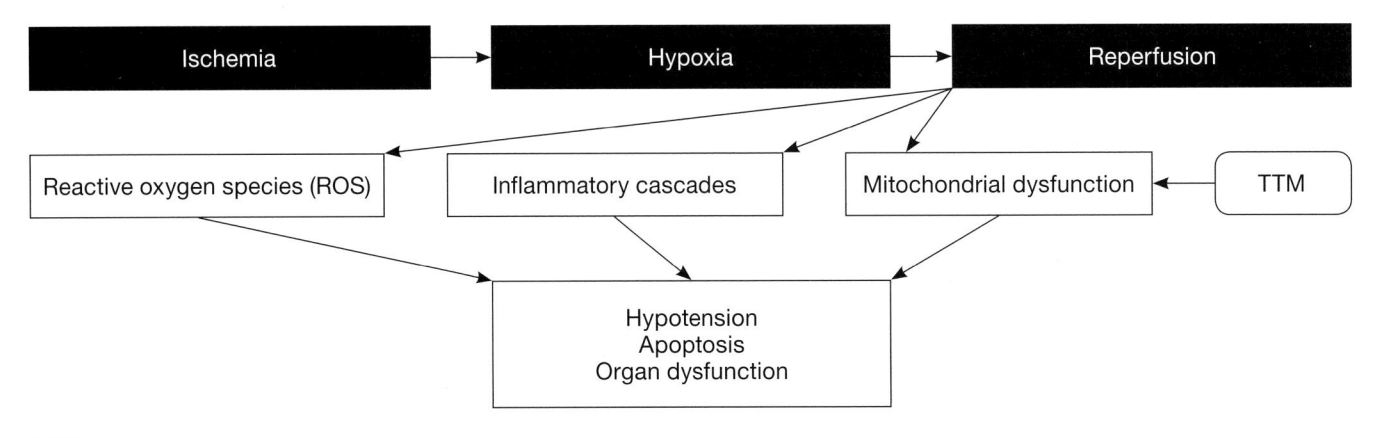

have suggested a beneficial role for dobutamine to address myocardial stunning.[3] If these measures fail to restore sufficient perfusion, mechanical circulatory support such as an intra-aortic balloon pump or extracorporeal membrane oxygenation circuit can be considered. The clinical value of these interventions following cardiac arrest resuscitation has not yet been determined, although initial studies of extracorporeal membrane oxygenation have been promising.

KEY POINTS

During emergency department care following cardiac arrest resuscitation, hemodynamic goals are as follows: mean arterial pressure, above 65 mm Hg; CVP, 8 to 12 mm Hg; Scvo$_2$, above 70%; urine output, more than 0.5 mL/kg/hr; and a normal or decreasing serum lactate concentration. Treat post–cardiac arrest hypotension initially with fluid boluses, then consider vasoactive and/or inotropic agents.

Continuous telemetry monitoring is essential to detect cardiac arrhythmias, such as new-onset atrial fibrillation or nonsustained ventricular tachycardia, which are common in the immediate postresuscitation period. Antiarrhythmic medications are often required to manage these arrhythmias, which could be a manifestation of ongoing myocardial ischemia. Recurrent episodes of post–cardiac arrest ventricular tachycardia should raise the possibility that the patient has an unrecognized coronary occlusion. An electrocardiogram (ECG) should be obtained as soon as possible after ROSC to determine whether there is new evidence of ST-segment elevation or the presence of new left bundle-branch block. If suspicion is high for recent coronary artery occlusion or significant coronary disease, the cardiac catheterization laboratory should be consulted promptly to consider percutaneous coronary intervention.[23] Consistent with the observation that a majority of out-of-hospital arrests are caused by myocardial ischemia with coronary obstruction, increasing evidence suggests that most out-of-hospital cardiac arrest patients benefit from early catheterization.[24-26] Studies have suggested that catheterization is underutilized following cardiac arrest resuscitation.[27] Therefore, emergency practitioners should aggressively advocate for cardiac catheterization for patients presenting after cardiac arrest when a noncardiac cause of arrest is not evident and should advocate for catheterization, especially when the initial arrest rhythm is ventricular tachycardia/ventricular fibrillation (VT/VF) or if the patient has a history of coronary artery disease.

KEY POINT

In the absence of complications, immediately activate the cardiac catheterization team, when institutionally available, for resuscitated patients with ST-elevation myocardial infarction or ST-elevation myocardial infarction equivalent. Most post–cardiac arrest patients should at least be considered for catheterization.

Postresuscitation Neurologic Injury

Given that most patients receive atropine, sedative agents, and/or neuromuscular blockade in the peri-arrest period, the initial neurologic examination might be limited. Electrical cerebral convulsive activity is present in 15% to 44% of patients in the first hours following cardiac arrest resuscitation.[28] Although recent reports suggest that not all post–cardiac arrest patients with seizures documented by electroencephalography have poor outcomes, the presence of seizures is a worrisome sign for marked neurologic injury.

Coma and impaired brain stem reflexes are common in the resuscitated cardiac arrest patient during emergency department evaluation. It is important to emphasize that abnormal neurologic reflexes such as fixed or dilated pupils or absence of the gag reflex within the first 72 hours following resuscitation are not predictive of cardiac arrest outcomes and should not be the basis for care decisions; this recommendation is supported by the American Academy of Neurology.[29] Many patients who do not exhibit coma after resuscitation still show a range of initial impairments such as inability to follow motor commands or make purposeful movements. They are likely suffering some degree of postresuscitation neurologic injury requiring PCAS treatment, as discussed below.

Another key neurologic assessment of the resuscitated cardiac arrest patient in the emergency department involves prompt computed tomography (CT) of the brain, which is useful in ruling out intracranial hemorrhage as the precipitating cause of the arrest.[30] Subdural or epidural bleeding can occur as a result of peri-arrest head trauma from falling and should be considered. Cerebral edema can be seen as well on the initial CT scan and, if present, might suggest a worsened prognosis[31] but does not preclude the use of TTM and aggressive care. Brain magnetic resonance imaging is logistically challenging in the emergency department setting for post–cardiac arrest patients and generally is not considered useful for acute evaluation.

KEY POINT

A noncontrast head CT scan should be obtained promptly in post–cardiac arrest patients when indicated (in those with head trauma, suspicion of stroke, or intracranial hemorrhage) and feasible. The scan can rule out subarachnoid hemorrhage as the cause of cardiac arrest. In the peri-arrest period, CT will also reveal subdural or epidural bleeding resulting from a traumatic injury.

Targeted Temperature Management

TTM represents the first clinically effective treatment for PCAS that is supported by randomized trial evidence. Two randomized controlled trials published in 2002 demonstrated that TTM substantially improves both survival and neurologic outcomes when implemented within hours after initial ROSC.[32,33] These trials included comatose post–cardiac arrest patients resuscitated from out-of-hospital VT/VF randomized to either an induced hypothermia intervention group (target core body temperature of 32°C-34°C) or to a control normothermic group in which temperature was not actively managed. Cerebral performance category scores were documented at hospital discharge. Good neurologic outcomes (as defined by a cerebral performance category score of 1 or 2) were significantly higher in the TTM arms of the studies. For example, the larger of the two trials found good neurologic outcome in 55% of TTM-treated patients versus 39% in the untreated group (*P*= .01). Although no randomized trials have been performed for cardiac arrest patients presenting with pulseless electrical activity or asystole as the initial rhythm of arrest, a growing body of clinical evidence suggests that TTM might improve outcomes for these patients as well.[34-36] The 2010 consensus resuscitation guidelines recommend TTM for resuscitated out-of-hospital VT/VF adult patients as a Class I indication; for patients resuscitated from cardiac arrest caused by nonshockable rhythms, TTM is a Class IIb indication.[2]

There is a growing consensus that almost all adult patients resuscitated from cardiac arrest who were not severely cognitively impaired prior to arrest and who remain unresponsive shortly after ROSC should be considered for TTM therapy. Resuscitated cardiac arrest patients who are awake and purposefully following commands can be excluded safely from TTM consideration. Relative exclusion criteria for TTM include the following: very poor pre-arrest cognitive status (bedbound nonverbal patients probably have little to gain from TTM) and cardiac arrest resulting from trauma or associated with significant bleeding. This latter exclusion criterion is typically invoked to minimize patient risk, as TTM is associated with a temperature-dependent coagulopathy and mild risk of increased bleeding.[37] However, use of anticoagulants and/or glycoprotein antagonists is not considered a contraindication to TTM, provided that clinically evident bleeding is not present (Table 13-1).

A Practical Approach to TTM

The emergency practitioner should ensure that post–cardiac arrest care, including TTM, is provided as part of a hospital-wide post–cardiac arrest care protocol. A comprehensive TTM protocol not only describes hypothermia care but also establishes lines of communication and coordination of care across the continuum of post–cardiac arrest care—from the emergency department, to the critical care setting, and often extending to the cardiac catheterization laboratory. Hospital TTM protocols should delineate the three phases of care inherent in the TTM process: induction, maintenance, and rewarming (Figure 13-2). In addition, TTM protocols should provide information regarding goals of treatment, adjunctive pharmacologic therapy (sedation, neuromuscular blockade), essential laboratory testing, and requisite monitoring. Incorporation of the protocol into electronic order sets standardizes the therapy, supports timely interventions, and serves as an educational resource for end-users. The development of a standing protocol is a vital step for hospital-based post–cardiac arrest care; examples are available on an internet resource page.[38]

TTM Induction

Induction represents the lowering of the core body temperature as quickly as possible to between 32°C and 34°C. The procedure requires preparation of the patient (intubation and sedation), mechanisms to prevent shivering, appropriate monitoring, intravenous and arterial cannulation, and baseline diagnostic testing. Each of these facets is discussed in this section (Table 13-2).

Commercial devices, including external wrap or pad systems and intravascular cooling catheters, can be used to initiate, maintain, and reverse the induced hypothermic state. Hypothermia can also be achieved by simple measures: ice packs, infusion of chilled intravenous fluids, or gastric lavage with chilled fluid. A combination of these methods is often used to achieve the target temperature promptly.

Induction of TTM is staff and task intensive. After intubation, patient care is optimized to set the stage for TTM. Appropriate levels of sedation/analgesia are essential in these patients, although no sedation regimen has been proved superior.[39]

TABLE 13-1.

Inclusion and Relative Exclusion Criteria for TTM

Eligibility criteria for post–cardiac arrest TTM
Coma following cardiac arrest and ROSC (does not follow commands)
Pre-arrest cognitive status not severely impaired (CPC not 4 or 5)
No other cause for coma
No uncontrolled bleeding
Absence of multisystem organ failure, severe sepsis
Less than 12 hours since return of ROSC
Relative exclusion criteria
Patient receiving oral or intravenous anticoagulants
Presentation with non-shockable rhythm
In-hospital location of arrest
Pregnancy
Peri-operative arrest

FIGURE 13-2.

The three phases of TTM, shown with an illustrative temperature curve for a post–cardiac arrest patient

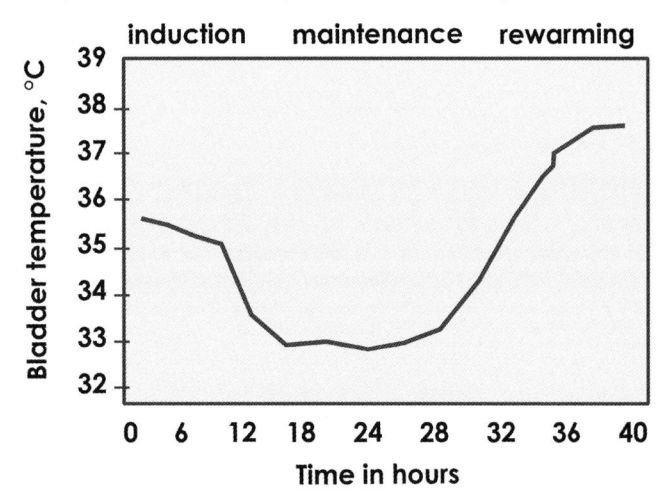

Bispectral index monitoring can be helpful to guide the use of sedation in patients treated with pharmacologic neuromuscular blockade.

Shivering is a challenge when core body temperature is manipulated. Shivering is detrimental because it can increase the basal metabolic rate.[40] It also increases the difficulty of achieving the target temperature in a timely fashion. Some hospitals favor the use of neuromuscular blockade, either as a bolus or infusion. Alternative methods to prevent shivering include surface counter warming, deeper sedation, and combinations of other pharmacologic agents. If paralytics are used, a baseline train-of-four assessment will help to guide the effectiveness of neuromuscular blockade therapy.

The patient undergoing TTM also requires core temperature monitoring, either by esophageal or urinary bladder probe. The use of tympanic membrane thermometers and other peripheral temperature devices is discouraged. An arterial line is necessary to manage hemodynamic status accurately, as blood pressure is often labile during the early hours of postresuscitation care. It is generally recommended that arterial cannulation be done prior to cooling, as induced hypothermia leads to some degree of peripheral vasoconstriction and increased bleeding, making the procedure somewhat more difficult. Central venous access is necessary as well for evaluation of volume status, assay of the $Scvo_2$, and fluid/medication administration. Baseline serologic testing should also be undertaken immediately following successful resuscitation, in addition to obtaining an ECG and chest radiographs.

Cooling should begin in conjunction with preparation of the patient. Immediately after sedating the patient and establishing core temperature monitoring, infuse 2 liters (approximately 30 mL/kg) of 4°C fluid over 30 minutes through a large peripheral intravenous line.[41] The cooling device is connected to the temperature sensor from the patient; the device is programmed to maintain the patient's temperature between 32°C and 34°C. Consider measures to counteract shivering according to hospital protocol. Acetaminophen administration, application of ice packs, and cool environment and respiratory circuits can hasten cooling.

TABLE 13-2.
TTM Preparation and Induction

Review of patient's eligibility, contraindications to TTM, advance directives
Intubation
Sedation, shivering control
Serologic testing, chest radiograph, ECG, and echocardiography
Core temperature monitoring (bladder, esophageal)
Arterial cannulation, central access placement
Peripheral infusion of 2 liters of cold (4°C) normal saline
Implementation of cooling device and temperature monitoring

TTM Maintenance and Rewarming

The target temperature is considered to be attained when the patient's temperature falls below 34°C; this cooled state is then maintained for 12 to 24 hours. It is vital that the temperature be sustained between 32°C and 34°C to avoid overcooling and the associated adverse effects from more profound hypothermia.[42] The maintenance phase typically represents a more stable period, although the patient's hemodynamic status must be monitored closely. A mean arterial blood pressure above 65 mm Hg is often considered to be the minimum needed to support cerebral perfusion.[20] Vigilant care is key in preventing the complications of artificial ventilation, complex pharmacologic therapies, and prolonged bedrest associated with this phase of TTM.

The rewarming phase of TTM begins 12 to 24 hours after the target temperature is reached. Rewarming can precipitate cardiovascular and cerebral stress by inducing hypotension secondary to vasodilation. Electrolyte shifts (especially hyperkalemia) and hypoglycemia are common during this period as well. It is generally recommended that rewarming be performed slowly, at a rate of 0.25°C to 0.5°C per hour, to minimize these potential adverse effects.

Managing Common Physiologic Effects of TTM

A number of potential side effects are associated with TTM (Table 13-3). Hypotension could be the result of a combination of mechanisms: systemic vascular resistance might be low secondary to the effects of PCAS, and a "cold diuresis"[37] could precipitate hypovolemia, requiring substantial amounts of fluid replacement. Electrolyte deficits (in particular, low levels of potassium and magnesium) are associated with cold diuresis as well; electrolyte repletion is often necessary. Hyperglycemia can

TABLE 13-3.
Potential Adverse Effects of TTM

More common
Bradycardia
Prolongation of QT interval
Coagulopathy with partial thromboplastin time prolongation, platelet dysfunction
Shivering
Electrolyte abnormalities
Hypokalemia and hyperglycemia during TTM induction
Hyperkalemia and hypoglycemia during rewarming
Hypotension associated with cold diuresis
Risk for infection (particularly pneumonia)
Less common
Arrhythmias
Significant bleeding
Skin injury from surface cooling methods

occur as a result of the patient's lack of sensitivity to intrinsic insulin and often requires insulin infusion. Bradycardia (heart rate <50 beats/min) is very common but often of little clinical consequence. Perfusion (evidenced by adequate blood pressure and a urine output of 1 mL/kg/hr) is usually well maintained despite bradycardia, so no intervention is required.[43] QT prolongation is frequently observed during cooling.[44] Post–cardiac arrest TTM has also been associated with a modestly increased risk of infection and coagulopathy with partial thromboplastin time prolongation.[37]

Among the less common effects of TTM are significant bleeding and arrhythmias. Investigators have reported bleeding complication rates of less than 5%.[43,45] Nonsustained VT and atrial fibrillation can occur, usually in association with lower core temperatures (<32°C).[37] Small boluses of warmed intravenous fluids can correct the temperature to above 32°C. The risk for skin injury is minimized by frequent skin assessment and repositioning of skin pads if external surface cooling systems are being used.

Readers should note that a recent randomized trial has called into question the ideal target temperature in TTM. Nielsen et al randomized 950 unconscious post-arrest patients to either 33°C or 36°C and found no difference in eventual mortality or neurologic outcome.[46] We anticipate that future studies will clarify the goal temperature in TTM.

Neuroprognostication

Although few practitioners are faced with predicting outcomes after initiating TTM in the emergency department, it is important for the physician to be familiar with neuroprognostication in the context of TTM when discussing expectations for the patient's recovery with family members. Neurologic assessment tools have varying degrees of utility in the TTM patient. Perman and colleagues[47] found few data supporting the optimal tools and time frame for neuroprognostication.[47] However, they found great variation in the timing of prognostic assessments and discrepancies in outcomes of patients assigned a poor prognosis prior to completion of TTM. The complex recovery patterns of TTM patients, influenced by the protracted metabolism of sedatives/neuromuscular blockade agents and the indeterminate effect of 24 hours of hypothermia on the brain, have prompted many resuscitation centers to recommend that neuroprognostication not occur before 72 hours after rewarming.[38]

Special Considerations

Unique Patient Populations

Although many hospitals do not cool pregnant patients after cardiac arrest, there are case reports describing good outcomes with the use of post–cardiac arrest TTM.[48,49] Patients with cardiac arrest induced by asphyxia or drug overdose might benefit from cooling.[50,51] A recent case report describes successful recovery in a soldier who was treated with TTM after suffering commotio cordis and pulmonary contusion on the battlefield, suggesting a role for TTM following traumatic cardiac arrest.[52]

Prehospital Cooling

Although multiple critical knowledge gaps exist regarding cooling (its timing, the technique for induction, the optimal target temperature, and the duration of cooling), preclinical data suggest that delaying induction of TTM might result in worse outcomes.[53,54] Some emergency medical services systems have explored prehospital TTM induction. This strategy seems logical, but the results of prehospital cooling trials have been discouraging. The impact on patient outcomes is not clear, so additional investigation is required.[55,56]

Pediatric Populations

Although children are more likely to survive to discharge after out-of-hospital and in-hospital cardiac arrest,[57] no randomized trial evidence exists to support TTM use in children, with the exception of TTM in neonatal hypoxic-ischemic encephalopathy.[58] A large randomized trial of TTM in pediatric cardiac arrest is currently under way in the United States.

Regionalization of Post–Cardiac Arrest Care/Patient Transfer

Mounting evidence indicates that multiple interventions, in addition to TTM, enhance the survival rate for patients who experience out-of-hospital cardiac arrest. Early cardiac intervention, mechanical and pharmacologic support of hemodynamics, and expert neurologic diagnosis and treatment are effective hospital-based interventions.[59] However, there is significant variability of post–cardiac arrest patient outcomes among hospitals.[60] In hospitals without a well-coordinated approach to post–cardiac arrest care, regionalization can be cost effective and might improve outcomes. Survivors of cardiac arrest and resuscitation, often critically ill, present significant challenges to medical practitioners in the postresuscitation period. These patients could benefit from transfer to a center that has developed expertise in treating this complex population.[61] Patients can be transferred in a safe and timely manner by immediate communication with the accepting hospital, preparation/stabilization of the patient, and initiation of TTM via infusion of cold fluids and application of ice packs. Efficient critical care ground or air transport will minimize time to cardiac intervention and target temperature. Vigilance during transport must include temperature monitoring and controlling the patient's response to rapid cooling.

Practice Guidelines

A number of resources are available on post–cardiac arrest care. The American Heart Association resuscitation guidelines were updated in 2010,[2] and guidelines regarding neurologic assessment related to cardiac arrest have been published by the American Academy of Neurology.[29] Numerous TTM protocols are listed on an internet site sponsored by the University of Pennsylvania.[38] Two organizations provide cardiac arrest resources for patient/family support: the Sudden Cardiac Arrest Association and the Sudden Cardiac Arrest Foundation.[62,63]

References

1. Moulaert VR, Verbunt JA, van Heugten CM, Wade DT. Cognitive impairments in survivors of out-of-hospital cardiac arrest: a systematic review. *Resuscitation.* 2009;80:297-305.
2. Peberdy MA, Callaway CW, Neumar RW, et al. Part 9: post-cardiac arrest care: 2010 American Heart Association Guidelines for Cardiopulmonary Resuscitation and Emergency Cardiovascular Care. *Circulation.* 2010;122(18 suppl 3):S768-S786.
3. Neumar RW, Nolan JP, Adrie C, et al. Post-cardiac arrest syndrome: epidemiology, pathophysiology, treatment, and prognostication. A consensus statement from the International Liaison Committee on Resuscitation (American Heart Association, Australian and New Zealand Council on Resuscitation, European Resuscitation Council, Heart and Stroke Foundation of Canada, InterAmerican Heart Foundation, Resuscitation Council of Asia, and the Resuscitation Council of Southern Africa); the American Heart Association Emergency Cardiovascular Care Committee; the Council on Cardiovascular Surgery and Anesthesia; the Council on Cardiopulmonary, Perioperative, and Critical Care; the Council on Clinical Cardiology; and the Stroke Council. *Circulation.* 2008;118:2452-2483.
4. Vanden Hoek TL, Qin Y, Wojcik K, et al. Reperfusion, not simulated ischemia, initiates intrinsic apoptosis injury in chick cardiomyocytes. *Am J Physiol Heart Circ Physiol.* 2003;284:H141-H150.
5. Beiser DG, Orbelyan GA, Inouye BT, et al. Genetic deletion of NOS3 increases lethal cardiac dysfunction following mouse cardiac arrest. *Resuscitation.* 2011;82:115-121.
6. Samborska-Sablik A, Sablik Z, Gaszynski W. The role of the immuno-inflammatory response in patients after cardiac arrest. *Arch Med Sci.* 2011;7:619-626.
7. Adrie C, Laurent I, Monchi M, et al. Postresuscitation disease after cardiac arrest: a sepsis-like syndrome? *Curr Opin Crit Care.* 2004;10:208-212.
8. Geocadin RG, Kowalski RG. Imaging brain injury after cardiac arrest resuscitation when it really matters. *Resuscitation.* 2011;82:1124-1125.
9. Kern KB. Postresuscitation myocardial dysfunction. *Cardiol Clin.* Feb 2002;20:89-101.
10. Gonzalez MM, Berg RA, Nadkarni VM, et al. Left ventricular systolic function and outcome after in-hospital cardiac arrest. *Circulation.* 2008;117:1864-1872.
11. Cerchiari EL, Safar P, Klein E, Diven W. Visceral, hematologic and bacteriologic changes and neurologic outcome after cardiac arrest in dogs: the visceral post-resuscitation syndrome. *Resuscitation.* 1993;25:119-136.
12. Chua HR, Glassford N, Bellomo R. Acute kidney injury after cardiac arrest. *Resuscitation.* 2012;83:721-727.
13. Domanovits H, Schillinger M, Mullner M, et al. Acute renal failure after successful cardiopulmonary resuscitation. *Intensive Care Med.* 2001;27:1194-1199.
14. Sharfuddin AA, Molitoris BA. Pathophysiology of ischemic acute kidney injury. *Nat Rev Nephrol.* 2011;7:189-200.
15. Adler C, Reuter H, Seck C, et al. Fluid therapy and acute kidney injury in cardiogenic shock after cardiac arrest. *Resuscitation.* 2013;84:194-199.
16. Pene F, Hyvernat H, Mallet V, et al. Prognostic value of relative adrenal insufficiency after out-of-hospital cardiac arrest. *Intensive Care Med.* 2005;31:627-633.
17. Kim JJ, Lim YS, Shin JH, et al. Relative adrenal insufficiency after cardiac arrest: impact on postresuscitation disease outcome. *Am J Emerg Med.* 2006;24:684-688.
18. Miller JB, Donnino MW, Rogan M, Goyal N. Relative adrenal insufficiency in post-cardiac arrest shock is under-recognized. *Resuscitation.* 2008;76:221-225.
19. Laver S, Farrow C, Turner D, Nolan J. Mode of death after admission to an intensive care unit following cardiac arrest. *Intensive Care Med.* 2004;30:2126-2128.
20. Gaieski DF, Band RA, Abella BS, et al. Early goal-directed hemodynamic optimization combined with therapeutic hypothermia in comatose survivors of out-of-hospital cardiac arrest. *Resuscitation.* 2009;80:418-424.
21. Rivers E, Nguyen B, Havstad S, et al. Early goal-directed therapy in the treatment of severe sepsis and septic shock. *N Engl J Med.* 2001;345:1368-1377.
22. Starodub R, Abella BS, Grossestreuer AV, et al. Association of serum lactate and survival outcomes in patients undergoing therapeutic hypothermia after cardiac arrest. *Resuscitation.* 2013;84:1078-1082..
23. O'Connor RE, Brady W, Brooks SC, et al. Part 10: acute coronary syndromes: 2010 American Heart Association Guidelines for Cardiopulmonary Resuscitation and Emergency Cardiovascular Care. *Circulation.* 2010;122(18 suppl 3):S787-S817.
24. Dumas F, Cariou A, Manzo-Silberman S, et al. Immediate percutaneous coronary intervention is associated with better survival after out-of-hospital cardiac arrest: insights from the PROCAT (Parisian Region Out of hospital Cardiac ArresT) registry. *Circ Cardiovasc Interv.* 2010;3:200-207.
25. Strote JA, Maynard C, Olsufka M, et al. Comparison of role of early (less than six hours) to later (more than six hours) or no cardiac catheterization after resuscitation from out-of-hospital cardiac arrest. *Am J Cardiol.* 2012;109:451-454.
26. Helton TJ, Nadig V, Subramanya SD, et al. Outcomes of cardiac catheterization and percutaneous coronary intervention for in-hospital ventricular tachycardia or fibrillation cardiac arrest. *Catheter Cardiovasc Interv.* 2012;80:E9-E14.
27. Merchant RM, Abella BS, Khan M, et al. Cardiac catheterization is underutilized after in-hospital cardiac arrest. *Resuscitation.* 2008;79:398-403.
28. Khot S, Tirschwell DL. Long-term neurological complications after hypoxic-ischemic encephalopathy. *Semin Neurol.* 2006;26:422-431.
29. Wijdicks EF, Hijdra A, Young GB, et al. Practice parameter: prediction of outcome in comatose survivors after cardiopulmonary resuscitation (an evidence-based review): report of the Quality Standards Subcommittee of the American Academy of Neurology. *Neurology.* 2006;67:203-210.
30. Skrifvars MB, Parr MJ. Incidence, predisposing factors, management and survival following cardiac arrest due to subarachnoid haemorrhage: a review of the literature. *Scand J Trauma Resusc Emerg Med.* 2012;20:75.
31. Metter RB, Rittenberger JC, Guyette FX, Callaway CW. Association between a quantitative CT scan measure of brain edema and outcome after cardiac arrest. *Resuscitation.* 2011;82:1180-1185.
32. Hypothermia after Cardiac Arrest Study Group. Mild therapeutic hypothermia to improve the neurologic outcome after cardiac arrest. *N Engl J Med.* 2002;346:549-556.
33. Bernard SA, Gray TW, Buist MD, et al. Treatment of comatose survivors of out-of-hospital cardiac arrest with induced hypothermia. *N Engl J Med.* 2002;346:557-563.
34. Sagalyn E, Band RA, Gaieski DF, Abella BS. Therapeutic hypothermia after cardiac arrest in clinical practice: review and compilation of recent experiences. *Crit Care Med.* 2009;37(7 suppl):S223-S226.
35. Lundbye JB, Rai M, Ramu B, et al. Therapeutic hypothermia is associated with improved neurologic outcome and survival in cardiac arrest survivors of non-shockable rhythms. *Resuscitation.* 2012;83:202-207.
36. Testori C, Sterz F, Behringer W, et al. Mild therapeutic hypothermia is associated with favourable outcome in patients after cardiac arrest with non-shockable rhythms. *Resuscitation.* 2011;82:1162-1167.
37. Polderman KH. Mechanisms of action, physiological effects, and complications of hypothermia. *Crit Care Med.* 2009;37(7 suppl):S186-S202.
38. Center for Resuscitation Science, Department of Emergency Medicine, University of Pennsylvania. Available at www.med.upenn.edu/resuscitation/index.shtml. Accessed on October 2, 2013.
39. Chamorro C, Borrallo JM, Romera MA, et al. Anesthesia and analgesia protocol during therapeutic hypothermia after cardiac arrest: a systematic review. *Anesth Analg.* 2010;110:1328-1335.
40. Polderman KH, Herold I. Therapeutic hypothermia and controlled normothermia in the intensive care unit: practical considerations, side effects, and cooling methods. *Crit Care Med.* 2009;37:1101-1120.
41. Kliegel A, Janata A, Wandaller C, et al. Cold infusions alone are effective for induction of therapeutic hypothermia but do not keep patients cool after cardiac arrest. *Resuscitation.* 2007;73:46-53.
42. Merchant RM, Abella BS, Peberdy MA, et al. Therapeutic hypothermia after cardiac arrest: unintentional overcooling is common using ice packs and conventional cooling blankets. *Crit Care Med.* 2006;34(12 suppl):S490-S494.
43. Nielsen N, Hovdenes J, Nilsson F, et al. Outcome, timing and adverse events in therapeutic hypothermia after out-of-hospital cardiac arrest. *Acta Anaesthesiol Scand.* 2009;53:926-934.
44. Nishiyama N, Sato T, Aizawa Y, et al. Extreme QT prolongation during therapeutic hypothermia after cardiac arrest due to long QT syndrome. *Am J Emerg Med.* 2012;30:638 e635-638.
45. Arrich J. Clinical application of mild therapeutic hypothermia after cardiac arrest. *Crit Care Med.* 2007;35:1041-1047.
46. Nielsen N, Wetterslev J, Cronberg T, et al. Targeted temperature management at 33°C versus 36°C after cardiac arrest. *N Engl J Med.* 2013;369:2197-2206.
47. Perman SM, Kirkpatrick JN, Reitsma AM, et al. Timing of neuroprognostication in postcardiac arrest therapeutic hypothermia. *Crit Care Med.* 2012;40:719-724.
48. Rittenberger JC, Kelly E, Jang D, et al. Successful outcome utilizing hypothermia after cardiac arrest in pregnancy: a case report. *Crit Care Med.* 2008;36:1354-1356.
49. Jacobs R, Honore PM, Hosseinpour N, et al. Sudden cardiac arrest during pregnancy: a rare complication of acquired maternal diaphragmatic hernia. *Acta Clin Belg.* 2012;67:198-200.
50. Lee BK, Jeung KW, Lee HY, Lim JH. Outcomes of therapeutic hypothermia in unconscious patients after near-hanging. *Emerg Med J.* 2012;29:748-752.
51. Cohen V, Jellinek SP, Stansfield L, et al. Cardiac arrest with residual blindness after overdose of Tessalon(R) (benzonatate) perles. *J Emerg Med.* 2011;41:166-171.
52. Carlson DW, Pearson RD, Haggerty PF, et al. Commotio cordis, Therapeutic hypothermia, and evacuation from a United States military base in Iraq. *J Emerg Med.* 2013;44:620-624.
53. Hicks SD, DeFranco DB, Callaway CW. Hypothermia during reperfusion after asphyxial cardiac arrest improves functional recovery and selectively alters stress-induced protein expression. *J Cereb Blood Flow Metab.* 2000;20:520-530.
54. Colbourne F, Sutherland GR, Auer RN. Electron microscopic evidence against apoptosis as the mechanism of neuronal death in global ischemia. *J Neurosci.* 1999;19:4200-4210.

55. Bernard SA, Smith K, Cameron P, et al. Induction of prehospital therapeutic hypothermia after resuscitation from nonventricular fibrillation cardiac arrest. *Crit Care Med.* 2012;40:747-753.
56. Hammer L, Vitrat F, Savary D, et al. Immediate prehospital hypothermia protocol in comatose survivors of out-of-hospital cardiac arrest. *Am J Emerg Med.* 2009;27:570-573.
57. Topjian AA, Nadkarni VM, Berg RA. Cardiopulmonary resuscitation in children. *Curr Opin Crit Care.* 2009;15:203-208.
58. Jacobs S. Whole-body hypothermia for neonatal hypoxic-ischemic encephalopathy reduces mortality into childhood. *J Pediatr.* 2012;161:968-969.
59. Nichol G, Aufderheide TP, Eigel B, et al. Regional systems of care for out-of-hospital cardiac arrest: A policy statement from the American Heart Association. *Circulation.* 2010;121:709-729.
60. Nichol G, Thomas E, Callaway CW, et al. Regional variation in out-of-hospital cardiac arrest incidence and outcome. *JAMA.* 2008;300:1423-1431.
61. Donnino MW, Rittenberger JC, Gaieski D, et al. The development and implementation of cardiac arrest centers. *Resuscitation.* 2011;82:974-978.
62. Sudden Cardiac Arrest Association. Available at: http://www.suddencardiacarrest.org/aws/SCAA/pt/sp/home_page. Accessed on October 1, 2013.
63. Sudden Cardiac Arrest Foundation. Available at: http://www.sca-aware.org. Accessed on October 1, 2013.

CHAPTER 14

Pericarditis, Myocarditis, and Endocarditis

Nikki Waller and Abhi Mehrotra

IN THIS CHAPTER

Clinical presentation
Clinical findings and diagnostic tools
Diagnostic imaging and laboratory studies
Management and treatment strategies

Pericarditis and Myocarditis

Nonspecific symptoms of chest pain, palpitations, dyspnea, and syncope are common presenting complaints in the emergency department. Although unstable coronary artery lesions and myocardial infarction (MI) are foremost in the differential diagnosis, inflammation/disease of the pericardium, myocardium, and valves must also be considered. To correctly diagnose these relatively uncommon conditions, the clinician must recognize clinical risk factors and distinguishing findings on the physical examination and electrocardiogram (ECG).

CASE ONE

A 26-year-old truck driver presents to the emergency department complaining of central chest pain that began yesterday. He recently had an upper respiratory tract infection. The pain occurs with inspiration and is exacerbated with lying down but is not affected by exertion. The physical examination is grossly unremarkable, with these vital signs: blood pressure, 121/87 mm Hg; heart rate, 96 beats/min; respiratory rate, 16 breaths/min; temperature, 37.3°C; and oxygen saturation, 99% on room air. The evaluating team develops a differential diagnosis and enacts a diagnostic plan, along with administration of ibuprofen for analgesia. They are thinking about causes of chest pain in a young person with a recent respiratory tract infection, which include pleurisy and pericarditis.

An ECG (Figure 14-1A) reveals patterns consistent with pericarditis. The patient is discharged home, being advised to continue the ibuprofen, to schedule a followup appointment with his primary care physician, and to return to the emergency department if his condition worsens.

CASE TWO

A 21-year-old man presents with complaints of left-sided chest pain that woke him from sleep at 2 AM. He recently saw a physician for a sore throat and was prescribed amoxicillin/clavulanic acid (Augmentin), despite a negative rapid strep test. He has been taking the antibiotic for 2 days. His examination is grossly unremarkable, with these vital signs: blood pressure, 135/87 mm Hg; heart rate, 71 beats/min; respiratory rate, 20 breaths/min; temperature, 35.9°C; and oxygen saturation, 98% on room air. The evaluating team develops a differential diagnosis that includes pneumonia, pleurisy, and costochondritis. They undertake a corresponding diagnostic plan and prescribe ibuprofen for analgesia. The patient's ECG is shown in Figure 14-2.

No further testing is performed. The patient is diagnosed with pericarditis and discharged home with a prescription for indomethacin and instructions to arrange followup care from

CARDIOVASCULAR EMERGENCIES

FIGURE 14-1A.

Initial ECG of patient in Case One. Interpretation: normal sinus rhythm, diffuse ST elevation, and PR depression in leads II, III, and aVF, which is consistent with pericarditis.

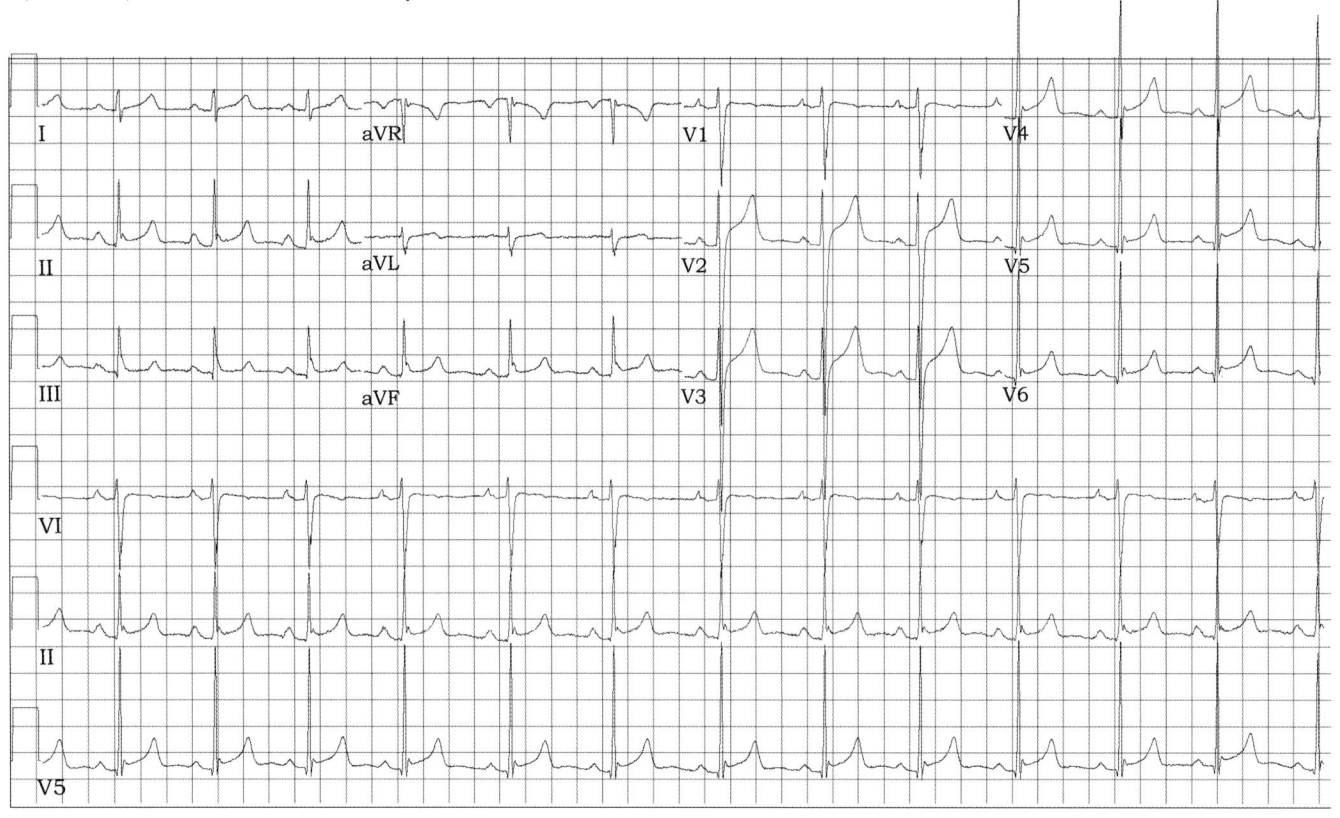

FIGURE 14-1B.

Patient's ECG 2 days later, demonstrating continued diffuse ST elevation.

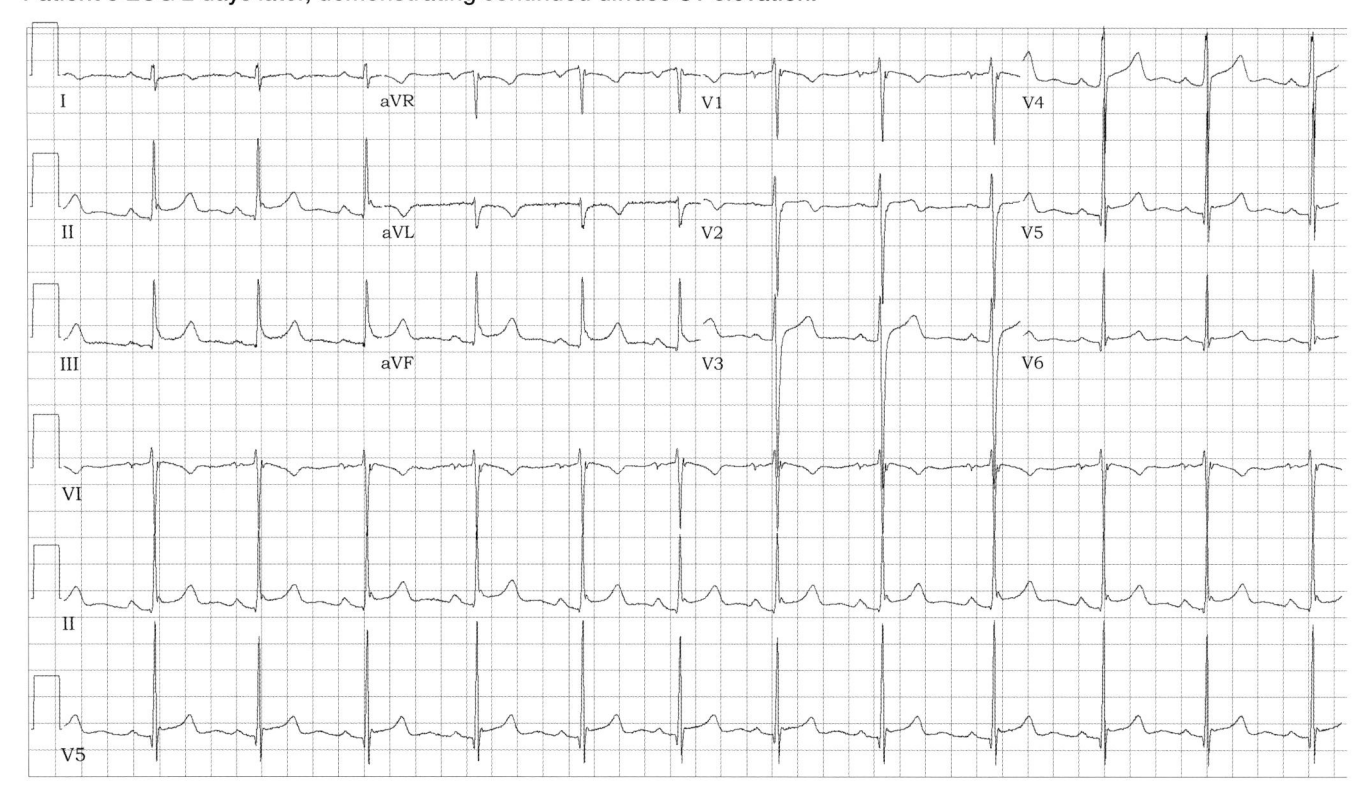

Pericarditis, Myocarditis, and Endocarditis

FIGURE 14-1C.
Patient's ECG 2 weeks later, demonstrating the ST segments moving toward the baseline, with development of anterolateral T-wave inversions.

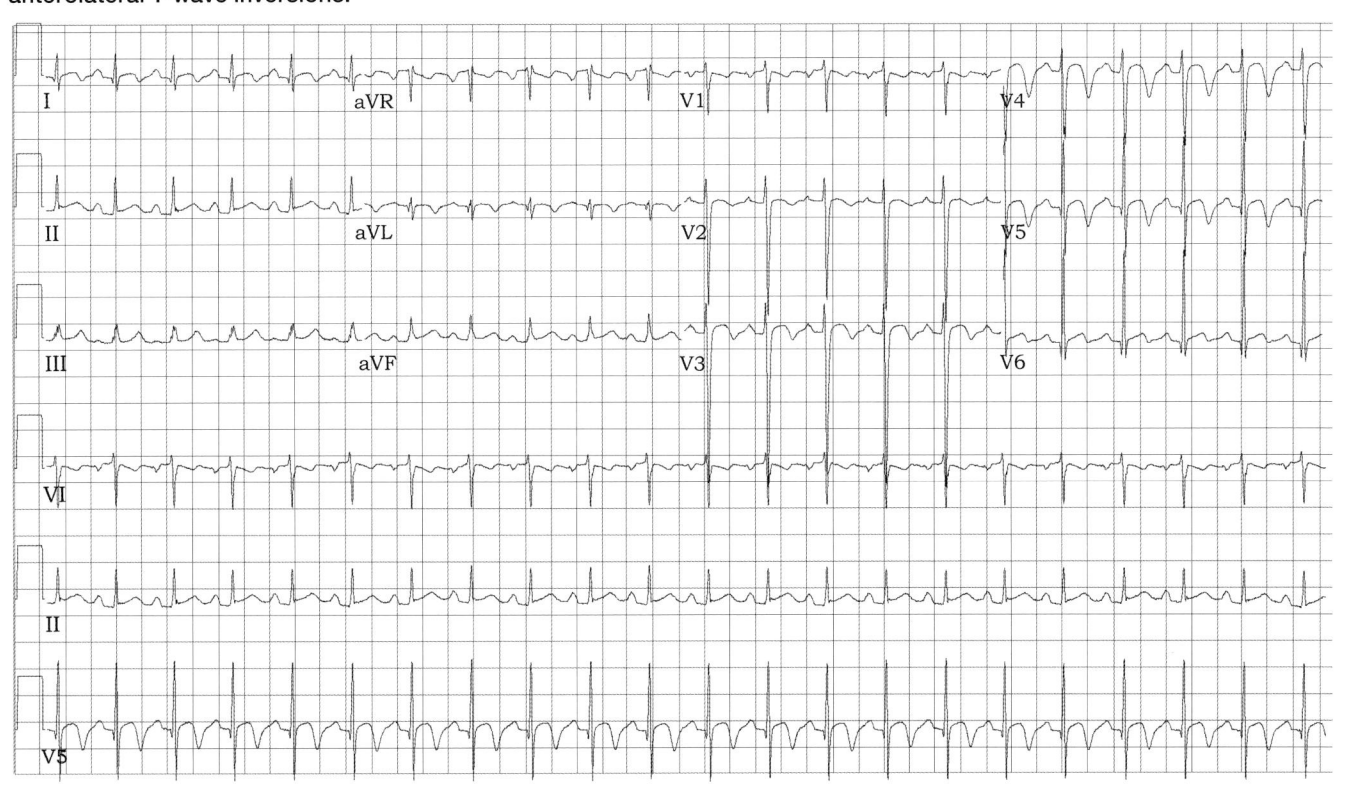

FIGURE 14-1D.
Patient's ECG 2 months later, showing ST segments returning to baseline and some persistent T-wave inversions.

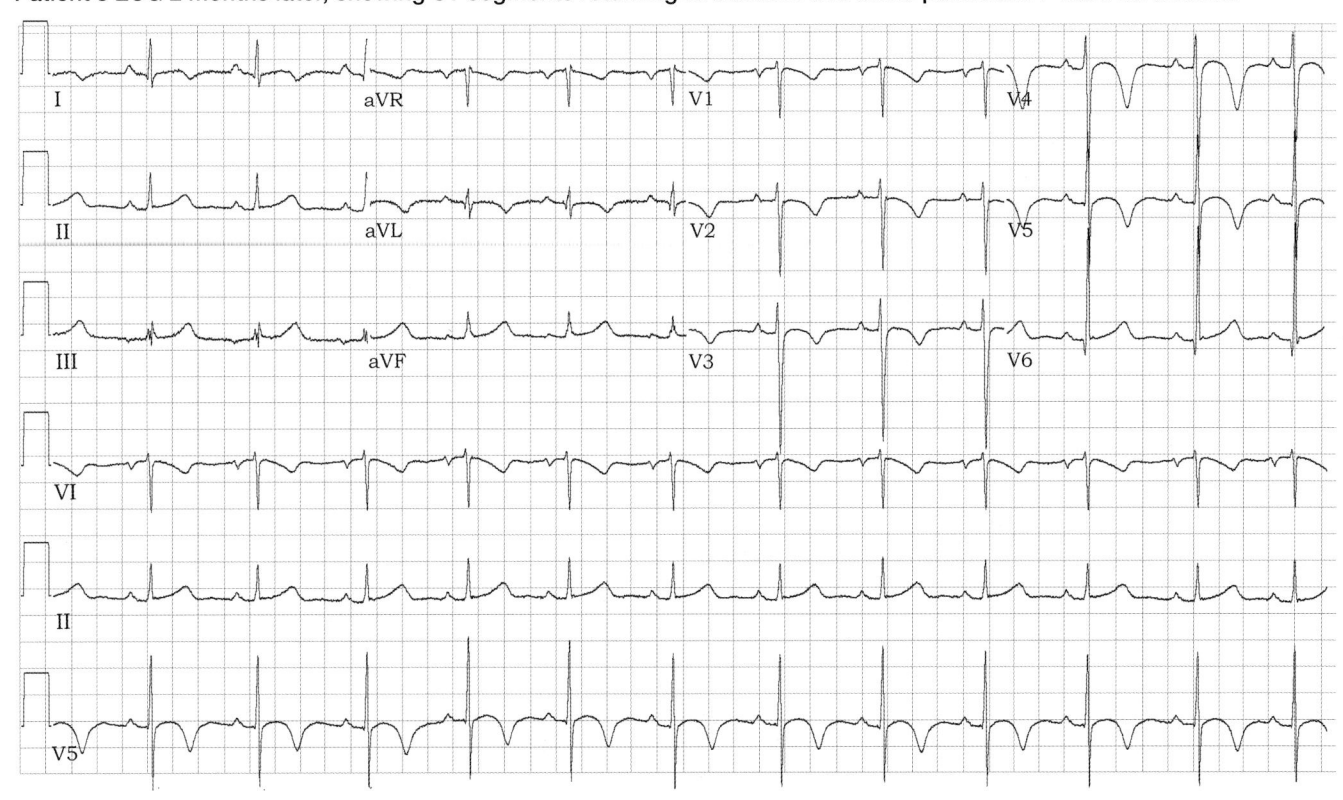

his primary care physician and to return to the emergency department if necessary.

Both of these cases involve young patients who presented to the emergency department with chest pain that caused enough concern to lead them to seek medical assistance. The differential diagnosis in both presentations includes pericarditis and myocarditis, which are frequently difficult to differentiate during an initial emergency department presentation.[1] Although these conditions are similar, their course of illness can be quite different. The outcomes of these patients will highlight the difficulty in identifying which patients will experience clinically important complications despite a relatively benign presentation. The patient in Case One ultimately required drainage of a pericardial effusion, and the patient in Case Two developed heart failure from myocarditis.

In this chapter, rather than silo the diseases, we present a typical approach for the undifferentiated patient in the emergency department. We discuss the disease processes, diagnostic approaches, and potential complications that emergency physicians need to understand.

A brief review of anatomy is important in order to understand the implications of the clinical presentation. The pericardium is divided into an inner layer—the visceral pericardium—and an outer layer—the parietal pericardium. The outer parietal layer is fibrous and helps to stabilize the heart within the chest cavity. These two layers are separated by a potential space, the pericardial sac, which usually contains a small amount of fluid.[2] Acute pericarditis is defined as inflammation affecting these layers. Myocarditis, on the other hand, is inflammation of the myocardium itself.

Acute pericarditis and myocarditis can be differentiated into infectious and noninfectious causes. In many instances, a specific cause is not elucidated in the emergency department but is later identified during inpatient workup. Causes of pericarditis are listed in Table 14-1. Even after extensive workups, most cases are categorized as idiopathic. Despite this fact, it is important to screen for causes that require specific interventions, have prognostic importance, and place the patient at risk for complications.[3] Common causes of myocarditis are listed in Table 14-2. In the developed world, viral causes such as adenovirus and parvovirus B19 are the most common.[4] Again, while identification of a source might not be integral to emergency department management, understanding the pathogenesis of the inflammation can facilitate treatment and anticipate complications.

Clinical Presentation and Evaluation

The presentations of pericarditis and myocarditis are often nonspecific (fatigue, chest pain, shortness of breath) and attributed to other more common diagnoses such as viral or acute coronary syndromes. The emergency physician is ultimately responsible for stabilizing the patient and making the correct diagnosis. Complications of pericarditis are closely linked to specific causes, so patients at risk should be screened appropriately. For example, patients with pericarditis due to malignancy are at increased risk for clinically significant effusions. Patients with bacterial pericarditis can go on to develop restrictive pericarditis if not treated aggressively.

Acute pericarditis is usually recognized from a combination of symptoms, the physical examination findings, and an ECG.

FIGURE 14-2.

ECG from Case Two. Interpretation: normal sinus rhythm with subtle ST elevation and PR depression in multiple leads.

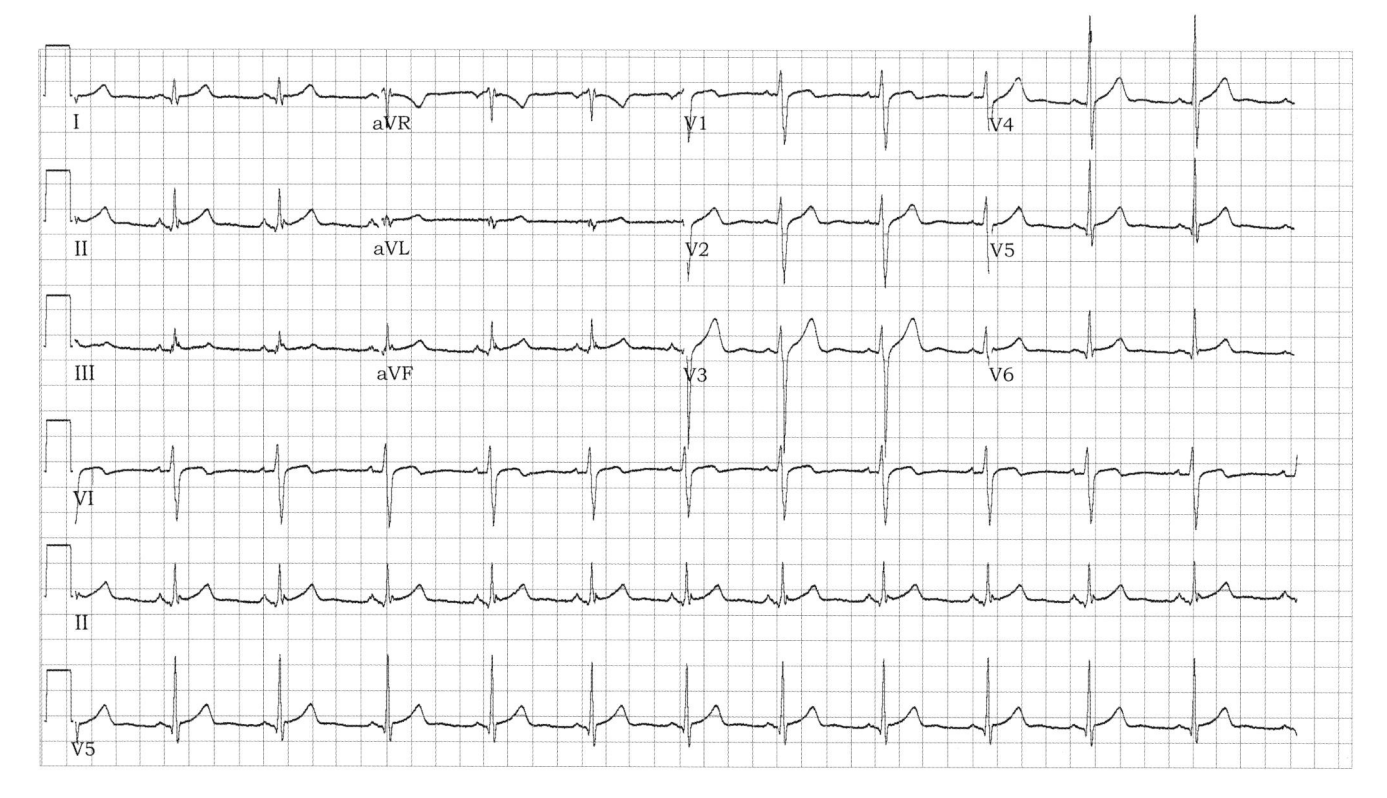

The classic presentation is pleuritic chest pain that is exacerbated by lying down and relieved by leaning forward. A pericardial friction rub might be heard during the physical examination. If the patient has progressed to tamponade, examination findings will include tachycardia, hypotension, and pulsus paradoxus. The ECG findings indicative of acute pericarditis vary depending on time since onset of symptoms. The stages evolve over days to weeks. The initial findings are diffuse ST elevation with PR depression, along with ST depression in leads aVR and V_1. As the disease progresses, the PR and ST segments normalize and the T waves flatten. This is followed by deep T-wave inversion, which can be permanent; however, eventually, the ECG usually normalizes. This progression point is illustrated in the ECGs for Case One (Figures 14-1A, B, and C).

KEY POINTS

Electrocardiographic findings associated with pericarditis:
    Stage 1: diffuse ST elevation; in leads that do not have ST elevation, look for PR deviation.
    Stage 2: normalization of ST and PR segments
    Stage 3: diffuse T-wave inversions
    Stage 4: normalization of the ECG, although T-wave inversions might persist

Pericarditis compared to acute MI on ECG[5]:
    ST elevation with an acute MI reflects an anatomic area of infarction with reciprocal changes in leads 180° from the elevation. With pericarditis, the ST changes are more generalized.

In pericarditis, ST elevation rarely exceeds 5 mm.

PR-segment elevation in lead aVR is an indication of an atrial current of injury and can occur in either acute pericarditis or acute MI. However, acute pericarditis is more likely to cause PR-segment depression in multiple leads, whereas acute MI typically produces ST-segment depression ("reciprocal depression") in some leads (Figures 14-3 and 14-4).

The role of further diagnostic studies in the emergency department for patients with suspected pericarditis is to identify causes and potential complications. A chest radiograph might identify a cause (eg, pneumonia, malignancy) or provide clues as to the presence of an effusion (eg, an altered cardiac silhouette). Bedside ultrasonography can provide an assessment of the pericardial space for an effusion, which can be very useful in planning the management of these patients. Echocardiography is virtually diagnostic for pericardial effusion and should be obtained in patients with hemodynamic instability (tachycardia and/or hypotension) or co-existing diseases that cause effusive pericarditis (malignancy, systemic inflammatory diseases, tuberculosis).

Laboratory evaluations in cases of suspected pericarditis are also directed at searching for a cause. The following tests can be considered:
- Complete blood count (CBC) to evaluate for leukocytosis
- Chemistries to evaluate for uremia
- Cardiac biomarkers to evaluate for myocardial cell

TABLE 14-1.
Causes of Pericarditis

Infectious
- Viral
  - Coxsackievirus A and B, echovirus, adenovirus, influenza, parvovirus, Epstein-Barr virus
- Bacterial
  - Tuberculosis, *Staphylococcus*, *Mycoplasma*, others
- Fungal and parasitic

Noninfectious
- Systemic diseases
  - System lupus erythematosus (SLE), rheumatoid arthritis, Sjögren syndrome, sarcoidosis
- Metabolic
  - Uremia, hypothyroidism
- Medication related
  - Phenytoin, isoniazid, procainamide, hydralazine
- Neoplastic

Traumatic
- Radiation, direct injury, Dressler syndrome

TABLE 14-2.
Causes of Myocarditis

Infectious
- Viral (eg, coxsackievirus A and B, adenovirus, cytomegalovirus, HIV, Epstein-Barr virus)
- Bacterial (eg, tuberculosis; *Mycoplasma*; *Staphylococcus*)
- Spirochetes (Lyme disease, syphilis)
- Protozoa (malaria; Chagas disease)

Noninfectious
- Systemic diseases
  - Autoimmune (sarcoidosis, giant cell, Wegener granulomatosis, SLE, celiac disease, Takayasu arteritis, Kawasaki disease)
  - Eosinophil related (Loeffler syndrome, Churg-Strauss syndrome)
- Toxin
  - Drug-induced (penicillin, cephalosporins, diuretics, sulfonamides, clozapine, lithium)
  - Cocaine
  - Snake bite

CARDIOVASCULAR EMERGENCIES

FIGURE 14-3.
ECG consistent with anterolateral MI demonstrates ST elevation in leads I, aVL, and V$_1$ through V$_6$ and reciprocal ST-segment depression in the inferior leads III and aVF.

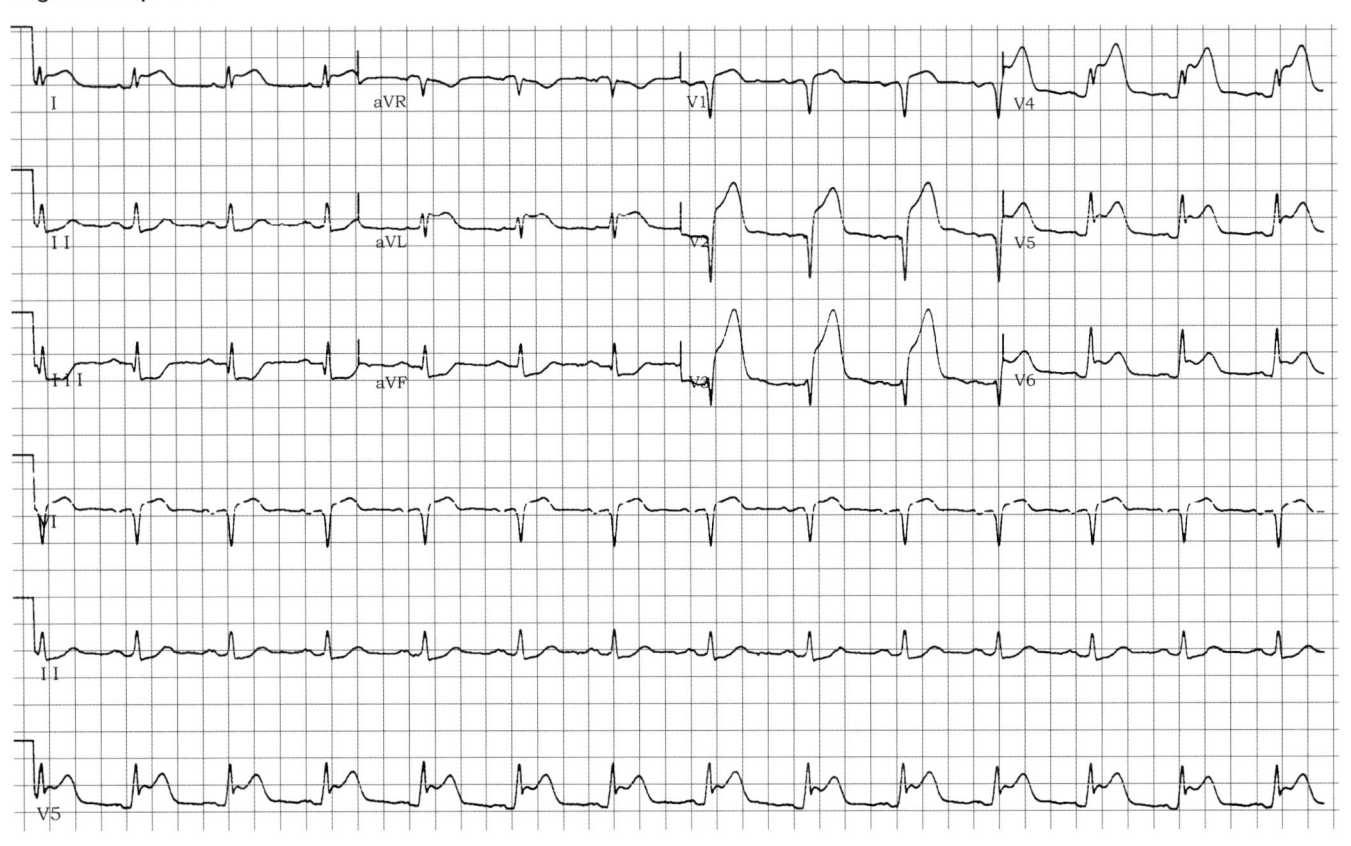

FIGURE 14-4.
ECG consistent with pericarditis demonstrates ST-segment elevations and PR-segment depressions in multiple leads.

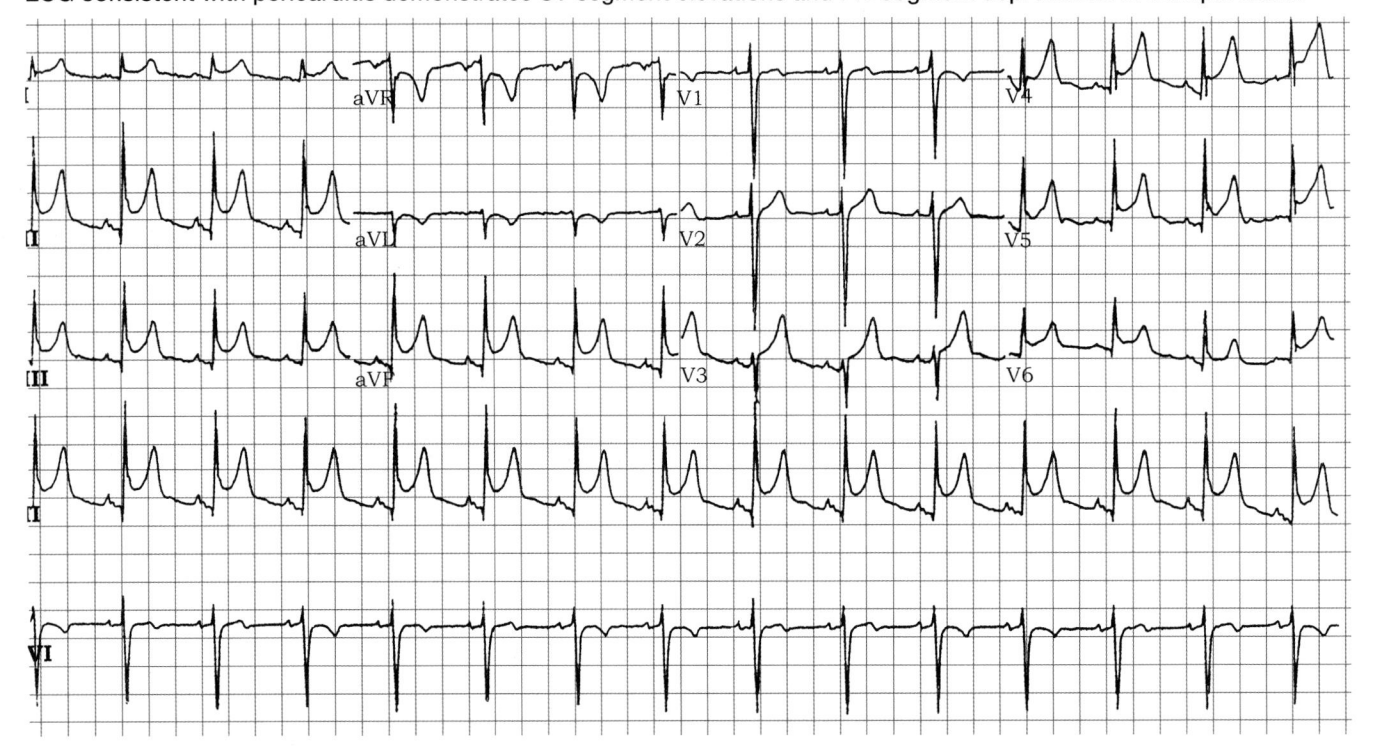

damage (Troponin might be mildly elevated; however, significant troponin elevations should prompt consideration of myocarditis.)
- Inflammatory markers such as the erythrocyte sedimentation rate (ESR) and C-reactive protein (CRP)

Patients with myocarditis usually present with symptoms consistent with a viral syndrome (fever, myalgia, headache, nausea/vomiting) but can also have signs of heart failure. Patient presentations vary according to the phase of the disease, as follows:
- Acute infection/inflammatory reaction—fever, myalgia, vague chest pain
- Myocardial inflammation—chest discomfort, arrhythmia, pulmonary congestion
- Progression to dilated cardiomyopathy—dyspnea, orthopnea, syncope.

Again, in the acute presentation, focusing on clinical stabilization and establishing the diagnosis are most important; searching for a cause usually requires a longer diagnostic workup. Understanding the causes (Table 14-2) can facilitate a more directed history and physical examination. The clinical evaluation is very similar to the approach used for pericarditis, including ECG analysis, chest radiograph, and laboratory studies. The most common ECG finding is sinus tachycardia, although ST-segment changes and arrhythmias could be noted. Recommended diagnostic laboratory studies for myocarditis include the following:
- CBC to evaluate for leukocytosis
- Chemistries to evaluate for uremia
- Cardiac biomarkers to evaluate for myocardial cell damage. Some studies have noted that the sensitivity of troponin to detect myocarditis is 35%, with a specificity of 89%.[6] B-type natriuretic peptide (BNP) gives an indication of heart failure as a result of the disease.
- Inflammatory markers—ESR and CRP—might be elevated but are nonspecific.[4]

Bedside echocardiography can be helpful in screening for findings supportive of the working diagnosis of myocarditis such as focal wall motion abnormalities, global hypokinesis, or pericardial effusion. Echocardiography can also demonstrate focal or diffuse edema associated with an inflammatory process. Although endomyocardial biopsy has been the diagnostic gold standard, its clinical applicability is limited, with only two Class I recommendations.[7] There are concerns about the number of samples necessary to obtain a diagnosis, along with interobserver variability. Given these limitations, diagnostic imaging has become significantly more prevalent in the evaluation of myocarditis. In fact, with utilization of specific techniques with cardiac magnetic resonance imaging (CMR), diagnostic accuracy approaches 78%.[8]

Three CMR sequences, as follows, can assist in the diagnosis:
- T2-weighted images (identify edema)
- T1-weighted images (identify hyperemia)
- Late gadolinium enhancement (identifies necrosis, fibrosis)

CMR provides the benefit of assessing the entire myocardium, as opposed to the individual areas that were selected for biopsy.

CASE ONE, CONTINUED

The patient returns to the emergency department 48 hours later with persistent pain and a new complaint of dyspnea. A repeat examination is unremarkable. His vital signs are as follows: blood pressure, 131/95 mm Hg; heart rate, 88 beats/min; respiratory rate, 18 breaths/min; temperature, 36.2°C; and oxygen saturation, 100% on room air.

The evaluating team orders a repeat ECG (Figure 14-1B), chest radiograph, and laboratory evaluation. His chest radiograph is unchanged from the previous visit. The cardiac biomarkers are negative, except for a mildly elevated troponin I (0.413 ng/mL). He is admitted to the hospital for telemetry monitoring and further evaluation. Another echocardiogram shows normal left ventricular ejection fraction (55% to 60%). The patient is discharged from the hospital on ibuprofen and colchicine, with instructions for close followup.

CASE TWO, CONTINUED

An echocardiogram demonstrates a low-normal ejection fraction and hypokinesis. The patient is started on carvedilol and lisinopril and then discharged 2 days later with no clinical symptoms. His discharge ECG shows T-wave abnormality in the inferior leads and flipped T waves developed laterally.

The patient returns to the emergency department approximately 12 hours after discharge with complaints of profound fatigue and persistent chest pain on exertion that had not been alleviated by a nonsteroidal anti-inflammatory drug (NSAID). His examination findings are unchanged, with the following vital signs: blood pressure, 155/89 mm Hg (lying down); heart rate, 76 beats/min; respiratory rate, 12 breaths/min; temperature, 36.7°C; oxygen saturation, 100% on room air.

Based on the results of his recent evaluation, the team pursues a more thorough workup, expanding the differential diagnosis to consider other conditions that can present as pericarditis. Repeat screening laboratory tests are significant for elevated cardiac markers—CK, 517 units/L; CK-MB, 39.9 ng/mL; and troponin, 12.30 ng/mL. The patient is admitted to the cardiology service for telemetry monitoring, and an echocardiogram is performed, which is also read as normal left ventricular function with an estimated ejection fraction of more than 55%.

The patient had further evaluation with serial cardiac markers and CMR (Figure 14-5). The markers continued to trend up, with a troponin peak of 16 ng/mL. He continued to take indomethacin and began feeling well.

Management

In both pericarditis and myocarditis, the prognosis is somewhat dependent on the inciting cause. The vast majority of patients with pericarditis may be treated with a 7- to 10-day course of high-dose aspirin, ibuprofen, or indomethacin, a Class I recommendation (Table 14-3). Colchicine has been shown to hasten resolution of symptoms and decrease recurrences and has a Class IIa recommendation.[9] Hospitalization is indicated for patients with pericarditis if interventions are necessary to address complications such as large effusions, cardiac tamponade, immunosuppression, and anticoagulation.[10] Recurrent pericarditis as well as constrictive pericarditis have significant associated morbidities.

The emergency department management of myocarditis is usually aimed at treating the systolic dysfunction and associated arrhythmias. Most patients are admitted to a telemetry unit for further evaluation of the cause, assessment of pump function, and telemetry monitoring. Although an array of therapies specific to individual causes of myocarditis is available (antivirals, anti-inflammatories, and immunoglobulin therapy), none requires administration in the emergency department.

Complications of Pericarditis

Complications of pericarditis include pericardial effusion and development of a constrictive pericardium. The likelihood of developing one of these complications largely depends on the underlying cause. The most common cause of pericarditis in an otherwise well patient is a viral infection, and the vast majority of these infections resolve without complications.[11] In contrast, bacterial pericarditis, although rare, is notable for a high rate of complications due to the exuberant inflammatory response that leads to effusions and subsequent constrictive pericarditis. Neoplastic and systemic diseases can also lead to the development of pericardial effusions. Clinically significant pericardial effusions are most often associated with diseases that involve the visceral serosa, (eg, adenocarcinomas of the breast and lung and systemic inflammatory conditions such as systemic lupus erythematosus [SLE]).

The clinical presentation of pericardial effusions depends on the etiology of the effusion and the rate at which the fluid has accumulated. The likelihood that an effusion will compromise cardiac output is related to the rate of accumulation and the size of the effusion. Rapidly collecting effusions, as seen after trauma, cause compensatory tachycardia and ultimately hypotension with relatively small volumes accumulated in the pericardium. In contrast, slowly developing effusions, as seen in neoplastic pericardial disease, can have minimal hemodynamic effects until a relatively large pericardial volume has collected. When the pericardium can stretch slowly, more than 1,000 mL of fluid can accumulate without a significant increase in pressure; in contrast, rapid accumulation of as little as 200 mL increases pericardial pressure, leading to hemodynamic compromise.

CASE THREE

A 35-year-old man with no relevant medical history presents with a sore throat, fever, and chest pain. His vital signs are as follows: blood pressure, 145/90 mm Hg; heart rate, 122 beats/min; respiratory rate, 24 breaths/min; and temperature, 38.3°C. His examination is notable for exudative pharyngitis, clear lungs, muffled heart sounds, and no rash. His ECG is consistent with pericarditis (Figure 14-4), and he is treated with naproxen and intravenous fluids. After infusion of 2 L of normal saline, the patient remains tachycardic and then develops shaking chills and a temperature of 39.4°C.

CASE FOUR

A 32-year-old woman with known metastatic breast cancer presents to the emergency department complaining of feeling light-headed and nearly passing out while climbing the stairs. Her vital signs are as follows: heart rate, 128 beats/min; blood pressure, 98/60 mm Hg; respiratory rate, 18 breaths/min, and temperature, 36.4°C. Her examination is notable for distended neck veins, muffled heart sounds, clear lungs, and 2+ pedal edema, which developed over the past 2 weeks. An ECG shows a sinus tachycardia with diffusely decreased voltage and electrical alternans (Figure 14-6).

FIGURE 14-5.

In the two- and four-chamber views (left and right, respectively), the blood pool is highlighted with contrast and healthy myocardium is dark. The patchy areas at the apex of the myocardium indicate myocarditis.

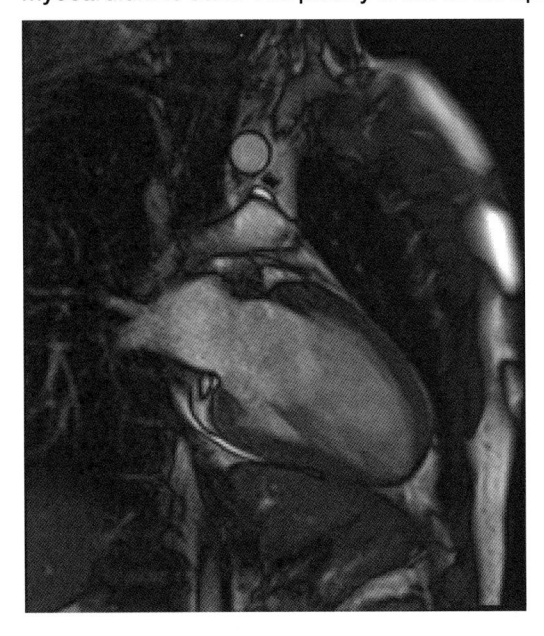

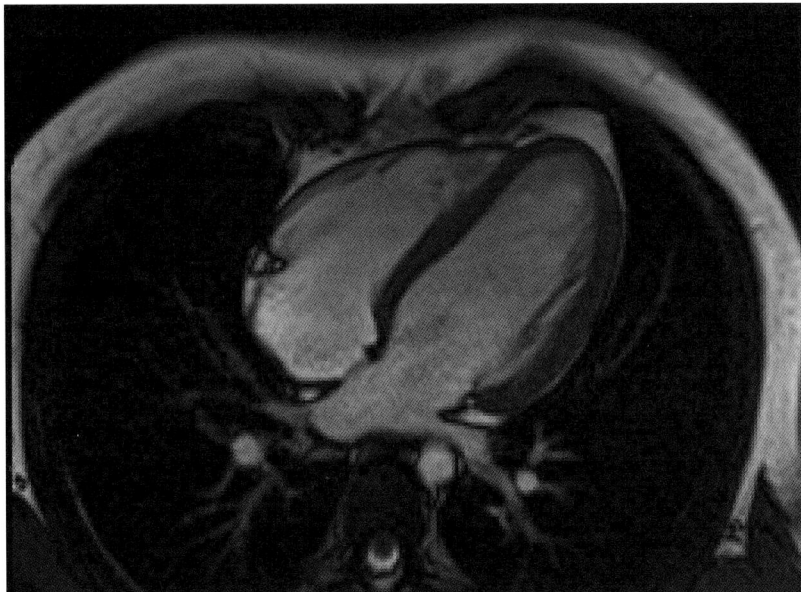

Both of these cases reveal findings that should raise the clinician's suspicion for a pericardial effusion. In the first case, the patient has sustained tachycardia in spite of a fluid bolus and antipyretics. Moreover, his clinical condition is deteriorating rapidly, with the development of shaking chills and a high fever, which is more consistent with a bacterial process than a viral infection. The chance that the pericardial effusion is bacterial, and hence purulent, should be of great concern, and mandates an entirely different treatment plan than nonsteroidal anti-inflammatory drugs and observation.

The second case causes even more concern because the patient has an underlying disease that puts her at high risk for effusive pericarditis. She is clearly hemodynamically compromised and has an ECG that demonstrates electrical alternans. Echocardiography will demonstrate the presence of a pericardial effusion, allow approximation of its volume, and, importantly, indicate whether it is hemodynamically significant.

KEY POINTS

Indications for urgent echocardiography in patients with pericarditis:

- Signs of hemodynamic instability (tachycardia, hypotension)
- Signs and symptoms of heart failure (dyspnea, presyncope/syncope, pedal edema)
- ECG clues such as low voltage or electrical alternans
- High-risk comorbidities such as lung or breast cancer or systemic diseases such as SLE, uremia, hypothyroidism
- Clinical presentations for which pericardiocentesis will be diagnostic/therapeutic, such as bacterial or mycobacterial disease

Pericardial Tamponade

Cardiac tamponade results from compression of the heart caused by the accumulation of fluid, pus, blood, clots, or gas within the pericardial space. The pericardium's ability to stretch varies with the rate of fluid accumulation. Rapidly accumulating collections create tamponade physiology at relatively small volumes. At some point, the intrapericardial pressure becomes high enough to impede cardiac filling, so cardiac output is impaired. The most common cause of cardiac tamponade is malignancy, particularly lung cancer, which is involved in more than 50% of all tamponade cases.[12,13]

The clinical findings associated with tamponade are often vague and nonspecific. They include dyspnea, hypotension, tachycardia, elevated jugular venous pressure, and pulsus paradoxus. A logical approach to making the diagnosis is to first suspect tamponade in patients with pericarditis and signs of hemodynamic compromise, specifically sustained tachycardia and/or hypotension. The second is to consider the diagnosis in patients presenting with tachycardia or hypotension of unclear cause, particularly those with comorbidities that would place them at risk for pericardial effusions. Finally, the clinician should have a low threshold for obtaining an echocardiogram in patients with an underlying disease that places them at risk for an effusive pericarditis. The diagnosis of cardiac tamponade is based on clinical suspicion, risk factors, clinical findings suggesting impaired cardiac output, and echocardiographic findings.

KEY POINTS

Sonographic diagnosis of a potentially hemodynamically compromising pericardial effusion is right atrial/ventricular diastolic collapse. Dilation of the inferior vena cava and a reduction of less than 50% in the diameter of the dilated inferior vena cava during inspiration (inferior vena cava plethora), reflecting a marked elevation in the central venous pressure, is seen frequently.[14]

Demonstration of at least 1 cm of pericardial fluid by echocardiogram suggests that pericardiocentesis can be performed safely.

Patients who are already hemodynamically unstable should have volume expansion. Positive-pressure ventilation should be avoided in these patients.[9]

CASE THREE, CONTINUED

Despite treatment with intravenous fluids and anti-inflammatory agents, the patient continues to appear ill, with sustained tachycardia. His temperature spikes to 39.4°C. Bedside echocardiography is performed and shows a pericardial effusion with fibrinous material within the effusion (Figure 14-7) without evidence of tamponade physiology. The patient is admitted for diagnostic pericardiocentesis; the pericardial fluid culture grew group A beta-hemolytic streptococci. A pericardial drain was inserted, and the patient was discharged 2 weeks later, following a course of intravenous antibiotics. Three months lat-

TABLE 14-3.

Medications for the Treatment of Acute Pericarditis

Medication	Dosage	Duration
Ibuprofen	300 to 800 mg every 6 to 8 hours	7 to 10 days
Aspirin	800 mg every 6 to 8 hours	7 to 10 days
Indomethacin	25 to 50 mg three times daily	Taper as symptoms improve
Colchicine	0.5 mg twice daily	3 months
Steroids	20 to 80 mg daily	For patients with connective tissue disease

er, he returned to the emergency department with signs and symptoms of heart failure. Echocardiography and right heart catheterization demonstrated the development of constrictive pericarditis.

CASE FOUR, CONTINUED

Bedside echocardiography shows a large pericardial effusion with right ventricular collapse (Figure 14-8). The patient is treated initially with intravenous fluids and is admitted to the hospital for a pericardial window. Subsequent pathology revealed a malignant effusion. She did well postoperatively, and the remainder of her course was determined by her primary malignancy.

KEY POINTS

Pericardiocentesis should be performed in the emergency department when a patient has a hemodynamically compromising effusion and hypotension or shock that is resistant to intravenous fluids.

Pericardiocentesis should be performed under sonographic guidance.

Sonography allows selection of the aspiration site closest to the effusion and minimizes the risk of inadvertent puncture of adjacent organs (heart, liver, lung).

Complications of Myocarditis

In the vast majority of patients, the disease course of myocarditis is self-limiting and resolves with minimal long-term effects. It is likely that most cases are never clinically recognized because the cardiac signs and symptoms are overshadowed by systemic manifestations of fever, myalgia, and fatigue. Patients who develop heart failure typically have an insidious onset of symptoms, and the diagnosis is often made when they present with fatigue, orthopnea, exertional dyspnea, and pedal edema. They are at risk for complications such as arrhythmia, sudden death, and stroke, similar to those of patients with heart failure from other causes. The mortality rate for patients with biopsy-proven myocarditis was as high as 19% in a population that was followed for more than 4 years.[15]

Myocarditis can also have a fulminant course, with the development of overt cardiac failure within days to weeks after a viral prodrome. Typically, patients report having had symptoms consistent with a recent viral infection (fevers, malaise, cough, gastroenteritis) and then become quite ill 1 to 2 weeks later. The classic presentation in the emergency department is a relatively healthy adult or child in cardiogenic shock. First-line treatment is supportive care and screening for reversible causes. This usually requires urgent myocardial imaging and cardiac catheterization to exclude coronary artery and valvular diseases. Most of these patients require inotropic support and, in many cases, an intra-aortic balloon pump. Given the severity of illness and the relative youth of many of these patients, extraordinary measures, including percutaneous extracorporeal membranous oxygenation, are often required to support life. The role of extracorporeal membranous oxygenation is to stabilize neurologic, pulmonary, and renal function while allowing time for ventricular recovery. If cardiac function does not improve, the patient can be bridged with a ventricular assist device, which has been shown to improve cardiac geometry and reduce wall

FIGURE 14-6.

Electrical alternans. This ECG demonstrates the low voltage that is prevalent when a pericardial effusion develops and the heart's position within the chest cavity varies on a beat-to-beat basis as it swings within the effusion.

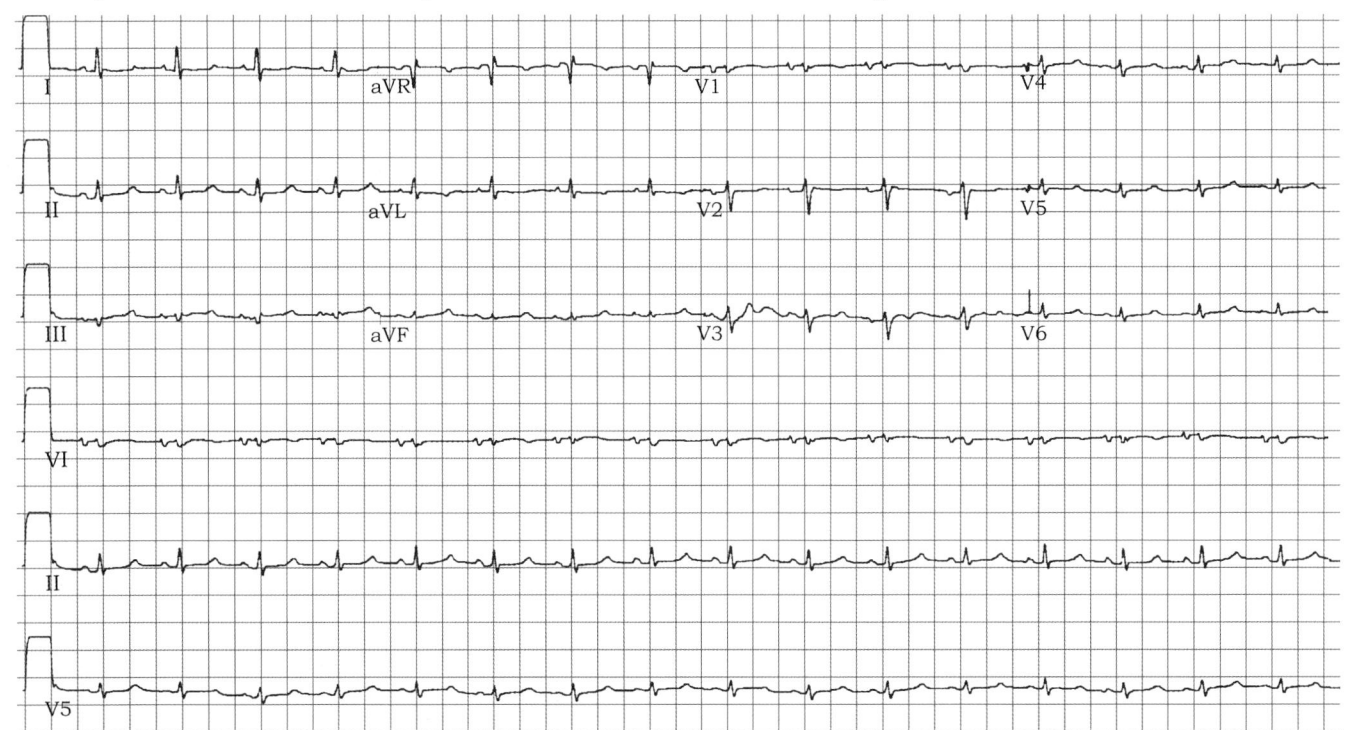

stress, thus improving cardiomyocyte function.[16,17]

Ironically, although presenting in extremis, patients diagnosed with fulminant myocarditis can make a full recovery without the long-term cardiac complications typically associated with acute myocarditis.[17] McCarthy and colleagues compared outcomes in 147 patients with myocarditis, classifying cases as either fulminant (patients with acute onset of symptoms and severe hemodynamic compromise requiring high-dose vasopressor agents or ventricular assist device support and positive biopsy results) or acute (patients with indistinct, prolonged onset of symptoms, less severe signs of heart failure, and positive biopsy results). Among the 15 patients with fulminant myocarditis, 2 required ventricular assist device support, and the 1- and 11-year transplant-free survival rates were both 93%. Patients with acute myocarditis had a 1-year transplant-free survival of 85% and an 11-year transplant-free survival of 45%.[17] Despite the catastrophic presentation of patients with fulminant presentations, full cardiac recovery is possible and even likely. Paradoxically, patients with more benign presentations often have a worse long-term prognosis.

KEY POINTS

Fulminant myocarditis is more likely to develop in infants and young adults than in older patients.

Patients with acute heart failure from fulminant myocarditis should be treated aggressively because they are likely to make a full recovery.

Pericarditis and myocarditis result from inflammation of the structures surrounding the heart and the muscle tissue.

FIGURE 14-7.

This subxiphoid view of the heart shows a pericardial effusion with echogenic fibrinous material contained within it. The effusion was aspirated for culture, which subsequently grew group A beta-hemolytic streptococci.

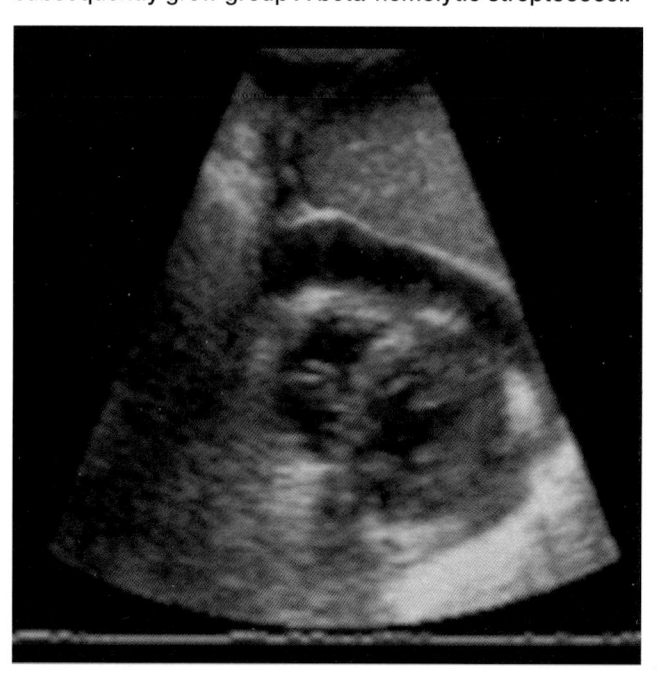

The clinical presentation of these conditions is often subtle and readily confused with other more commonly encountered conditions. So far, this chapter has described the clinical presentation, role of diagnostic studies, treatment plans, and complications of inflammatory conditions affecting the pericardium and myocardium. We will now discuss inflammation of the valves, which can present with equally subtle and nonspecific complaints.

Endocarditis

The diagnosis of infective endocarditis is rarely made in the emergency department because it is relatively uncommon and presenting signs and symptoms are similar to other more commonly encountered clinical conditions. Furthermore, there are no studies or data specific to emergency department patients that are available to guide emergency physicians in identifying and treating patients with this condition. Therefore, physicians must understand the various ways patients can present, as well as the disease process, the patients it tends to affect, and the bacteria that are commonly involved.

CASE FIVE

A 55-year-old man presents to the emergency department after experiencing 3 weeks of fever, fatigue, myalgia, and weight loss. He had been seen twice before at another emergency department and was diagnosed each time with a viral infection. He has had fever, chills, and night sweats daily. He reports no relevant medical history, except having "a heart murmur as a child." The physical examination is significant for a fever and a holosystolic ejection murmur, loudest at the apex.

CASE SIX

A 30-year-old man presents to the emergency department

FIGURE 14-8.

This subxiphoid view of the heart shows a large circumferential pericardial effusion. The right ventricle is completely collapsed. The patient was taken to the operating room for a pericardial window.

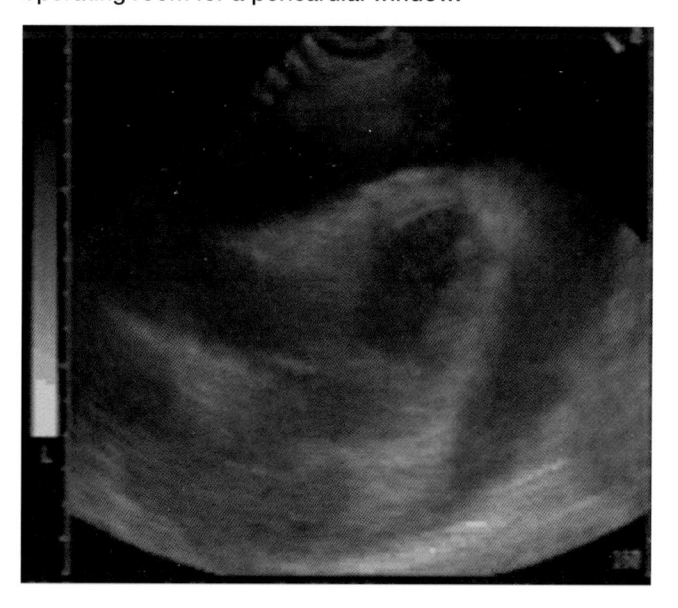

with fever, shortness of breath, and a painful left arm. He admits to intravenous drug use. His physical examination is significant for stable vital signs, except for a temperature of 38.9°C, basilar crackles on lung auscultation, a soft systolic cardiac murmur, and a large fluctuant mass in his left antecubital region. The abscess is drained by simple incision in the emergency department, and the patient is admitted for intravenous antibiotics and hemodynamic monitoring. An admission ECG (Figure 14-9) shows a type I second-degree atrioventricular heart block. Stat echocardiography and cardiothoracic surgery consultation are ordered.

Both of these patients were ultimately diagnosed with infective endocarditis.

Clinical Presentation

As demonstrated in Case Five, many patients with subacute infective endocarditis present with nonspecific symptoms that are common among emergency department patients—fever, fatigue, chills, nausea, night sweats, arthralgia, myalgia, and weight loss. So, how can emergency physicians identify patients with infective endocarditis? The possibility of infective endocarditis should be considered in any patient who has had a fever of unexplained origin for more than 1 week. A murmur or other evidence of valvular disease is the second most common sign. Acute infective endocarditis usually involves left-sided heart valves and often presents as severe sepsis with fever and shock. An increasing number of patients are presenting with more acute illness and without classic signs of infective endocarditis because of a shift in etiology (host factors) and microbiology (infectious causes).

KEY POINTS

Fever is the single most common feature of infective endocarditis.

Approximately 75% of all patients with infective endocarditis have a preexisting structural abnormality of the valve involved; therefore, the clinician should have a higher suspicion for infective endocarditis in patients who report a history of a heart murmur.

Other common findings relate to the infection itself or embolism. These include splenomegaly, microscopic hematuria, anemia, leukocytosis, and elevated ESR. Cutaneous signs, caused by microemboli or focal vasculitis, are observed less frequently today. Subungual or splinter hemorrhages are 1- to 2-mm brown streaks under the nails. Petechiae can be seen on mucosal surfaces or the extremities. Osler nodes are red, painful lesions on the palms and soles. Janeway lesions are nontender erythematous macules on the palms and soles.[18]

Most patients initially present with complications of endocarditis, both cardiac and noncardiac. Acute heart failure is the most frequent complication, exemplified by the patient in Case Six, with his shortness of breath and crackles on pulmonary examination. Infective endocarditis should always be considered in patients with new and unexplained heart failure. It is usually the result of valvular insufficiency of the aortic or mitral valves and occurs in 20% to 60% of cases.[19,20] It can be insidious or develop acutely from perforation of a valve leaflet, chordae rupture, or valve obstruction from large vegetations. The presence of "new" heart failure has the greatest impact on prognosis, as it is the most common cause of death.[19,21] Exten-

FIGURE 14-9.

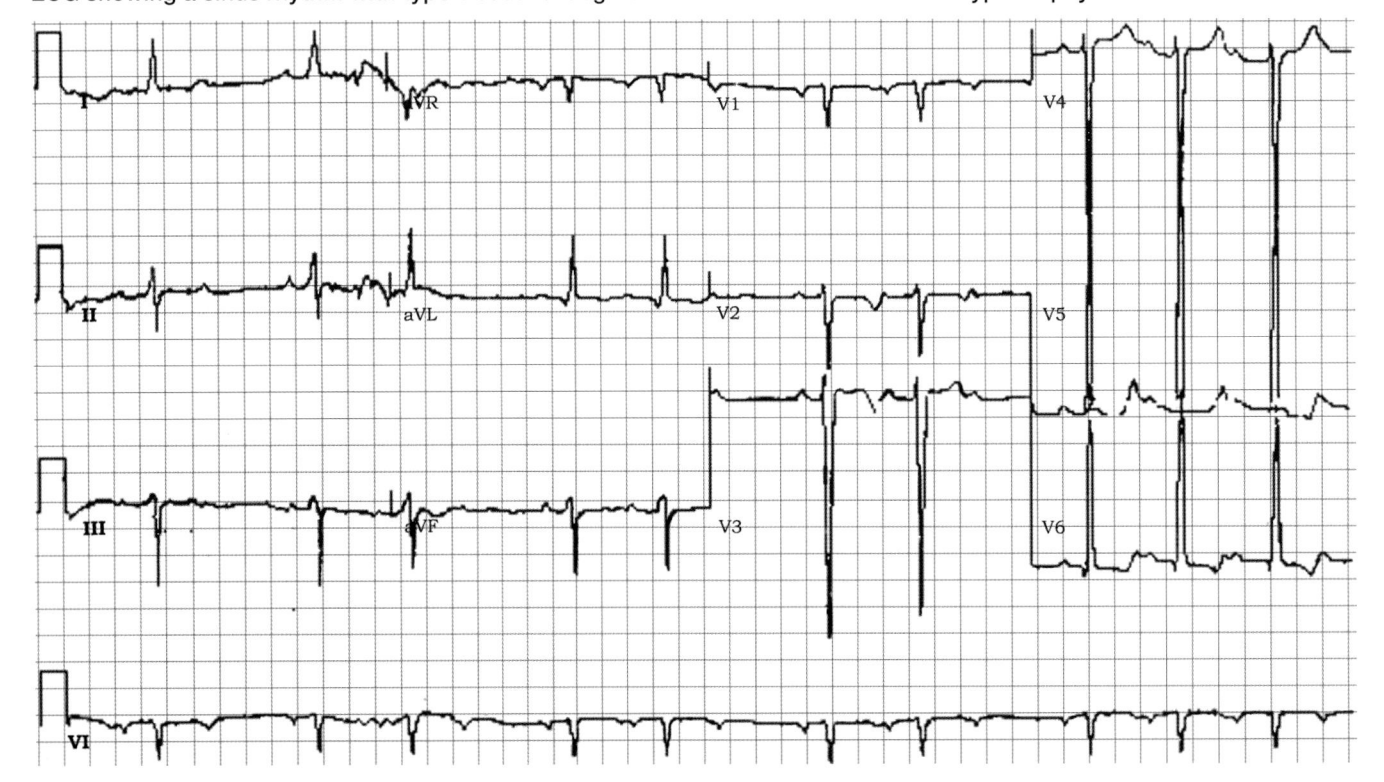

ECG showing a sinus rhythm with type 1 second-degree AV block and left ventricular hypertrophy

sion of infective endocarditis beyond the valve annulus predicts a higher mortality rate, more frequent development of heart failure, and the need for cardiac surgery. Extension of the infection into the perivalvular tissue is common, occurring in 10% to 40% of all cases of native-valve infective endocarditis.[22] In native aortic-valve infective endocarditis, the extension generally occurs through the weakest portion of the annulus, which is near the membranous septum and atrioventricular node. This area is particularly vulnerable to abscess formation and explains why heart block is a frequent sequela. As seen in Case Six, the presence of a Wenckebach conduction abnormality should raise concern for infective endocarditis with perivalvular extension in the region of the heart around the atrioventricular node. Any newly acquired conduction deficit in a febrile patient should be assumed to be secondary to abscess formation, prompting emergent echocardiography and cardiothoracic consultation.

KEY POINTS

The ECG can provide clues to the presence of myocardial abscess/infiltration, including heart block and conduction delays.

The ECG in Figure 14-9 shows type I second-degree heart block, which suggests a perivalvular abscess in the setting of infective endocarditis. A cardiothoracic surgeon should be consulted emergently because the patient is at risk for acute valvular insufficiency.

The second most frequent complication is embolization of cardiac vegetation. Central nervous system complications from emboli occur most frequently in left-sided infective endocarditis and are the first sign in 47% of cases.[23] In 20% of cases, infective endocarditis presents as stroke but can also manifest as transient ischemic attacks and meningitis.[20,23] Mycotic aneurysms result from septic embolization to arterial cerebral vessels and cause intracranial hemorrhages. Intravenous drug users are at risk for right-sided (tricuspid and pulmonary) valvular infections that often initially present as septic emboli in the lung. These appear as infiltrates that are easily misdiagnosed as pneumonia; they can disappear and reappear on serial radiographs or progress to cavitation. Emboli also affect many other organ systems, causing various presentations and symptoms such as emboli to the kidneys presenting as flank pain, hematuria, and renal failure; splenic emboli causing abdominal pain and abscess formation; and coronary emboli causing myocardial infarctions. Emboli can also lead to extremity vascular occlusion, which presents as ischemia of the digits or, rarely, limbs.[24]

KEY POINTS

Thrombolytic therapy for MI in the setting of infective endocarditis is not recommended because of the risk of intracerebral hemorrhage.[18,25]

Infective endocarditis should be considered in any patient who has had a fever of unexplained origin for more than 1 week.

Many cases of infective endocarditis initially present as one of its many complications, including heart failure, pericarditis, heart block, and stroke.

An Evolving Disease

Over the past 30 years, infective endocarditis has remained relatively uncommon, with an overall incidence between 2 and 6 per 100,000 individuals per year.[26-31] The high mortality rate has not changed either, despite medical advances, remaining as high as 20% to 40% at 1 year.[32,33] This apparent lack of progress stems from an evolving disease process. Historically, infective endocarditis affected children and young adults with chronic rheumatic heart disease and poor dentition. However, over the past 20 years, the prevalence of rheumatic heart disease has decreased, while the prevalence of chronically ill patients receiving invasive care has increased.[32] New at-risk populations have emerged—intravenous drug users, hemodialysis patients, the elderly, the immunosuppressed, and patients with medical devices such as prosthetic valves and intravenous catheters.[32,34] These patients commonly present to the emergency department, frequently for concerns about infection, which is why emergency physicians must be able to identify and treat infective endocarditis and its complications.

Along with this change in risk factors, the microbiology has shifted. The three major bacterial causes of infective endocarditis—streptococci, staphylococci, and enterococci—have remained constant over the decades. However, their percentages in the causation of infective endocarditis have changed drastically. Multiple studies have demonstrated that *Staphylococcus aureus* has surpassed viridans group streptococci as the leading cause of infective endocarditis in industrialized countries,[28,29,35] but the viridans group remains the most common source of among children. An increase in the prevalence of multidrug-resistant pathogens has contributed to the stagnant mortality rate.[32] In rare cases, infective endocarditis is caused by other microbes such as the HACEK group, gram-negative bacilli, anaerobes, and fungi. These cases tend to be more difficult to diagnose and treat.

KEY POINTS

Endocarditis remains relatively uncommon but deadly.

The three major bacterial causes of infective endocarditis are streptococci, staphylococci, and enterococci.

Pathophysiology

Infective endocarditis results from colonization of damaged valves by bacteria circulating in the blood. These abnormal valves cause a local thrombotic endocarditis as part of the normal healing process, which serves as an ideal location for bacterial infection. Endothelial damage can be caused by turbulent blood flow and inflammation associated with congenital heart disease or prosthetic valves, as well as medical devices and cardiac implantables. Medical equipment is prone to biofilm and thrombus formation, the necessary environment for bacterial infection.

Classification

The clinical presentation, complications, and treatment of infective endocarditis are heavily influenced by the valve involved and whether it is native or prosthetic. For this reason, it can best be classified into four categories: left sided native-valve infective endocarditis, left-sided prosthetic-valve infective endocarditis, right-sided infective endocarditis, and health-care–associated infective endocarditis.

Left-sided native-valve infective endocarditis is the most common form, representing 70% of cases.[34] Congenital heart disease can lead to development of abnormal endothelium and lesions, favoring attachment of circulating bacteria and promoting the disease. Mitral valve prolapse can increase the risk of infective endocarditis 10- to 100-fold and is found in about a quarter of all cases.[36,37] Chronic rheumatic heart disease is still a contributing risk factor in developing countries.

Left-sided prosthetic-valve infective endocarditis is the most severe form, with the highest mortality rate, 1% to 3% at 1 year and 2% to 6% at 5 years after valve implanation.[34] Early prosthetic-valve infective endocarditis is classified as occurring within 2 months after surgery (although European guidelines have changed this timeframe to 12 months) and usually is caused by hospital-related microbes such as methicillin-resistant *S. aureus* (MRSA). Late prosthetic-valve infective endocarditis is similar to native-valve disease.[38]

Right-sided infective endocarditis is most common in intravenous drug users and typically affects the tricuspid valve. It can also occur in patients with congenital heart disease and cardiac implantables such as pacemakers, defibrillators, and central venous catheters. Right-sided infective endocarditis has a much better prognosis than left-sided infective endocarditis, with a mortality rate below 10%.[19,28] *S. aureus* and viridans streptococci are the most common microbes in intravenous drug users; coagulase-negative staphylococci are commonly associated with cardiac devices.[19,26]

Health-care–associated infective endocarditis is occurring more frequently in industrialized countries. Most cases occur in patients without underlying valvular disease. Risk factors include hemodialysis, immunosuppressive therapy, diabetes mellitus, and cancer. *S. aureus* is the most common microbe, but enterococci are also common.[26]

Diagnosis

The single most important factor in the diagnosis of infective endocarditis is a high clinical suspicion for the disease. Often, the presenting features are not classic. Patients are often misdiagnosed with viral illnesses, rheumatologic conditions, or suspected malignancies. Suspicion for endocarditis requires hospital admission to confirm the diagnosis, after blood cultures reveal an infectious organism and echocardiogram reveals a source. When infective endocarditis is clinically suspected in the emergency department, the initial evaluation should include CBC, chemistries, blood cultures, a chest radiograph, and an ECG and echocardiogram, if available.

> **KEY POINT**
>
> Laboratory tests for those with infective endocarditis can reveal leukocytosis, anemia, elevated ESR and/or CRP, and microscopic hematuria; however, the absence of these findings cannot rule out the diagnosis.

The Duke criteria for the diagnosis of infective endocarditis were developed in 1994 and later modified (Table 14-4).[39] Blood cultures are positive in 85% of infective endocarditis cases. Blood cultures can be negative because of prior antibiotic treatment, fastidious organisms such as the HACEK group and fungi, or intracellular bacteria. Transesophageal echocardiography has a sensitivity of 90% to 100% for detecting vegetations, and the sensitivity of transthoracic echocardiography ranges from 40% to 63%.[40]

> **KEY POINT**
>
> Echocardiography is crucial in the diagnosis of infective endocarditis; however, a negative transthoracic echocardiographic examination does not rule it out. Sensitivities for detecting vegetations range from 90% to 100% for transesophageal echocardiography and 40% to 63% for transthoracic echocardiography.[41]

CASE FIVE, CONTINUED

After admission to the hospital, the patient's blood cultures grew *Streptococcus viridans*. His echocardiogram (Figure 14-10) showed a vegetation on the mitral valve, with severe regurgitation.

> **KEY POINTS**
>
> Endocarditis is difficult to diagnose in the emergency department.
>
> Diagnosis requires a high degree of clinical suspicion from the emergency physician.
>
> Admit patients to the hospital for definitive testing, including an echocardiogram.

Treatment

When infective endocarditis is suspected, empiric antibiotic treatment should be initiated quickly, preferably after cultures are obtained. Antibiotic selection should be based on the patient's history and the likely cause of the infection. In patients with native valves, an empiric treatment regimen with a beta-lactam antibiotic, either a penicillin (eg, nafcillin or ampicillin-sulbactam) or a cephalosporin (eg, ceftriaxone), vancomycin, and gentamicin will give synergistic coverage for more than 80% of the causes of infective endocarditis, given that most are staphylococci (including MRSA), streptococci, or enterococci. In patients with prosthetic valves, add rifampin to vancomycin and gentamicin because it helps eradicate bacteria attached to foreign materials. Most patients require 4 to 6 weeks of therapy.

> **KEY POINT**
>
> Antiplatelet therapy and anticoagulation are not indicated and do not reduce the risk of embolism,[42] but initiation of antibiotics does. Embolic rates decrease after only 1 week of antibiotic treatment.

CASE FIVE, CONTINUED

The patient was treated with intravenous ceftriaxone and gentamicin and underwent mitral valve repair surgery. He also had total dental extraction, as poor dental hygiene was thought to be the source of infection. He was discharged on hospital day 18 and completed 6 weeks of antibiotics.

CASE SIX, CONTINUED

The presence of type I second-degree heart block raised immediate concern about a perivalvular abscess. Urgent echocardiography was ordered, and cardiothoracic surgery was consulted. Over the next 2 hours, the patient became restless and then acutely short of breath and hypotensive. He was intubated, started on vasopressors, and transferred to an operating room, where he died. Autopsy revealed aortic valve rupture from an aortic ring abscess.

In-hospital mortality rates range from 10% to 25%.[28,43] Predictors of poor outcome include older age; prosthetic valve involvement; diabetes mellitus; complications such as heart failure, renal failure, or stroke; *S. aureus* as the causative organism; and severe aortic or mitral valve regurgitation. Surgical management is required in about 50% of infective endocarditis cases. No randomized controlled trials have been published to confirm the role of surgical management; therefore, the choice of this treatment plan is largely based on observational series and expert opinion. However, multiple studies have confirmed the benefit of surgery in complicated infective endocarditis.[39]

TABLE 14-4.

Modified Duke Criteria for Diagnosis of Infective Endocarditis. From: Li JS, Sexton DJ, Mick N, et al. Proposed modifications to the Duke criteria for the diagnosis of infective endocarditis. *Clin Infect Dis.* 2000;30:633-638. Copyright Oxford University Press, 2000. Used with permission.

Major criteria

- Blood cultures
  - At least two separate positive blood cultures infected with typical infective endocarditis microorganisms
  - Persistently positive blood cultures
  - Single positive culture for *Coxiella burnetii* or anti-phase I antibody titer >1:800
- Imaging showing endocardial involvement
  - New valve regurgitation
  - Oscillating intracardiac mass on the valve or supporting structure
  - Abscess
  - New partial dehiscence of prosthetic valve

Minor criteria

- Predisposing cardiac condition or intravenous drug use
- Fever (≥38°C or 100.4°F)
- Positive blood cultures, but not meeting major criteria
- Vascular phenomena: arterial emboli, mycotic aneurysms, petechiae, and/or Janeway lesions
- Immunologic phenomena: glomerulonephritis, Osler nodes, Roth spots, and/or rheumatoid factor

Diagnosis

- Definite
  - Pathology or bacteriology of vegetations *or*
  - 2 major criteria *or*
  - 1 major and 3 minor criteria *or*
  - 5 minor criteria
- Possible
  - 1 major and 1 minor criterion *or*
  - 3 minor criteria

Heart failure is the major indication for surgical intervention. Specific indications for emergent surgery include severe aortic or mitral regurgitation, valve obstruction causing pulmonary edema or cardiogenic shock, and fistula formation. Urgent surgical consultation is also required for patients with abscess formation and prosthetic valve obstruction or dehiscence.

KEY POINTS

Empiric antibiotic therapy, including a beta-lactam or cephalosporin, vancomycin, and gentamycin, should be initiated in the emergency department for patients for whom there is a high clinical suspicion of infective endocarditis.

Rifampin should be included in the treatment of patients with prosthetic valves.

Obtain emergent surgical consultation in cases with evidence of conduction defects, acute valvular insufficiency causing pulmonary edema or cardiogenic shock, or myocardial abscess and/or fistula formation on echocardiogram.

Noninfective Endocarditis

Endocarditis can also result from mechanical irritation, neoplastic processes, and autoimmune disorders. These causative mechanisms also induce inflammation of the endocardium and heart valves as the result of physical trauma rather than infection. Noninfective endocarditis commonly affects healthy, undamaged valves. The vegetations tend to be smaller compared with those in infective endocarditis. It usually occurs in a hypercoagulable state such as pregnancy, cancer, or sepsis. It can also occur in autoimmune disorders such as SLE, or Libman-Sacks endocarditis. Presenting symptoms result from embolization, since the vegetations themselves are asymptomatic. Patients may have a murmur, but the absence of one does not preclude the diagnosis. Treatment is aimed at the predisposing disorder and supportive care but may include anticoagulation.

Conclusion

Inflammatory diseases of the heart have a variety of presentations in the emergency department, including chest pain, shortness of breath, fever, and other nonspecific complaints. Although acute coronary syndrome assessment frequently assumes a predominant role in the differential diagnosis, emergency physicians must have a high degree of suspicion for these conditions in order not to miss or delay the correct diagnosis. This often is dependent on recognition of patients who may be at risk and of those with presentations that deviate from more commonly encountered conditions, as well as a heightened awareness for patients presenting for care after protracted illnesses without a clear diagnosis.

References

1. Kindermann I, Barth C, Mahfoud F, et al. Update on myocarditis. *J Am Coll Cardiol*. 2012;59:779-792.
2. Dudzinski DM, Mak GS, Hung JW. Pericardial diseases. *Curr Probl Cardiol*. 2012;37:75-118.
3. Imazio M. Contemporary management of pericardial diseases. *Curr Opin Cardiol*. 2012;27:308-317.

FIGURE 14-10.

Four-chamber view on transthoracic echocardiography. Vegetation can be seen on the atrial side of the mitral valve.

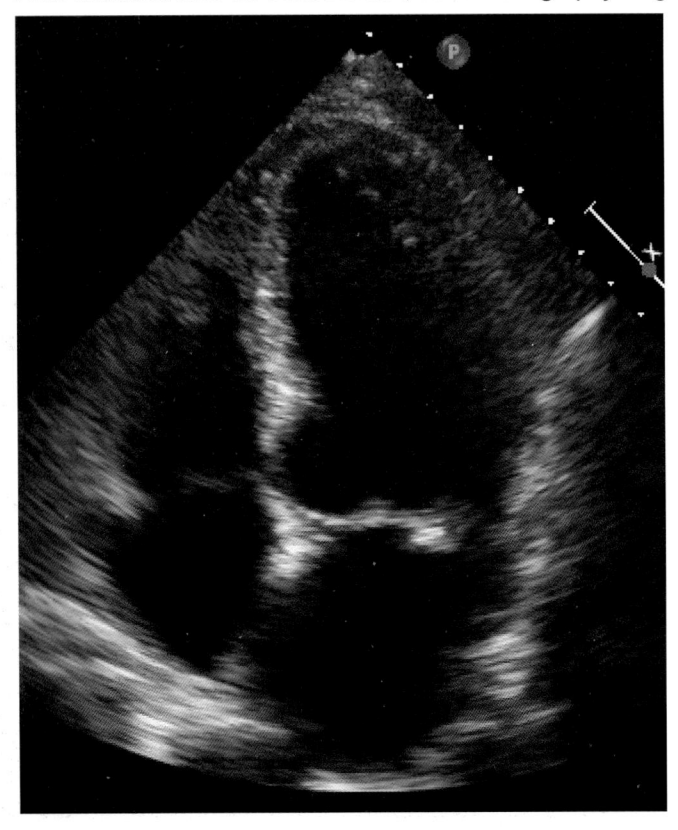

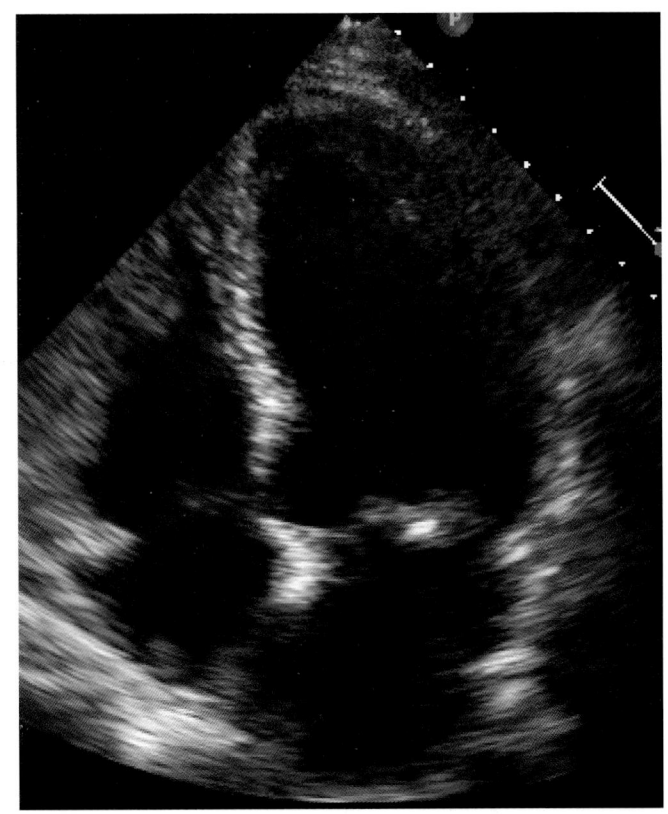

4. Elamm C, Fairweather D, Cooper LT. Pathogenesis and diagnosis of myocarditis. *Heart.* 2012;98:835-840.
5. Huang HD, Birnbaum Y. ST elevation: differentiation between ST elevation myocardial infarction and nonischemic ST elevation. *J Electrocardiol.* 2011;44:494.e1-494.e12.
6. Smith SC, Ladenson JH, Mason JW, et al. Elevations of cardiac troponin I associated with myocarditis: experimental and clinical correlates. *Circulation.* 1997;95:163-168.
7. Guglin M, Nallamshetty L. Myocarditis: diagnosis and treatment. *Curr Treat Options Cardiovasc Med.* 2012;14:637-651.
8. American College of Cardiology Foundation Task Force on Expert Consensus Documents, Hundley WG, Bluemke DA, et al. ACCF/ACR/AHA/NASCI/SCMR 2010 expert consensus document on cardiovascular magnetic resonance: a report of the American College of Cardiology Foundation Task Force on Expert Consensus Documents. *J Am Coll Cardiol.* 2010;55:2614-2662.
9. Sparano DM, Ward RP. Pericarditis and pericardial effusion: management update. *Curr Treat Options Cardiovasc Med.* 2011;13:543-555.
10. Htwe TH, Khardori NM. Cardiac emergencies: Infective endocarditis, pericarditis, and myocarditis. *Med Clin North Am.* 2012;96:1149-1169.
11. Imazio M, Brucato A, Maestroni S, et al. Risk of constrictive pericarditis after acute pericarditis. *Circulation.* 2011;124:1270-1275.
12. Little WC, Freeman GL. Pericardial disease. *Circulation.* 2006;113:1622-1632.
13. Spodick DH. Acute cardiac tamponade. *N Engl J Med.* 2003;349:684-690.
14. Goodman A, Perera P, Mailhot T, Mandavia D. The role of bedside ultrasound in the diagnosis of pericardial effusion and cardiac tamponade. *J Emerg Trauma Shock.* 2012;5:72-75.
15. Grun S, Schumm J, Greulich S, et al. Long-term follow-up of biopsy-proven viral myocarditis: predictors of mortality and incomplete recovery. *J Am Coll Cardiol.* 2012;59:1604-1615.
16. Acker M. Mechanical circulatory support for patients with acute-fulminant myocarditis. *Ann Thorac Surg.* 2001;71 (suppl 1):S73-S76.
17. McCarthy RE 3rd, Boehmer JP, Hruban RH, et al. Long-term outcome of fulminant myocarditis as compared with acute (nonfulminant) myocarditis. *N Engl J Med.* 2000;342:690-695.
18. Overend L, Rose E. Uncertainties in managing myocardial infarction associated with infective endocarditis. *Exp Clin Cardiol.* 2012;17:144-145.
19. Baddour LM, Wilson WR, Bayer AS, et al. Infective endocarditis: diagnosis, antimicrobial therapy, and management of complications. *Circulation.* 2005;111:e394-e434.
20. Bashore TM, Cabell C, Fowler V. Update on infectious endocarditis. *Curr Probl Cardiol.* 2006;31:274-352.
21. Sexton D, Spelman D. Current best practices and guidelines: assessment and management of complications in infective endocarditis. *Cardiol Clin.* 2003;21:273-282.
22. Bayer AS, Bolger AF, Taubert KA, et al. Diagnosis and management of infective endocarditis and its complications. *Circulation.* 1998;98:2936-2948.
23. Heiro M, Nikoskelainem J, Engblom E, et al. Neurologic manifestations of infective endocarditis. *Arch Intern Med.* 2000;160:2781-2787.
24. Crawford MH, Durack DT. Clinical presentation of infective endocarditis. *Cardiol Clin.* 2003;21:159-166.
25. Khan F, Khakoo R, Failinger C. Managing embolic myocardial infarction in infective endocarditis: current options. *J Infect.* 2005;51:e101-e105.
26. Que YA, Moreillon P. Infective endocarditis. *Nat Rev Cardiol.* 2011;8:322-336.
27. Moreillon P, Que YA. Infective endocarditis. *Lancet.* 2004;363:139-149.
28. Hoen B, Alla F, Selton-Suty C, et al. Changing profile of infective endocarditis: results of a 1-year survey in France. *JAMA.* 2002;288:75-81.
29. Tleyjeh IM, Abdel-Latif A, Rahbi H, et al. A systematic review of population-based studies of infective endocarditis. *Chest.* 2007;132:1025-1035.
30. Correa de Sa DD, Tleyjeh IM, Anavekar NS, et al. Epidemiological trends of infective endocarditis: a population-based study in Olmsted County, Minnesota. *Mayo Clin Proc.* 2010;85:422-426.
31. Delahaye F, Goulet V, Lacassin F, et al. Characteristics of infective endocarditis in France in 1991: a 1-year survey. *Eur Heart J.* 1995;16:394-401.
32. Cabell CH, Jollis JG, Peterson GE, et al. Changing patient characteristics and the effect on mortality in endocarditis. *Arch Intern Med.* 2002;162:90-94.
33. Thuny F, Grisoli D, Collart F, et al. Management of infective endocarditis: challenges and perspectives. *Lancet.* 2012;379:965-975.
34. Murdoch DR, Corey GR, Hoen B, et al. Clinical presentation, etiology, and outcome of infective endocarditis in the 21st century. *Arch Intern Med.* 2009;169:463-473.
35. Fowler VG, Miro JM, Hoen B, et al. *Staphylococcus aureus* endocarditis: a consequence of medical progress. *JAMA.* 2005;293:3012-3021.
36. Kim S, Kuroda T, Nishinaga M, et al. Relationship between severity of mitral regurgitation and prognosis of mitral valve prolapse: echocardiographic follow-up study. *Am Heart J.* 1996;132:348-355.
37. Weinberger I, Rotenberg Z, Zacharovitz D, et al. Native valve infective endocarditis in the 1970s versus 1980s: underlying cardiac lesions and infecting organisms. *Clin Cardiol.* 1990;13:94-98.
38. Wang A, Athan E, Pappas PA, et al. Contemporary clinical profile and outcome of prosthetic valve endocarditis. *JAMA.* 2007;297:1354-1361.
39. Li JS, Sexton DJ, Mick N, et al. Proposed modifications to the Duke criteria for the diagnosis of infective endocarditis. *Clin Infect Dis.* 2000;30:633-638.
40. Evangelista A, Gonzalez-Alujas MT. Echocardiography in infective endocarditis. *Heart.* 2004;90:614-617.
41. Mylonakis E, Calderwood SB. Infective endocarditis in adults. *N Engl J Med.* 2001;345:1318-1330.
42. Chan KL, Dumesnil JG, Cujec B, et al. A randomized trial of aspirin on the risk of embolic events in patients with infective endocarditis. *J Am Coll Cardiol.* 2003;42:775-780.
43. Habib G, Hoen B, Tornos P, et al. Guidelines on the prevention, diagnosis, and treatment of infective endocarditis. *Eur Heart.* 2009;30:2369-2413.

Additional Reading

Algalarrondo V, Boycott H, Eliahou L, et al. Indications of anti-inflammatory drugs in cardiac diseases. *Antiinflamm Antiallergy Agents Med Chem.* 2013;12:3-13.

Brown JL, Hirsh DA, Mahle WT. Use of troponin as a screen for chest pain in the pediatric emergency department. *Pediatr Cardiol.* 2012;33:337-342.

Caforio AL, Marcolongo R, Jahns R, et al. Immune-mediated and autoimmune myocarditis: clinical presentation, diagnosis and management. *Heart Fail Rev.* 2013;18:715-732.

Eppert A. Towards evidence-based emergency medicine: best BETs from the Manchester Royal Infirmary. BET 3: Colchicine as an adjunct to nonsteroidal anti-inflammatory drugs for the treatment of acute pericarditis. *Emerg Med J.* 2011;28:244-245.

Gallagher S, Jones DA, Anand V, et al. Diagnosis and management of patients with acute cardiac symptoms, troponin elevation and culprit-free angiograms. *Heart.* 2012;98:974-981.

Hooper AJ, Celenza A. A descriptive analysis of patients with an emergency department diagnosis of acute pericarditis. *Emerg Med J.* 2013;30:1003-1008.

Imazio M. Treatment of recurrent pericarditis. *Expert Rev Cardiovasc Ther.* 2012;10:1165-1172.

Imazio M. Evaluation and management of pericarditis. *Expert Rev Cardiovasc Ther.* 2011;9:1221-1233.

Imazio M, Adler Y. Treatment with aspirin, NSAID, corticosteroids, and colchicine in acute and recurrent pericarditis. *Heart Fail Rev.* 2012;18:355-360.

Imazio M, Brucato A, Forno D, et al. Efficacy and safety of colchicine for pericarditis prevention. systematic review and meta-analysis. *Heart.* 2012;98:1078-1082.

Johnen J, Radermecker MA, Defraigne JO. Constrictive pericarditis: case report and review. *Rev Med Liege.* 2012;67:107-112.

Khandaker MH, Schaff HV, Greason KL, et al. Pericardiectomy vs medical management in patients with relapsing pericarditis. *Mayo Clin Proc.* 2012;87:1062-1070.

Maisch B, Pankuweit S. Standard and etiology-directed evidence-based therapies in myocarditis: state of the art and future perspectives. *Heart Fail Rev.* 2013;18:761-795.

Marchant DJ, Boyd JH, Lin DC, et al. Inflammation in myocardial diseases. *Circ Res.* 2012;110:126-144.

Mehrzad R, Spodick DH. Pericardial involvement in diseases of the heart and other contiguous structures: Part II: Pericardial involvement in noncardiac contiguous disorders. *Cardiology.* 2012;121:177-183.

Mehrzad R, Spodick DH. Pericardial involvement in diseases of the heart and other contiguous structures: Part I: Pericardial involvement in infarct pericarditis and pericardial involvement following myocardial infarction. *Cardiology.* 2012;121:164-176.

Molina KM, Garcia X, Denfield SW, et al. Parvovirus B19 myocarditis causes significant morbidity and mortality in children. *Pediatr Cardiol.* 2013;34:390-397.

Mookadam F, Jiamsripong P, Raslan SF, et al. Constrictive pericarditis and restrictive cardiomyopathy in the modern era. *Future Cardiol.* 2011;7:471-483.

Ratnapalan S, Brown K, Benson L. Children presenting with acute pericarditis to the emergency department. *Pediatr Emerg Care.* 2011;27:581-585.

Riera AR, Ferreira C, Ferreira Filho C, et al. Clinical value of lead aVR. *Ann Noninvasive Electrocardiol.* 2011;16:295-302.

Rigante D, Cantarini L, Imazio M, et al. Autoinflammatory diseases and cardiovascular manifestations. *Ann Med.* 2011;43:341-346.

Sabbatani S, Manfredi R, Ortolani P, et al. Myopericarditis during a primary Epstein-Barr virus infection in an otherwise healthy young adult: an unusual and insidious complication. Case report and a 60-year literature review. *Infez Med.* 2012;20:75-81.

Sagar S, Liu PP, Cooper LT Jr. Myocarditis. *Lancet.* 2012;379:738-747.

Sagristà-Sauleda J, Mercé AS, Soler-Soler J. Diagnosis and management of pericardial effusion. *World J Cardiol.* 2011;3:135-143.

Takahashi H, Nagao K. Post-myocardial infarction syndrome. *Nihon Rinsho.* 2011;69 (suppl 9):226-229.

Yilmaz A, Ferreira V, Klingel K, et al. Role of cardiovascular magnetic resonance imaging (CMR) in the diagnosis of acute and chronic myocarditis. *Heart Fail Rev.* 2013;18:747-760.

Yusuf SW, Sharma J, Durand JB, et al. Endocarditis and myocarditis: a brief review. *Expert Rev Cardiovasc Ther.* 2012;10:1153-1164.

CHAPTER 15

Hypertensive Emergencies and Elevated Blood Pressure

Michael Jay Bresler

IN THIS CHAPTER

The scope of the problem

The role of the emergency physician in managing hypertension

Pathophysiology of hypertension

Pharmacologic treatment modalities

Specific emergencies that could require blood pressure reduction in the emergency department

Outpatient therapy

CASE ONE
You have evaluated a 64-year-old woman with a cough. You've diagnosed her with bronchitis, and she is now ready for discharge. Her blood pressure was 250/130 initially but is now down to 210/110. She is not taking any medication and has no history of hypertension. "Hey, Doc," asks the nurse, "What do you want to give her?"

CASE TWO
Same patient, but her discharge blood pressure is 250/140. "Hey, Doc," asks the nurse, "What do you want to give her?"

CASE THREE
You are evaluating a 64-year-old man who has had 3 hours of severe chest pain radiating to his back. His initial blood pressure is 230/110. His electrocardiogram (ECG) is normal, but a chest radiograph and computed tomography (CT) angiogram reveal an acute aortic dissection. "Hey, Doc," says the nurse, "The surgeon will be here in an hour."

These are typical scenarios for emergency physicians. What, if anything, should be done about these blood pressures? By the end of this chapter, the answers should be clear.

This chapter addresses the following questions related to emergency department care:
- When should elevated blood pressure be treated?
- When should elevated blood pressure not be treated?
- When should outpatient therapy be started?
- What agents should be used? For what conditions?

The Scope of the Problem
Historically, physicians have not been concerned about blood pressures below 140 mm Hg systolic or 90 mm Hg diastolic. However, we now recognize that levels between 130 and 139 systolic and 80 to 90 diastolic should raise concern. Patients with sustained blood pressures in this range (called prehypertension) have double the risk of eventually developing hypertension, so lifestyle and diet intervention are indicated.[1]

The Framingham Heart Study found that systolic blood pressures (SBPs) in the 130 to 139 range and diastolic blood pressures (DBPs) in the 85 to 89 range are associated with more than a two-fold increase in the relative risk of cardiovascular disease compared with levels below 120/80 mm Hg. One in four Americans is hypertensive, including two of every three over the age of 65. People who are normotensive at age 55 have a 90% lifetime risk of eventually developing hypertension.[1,2]

Twenty-seven percent of American adults have abnormally elevated blood pressure (above 140/90 mm Hg). When prehypertension is also considered, this number increases to 60%, which includes 88% of people over age 60 and 40% of those between 18 and 39 years of age.[3]

A metaanalysis of 12 prehypertension studies involving 518,520 people over various years of followup found a significant long-term risk of stroke associated with prehypertension. Seven of the 12 studies stratified prehypertension. They found no increased risk of stroke for those with SBP between 120 and 129 *and* DBP between 80 and 84 mm Hg. However, for people with SBP of 130 to 139 *or* DBP of 85 to 90, the long-term relative risk of stroke was 1.79 (95% CI, 1.49-2.16).[4]

Men typically develop hypertension earlier than women; however, after menopause, women catch up and may even surpass men in the incidence of hypertension.[5]

Ethnicity is also a factor. While approximately one in four adult Caucasian and Hispanic Americans is hypertensive, this proportion increases to one in three among African Americans. Hypertension develops earlier and tends to cause more organ damage in African Americans.[6]

Should blood pressure increase with age? The answer is "No." In societies with natural diet, less salt, less obesity, and more exercise, blood pressure does not rise with age. Hypertension is a "disease" that is rampant in our modern Western society. The well-known atherosclerotic risk factors such as diet and lack of exercise and the metabolic syndrome are all contributing factors. The result is replacement of arterial wall elastin with collagen and fibrous tissue, leading to decreased compliance and increased resistance.

Both SBP and DBP tend to rise with age in our society. Below age 50, combined systolic and diastolic hypertension is most common. Over age 50, isolated systolic hypertension predominates.[1] Isolated systolic hypertension is of particular concern. In persons older than 50 years, SBP over 140 mm Hg is a more important cardiovascular disease risk factor than elevations of DBP.[1] This is because the increased pulse pressure causes a repetitive pounding of a jet of blood against the arterial walls. Cardiovascular risk increases when increased systolic pressure is combined with decreased diastolic pressure. This may seem counterintuitive, but a chronic blood pressure of 170/70 could present a greater cardiovascular risk than 170/100.[1] For every 20 mm Hg above a systolic pressure of 115, or 10 mm Hg above a diastolic pressure of 70, the mortality rate from both ischemic heart disease and stroke *doubles*.[7,8]

Hypertension is often classified as either "essential" or "secondary." Essential hypertension, which characterizes about 95% of cases, has no specific identifiable cause and is thought to be associated with the general risk factors for cardiovascular disease. Those factors include atherosclerosis, obesity, the metabolic syndrome, salt intake, sleep apnea, and heredity. The remaining 5% of hypertensive people have secondary hypertension caused by specific identifiable conditions such as renal failure, renal artery stenosis, endocrine abnormalities, coarctation of the aorta, drugs, or drug withdrawal.[1]

In addition to being associated with atherosclerosis in many patients, obesity can cause high blood pressure directly by several mechanisms, including activation of the renin-angiotensin-aldosterone system (RAAS), which leads to increased blood volume, increased sympathetic nervous system activity, and vascular inflammation.

Chronic renal failure causes hypertension in 80% of patients as a result of volume overload and vasoconstriction via the RAAS. Chronic renal failure is a major cause of cardiovascular complications.[9]

Renal artery stenosis is the cause of secondary hypertension in a small percentage of people with high blood pressure. The stenosis is usually caused by atheroma, though in a small percentage it is associated with fibromuscular dysplasia, particularly in younger female patients.[10]

Endocrine abnormalities leading to hypertension include those associated with aldosterone, glucocorticoids, pheochromocytoma, thyroid hormone, and pregnancy.

Medications can elevate blood pressure. Examples include glucocorticoids, immunosuppressants such as cyclosporine, and monoamine oxidase inhibitors associated with tyramine ingestion from certain cheeses. In emergency departments, acutely elevated blood pressure resulting from abuse of stimulants such as cocaine or amphetamines is not uncommon. Drug withdrawal can also cause acutely elevated blood pressure. This can be seen with abrupt withdrawal from beta-blockers, clonidine, or addictive drugs such as alcohol or narcotics.

Regardless of the cause, chronic hypertension is a major risk factor for stroke, myocardial infarction, aortic dissection, peripheral vascular disease, and renal failure.[1-4] Therefore, chronic hypertension must be controlled.

The Role of the Emergency Physician in Managing Hypertension

Acute elevation of blood pressure in emergency department patients might be a life-threatening event. However, since chronic hypertension in many of our patients is either undiagnosed or undertreated, we have the opportunity to intervene in the long-term progression to disability or death that is often the result of this disease process.

KEY POINT

Assessing elevated blood pressure, both acute and chronic, is part of the practice of emergency medicine.

A question that emergency physicians often face when confronted with an elevated blood pressure reading is: "Does this reading reflect true hypertension?" Blood pressure readings are often elevated in the emergency department in response to pain or fear (the "white coat syndrome")[8,11,12] and often decline during the course of a visit, so it important to recheck an initially high reading prior to discharge.[11]

A common cause of falsely diagnosed high blood pressure is an ill-fitting cuff. The sphygmomanometer cuff should fit the arm properly. Larger cuffs should be used on patients with larger arms.

Up to 25% of patients in some emergency department populations have true chronic hypertension. In a study of asymptomatic emergency department patients with blood pressure above 140/90 mm Hg who agreed to followup at home, more than half continued to experience elevated pressures. Most of the other patients remained at prehypertension levels. The elevated pressures were found to be independent of pain or anxiety in the emergency department.[11] Another study followed emergency department patients with blood pressure readings above 140/90 mm Hg and found that 54% continued to have an elevated pressure when they were later evaluated as outpatients.[12]

Many patients who have elevated blood pressure in the emergency department are not made aware of the finding or of the importance of outpatient followup. A prospective study of 991 emergency department patients found that 45% of them had a blood pressure of 140/90 mm Hg or higher. One third (105) had no history of hypertension, yet only 33% of those with no history of hypertension and only half of those with a known history of it were informed of their elevated blood pressure while they were in the emergency department. Additionally, only 13% of those with no history of hypertension and 31% of those with a known history of hypertension were advised to have their pressures checked later.[13]

> **KEY POINT**
>
> Consistently elevated blood pressure in the emergency department reflects true hypertension roughly half the time.

It is useful to separate elevated blood pressure into the two general categories of "hypertensive emergencies" and "asymptomatic presentations of markedly elevated blood pressure," because our approach to them is different.

Hypertensive Emergencies

By definition, patients with a hypertensive emergency have evidence of *acute* organ injury caused by the elevated blood pressure. The organs affected are typically the brain, heart, or kidney. In hypertensive emergencies, systolic pressures are generally above 180 mm Hg and diastolic pressures are above 120 mm Hg. However, the diagnosis of hypertensive emergency is based on evidence of acute organ injury rather than the specific pressure. Patients with a hypertensive emergency typically receive intravenous medications and are admitted to the hospital.[14,15]

Asymptomatic Markedly Elevated Blood Pressure

In contrast to patients with hypertensive emergencies, patients with asymptomatic markedly elevated blood pressure have no evidence of *acute* organ injury caused by the elevated pressure.[16] The definition depends not on the blood pressure value *per se*, but on the absence of acute organ injury. In a clinical policy recently adopted by the American College of Emergency Physicians (ACEP),[16] asymptomatic markedly elevated blood pressure is defined as a systolic pressure of 160 mm Hg or more or a diastolic pressure of 100 mm Hg or more.

> **KEY POINT**
>
> The term *hypertensive urgency* has traditionally been used to define a condition of sustained, acutely elevated blood pressure in a range similar to that of hypertensive emergency, but without evidence of acute organ injury.

Asymptomatic elevated blood pressure generally does not require treatment in the emergency department. The 2013 ACEP clinical policy[16] uses the term *asymptomatic markedly elevated blood pressure* to differentiate the condition that does not require emergency department treatment from hypertensive emergency, which does require emergency department treatment.

Emergency physicians confronted with an asymptomatic patient with markedly elevated pressure must consider whether or not to initiate a workup and whether or not to treat the blood pressure. ACEP addressed both of these issues with Level C recommendations in its 2013 clinical policy, *Critical Issues in the Evaluation and Management of Adult Patients in the Emergency Department With Asymptomatic Elevated Blood Pressure*[16] (Table 15-1). According to that policy, routine screening of these patients for target organ injury does not reduce the rate of adverse outcomes and is not required. In selected patients, such as those with poor likelihood of followup, screening for an elevated serum creatinine level could identify kidney injury that affects disposition (eg, hospital admission).[16] ACEP policy advises that, although such patients should be referred for outpatient followup, medical intervention in the emergency department does not reduce the rate of adverse outcomes and is not required. However, for some patients, such as those with poor followup resources, markedly elevated pressure may be treated in the emergency department or therapy may be initiated for long-term control.[16]

> **KEY POINTS**
>
> In patients with hypertensive emergencies, acute organ injury is caused by the acutely elevated blood pressure. Treatment typically includes parenteral medication and hospital admission.[14,15]
>
> In emergency department patients with asymptomatic markedly elevated blood pressure, does screening for target organ injury reduce the rate of adverse outcomes?
>
>   Routine screening for acute target organ injury is not required.
>
>   In selected patients, serum creatinine screening may identify patients appropriate for hospital admission.[16]
>
> In patients with asymptomatic markedly elevated blood pressure, does medical intervention in the emergency department reduce the rate of adverse outcomes?
>
>   Medical intervention is not required in the emergency department.
>
>   In selected patients, markedly elevated pressure can be treated in the emergency department or therapy can be initiated for long-term control.
>
>   Patients should be referred for outpatient followup.[16]

Pathophysiology of Hypertension

Contraction and relaxation of the muscles in the walls of the blood vessels determine the degree of vasoconstriction and vasodilation. These factors are affected by the inherent stiffness (resistance to distension) of the vessel wall. In Western society, chronic hypertension is usually the result of the replacement of distensible elastin fibers in the vessel walls with rigid collagen and fibrous tissue. While heredity, of course, has a role, in most people this process is largely caused by the risk factors for cardiovascular disease. Over time, these cardiovascular risk factors increase vascular resistance not only by replacement of elastin by collagen and fibrous tissue in the vessel walls but also by precipitating endothelial dysfunction.

Endothelial dysfunction has a number of deleterious effects. It leads to capillary permeability and depletion of nitric oxide, a potent mediator of vasodilation. It also causes inflammation with release of proinflammatory cytokines and white cell adhesion molecules, leading to further inflammation. Endothelial dysfunction also stimulates release of endothelin 1 and other vasoconstrictor agents.[17-21] Finally, this process triggers the RAAS, resulting in production of angiotensin II, a powerful vasoconstrictor with additional effects that are discussed below. In the emergency department, we cannot alter the inherent stiffness of the arterial walls, but we can affect vascular muscle tone.

Vasoconstriction is caused by a number of factors, including alpha$_1$-adrenergic innervation of the vascular muscles, circulating catecholamines, angiotensin II, and arginine vasopressin (AVP), also known as antidiuretic hormone (ADH). AVP/ADH has a direct vasoconstrictive action in addition to its effect on intravascular volume.

Vasodilation typically results from inhibition of alpha$_1$-adrenergic effects, alpha$_2$-adrenergic stimulation, beta$_2$-adrenergic stimulation, and the effects of nitric oxide.

Blood pressure is determined by cardiac output and arterial vascular resistance. Since cardiac output consists of the product of heart rate multiplied by stroke volume, we can say that blood pressure equals stroke volume (SV) times heart rate (HR) times peripheral (arterial) vascular resistance (PVR).

KEY POINT

Blood pressure = SV × HR × PVR

The only way blood pressure can change is by alteration of one or more of these parameters. We will soon discuss the various pharmacologic agents that can be used to treat elevated blood pressure in the emergency department. Most of them reduce PVR. However, before we delve into the medications, it is important to understand the concept of autoregulation.

Autoregulation

Systemic blood pressure can vary widely, depending on exertion, fear, or other factors. However, the pressure in certain vital organs is more finely tuned. Cerebral blood flow is particularly important in this regard. Major elevations of systemic blood pressure are "damped out" by constriction of the precap-

TABLE 15-1.

ACEP Clinical Policy: Critical Issues in the Evaluation and Management of Adult Patients in the Emergency Department with Asymptomatic Elevated Blood Pressure. From: Wolf SJ, Lo B, Shih RD, et al; American College of Emergency Physicians Clinical Policies Committee. Clinical policy: critical issues in the evaluation and management of adult patients in the emergency department with asymptomatic elevated blood pressure. *Ann Emerg Med.* 2013;62(1):59-68.

1. In emergency department patients with asymptomatic elevated blood pressure, does screening for target organ injury reduce rates of adverse outcomes?

   Level A recommendations. None specified.

   Level B recommendations. None specified.

   Level C recommendations.

   1) In emergency department patients with asymptomatic markedly elevated blood pressure, routine screening for acute target organ injury (eg, serum creatinine, urinalysis, ECG) is not required.

   2) For select patients (eg, those with poor followup likelihood), screening for an elevated serum creatinine level might identify kidney injury that influences disposition (eg, hospital admission).

2. In patients with asymptomatic markedly elevated blood pressure, does emergency department medical intervention reduce rates of adverse outcomes?

   Level A recommendations. None specified.

   Level B recommendations. None specified.

   Level C recommendations.

   1) In patients with asymptomatic markedly elevated blood pressure, routine emergency department medical intervention is not required.

   2) For select patients (eg, those with poor followup resources), emergency physicians may treat markedly elevated blood pressure or initiate therapy for long-term control. [Consensus recommendation]

   3) Patients with asymptomatic markedly elevated blood pressure should be referred for outpatient followup. [Consensus recommendation]

illary cerebral vasculature, so that cerebral perfusion pressure is maintained within acceptable limits. Adjustment occurs in the opposite direction with systemic hypotension. The cerebral vasculature dilates to allow increased cerebral flood flow.[22]

In the setting of a hypertensive emergency, autoregulation can fail, leading to endothelial dysfunction and a cascade of deleterious processes resulting in cellular necrosis. The brain is particularly at risk. Among those harmful sequelae of endothelial dysfunction are capillary permeability and edema, inflammation, thrombosis, decreased nitric oxide production, and release of various vasoconstricting agents such as endothelin 1.[18]

KEY POINT

Autoregulation of cerebral blood flow can fail in hypertensive crisis, leading to endothelial dysfunction and a number of deleterious sequelae, ultimately resulting in cell death.

In patients with chronic hypertension, the "set point" at which autoregulation triggers cerebrovascular constriction or dilation rises. In other words, the cerebral circulation adjusts to the chronically elevated pressure. If the blood pressure is reduced rapidly to a normal level in such patients, cerebral perfusion pressure might fall below levels sufficient to maintain adequate cerebral tissue oxygenation (Figure 15-1).

For this reason, blood pressure should almost never be lowered rapidly and should almost never be lowered to a normal level in the emergency department. The goal of managing elevated blood pressure in a hypertensive emergency is to gradually reduce the mean arterial pressure (MAP) over about an hour by approximately 10% to 20%, with the diastolic pressure generally no lower than about 110 mm Hg. Further reduction can be achieved slowly over the ensuing hours in the hospital. The one exception to this rule is thoracic aortic dissection, when rapid reduction to near normal, or slightly below normal, pressure might be indicated. This scenario is discussed later in this chapter.

KEY POINT

With the exception of aortic dissection, the goal in reducing blood pressure in hypertensive crisis is a 10% to 20% reduction of MAP, with the diastolic pressure generally no lower than about 110 mm Hg.

The Renin-Angiotensin-Aldosterone System[23,24]

Homeostasis of blood pressure is in large part mediated by the RAAS. When blood pressure, and thus renal blood flow, falls, the juxtaglomerular cells of the kidney release *renin*. Renin catalyzes the conversion of *angiotensinogen* produced by the liver to *angiotensin I*. Angiotensin I is then converted to *angiotensin II* by the catalytic effect of *angiotensin-converting enzyme* (ACE) (Figure 15-2).

Angiotensin II is an extremely important agent in main-

FIGURE 15-1.

Cerebral autoregulation, hypertension, and excessive correction. Rapid reduction of blood pressure to normal in patients with chronically elevated pressure can result in a disproportionate reduction of cerebral blood flow to ischemic levels. Adapted from: Elliott WJ. Hypertensive emergenices. *Crit Care Clin.* 2001;17:435.

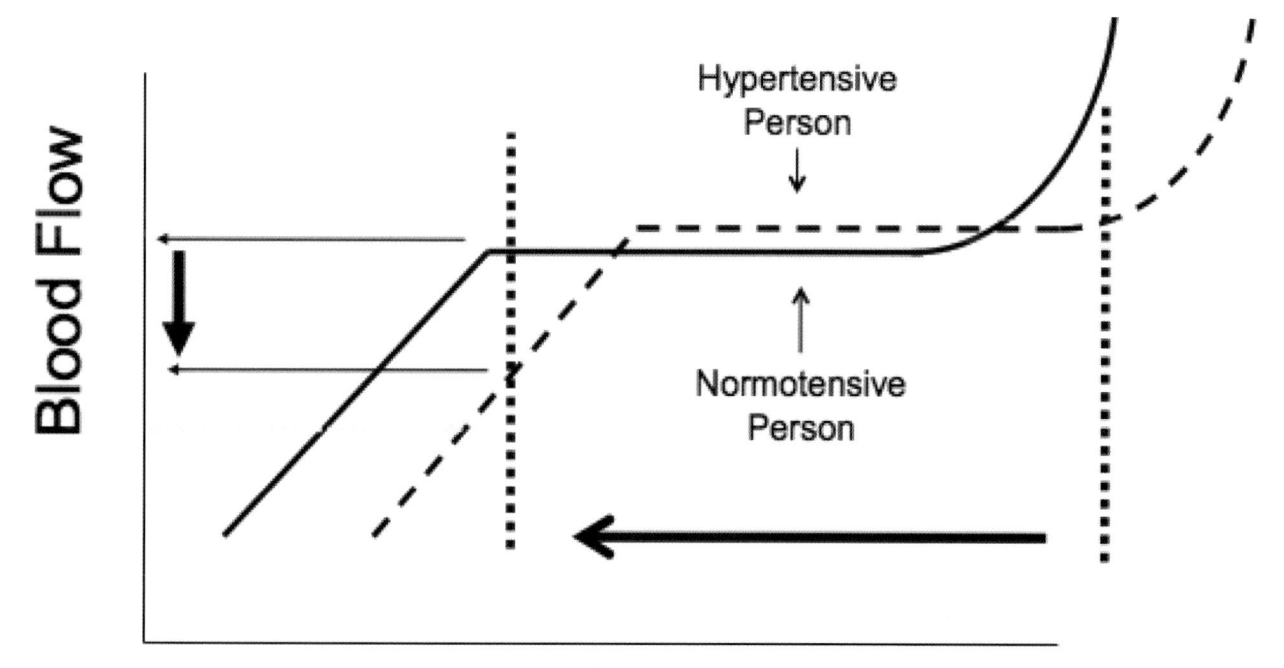

taining blood pressure. It is a powerful vasoconstrictor, and it stimulates the release of aldosterone from the adrenal glands. Aldosterone then leads to increased sodium and water retention by the kidneys, thereby increasing intravascular volume. Angiotensin II stimulates release of antidiuretic hormone from the pituitary, leading to further water retention by the kidneys. Excess angiotensin II is thought to stimulate an inflammatory response in the smooth muscle of the vasculature and the heart, leading over time to stiffening of the arterial walls, increased vascular resistance, and ventricular hypertrophy. Angiotensin II also leads to decreased production of nitric oxide, a principal agent of vasodilation (Table 15-2).

The crucial role that angiotensin II plays in the regulation of blood pressure provides an excellent target for blood pressure reduction, by interfering with either its production or its action at the receptor site. Angiotensin II activity can be reduced by blocking the renin-mediated conversion of angiotensinogen to angiotensin I, by blocking the ACE-mediated conversion of angiotensin I to angiotensin II, or by blocking the end-organ action of angiotensin II at the receptor site. Thus, we have three categories of pharmacologic agents to lower blood pressure by altering the RAAS.

Pharmacologic Treatment Modalities

As mentioned, the only way blood pressure can be affected is by altering stroke volume, heart rate, or peripheral arterial vascular resistance—or some combination of these elements. The effect of all antihypertensive medications is governed by this principle. The agents that are available for treatment of elevated blood pressure[25-29] fall into several pharmacologic groups, which are discussed in this section.

Parenteral Vasodilators (Table 15-3)

Nitroprusside[30,31]

Nitroprusside has long been the standard parenteral agent used to lower blood pressure in the emergency department. It generates nitric oxide, a potent vasodilator. Although nitroprusside dilates both the arterial and venous circulation, it predominantly affects the arterial vasculature and is a very potent antihypertensive agent. Nitroprusside has a very short half-life, and its action can be terminated rapidly by discontinuing the infusion should the blood pressure drop excessively.

However, nitroprusside does have some negative attributes. It is unstable to ultraviolet light and must be wrapped in opaque foil. Additionally, overshooting the intended reduction in blood pressure is not uncommon, so the patient should remain supine. During nitroprusside infusion, continuous monitoring of the blood pressure via an arterial line is typically recommended. Nitroprusside is metabolized to cyanide and then to thiocyanate, both of which are toxic. Nitroprusside crosses into the fetal circulation and is potentially toxic to the fetus. If it extravasates, it can cause tissue necrosis. Finally, at least theoretically, it can increase intracranial pressure.

Nitroglycerin[32]

Like nitroprusside, *nitroglycerin* is a nitric oxide generator that induces both arterial and venous dilation. However, unlike nitroprusside, venodilation predominates. This means that nitroglycerin is not an ideal drug for the purpose of lowering arterial blood pressure. It serves well, however, as the basis of therapy for acute heart failure and acute coronary syndromes, due to its preload-reducing effect via venodilation and its effect on coronary artery resistance.[33] Because nitroglycerin can cause arterial vasodilation and induce hypotension, the patient's blood pressure should be monitored carefully.

Fenoldopam[34-36]

Fenoldopam is an alternative to nitroprusside. It is a dopamine-1 (DA-1) receptor agonist. DA-1 receptors cause dilation of the vasculature of the renal, cerebral, coronary, and mesenteric circulation. Unlike nitroprusside, it is not metabolized to cyanide and thiocyanate.

Fenoldopam has a rapid onset and offset of action but, compared with nitroprusside, it presents less chance of overshooting the intended clinical effect and causing lower-than-intended blood pressure. Because it dilates the renal vasculature, it has a beneficial effect on kidney function. It is not a light-sensitive drug. It should be used with caution in patients with glaucoma, because it raises intraocular pressure.

FIGURE 15-2.

Synthesis of angiotensin II: part of the renin-angiotensin-aldosterone system.

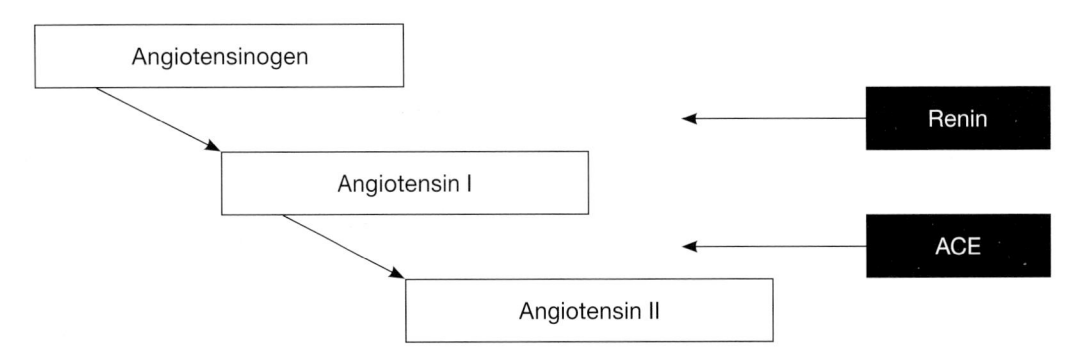

Renin and angiotensin-converting enzymes catalyze the systhesis of angiotensin I and angiotensin II, respectively.

KEY POINTS

Nitroprusside is a very effective antihypertensive agent, but it has a number of negative attributes, including photosensitivity, the production of toxic metabolites, and its tendency to drop the blood pressure beyond the intended target.

Nitroglycerin is not an ideal drug to lower blood pressure directly, but it is the basis of treatment of acute heart failure and acute cardiac syndromes.

Fenoldopam is an effective parenteral antihypertensive that dilates the renal vasculature.

Beta-Blockers (Table 15-4)

Beta$_1$-adrenergic stimulation increases heart rate as well as myocardial contractility. Thus, beta-blocking agents are ideal for lowering blood pressure by decreasing all three parameters: heart rate (bradycardic effect), stroke volume (lusitropic effect), and, with some preparations, peripheral vascular resistance (vasodilation). They also decrease renin output from the kidneys, which decreases angiotensin II, leading to a number of additional antihypertensive effects that are discussed later in this chapter.

Beta-blockers are particularly useful in patients with coronary artery disease, because they decrease myocardial oxygen demand. Potential disadvantages caused by excessive beta-blockade include bradycardia, heart block, heart failure, and bronchospasm (by inhibiting the bronchodilating effect of beta$_2$-stimulation). Therefore, beta-blockers should be used with caution in patients with underlying cardiac conduction or bronchospastic disorders.

Beta-blockers commonly used in emergency medicine are metoprolol, labetalol (which is also an alpha-blocker), and esmolol. Esmolol is a parenteral beta-blocker that is both short acting and cardioselective. Esmolol is thus preferred in patients with relative contraindications to beta-blockade, such as those with cardiac conduction or bronchospastic disorders. In such patients, discontinuation of the esmolol infusion leads to rapid termination of its effect.

KEY POINTS

Beta-blockers (generic names often end in "-lol"):

TABLE 15-2.

Actions of angiotensin II

Decreased nitric oxide leads to further vasoconstriction
Hypertrophy of smooth muscle cells leads to increased vascular resistance and ventricular hypertrophy
Inflammatory response
Powerful vasoconstrictor
Release of aldosterone
Release of antidiuretic hormone

Advantage—especially useful in patients with coronary artery disease

Precautions—bradycardia, heart block, bronchospasm

Calcium Channel Blockers[26,37-41] (Table 15-5)

By blocking the calcium channels in the musculature of the arterial walls and the heart, as well as by slowing atrioventricular conduction and sinuatrial node automaticity, the medications in this category are quite effective as antihypertensive and antiarrhythmic agents, depending on their individual properties.

There are two subtypes of calcium channel blockers. In the dihydropyridine group, the vascular effect predominates, whereas in the nondihydropyridine group, the cardiac effect predominates. Dihydropyridine agents such as *nifedipine, amlodipine, felodipine, nicardipine,* and *clevidipine* are most effective in lowering blood pressure. The nondihydropyridines, such as *verapamil* and *diltiazem*, are used in the emergency department to decrease the heart rate in patients with supraventricular tachycardias such as atrial fibrillation.

The parenteral dihydropyridine agents have several advantages over nitroprusside in treating hypertensive emergencies. They are as effective as nitroprusside in reducing blood pressure, but they have no toxic metabolites and are not light sensitive. Additionally, they are less likely to overshoot the target blood pressure, so there is less need for frequent rate adjustment. Arterial lines are often considered unnecessary.

The calcium channel blockers that are most useful for treating hypertensive emergencies in the emergency department are *nicardipine and clevidipine*. In conditions associated with tachycardia such as atrial fibrillation with rapid ventricular response *diltiazem* and *verapamil* are more appropriate.

KEY POINT

Dihydropyridine calcium channel blockers have no toxic metabolites, are not light sensitive, and require less frequent rate adjustments when compared to nitroprusside.

Angiotensin-Converting Enzyme Inhibitors

The first drugs developed to affect the production of angiotensin II were the ACE inhibitors (Figure 15-2). They effectively control blood pressure for millions of patients and are widely prescribed. In addition to their direct inhibition of angiotensin II synthesis, ACE inhibitors block the metabolism of bradykinin, a powerful vasodilator, which enhances their effect.

However, the blocking of bradykinin metabolism by ACE

TABLE 15-3.

Parenteral vasodilators

Fenoldopam
Nitroglycerine
Nitroprusside

inhibitors also limits their use in many patients. Increased bradykinin may be associated with a bothersome chronic cough, necessitating discontinuation of the ACE inhibitors. More importantly, inhibition of bradykinin metabolism can cause life-threatening angioedema.[42]

KEY POINT

When evaluating patients with angioedema, it is important to ask if they are taking an ACE inhibitor.

The ACE inhibitors are not commonly used in the emergency department, with the exception of *enalaprilat,* which can be helpful in treating acute heart failure. However, the oral forms are prescribed for millions of patients and are particularly useful in diabetic patients and those with renal disease or heart failure.

Angiotensin II Receptor Blockers (ARBs)

Because of the cough that is experienced by many patients who take an ACE inhibitor and the drug's potentially fatal, though rare, association with angioedema, many patients are now prescribed one of the more recently developed ARBs. Rather than decreasing production of angiotensin II, ARBs achieve an effect similar to that of ACE inhibitors by blocking its action downstream at the receptor site (Figure 15-2). Unlike the ACE inhibitors, they do not inhibit metabolism of bradykinin and thus do not cause coughing. The incidence of angioedema in patients taking ARBs is significantly lower than in those taking ACE inhibitors.[43] As with the ACE inhibitors, there is not much use for ARBs in the emergency department, but these medications are increasingly prescribed for oral use, so it is important for emergency physicians to be aware of their properties.

Direct Renin Inhibitors

The newest agents that affect the RAAS are the direct renin inhibitors. Similar to the ACE inhibitors, which catalyze the conversion of angiotensin I to angiotensin II, the direct renin inhibitors act upstream by inhibiting the renin-mediated conversion of angiotensinogen to angiotensin I (Figure 15-2).

Like the ARBs and unlike the ACE inhibitors, the renin inhibitors do not interfere directly with the metabolism of bradykinin, so the cough and angioedema associated with increased levels of bradykinin would not be expected. However, these agents only recently became available, and reports of both cough and angioedema associated with their use are beginning to emerge. Still, their adverse effects are probably less frequent than those associated with ACE inhibitors.[43]

KEY POINT

In the emergency department, ACE inhibitors, ARBs, and renin inhibitors generally have no role in the acute lowering of blood pressure. However, they are excellent agents for the outpatient management of hypertension.

Diuretics[25,29,44]

Similar to the mediators of the RAAS, diuretics play a significant role in the outpatient treatment of hypertension; however, they are not very effective in treating acutely elevated blood pressure. Because many patients take diuretics on a long-term basis, it is relevant that we discuss them in this chapter.

Diuretics reduce blood volume, and they can dilate blood vessels. There are four main classes of diuretics:
- *Loop diuretics,* such as *furosemide* and *bumetanide,* are best for diuresis. They are quite potent because they block sodium/potassium exchange in the ascending loop of Henle, where most of the sodium is resorbed.
- *Thiazide diuretics,* such as *hydrochlorothiazide, chlorthalidone,* and *indapamide,* are best for treating chronic hypertension. They are less potent than the loop diuretics, but they have a longer half-life and are thus better for controlling chronic hypertension. They block ion exchange in the distal loop, where less sodium is resorbed.
- *Potassium-sparing diuretics,* such as *spironolactone* and *triamterene,* are the weakest diuretics. They act in the collecting system.
- *Carbonic anhydrase inhibitors,* such as *acetazolamide,* have little use in treating hypertension. They are weak diuretics and are used for conditions such as glaucoma and altitude illness. They exchange hydrogen ions for sodium ions in the proximal tubule.

The diuretics have a number of advantages for treating chronic hypertension. They are inexpensive, and they are effective in preventing the cardiovascular complications of chronic hypertension.[25,29]

The side effects of diuretics include hypokalemia, hypomagnesemia, hyponatremia, and hyperuricemia. Patients who are allergic to sulfonamide antibiotics might be allergic to certain

TABLE 15-4.

Beta-blockers most useful in the emergency department

Esmolol—short acting, particularly appropriate in patients with relative contraindications for beta-blockade
Labetalol—induces both alpha- and beta-blockade
Metoprolol

TABLE 15-5.

Calcium channel blockers most useful in the emergency department

Dihydropyridines to treat lower blood pressure in hypertensive crisis
Clevidipine
Nicardipine
Nondihydropyridines to lower heart rate in supraventricular tachycardias
Diltiazem
Verapamil

diuretics; however, this concern is controversial. Diuretics are often used in patients with an allergy to sulfonamides as long as their reaction has never been anaphylactic.

> **KEY POINTS**
>
> There are two classes of sulfonamides—those with an aromatic amine (the antimicrobial sulfonamides) and those without an aromatic amine (eg, the diuretics acetazolamide, furosemide, hydrochlorothiazide, and indapamide). Hypersensitivity reactions occur when the aromatic amine group is oxidized into hydroxylamine metabolites by the liver. Sulfonamides that do not contain this aromatic amine group undergo different metabolic pathways, suggesting that allergic reactions in this group are not linked to cross-reactivity in sulfa-allergic patients. That point is far from settled at this time.[45]
>
> Diuretics have no significant role in the emergency department to lower blood pressure; however, they are effective as outpatient therapy for many patients.

Alpha-Adrenergic Blockers and Agonists

Stimulation of the alpha$_1$-adrenergic receptors in the muscles of the walls of the blood vessels causes vasoconstriction. Stimulation of the alpha$_2$-receptors has a number of effects, among them inhibition of vasoconstriction and thus vasodilation. We can therefore modulate peripheral arterial vascular resistance and blood pressure by manipulating either portion of the alpha-adrenergic system.

Alpha$_1$-adrenergic blocking agents have a very limited role in the emergency department, but intravenous *phentolamine*, along with a beta-blocker to block tachycardia, may be used to lower blood pressure in patients with pheochromocytoma. It can also be used to treat acutely elevated blood pressure in patients with monoamine oxidase inhibitor toxicity. In the outpatient setting, oral *phenoxybenzamine*, and the newer generation of alpha$_1$-blockers such as *prazosin, doxazosin,* and *terazosin* can also be useful for treating hypertension related to pheochromocytoma.

The alpha$_2$-adrenergic agonist *clonidine* is one of many drugs used in the past to lower blood pressure in patients with hypertensive urgency when treatment was considered necessary.[46] However, in recent years, practice has changed toward not treating asymptomatic hypertension in the emergency department (Table 15-1).[16] Clonidine should not be prescribed for outpatient therapy. It is not a good drug for long-term blood pressure control. Its discontinuation after chronic use can cause rebound hypertension.

Miscellaneous Agents

A number of older medications have been superseded by newer agents. Medications that no longer have much, if any, role in emergency medicine include the ganglionic blocker *trimethaphan* and centrally acting sympatholytic agents such as *reserpine* and *alpha methyldopa*. While *hydralazine*, a direct muscle relaxant, has traditionally been used to treat hypertensive crisis in pregnancy, newer agents such as *labetalol* are used increasingly by obstetricians and emergency physicians to treat this disorder.[47,48]

Specific Emergencies That Could Require Blood Pressure Reduction in the Emergency Department

In the previous section, we discussed pharmacologic agents. We now apply these medications to the specific disorders in which acutely elevated blood pressure might require treatment in the emergency department (Table 15-6).[49-51] In many of these conditions, treatment of the underlying disorder obviates the need to address the secondary effect of elevated blood pressure.

Hypertensive Encephalopathy

In this disorder, acutely elevated blood pressure overwhelms cerebral autoregulation, leading to arteriolar spasm and resultant cerebral ischemia, vascular permeability with resultant cerebral edema, and possible hemorrhage.

Symptoms are generally global, such as headache, nausea, blurred vision, or altered level of consciousness. Symptoms may occasionally be focal, but generally they do not correspond to a single anatomic vessel, as occurs with stroke. A CT scan might show cerebral edema or small focal hemorrhages, or it could be unremarkable in the early stages.

Treatment involves the slow and controlled reduction of blood pressure over about an hour. As discussed in the section on autoregulation above, to avoid cerebral hypoperfusion, rapid reduction of blood pressure (and reduction to a normal level) should never be achieved in the emergency department except in cases of aortic dissection. In all other hypertensive emergencies, blood pressure should generally remain above a diastolic pressure of 110 mm Hg during the emergency department phase of care.

Several agents can be used to lower the blood pressure in a patient with hypertensive encephalopathy. Nitroprusside is effective, but it can easily overshoot the target blood pressure

TABLE 15-6.

Conditions in which acutely elevated blood pressure may need to be treated in the emergency department

Acute coronary syndromes and myocardial infarction
Acute heart failure/pulmonary edema
Acute renal failure
Aortic dissection
Cocaine and amphetamine toxicity
Hypertensive encephalopathy
Microangiopathic hemolytic anemia
Pheochromocytoma
Preeclampsia and eclampsia
Stroke
Uncontrolled epistaxis or other hemorrhage

and, at least theoretically, increase intracranial pressure.[49] Nitroprusside also impairs cerebrovascular reactivity to changes in carbon dioxide levels and exacerbates the drop in cerebral perfusion pressure in response to a given decrease in peripheral blood pressure.[42]

Labetalol, which has both alpha- and beta-blocking properties, is an ideal drug for acute cerebral hypertensive emergencies. It shifts the cerebral autoregulation set point to a lower level, thereby preserving cerebral blood flow at lower blood pressures[52,53] (Figure 15-1). Unlike nitroprusside, it preserves cerebrovasculature reactivity to carbon dioxide.

The calcium channel blocker *nicardipine* is favored by many stroke neurologists for acute and titratable control of elevated blood pressure. It is being used increasingly in patients with hypertensive encephalopathy and, when necessary, acute stroke.[54] A recently introduced calcium channel blocker, *clevidipine*, could also prove useful in this disorder.[40]

KEY POINT

Recommended treatment options for hypertensive encephalopathy[40,49,54]:

- Labetalol
- Nicardipine
- Fenoldopam or clevidipine may be considered.

Ischemic and Hemorrhagic Stroke

Many stroke patients present to the emergency department with acutely elevated blood pressure. It is now thought that this elevation is generally a beneficial, transient response, particularly in ischemic stroke, that increases cerebral blood flow to the area of ischemia. In most cases, elevated blood pressure associated with ischemic stroke should not be treated in the emergency department unless the pressure remains extremely elevated.[54] As with other emergency department patients, the initial blood pressure generally declines after the patient is reassured and painful procedures such as intravenous line insertion and blood draws have been completed.[11] However, persistent, severe hypertension in stroke patients should be reduced gently, especially in those with hemorrhagic stroke.[54-57] For *ischemic* stroke, the 2007 guidelines from the American Academy of Neurology state: "The level of blood pressure that would mandate such treatment is not known, but consensus exists that medications should be withheld unless the systolic blood pressure is >220 mm Hg or the diastolic blood pressure is >120 mm Hg" (Class I, Level of Evidence: C).[54]

The goal is an approximate 10% to 20% reduction of the MAP without reducing the DBP below 110 mm Hg. If treatment of the elevated blood pressure is deemed appropriate, the target of 185/110 to meet criteria for administration of tissue plasminogen activator (tPA) in ischemic stroke is reasonable, even in patients who are not tPA candidates.

For *hemorrhagic* stroke, the 2010 American Heart Association/American Stroke Association guidelines recommend lowering blood pressure if the SBP is above 180 or the MAP is above 130. A target of approximately 160/90 or an MAP of 110 might be appropriate (Level of Evidence: C). The guidelines also state that for patients presenting with SBP of 150 to 220 mm Hg, acute lowering to 140 mm Hg is probably safe (Class IIa; Level of Evidence: B).[56]

The agents most often used for blood pressure reduction in stroke are, as in hypertensive encephalopathy, *labetalol* and *nicardipine*.

KEY POINTS

In *ischemic* stroke, consider blood pressure reduction if the SBP is above 220 or the DBP is above 120 mm Hg. The tPA target of 185/110 is a reasonable goal.[54]

In *hemorrhagic* stroke, a target of approximately 160/90 or an MAP of 110 mm Hg might be appropriate. The reduction of SBP to 140 mm Hg is also probably safe in patients who have an initial SBP between 150 and 220 mm Hg.[56]

Recommended treatment options for severe hypertension associated with acute stroke[40,49,54,56]:

- Labetalol
- Nicardipine
- Fenoldopam or clevidipine may also be considered.

Acute Aortic Dissection[27,49]

The goal in the initial treatment of acute aortic dissection is to prevent extension of the dissection and/or rupture, most commonly into the pericardial space. This is accomplished by rapidly lowering blood pressure to a normal or even subnormal level. Aortic dissection is the only condition for which rapid reduction, as well as reduction to a normal or subnormal level, is indicated. In addition, reflex tachycardia must be prevented to reduce aortic wall stress. Several therapeutic choices are available.

One option is to lower the blood pressure with *nitroprusside* and prevent reflex tachycardia with a beta-blocker such as *metoprolol* or *esmolol*. Nitroprusside is the most rapidly acting agent; alternatives include nicardipine and fenoldopam. The beta-blocker should be started first to prevent reflex tachycardia.

Another option is to use the alpha-blocking effect of *labetalol* to lower blood pressure as well as its beta-blocking effect to prevent tachycardia. However, it should be noted that intravenous labetalol has approximately seven times more beta- than alpha-blocking effect; therefore a second agent for blood pressure lowering is still usually required.

KEY POINT

Recommended treatment for acute aortic dissection (both blood pressure and heart rate should be lowered):

- To lower heart rate: administer a beta-blocker such as metoprolol or esmolol prior to medications that solely reduce blood pressure
- To lower blood pressure: nitroprusside, nicardipine, or fenoldopam
- To lower blood pressure and heart rate: labetalol

Unstable Angina, Non–ST-Elevation Myocardial Infarction, and ST-Elevation Myocardial Infarction

Although acutely elevated blood pressure can precipitate angina or myocardial infarction, elevated blood pressure in these conditions is usually the result of the acute cardiac event. Treatment of the acute coronary syndrome (ACS) or myocardial infarction (MI), and especially pain control, usually lowers blood pressure to a satisfactory level. Thus, the acutely elevated blood pressure generally does not need to be addressed specifically, because it will usually respond to nitroglycerin, opioids, beta-blockers, and other interventions appropriate for these conditions.

KEY POINT

Treatment of the underlying disorder (ACS or MI) usually lowers blood pressure satisfactorily.

Acute Heart Failure/Pulmonary Edema

Patients presenting to the emergency department with acute pulmonary edema commonly have acutely elevated blood pressure. As with ACS or MI, the blood pressure rarely needs to be addressed directly. As hypoxia and the sensation of dyspnea respond to oxygen and vasodilation with nitroglycerin, the blood pressure usually declines to an acceptable level.[58-60]

If the blood pressure remains significantly elevated despite adequate nitroglycerin and relief of hypoxia, acute hypertension might be the cause of the acute heart failure, rather than the opposite. In this rare situation, reduction of blood pressure using *nitroprusside* is considered an option.

KEY POINT

Administration of oxygen and a vasodilator such as nitroglycerin usually lowers blood pressure satisfactorily in patients with hypertension associated with acute heart failure/pulmonary edema.

Preeclampsia and Eclampsia

Blood pressure typically declines during pregnancy—SBP above 140 mm Hg and DBP over 90 mm Hg are abnormal. Signs of pathology associated with hypertension in pregnancy include hyperreflexia, proteinuria, abnormal renal or hepatic function, and seizures. Emergent treatment is indicated if the SBP is over 160 or the DBP is over 110. As with other hypertensive emergencies, the pressure should be lowered gradually over about an hour and maintained at an elevated level in the emergency department, in this case, to avoid placental hypoperfusion. The DBP should not be dropped below 90 mm Hg.[27,48,61]

Intravenous *hydralazine* has been used traditionally to treat hypertension associated with preeclampsia and eclampsia, and this is still an acceptable choice. However, *labetalol* or *nicardipine* is used more commonly by emergency physicians, and the American College of Obstetrics and Gynecology endorses both hydralazine and labetalol as acceptable alternatives.[47,48]

Nitroprusside is effective in lowering blood pressure, but it crosses the placental barrier, raising concern for fetal cyanide poisoning. Magnesium should be added to prevent seizures.

KEY POINT

Recommended treatment options for hypertension in preeclampsia/eclampsia are labetalol, nicardipine, and hydralazine. Magnesium is used to prevent seizures.

Cocaine and Amphetamine Toxicity

Benzodiazepines are the treatment of choice. They act as a competitive inhibitor at the receptor site. A danger of treating these disorders with a beta-blocker alone is that their alpha-adrenergic toxicity remains and manifests as reflex vasoconstriction in the setting of isolated beta-blockade.

KEY POINT

Benzodiazepines are recommended for treatment of hypertension associated with cocaine and amphetamine toxicity.

Pheochromocytoma

Treatment of this disorder is similar to that of aortic dissection. Both blood pressure and heart rate must be addressed, as pheochromocytoma causes a mixed alpha- and beta-adrenergic toxicity.

The traditional treatment for hypertension associated with pheochromocytoma has been *phentolamine (an alpha-blocker)* or *nitroprusside* to lower blood pressure, together with a beta-blocker such as *metoprolol* to lower the heart rate. Since labetalol has both alpha- and beta-blocking properties, it would seem to be an option for pheochromocytoma. However, it is a more powerful beta-blocker than alpha-blocker, so its administration could lead to paradoxic vasoconstriction and increased blood pressure. It has not been used extensively to treat pheochromocytoma.

KEY POINT

Recommended treatments for hypertension associated with pheochromocytoma:

To lower blood pressure: phentolamine or nitroprusside

To lower heart rate: a beta-blocker such as metoprolol

Acute Renal Failure

Elevated blood pressure in association with acute renal failure is often treated by dialysis. When additional medications are needed, *nitroprusside* is quite effective; however, nitroprusside is metabolized to cyanide and then to thiocyanate, both of which are toxic. Thiocyanate levels increase higher than usual in renal failure.[62] Safer alternatives for the treatment of hypertension associated with renal failure are *nicardipine* and *fenoldopam*.[27]

KEY POINT

Recommended treatment for hypertension in association with acute renal failure:

TABLE 15-7.

Examples of outpatient antihypertensive medications

Angiotensin-converting enzyme inhibitors
Benazepril
Captopril
Enalapril
Lisinopril
Quinapril
Ramipril
Angiotensin receptor blockers
Losartan
Olmesartan
Telmisartan
Valsartan
Beta-blockers
Atenolol
Bisoprolol
Carvedilol
Labetalol
Metoprolol
Nadolol
Pindolol
Propranolol
Timolol
Calcium channel blockers (dihydropyridines)
Amlodipine
Felodipine
Isradipine
Nicardipine
Nifedipine
Diuretics
Chlorthalidone
Hydrochlorothiazide
Spironolactone
Triamterene
Renin inhibitor
Aliskiren

Dialysis
Nicardipine
Fenoldopam

Asymptomatic Markedly Elevated Blood Pressure

As discussed earlier,[16] this condition is defined as a sustained, acutely elevated blood pressure in a potentially dangerous range, but without evidence of acute organ injury. Although treatment of elevated blood pressure over the long term is of course important, there has been no convincing evidence that treatment of asymptomatic elevated blood pressure in the emergency department is warranted.[63] According to the 2013 ACEP clinical policy on the management of adult patients with asymptomatic elevated blood pressure,[16] patients with this condition should be referred for outpatient followup, but treatment in the emergency department is not required.[16]

The ACEP clinical policy does state that in select patient populations, such as those with poor followup potential, emergency physicians may treat markedly elevated blood pressure in the emergency department and/or initiate therapy for long-term control.[16] A number of agents have been utilized in this situation, including beta-blockers, calcium channel blockers, and ACE inhibitors.[64-66]

Outpatient Therapy

Patients who present to emergency departments take a myriad of prescription blood pressure medications. Table 15-7 lists some of them.

Over the past few years, many combination drugs have become available. Some preparations combine an antihypertensive

TABLE 15-8.

Summary of the treatment recommendations of the Eighth Joint National Committee (JNC-8)[69]

In the general nonblack population, including those with diabetes, initial antihypertensive treatment should include either
A thiazide-type diuretic or
A calcium channel blocker or
An angiotensin-converting enzyme (ACE) inhibitor or
An angiotensin receptor blocker (ARB)
In the general black population, including those with diabetes, initial antihypertensive treatment should include either
A thiazide-type diuretic or
A calcium channel blocker
In the population aged 18 years with chronic kidney disease, initial (or add-on) antihypertensive treatment should include either
An ACE inhibitor or
An ARB
This applies to all patients with chronic kidney disease and hypertension regardless of race or diabetes status.

medication with a statin. Many combine an antihypertensive with a low-dose diuretic. And still others combine antihypertensive medications from two or even three classes.

Although outpatient therapy for high blood pressure is not generally considered a part of an emergency physician's practice, initiation of therapy, or adjustment of existing therapy, is sometimes deemed appropriate. It is difficult to delineate the exact blood pressure parameters that warrant a prescription written by an emergency physician. This is a judgment call and must be tailored to the individual patient. However, if the blood pressure remains significantly elevated by the time of emergency department discharge, initiation or adjustment of outpatient therapy by the emergency physician might be indicated. This may be particularly appropriate in patients with heart failure, coronary artery disease, renal failure, or diabetes.

Many classes of antihypertensive medication are effective. A review that combined data from 42 clinical trials involving 192,478 patients randomized to 7 major treatment strategies, including placebo, found significant benefit from low-dose diuretics. Compared with placebo, low-dose diuretics were effective in reducing the relative risk of coronary heart disease, congestive heart failure, stroke, cardiovascular disease events, cardiovascular disease mortality, and total mortality. None of the first-line treatment strategies employing either beta-blockers, ACE inhibitors, calcium channel blockers, alpha-blockers, or angiotensin receptor blockers (ARBs) was significantly better than low-dose diuretics for any outcome.[66] Contrary to the results of the large studies cited above, however, a relatively small study with approximately 6,000 patients found ACE inhibitors to be superior to diuretic alone.[67]

So what drug might be appropriate for an emergency physician to prescribe as outpatient antihypertensive therapy? The long-awaited "2014 Evidence-Based Guideline for the Management of High Blood Pressure in Adults: Report From the Panel Members Appointed to the Eighth Joint National Committee (JNC-8)" was published as this book was going to press.[68] Whereas the 2003 JNC-7 report[1] recommended beginning outpatient therapy with a low-dose diuretic, and included beta-blocking agents as one of the choices, the JNC-8 report states that therapy in the nonblack general population should be initiated with any of the following: thiazide diuretic, calcium channel blocker, ACE inhibitor, or ARB. Black patients should receive only a diuretic or a calcium channel blocker. Regardless of race, therapy in patients with chronic kidney disease should include an ACE inhibitor or ARB.[67] Table 15-8 summarizes the medication recommendations of the JNC-8.

The JNC-8 recommendations also include the baseline blood pressures at which outpatient pharmacologic therapy of chronic hypertension should begin as well as the targeted goals of therapy.[68] However, these aspects of the report are not only controversial[69-71] but are also more applicable to primary care physicians than to the practice of emergency medicine.

CASE ONE RESOLUTION

You have evaluated a 64-year-old woman with a cough. You've diagnosed her with bronchitis, and she's now ready for discharge. Her blood pressure was 250/130 initially but is now down to 210/110. She's not taking any medication and has no history of hypertension. "Hey, Doc," asks the nurse, "What do you want to give her?"

This patient has asymptomatic markedly elevated blood pressure, which by definition is not accompanied by evidence of acute organ dysfunction. According to the 2013 ACEP clinical policy on asymptomatic elevated blood pressure,[16] neither diagnostic studies nor emergency department treatment to lower the blood pressure is required. However, referral for outpatient evaluation and treatment is warranted.[16]

CASE TWO RESOLUTION

Same patient, but her discharge blood pressure is 250/140 mm Hg. "Hey, Doc," asks the nurse, "What do you want to give her?"

Although routine medical intervention in the emergency department for asymptomatic markedly elevated blood pressure is not required according to the ACEP clinical policy,[16] many emergency physicians feel uncomfortable not addressing a pressure of this magnitude. Diagnostic studies, especially measurement of serum creatinine, could be appropriate. Treatment of the elevated pressure in the emergency department and initiation of outpatient therapy might also be appropriate, particularly if the patient might have a problem with outpatient followup.[16]

CASE THREE RESOLUTION

You're evaluating a 64-year-old man who has had severe chest pain radiating to his back for the past 3 hours. His initial blood pressure is 230/110 mm Hg. His ECG is normal but a chest radiograph and CT angiogram reveal an acute aortic dissection. "Hey, Doc," the nurse says, "The surgeon will be here in an hour."

Elevated blood pressure in the setting of acute aortic dissection must be addressed emergently. Rapid lowering of the patient's blood pressure is indicated, along with prevention of reflex tachycardia. Appropriate therapy includes initiation of a beta-blocker such as metoprolol prior to nitroprusside or single therapy with labetalol.

References

1. Chobanian AV, Bakris GL, Black HR, et al. and the National High Blood Pressure Education Program Coordinating Committee. The Seventh Report of the Joint National Committee on Prevention, Detection, Evaluation, and Treatment of High Blood Pressure. The JNC 7 Report. *JAMA*. 2003;289:2560-2572. Erratum in: *JAMA*. 2003;290:197.
2. Vasan RS, Larson MG, Leip EP, et al. Impact of high-normal blood pressure on the risk of cardiovascular disease. *N Engl J Med*. 2001;345:1291-1297.
3. Wang Y, Wang QJ. The prevalence of prehypertension and hypertension among US adults according to the new Joint National Committee guidelines. *Arch Intern Med*. 2004;164:2126-2134.
4. Lee M, Saver JL, Chang B, et al. Presence of baseline prehypertension and risk of incident stroke: a meta-analysis. *Neurology*. 2011;77:1330-1337.
5. Vasan RS, Beiser A, Seshadri S, et al. Residual lifetime risk for developing hypertension in middle-aged women and men: the Framingham Heart Study. *JAMA*. 2002;287:1003-1010.
6. Wright JT Jr, Agodoa L, Contreras G, et al. Successful blood pressure control in the African American Study of Kidney Disease and Hypertension. *Arch Intern Med*. 2002;162:1636-1643.
7. Lewington S, Clarke R, Qizilbash N, et al. Age-specific relevance of usual blood pressure to vascular mortality. *Lancet*. 2002;360:1903-1913.

8. Staessen JA, Gasowski J, Wang JG, et al. Risks of untreated and treated isolated systolic hypertension in the elderly: meta-analysis of outcome trials. *Lancet.* 2000;355:865-872.
9. Santos PC, Krieger JE, Pereira AC. Renin-angiotensin system, hypertension, and chronic kidney disease: pharmacogenetic implications. *J Pharmacol Sci.* 2012;120:77-88.
10. Geavlete O, Calin C, Croitoru M, Lupescu I, et al. Fibromuscular dysplasia - a rare cause of renovascular hypertension. Case study and overview of the literature data. *J Med Life.* 2012;5:316-320.
11. Tanabe P, Persell SD, Adams JG, et al. Increased blood pressure in the emergency department: pain, anxiety, or undiagnosed hypertension? *Ann Emerg Med.* 2008;51:221-229.
12. Cline DM, Selvin V, Ferrario CM, et al. Emergency department versus clinic followup blood pressures. *Acad Emerg Med.* 2006;13:S188.
13. Baumann BM, Abate NL, Cowan RM, Boudreaux emergency department. Differing prevalence estimates of elevated blood pressure in emergency department patients using 4 methods of categorization. *Am J Emerg Med.* 2008;26:561-565.
14. Decker WW, Godwin SA, Hess EP, et al. Clinical policy: critical issues in the evaluation and management of adult patients with asymptomatic hypertension in the emergency department. *Ann Emerg Med.* 2006;47:237-249.
15. Mancia G, De Backer G, Dominiczak A, et al. 2007 Guidelines for the management of arterial hypertension: the Task Force for the Management of Arterial Hypertension of the European Society of Hypertension (ESH) and of the European Society of Cardiology (ESC). *J Hypertens.* 2007;25:1105-1187.
16. Wolf SJ, Lo B, Shih RD, et al; American College of Emergency Physicians Clinical Policies Committee. Clinical policy: critical issues in the evaluation and management of adult patients in the emergency department with asymptomatic elevated blood pressure. Ann Emerg Med. 2013;62(1):59-68. Available at www.acep.org/clinicalpolicies. Accessed on October 7, 2013.
17. Beevers G, Lip GY, O'Brien E. The pathophysiology of hypertension. *BMJ.* 2001;322:912-916.
18. Bautista LE. Inflammation, endothelial dysfunction, and the risk of high blood pressure: epidemiologic and biological evidence. *J Hum Hypertens.* 2003;17:223-230.
19. Ault MJ, Ellrodt AG. Pathophysiologic events leading to the end organ effects of acute hypertension. *Am J Emerg Med.* 1985;3:10-15.
20. Okada M, Matsumori A, Ono K, et al. Cyclic stretch upregulates production of interleukin-8 and monocyte chemotactic and activating factor/monocyte chemoattractant protein-1 in human endothelial cells. *Arterioscler Thromb Vasc Biol.* 1998;18:894-901.
21. Verhaar MC, Beutler JJ, Gaillard CA, et al. Progressive vascular damage in hypertension is associated with increased levels of circulating P-selectin. *J Hypertens.* 1998;16:45-50.
22. Strandgaard S, Paulson OP. Cerebral autoregulation. *Stroke.* 1984;709:413-416.
23. üsing R, Sellers F. ACE inhibitors, angiotensin receptor blockers and direct renin inhibitors in combination: a review of their role after the ONTARGET trial. *Curr Med Res Opin.* 2009;25:2287-2301.
24. Musini VM, Fortin PM, Bassett K, Wright JM. Blood pressure lowering efficacy of renin inhibitors for primary hypertension. *Cochrane Database Syst Rev.* 2008 Oct 8;(4):CD007066
25. The ALLHAT Officers and Coordinators for the ALLHAT Collaborative Research Group: The major outcomes in high risk hypertensive patients randomized to angiotensin-converting enzyme inhibitor or calcium channel blocker vs. diuretic. The Antihypertensive and Lipid-Lowering Treatment to Prevent Heart Attack Trial (ALLHAT). *JAMA.* 2002;288:2981-2997.
26. aron J. Treatment of acute severe hypertension: current and newer agents. *Drugs.* 2008;68:283-297.
27. Johnson W, Nguyen ML, Patel R. Hypertension crisis in the emergency department. *Cardiol Clin.* 2012;30:533-543.
28. Patel HP, Mitsnefes M. Advances in the pathogenesis and management of hypertensive crisis. *Curr Opin Pediatr.* 2005;17:210-214.
29. Moser M, Oparil S, Cushman W, Papademetriou V. The ALLHAT study revisited: do newer data from this trial and others indicate changes in treatment guidelines? *J Clin Hypertens.* 2007;9:372-380.
30. Kowaluk EA, Seth P, Fung HL. Metabolic activation of sodium nitroprusside to nitric oxide in vascular smooth muscle. *J Pharmacol Exp Ther.* 1992;262:916-922.
31. Kowaluk EA, Fung HL. Vascular nitric oxide-generating activities for organic nitrites and organic nitrates are distinct. *J Pharmacol Exp Ther.* 1991;259:519-525.
32. Agvald P, Adding LC, Artlich A, et al. Mechanisms of nitric oxide generation from nitroglycerin and endogenous sources during hypoxia in vivo. *Br J Pharmacol.* 2002;135:373-382.
33. Kalweit GA, Schipke JD, Godehardt E, Gams E. Changes in coronary vessel resistance during postischemic reperfusion and effectiveness of nitroglycerin. *J Thorac Cardiovasc Surg.* 2001;122:1011-1018.
34. Murphy MB, Murray C, Shorten GD. Fenoldopam: a selective peripheral domapine-receptor agonist for the treatment of severe hypertension. *N Engl J Med.* 2001;345:1548-1557.

35. Tumlin JA, Dunbar LM, Oparil S, et al. Fenoldopam, a dopamine agonist, for hypertensive emergency: a multicenter randomized trial. Fenoldopam Study Group. *Acad Emerg Med.* 2000;7:653-662.
36. Devlin JW, Seta ML, Kanji S, et al. Fenoldopam versus nitroprusside for the treatment of hypertensive emergency. *Ann Pharmacother.* 2004;38:755-759.
37. Wallin JD. Intravenous nicardipine hydrochloride: treatment of patients with severe hypertension. *Am Heart J.* 1990;119(2 pt 2):434-437.
38. Neutel JM, Smith DH, Wallin D, et al. A comparison of intravenous nicardipine and sodium nitroprusside in the immediate treatment of severe hypertension. *Am J Hypertens.* 1994;7:623-628.
39. Yang HJ, Kim JG, Ryoo E, et al. Nicardipine versus nitroprusside infusion as antihypertensive therapy in hypertensive emergencies. *J Int Med Res.* 2004;32:118-123.
40. Deeks emergency department, Keating GM, Keam SJ. Clevidipine: a review of its use in the management of acute hypertension. *Am J Cardiovasc Drugs.* 2009;9:117-34.
41. Aronson S, Dyke CM, Stierer KA, et al. The ECLIPSE trials: comparative studies of clevidipine to nitroglycerin, sodium nitroprusside, and nicardipine for acute hypertension treatment in cardiac surgery patients. *Anesth Analg.* 2008;107:1110-1121.
42. Cross-Reactivity of ACE Inhibitor-Induced Angioedema with ARBs. Available at www.uspharmacist.com/content/c/10394/?t=women's_health. Accessed on October 2, 2013.
43. Toh S, Reichman ME, Houstoun M, et al. Comparative risk for angioedema associated with the use of drugs that target the renin-angiotensin-aldosterone system. *Arch Intern Med.* 2012;172:1582-1589.
44. Cushman WE, Ford CE, Cutler JA, et al. Success and predictors of blood pressure control in diverse North American settings: the Antihypertensive and Lipid-Lowering Treatment to Prevent Heart Attack Trial (ALLHAT). *J Clin Hypertens.* 2002;4:393-404.
45. Healy R, Jankowski TA. Which diuretics are safe and effective for patients with a sulfa allergy? *J Fam Pract.* 2007;56:488-490.
46. Bender SR, Fong MW, Heitz S, Bisognano JD. Characteristics and management of patients presenting to the emergency department with hypertensive urgency. *J Clin Hypertens* (Greenwich). 2006;8:12-18.
47. Emergent therapy for acute-onset, severe hypertension with preeclampsia or eclampsia. Committee Opinion No. 514. American College of Obstetricians and Gynecologists. *Obstet Gynecol.* 2011;118:1465-1468.
48. Vidaeff AC, Carroll MA, Ramin SM. Acute hypertensive emergencies in pregnancy. *Crit Care Med.* 2005;33(10 suppl):S307-S312.
49. Varon J. Diagnosis and management of labile blood pressure during acute cerebrovascular accidents and other hypertensive crises. *Am J Emerg Med.* 2007;25:949-959.
50. Abstracts of the 23rd Annual Scientific Meeting, American Society of Hypertension, New Orleans, Louisiana, May 14-17, 2008. *J Clin Hypertens.* 2008;10(5 suppl A):A1-A169.
51. Flanigan JS, Vitberg D. Hypertensive emergency and severe hypertension: what to treat, who to treat, and how to treat. *Med Clin North Am.* 2006;90:439-451..
52. Adams RE, Powers WJ. Management of hypertension in acute intracerebral hemorrhage. *Crit Care Clin.* 1997;13:131-161.
53. Olsen KS, Svendsen LB, Larsen FS, et al. Effect of labetalol on cerebral blood flow, oxygen metabolism and autoregulation in health humans. *Br J Anaesth.* 1995;75:51-54.
54. Adams HP Jr, del Zoppo G, Alberts MJ, et al. Guidelines for the early management of adults with ischemic stroke: a guideline from the American Heart Association/American Stroke Association Stroke Council, Clinical Cardiology Council, Cardiovascular Radiology and Intervention Council, and the Atherosclerotic Peripheral Vascular Disease and Quality of Care Outcomes in Research Interdisciplinary Working Groups: The American Academy of Neurology affirms the value of this guideline as an educational tool for neurologists. *Circulation.* 2007;115:e478-e534.
55. Arima H, Anderson CS, Wang JG, et al. Lower treatment blood pressure is associated with greatest reduction in hematoma growth after acute intracerebral hemorrhage. *Hypertension.* 2010;56:852-858.
56. Morgenstern LB, Hemphill JC 3rd, Anderson C, et al. Guidelines for the management of spontaneous intracerebral hemorrhage: a guideline for healthcare professionals from the American Heart Association/American Stroke Association. *Stroke.* 2010;41:2108-2129.
57. Anderson CS, Huang Y, Arima H, et al. Effects of early intensive blood pressure lowering treatment on the growth of hematoma and perihematomal edema in acute intracerebral hemorrhage: the Intensive Blood Pressure Reduction in Acute Cerebral Haemorrhage Trial (INTERACT). *Stroke.* 2010;41:307-312.
58. Cotter G, Metzkor E, Kaluski E, et al. Randomised trial of high-dose isosorbide dinitrate plus low-dose furosemide versus high-dose furosemide plus low-dose isosorbide dinitrate in severe pulmonary oedema. *Lancet.* 1998;351:389-393.
59. Vasodilation in the Management of Acute CHF (VMAC) Investigators. Intravenous nesiritide vs nitroglycerin for treatment of decompensated congestive heart failure: a randomized controlled trial. *JAMA.* 2002;287:1531-1540.

60. Abraham WT, Adams KF, Fonarow GC, et al. In-hospital mortality in patients with acute decompensated heart failure requiring intravenous vasoactive medications: an analysis from the Acute Decompensated Heart Failure National Registry (ADHERE). *J Am Coll Cardiol.* 2005;46:57-64.
61. Savvidou MD, Hingorani AD, Tsikas D, et al. Endothelial dysfunction and raised plasma concentrations of asymmetric dimethylarginine in pregnant women who subsequently develop pre-eclampsia. *Lancet.* 2003;361:1511-1517.
62. Cailleux A, Subra JF, Riberi P, et al. Cyanide and thiocyanate blood levels in patients with renal failure or respiratory disease. *J Med.* 1988;19:345-351.
63. Perez MI, Musini VM. Pharmacological interventions for hypertensive emergencies: a Cochrane systematic review. *J Hum Hypertens.* 2008;22:596-607.
64. Grassi D, O'Flaherty M, Pellizzari M, et al. Hypertensive urgencies in the emergency department: evaluating blood pressure response to rest and to antihypertensive drugs with different profiles. *J Clin Hypertens.* 2008;10:662-667.
65. Bakris GL, Kaplan NM, Forman JP. Management of severe asymptomatic hypertension (hypertensive urgencies). UpToDate. October 2012;Topic 3830. Version 8.0.
66. Psaty BM, Lumley T, Furberg CD, et al. Health outcomes associated With various antihypertensive therapies used as first-line agents: a network meta-analysis. *JAMA.* 2003;289:2534-2544.
67. Wing LM, Reid CM, Ryan P, et al. for the Second Australian National Blood Pressure Study. A comparison of outcomes with angiotensin-converting-enzyme inhibitors and diuretics for hypertension in the elderly. *N Engl J Med.* 2003;348:583-592.
68. James PA, Oparil S, Carter BL, et al. 2014 evidence-based guideline for the management of high blood pressure in adults: report from the panel members appointed to the Eighth Joint National Committee (JNC 8). *JAMA.* 2014;311(5):507-520. doi:10.1001/jama.2013.284427.
69. Sox HC. Assessing the trustworthiness of the guideline for management of high blood pressure in adults. *JAMA.* 2014;311(5):472-474.
70. Peterson ED, Gaziano JM, Greenland P. Recommendations for treating hypertension: what are the right goals and purposes? *JAMA.* 2014;311(5):474-476.
71. Bauchner H, Fontanarosa PB, Golub RM. Updated guidelines for management of high blood pressure: recommendations, review, and responsibility. *JAMA.* 2014;311(5):477-478.

Additional Reading

General Reviews

Elliott WJ. Clinical features in the management of selected hypertensive emergencies. *Progr Cardiovasc Dis.* 2006;48:316-325.

Elliott WJ. Management of hypertension emergencies. *Curr Hypertens* Rep. 2003;5:486-492.

Fenves AZ, Ram CV. Drug treatment of hypertensive urgencies and emergencies. *Semin Nephrol.* 2005;25:272-280.

Lehrmann JF, Tanabe P, Baumann BM, et al. Knowledge translation of the American College of Emergency Physicians clinical policy on hypertension. *Acad Emerg Med.* 2007;14:1090-1096.

Marik PE, Rivera R. Hypertensive emergencies: an update. *Curr Opin Crit Care.* 2011;17:569-580.

Vaughn CJ, Delanty N. Hypertensive emergencies. *Lancet.* 2000;356:411-417.

Yan C, Kim D, Aizawa T, et al. Functional interplay between angiotensin II and nitric oxide. *Arterioscler Thromb Vasc Biol.* 2003;23:26 36.

Specific Treatment Modalities

Bahadur, MM, Aggarwal VD, Mali M, et al. Novel therapeutic option in hypertensive crisis: sildenafil augments nitroprusside-induced hypotension. *Nephrol Dial Transplant.* 2005;20:1254-1256.

Elliott WJ, Weber RR, Nelson KS, et al. Renal and hemodynamic effects of intravenous fenoldopam versus nitroprusside in severe hypertension. *Circulation.* 1990;81:970-977.

Olsen KS, Svendsen LB, Larsen FS, et al. Effect of labetalol on cerebral blood flow, oxygen metabolism and autoregulation in health humans. *Br J Anaesth.* 1995;75:51-54.

Oparil S, Aronson S, Deeb GM, et al. Fenoldopam: A new parenteral antihypertensive: consensus roundtable on the management of perioperative hypertension and hypertensive crisis. *Am J Hypertens.* 1999;12:653-654.

Panacek EA, Bednarczyk EM, Dunbar LM, et al. Fenoldopam Study Group. Randomized, prospective trial of fenoldopam vs. sodium nitroprusside in the treatment of acute severe hypertension. *Acad Emerg Med.* 1995;2:959-965.

Pollack CV, Varon J, Garrison NA, et al. Clevidipine, an intravenous dihydropyridine calcium channel blocker, is safe and effective for the treatment of patients with acute severe hypertension. *Ann Emerg Med.* 2009;53:329-338.

Post JB, Frishman WH. Fenoldopam: A new dopamine agonist for the treatment of hypertensive urgencies and emergencies. *J Clin Pharmacol.* 1998;38:2-13.

Reisin E, Huth MM, Nguyen blood pressure, et al. Intravenous fenoldopam versus sodium nitroprusside in patients with severe hypertension. *Hypertension.* 1990;15(2 suppl):159-162.

Shusterman NH, Elliott WH, White WB. Fenoldopam, but not nitroprusside, improves renal function in severely hypertensive patients with normal or impaired baseline renal function. *Am J Med.* 1993;95:161-168.

Vincent JL, Berlot G, Preiser JC, et al., Intravenous nicardipine in the treatment of postoperative arterial hypertension. *J Cardiothorac Vasc Anesth.* 1997;11:160-164.

White WB, Halley SE. Comparative renal effects of intravenous administration of fenoldopam myselate and sodium nitroprusside in patients with severe hypertension. *Arch Intern Med.* 1989;149:870-874.

Outpatient Therapy

Aliskiren/Valsartan (Valturna) for Hypertension. *Med Lett.* 2009;51:94-95.

Blood Pressure Lowering Treatment Trialists' Collaboration: Effects of ACE inhibitors, calcium antagonists, and other blood-pressure-lowering drugs: results of prospectively designed overviews of randomized trials. *Lancet.* 2000;356:1955-1964.

Cook NR, Cutler JA, Obarzanek E, et al. Long term effects of dietary sodium reduction on cardiovascular disease outcome: observational followup of the Trials of Hypertension Prevention (TOHP). *BMJ.* 2007;334(7599):885-888.

Cutler JA, Roccela A. Salt reduction for preventing hypertension and cardiovascular disease. *Hypertension.* 2006;48:818-819.

Davis BR, Piller LB, Cutler JA. Role of diuretics in the prevention of heart failure: the antihypertensive and lipid-lowering treatment to prevent heart attack trial. *Circulation.* 2006;113:2201-2210.

Frank J. Managing hypertension using combination therapy. *Am Fam Phys.* 2008;77:1279-1286.

Gu Q, Burt VL, Dillon CF, et al. Trends in antihypertensive medication use and blood pressure control among United States adults with hypertension. The National Health and Nutrition Examination Survey, 2001 to 2010. *Circulation.* 2012;126:2105-2114.

Julius S, Kjeldsen SE, Weber M, et al. Outcomes in hypertensive patients at high cardiovascular risk treated with regimens based on valsartan or amlodipine: the VALUE trial. *Lancet.* 2004;363:2022-2031.

Law MR, Morris JK, Wald NJ. Use of blood pressure lowering drugs in the prevention of cardiovascular disease: meta-analysis of 147 randomised trials in the context of expectations from prospective epidemiological studies. *BMJ.* 2009;338:b1665.

Mitka M. Consumer group asks FDA to warn patients about hypertension combination therapy. *JAMA.* 2012;308:270-271.

Moser M, Cushman WC, Kaplan NM. Control of blood pressure: does it matter which agent you use? *J Clin Hypertens.* 2007;9:964-973.

Neutel JM, Sica DA, Franklin SS. Hypertension control: still not there-how to select the right add-on therapy to reach goal blood pressures. *J Clin Hypertens.* 2007;9:889-896.

Wald DS, Law M, Morris JK, et al. Combination therapy versus monotherapy in reducing blood pressure: meta-analysis on 11,000 participants from 42 trials. *Am J Med.* 2009;122:290-300.

CARDIOVASCULAR EMERGENCIES

CHAPTER 16

Cardiac Disease in Special Populations: HIV, Pregnancy, and Cancer

Siamak Moayedi and Mercedes Torres

IN THIS CHAPTER

Cardiac disease and HIV infection
Cardiac disease in pregnancy
Cardiac disease in cancer patients

Although cardiac disease affects all segments of the population, certain patients demonstrate unique risk factors and manifestations and require unique treatment plans based on concurrent medical issues. The diagnosis and treatment of cardiac disease can be complex in people infected with the human immunodeficiency virus (HIV), pregnant women, and cancer patients. The pathophysiology of cardiac disease in these groups is often directly related to the physiologic changes occurring as a result of their underlying state of health. A focus on the distinct features of each situation as they relate to the development of myocardial disease, pericardial disease, acute coronary syndrome, arrhythmias, and pulmonary hypertension provides the necessary background for optimal emergency care for these patients.

Cardiac Disease and HIV Infection

Since the 1980s, the field of medicine has made significant strides in understanding the pathophysiology of HIV infection and its clinical implications. These discoveries led to the introduction of highly active antiretroviral therapy (HAART) in the 1990s and dramatically improved the survival of HIV-infected people. As a result, the characteristics of cardiac disease in HIV-infected patients have changed. In the pre-HAART era, pericarditis, myocarditis, and cardiomyopathy were the most common cardiac complications of HIV infection.[1] In areas with poor access to medical care and HAART, these illnesses are still prevalent. Coronary artery disease (CAD) and acute coronary syndrome (ACS) are increasingly prevalent among HIV-infected patients in the developed world.[1] They have become the third most common cause of death in HIV-infected patients in the United States.[2] Emergency physicians caring for HIV-infected patients have experienced these changes firsthand. It is critical to understand the unique features of CAD and ACS in HIV-infected patients and the cardiac complications associated with antiretroviral (ARV) therapy. Simultaneously, the medical community's understanding of pericardial and myocardial disease continues to expand and remains relevant to the emergency care of patients with advanced HIV infection in resource-limited settings.

Acute Coronary Syndrome and Myocardial Infarction

CAD and ACS have become a common cause of morbidity and mortality among HIV-infected patients. The cause of this shift in the cardiac disease profile of HIV-infected patients appears to be multifactorial. ARVs such as protease inhibitors have been shown to cause hyperlipidemia, insulin resistance, and the metabolic syndrome, thereby creating multiple risk factors for the development of CAD. In addition, the virus itself has been shown to have direct effects on endothelial cells, leading to atherogenesis.[1] Furthermore, HIV-infected patients can present with multiple risk factors for ACS unrelated to their HIV-infection, such as a history of smoking, cocaine use, hypertension, and preexisting diabetes or hyperlipidemia. HIV-infected patients with ACS tend to present at a younger age, with a higher proportion of women affected, than is the case with non–HIV-infected patients.[3]

Multiple observational studies have demonstrated the association between the risk of ACS and the amount of time an HIV-infected patient has been taking ARVs. In 2008, members of the Data Collection on Adverse Events of Anti-HIV Drugs (DAD) study group published the results of an international collaboration involving 23,437 HIV-1–infected patients from 21 countries and their risk of ACS.[4] Their results confirmed previous observations. They documented an increased relative risk of myocardial infarction (MI) in HIV-infected patients taking ARVs and further demonstrated that the relative risk of MI doubled over a 5-year period of exposure to protease inhibitors. Protease inhibitors were independently associated with an increased risk of MI, while other classes of ARVs were not.[4] Protease inhibitors have been shown to cause elevated total cholesterol, triglyceride, and low-density lipoprotein (LDL) levels while decreasing high-density lipoprotein (HDL) levels. In addition, they cause central obesity, insulin resistance, and the metabolic syndrome. All of these metabolic changes contribute to CAD.[1,3] However, the authors of the DAD study noted that these metabolic changes alone could not account for the increased risk observed in HIV-infected patients taking protease inhibitors. They postulated that there might be direct cellular mechanisms, not yet identified, by which protease inhibitors promote atherogenesis.[4] Overall, the DAD results demonstrated that protease inhibitor use is a risk factor for CAD comparable in magnitude to a history of smoking or diabetes.[4]

KEY POINT

Protease inhibitor use is a risk factor for the development of CAD comparable to a history of diabetes or tobacco use and greater than a family history of CAD.[4]

While treatment with protease inhibitors confers an increased risk of ACS for HIV-infected patients, uncontrolled viral replication is even more detrimental.[1,3,5] HIV causes a chronic inflammatory state affecting the endothelium and vascular structures of the heart. In a recent comparison with non–HIV-infected controls, HIV-infected patients who had never received ARVs demonstrated endothelial dysfunction and carotid intima-media thickening.[6] Furthermore, when the data were divided based on viral load, the HIV-infected patients with high viral loads had significantly increased degrees of endothelial dysfunction. On a molecular level, several cytokines and proteins have been implicated in the process of HIV-related inflammation and atherogenesis.[3,6,7] The Strategies for Management of Antiretroviral Therapy (SMART) study group examined this issue on the clinical level.[5] Over 5,000 HIV-infected patients were randomized between continuous ARV exposure and interrupted therapy for an average of 16 months. Multiple end points were used to compare the risks of continuous exposure to ARVs versus CD4-guided interrupted ARV exposure. Patients in the interrupted treatment arm were taken off ARVs when their CD4 counts rose above 350 cells/mm^3 and placed back on ARVs when the CD4 count fell below 250 cells/mm^3. This allowed times of uncontrolled viral replication when no ARVs were being prescribed. Results demonstrated significantly increased morbidity and mortality in the interrupted treatment arm, as well as higher rates of new cardiovascular, renal, and hepatic disease. The hazard ratio of fatal or nonfatal cardiovascular disease in these patients was 1.6.[5] These results demonstrated that the cardiovascular risks of ARVs are outweighed by the risk of uncontrolled viral replication of HIV.

In the emergency department, when HIV-infected patients present with symptoms consistent with a possible diagnosis of ACS, practitioners should maintain a lower threshold for evaluation and treatment. HIV-infected patients on protease inhibitors, as well as those not currently on ARVs, are at significantly increased risk of ACS and MI. Based on the SMART trial results, HIV-infected patients who have had periods of non-compliance with their ARV regimens may be at highest risk of ACS because of their exposure to uncontrolled viral replication. The evaluation and treatment of HIV-infected patients presenting with symptoms that raise concern about ACS should be similar to those for the non–HIV-infected population. HIV-infected patients with acute MI have lower thrombolysis rates, lower percutaneous coronary intervention (PCI) rates, and higher mortality rates.[8] The cause of this disparity is not clear, as HIV-infected patients are equally as eligible for PCI and coronary artery bypass grafting as their non–HIV-infected counterparts.[1,8] However, relative contraindications to fibrinolytics such as acute pericarditis, infective endocarditis, acute cavitating pulmonary tuberculosis, and thrombocytopenia should be considered in this special population.[7] HIV-infected patients who undergo PCI have no difference in terms of adverse events, but they demonstrate a higher rate of restenosis.[1,2] As such, when HIV-infected patients with a history of PCI present to an emergency department with symptoms of ACS, the threshold for evaluation for restenosis should be lower.[1]

KEY POINT

In the emergency department, practitioners should maintain a low threshold for evaluation and treatment of HIV-infected patients for ACS. Patients who are noncompliant with their HAART are at greater risk of CAD and ACS than their HAART-compliant HIV-infected counterparts.

QTc Prolongation

A common ECG finding in HIV-infected patients is QTc prolongation. Patients with QTc intervals greater than 500 msec demonstrate a significantly increased risk of malignant arrhythmias, namely torsade de pointes.[9,10] The exact mechanism of the development of QTc prolongation in HIV-infected individuals is unknown. In many cases, it can be explained by a combination of the factors outlined in Table 16-1. Recent studies have shown that HIV-infected patients' risk for developing QTc prolongation increases significantly after the fourth year of infection.[11]

Although the mechanism of QTc prolongation among HIV-infected patients is unclear, a relationship with the use of ARVs, namely protease inhibitors, has been observed.[10] Given that protease inhibitors are one of the most frequently prescribed drugs for HIV-infected patients worldwide, determining their arrhythmogenic potential is paramount. It is postulated that protease inhibitors block specific potassium channels, leading to QTc prolongation. A handful of studies have attempted to determine the validity of this observation. Their results have been mixed.[10] Studies that demonstrated a relationship between protease inhibitor use and QTc prolongation have been criticized for their inability to account for potential confounders of their results.

Larger studies suggest that QTc prolongation is not related to protease inhibitor use. SMART trial data from 3,719 HIV-infected patients showed no relationship between protease inhibitor-based drug regimens and QTc prolongation compared with non–protease inhibitor drug regimens.[12] In addition, a prospective cross-sectional study of over 900 HIV-infected patients, in which the researchers accounted for possible confounders, demonstrated no association between ARV use and QTc prolongation.[11] Instead, researchers demonstrated an increased risk of QTc prolongation in women, whites, and patients of advanced age. Electrocardiographic findings associated with an increased risk of developing QTc prolongation included an incomplete right bundle-branch block and ventricular hypertrophy.[11] These results demonstrate that other factors such as underlying cardiac disease are more likely to contribute to the development of QTc prolongation in HIV-infected patients.

Therefore, QTc prolongation among HIV-infected patients is likely multifactorial.[10] The theoretic link between protease inhibitors and QTc prolongation through potassium channel blockage and P450 metabolism has not been established in the clinical setting. In addition, other factors (eg, concurrent use of other QTc-prolonging medications; age; gender; and coexisting cardiac, renal, or hepatic disease) contribute to an overall increased risk of QTc prolongation in HIV-infected patients, leading to an increased risk of torsade de pointes.

In the emergency department, the ECG of an HIV-infected patient should be scrutinized for QTc prolongation. Any known QTc-prolonging medications should be discontinued if it is found. Protease inhibitors should not be discontinued, because their role in prolongation of the QTc interval has not been established. Close consultation with an infectious disease specialist should guide any decision making regarding modification of the ARV regimen. Emergency practitioners prescribing new medications to HIV-infected patients should consider obtaining an ECG if those new medications are known to cause QTc prolongation (polypharmacy clearly increases the risk of the development of torsade de pointes in this high-risk population). If torsade de pointes develops, the treatment is the same as for non–HIV-infected patients, including administration of intravenous magnesium, tight control of potassium levels above 4.5 mEq/L, and overdrive transvenous pacing in refractory cases.[10]

KEY POINT

In the emergency department, if the ECG of an HIV-infected patient demonstrates QTc prolongation, the medication regimen should be reviewed and QTc-prolonging drugs, with the exception of ARVs, should be eliminated or avoided.

Pericardial Disease

Pericardial disease in HIV-infected patients can manifest as an asymptomatic effusion, effusion with pericarditis, constrictive pericarditis, or neoplastic infiltration.[13] The most common among these is an asymptomatic pericardial effusion, which occurs in 22% of patients with the acquired immunodeficiency syndrome (AIDS). The incidence of symptomatic pericarditis among AIDS patients is 11% per year.[14] Although decreasing in prevalence since the introduction of HAART, pericarditis is still a major factor in the morbidity and mortality of HIV-infected patients in resource-limited settings without access to ARVs. In one study, AIDS patients with effusions had a 6-month mortality rate of 62% compared with a 7% mortality rate among those without effusions.[15]

KEY POINTS

Since the introduction of HAART, pericardial disease and cardiomyopathy are less frequently encountered in the HIV-infected population of the developed world. However, they remain the most common cardiac complications of the disease in resource-limited settings without access to HAART.

AIDS patients with pericardial effusions have a 6-month mortality rate of 62% compared with 7% among AIDS patients without effusions.[15]

The causes of pericarditis or asymptomatic pericardial effusions in HIV-infected patients are often elusive. Even in patients with clinical deterioration requiring pericardial drainage or window, most effusions prove idiopathic.[14,16] The causes that have been identified are listed in Table 16-2. Pathologic analysis

TABLE 16-1.
Causes of QTc Prolongation in HIV-Infected Patients[9,10]

Exposure to QTc-prolonging medications
Pentamidine
Methadone
Antiemetics
Clarithromycin
Exposure to ARVs
Electrolyte abnormalities
Preexisting cardiac or hepatic disease
HIV-related autonomic dysfunction

of idiopathic effusions has suggested the possibility of HIV itself causing increased cytokine expression, leading to a capillary leak syndrome and subsequent effusion formation.[14,15] In addition, some cases of idiopathic pericardial effusion have been associated with concurrent myocarditis.[16,17]

The clinical presentation and overall management of HIV-infected patients with pericarditis is similar to that of the non–HIV-infected population. Asymptomatic HIV-infected patients who are incidentally found to have small to moderate-sized effusions do not require emergent diagnostic evaluation and can follow up for further outpatient monitoring. Those who are not on ARVs and demonstrate other evidence of opportunistic infection or AIDS-defining illness should be started on ARVs as soon as possible, with consultation by an infectious disease specialist, given the increased mortality associated with the presence an effusion.[13,14]

Symptomatic patients with pericardial effusions most commonly present to the emergency department complaining of dyspnea and are found to be tachycardic.[13,16] If the patient's clinical symptoms can be managed on an outpatient basis, he or she can be discharged with close followup for monitoring and initiation of ARVs as indicated. Even in symptomatic patients who require admission for supportive care, small to moderate effusions typically resolve without requiring invasive diagnostic evaluation or drainage.[13] Echocardiography is the diagnostic study of choice for patients with symptoms to determine the size and hemodynamics of the effusion. In rare cases, cardiac tamponade physiology develops, requiring emergent intervention with pericardiocentesis or pericardial window. In these instances, samples should be sent for culture, cytology, and gram stain.[14]

KEY POINT

Even symptomatic patients with small or moderate-sized pericardial effusions rarely require drainage.

In sub-Saharan Africa and other less developed parts of the world, tuberculosis (TB) pericarditis is the most common cause of pericardial effusion in HIV-infected patients.[17,18] For those who live in TB-endemic regions of Africa, more than 90% of pericardial effusions in HIV-infected patients are associated with TB.[17,18] Studies in these areas have shown that the 1-year mortality rate is increased from 12% among non–HIV-infected patients with TB pericarditis to 22% among HIV-infected patients with TB pericarditis.[17]

Treatment of TB pericarditis in HIV-infected patients is similar to that for non–HIV-infected patients, based on a multidrug regimen for 6 to 12 months. In patients not already on ARVs, the timing of ARV initiation is variable and should be determined by an infectious disease specialist. Although some articles support the initiation of a 6- to 8-week regimen of corticosteroids for patients with TB pericarditis, the benefits are still being debated.[19] The decision to initiate corticosteroid treatment for TB pericarditis should be made in conjunction with an infectious disease specialist. Notably, if prescribed, prednisone dosing should be high (1 to 2 mg/kg), given that concurrent rifampin therapy will increase its metabolism.[19]

KEY POINT

Tuberculosis is a leading cause of pericarditis in HIV-infected patients in the developing world.

TABLE 16-2.

Causes of Pericarditis in HIV-Infected Patients[13,14,16]

Bacterial infection	*Mycobacterium tuberculosis*
	Mycobacterium avium intracellulare
	Nocardia asteroids
	Staphylococcus aureus
Viral infection	Coxsackievirus
	Herpes simplex virus
	Cytomegalovirus
	Epstein-Barr virus
Fungal infection	*Cryptococcus neoformans*
	Histoplasma capsulatum
Neoplasm	Kaposi sarcoma
	Lymphoma
Other	Uremia
	Autoimmune

Myocardial Disease and Dilated Cardiomyopathy

Since the advent of HAART, myocarditis and cardiomyopathy have become less prominent in the developed world. A large proportion of HIV-infected patients in sub-Saharan Africa and other less developed areas still suffer from these illnesses.[20] In the largest study of cardiac manifestations of advanced HIV infection in sub-Saharan Africa, HIV-related cardiomyopathy was the most common diagnosis, occurring in 38% of the more than 500 enrolled patients.[20,21]

Several factors contribute to the development of cardiomyopathy in HIV-infected patients. First, although myocardial cells do not have CD4 receptors, the HIV virus has been shown to enter these cells and impair their function. HIV-1 can be present in myocardial cells for extended periods, regardless of ARV use, causing the release of cytotoxic cytokines and progressive tissue damage due to the chronic inflammatory state.[13,14] In addition, many of the common opportunistic infections that arise in HIV-infected patients can cause subclinical myocarditis or manifestations consistent with dilated cardiomyopathy. These include infections of coxsackievirus, Epstein Barr virus, cytomegalovirus, toxoplasmosis, and *Mycobacterium avium intracellulare*. Other common causes in patients with untreated HIV include autoimmune disease, Kaposi sarcoma, lymphoma, drug toxicities, and malnutrition.[20,22,23] Notably, the use of zidovudine in HAART regimens has been associated with the development of dilated cardiomyopathy.[13]

Most HIV-infected patients with myocarditis remain asymptomatic. They tend to have significantly higher viral loads and lower CD4 counts.[21,23] Those who are symptomatic typically present with evidence of left ventricular dysfunction.[16] The severity of heart failure varies; however, once patients develop clinically evident heart failure, they progress rapidly, with increased mortality rates.[13,14,23] The emergency department evaluation of these patients is the same as that of non–HIV-infected patients presenting with symptoms of cardiomyopathy and heart failure. An echocardiogram is essential to determine the extent of disease and is typically obtained during the inpatient or subsequent outpatient evaluation.[14]

KEY POINT

By the time HIV-infected patients develop clinically evident heart failure, they progress rapidly and have significantly increased mortality rates.[13,14,23]

TABLE 16-3.

Risk Factors for Myocardial Infarction Specific to Pregnancy[28]

Age older than 30
Multigravidas
Thrombophilia
Preeclampsia and eclampsia
Transfusions
Postpartum infections

The treatment of myocarditis and dilated cardiomyopathy in HIV-infected patients in the emergency department is similar to that of non–HIV-infected patients. In addition to providing supportive care to improve patients' hemodynamics, practitioners caring for HIV-infected patients presenting with symptoms of myocardial disease should expedite infectious disease intervention for the initiation of ARVs.

Cardiac Disease in Pregnancy

Cardiac disease complicates more than 1% of pregnancies in the United States and causes 20% of nonobstetric deaths.[24,25] The increase in heart disease during pregnancy is attributed to increased rates of obesity, hypertension, and diabetes in addition to the survival of women with congenital heart disease to maternal age. Furthermore, women are increasingly postponing pregnancy until the fourth decade of life. In developed countries, cardiomyopathies, structural heart diseases, pulmonary hypertension, acute myocardial infarction (AMI), and conduction abnormalities are the leading cardiac causes of maternal death.[26]

The physiologic changes that occur during pregnancy lead to increases in preload, cardiac output, blood volume, and oxygen consumption. Such changes can unmask, worsen, or induce cardiac dysfunction. In obstetric patients presenting to the emergency department, cardiac decompensation is often difficult to diagnose because complaints of shortness of breath, peripheral edema, and chest pain can be attributed to normal pregnancy. The times of greatest risk for cardiac disease during pregnancy are the third trimester and the peripartum and immediate postpartum periods.[27]

Acute Myocardial Infarction in Pregnancy

ACS is a rare event in women of childbearing age. The incidence of AMI is estimated to be 6.2 per 100,000 pregnancies, with a case fatality rate of 5.1%.[28] This represents a three- to four-fold increase over the rate among nonpregnant women. The incidence of AMI increases with maternal age and is 30 times higher for women older than 40 years of age.[28] Risk factors associated with AMI are consistent with traditional risk factors, including chronic hypertension, diabetes mellitus, and smoking. Additional risk factors specific to pregnancy are listed in Table 16-3.[28] AMI can occur at any stage of pregnancy but is most common in the third trimester and within the first 6 weeks of the postpartum period.[29]

In a review of 103 obstetric patients diagnosed with AMI between 1995 and 2005, coronary angiography and postmortem evaluation demonstrated that 40% had stenosis from atherosclerosis, 27% had coronary artery dissection, and the remaining 33% showed thrombus without stenosis, vasospasm, or normal angiography.[29] Coronary artery dissection is a rare cause of AMI in nonpregnant women; however, it represents the majority of cases of MI in the peripartum period. It is postulated that the elevated level of progesterone during pregnancy induces structural changes in the vessel wall. This, in combination with the increased cardiac output and blood volume of pregnancy, may lead to greater shear forces, causing coronary dissection.[29]

> **KEY POINT**
>
> The major cause of AMI in pregnant women in the peripartum period is coronary artery dissection.

The emergency department approach to diagnosis and treatment of AMI in pregnant women is similar to that in nonpregnant patients. Beyond the history and physical examination, particular attention should be given to the risk factors listed above. Electrocardiography and cardiac biomarker assessments should be performed. As with nonpregnant patients, troponin levels are more useful than creatine kinase and myoglobin.[30] Both aspirin and heparin are safe in pregnancy. Intravenous infusion of heparin is preferred because of the relative ease of anticoagulation reversal if bleeding complications arise. Nitroglycerine may be used for the treatment of anginal pain and demonstrates tocolytic properties. However, maternal hypotension should be avoided, so careful titration is necessary.[31] In the setting of ST-elevation MI, PCI is recommended over fibrinolytic therapy.[32] PCI is considered safe for maternal and fetal survival and is preferred over fibrinolytics because of the decreased risk of bleeding in pregnancy and the increased incidence of coronary dissection as a cause of AMI.[31] The fetus should be monitored, and a plan for urgent delivery of a viable fetus should be established in case of the clinical deterioration of the mother.

Heart Failure

Causes of heart failure in pregnancy include underlying structural heart disease, cardiomyopathy, hypertensive disorders, arrhythmias, and ACS. In the developed world, congenital heart disease has surpassed rheumatic fever as a major cause of maternal heart disease in pregnancy.[27] Predictors of cardiac complications during pregnancy include previous cardiac events, previous symptomatic sustained arrhythmia, New York Heart Association functional class II or higher, aortic or mitral valve obstruction, and a left ventricular ejection fraction less than 40%.[33]

Pregnant women present with new-onset heart failure as a result of the increasing demands on the heart during pregnancy or as an exacerbation of primary heart disease. Typically, patients exhibit dyspnea on exertion, orthopnea, and lower extremity edema. The diagnosis is confirmed based on the patient's history, physical examination, an electrocardiogram, and echocardiography. Brain natriuretic peptide (BNP) levels are helpful in ruling out the diagnosis of decompensated heart failure. A value less than 100 pg/mL is considered normal. Although pregnant patients demonstrate elevated BNP levels because of increased blood volumes, the absolute value is expected to remain less than 100 pg/mL in nonpathologic cases.[34] There is no significant physiologic change in BNP levels throughout pregnancy or in the postpartum period.[34]

> **KEY POINT**
>
> The BNP level does not change significantly throughout pregnancy or in the postpartum period.

Pulmonary Hypertension

Pulmonary hypertension of any cause is considered a contraindication to pregnancy and poses a significant risk of maternal death.[26] This condition is diagnosed in some women during pregnancy, and others refuse to follow their obstetrician's advice, so they might present to the emergency department with an exacerbation during pregnancy. Normally in pregnancy, decreased peripheral vascular resistance accommodates for increased plasma volume. However, pulmonary vascular disease halts this normal response, resulting in a progressive increase in lung plasma volume, increased right ventricular load, and ultimately right heart failure. Patients present with hypoxia, edema, chest pain, and syncope. They are at risk of sudden death from severe right heart failure and arrhythmias, leading to a 52% maternal mortality rate.[35] Medical therapy is focused on avoiding increased pulmonary vascular resistance and maintaining right ventricular preload.

Cardiomyopathy

Peripartum cardiomyopathy is defined as the development of heart failure from the end of the third trimester until 5 months postpartum in the absence of underlying cardiac disease or other identifiable cause. Peripartum cardiomyopathy occurs in 1 of 1,500 to 3,000 pregnancies.[27] Its cause is unclear but might include myocarditis, immunologic dysfunction, genetic predisposition, and increased myocyte apoptosis.[36] Multiparity, advanced maternal age, multiple gestations, and preeclampsia are predisposing factors. Patients with cardiomyopathy present with symptoms of left and right heart failure, including marked dyspnea, orthopnea, and peripheral edema. The risk of intracardiac thrombus and the potential for embolism increases with ejection fractions less than 35%; anticoagulation could be required in these cases.[37] Approximately half of patients with peripartum cardiomyopathy recover systolic function within 6 months.[36] Unfortunately, 20% die or deteriorate to the point of requiring heart transplantation.

> **KEY POINT**
>
> Peripartum cardiomyopathy can occur up to 5 months post partum.

In general, the treatment of pregnant patients with heart failure is the same as that of nonpregnant patients. Severe failure may require either noninvasive or invasive ventilation. Medication strategies are similar, with the notable exception of angiotensin-converting enzyme (ACE) inhibitors, which are teratogenic. There is extensive experience with digoxin, and it is considered a safe drug to use during pregnancy.[38] Nitrates, hydralazine, and furosemide have all been used safely during pregnancy. Medications that are unsafe during pregnancy are listed in Table 16-4.

Hypertension

Hypertension during pregnancy is an important cause of maternal morbidity and mortality. Chronic hypertension, gestational hypertension, and preeclampsia complicate 12% to 22% of pregnancies.[27] Pregnancy-induced (gestational) hypertension is distinguished from preeclampsia by a lack of proteinuria; the blood pressure usually returns to normal within 3 weeks after delivery. Gestational hypertension complicates 6% to 7% of pregnancies, leading to preterm delivery, preeclampsia, placental abruption, and intrauterine growth retardation.[39] Diabetes, cardiac disease, renal disease, advanced maternal age, obesity, and multiple gestations are risk factors for the development of gestational hypertension.[39] The cause of gestational hypertension is not known, but it is likely similar to that of essential hypertension, as affected women frequently develop hypertension and cardiovascular disease later in life.[40]

The management of pregnant patients presenting to the emergency department with incidental hypertension varies depending on the trimester. In general, asymptomatic women who present for nonobstetric complaints early in their pregnancies should be referred to their obstetrician for further evaluation and management. Patients presenting beyond the second trimester (and up to 6 weeks post partum) with hypertension should be tested for preeclampsia, including complete blood count, comprehensive metabolic panel, urinalysis, lactate dehydrogenase, and uric acid levels. These women need obstetric consultation and likely transfer to an obstetrics unit for fetal monitoring. Patients with mild hypertension and no evidence of end-organ damage or laboratory test abnormalities might not require any medications.

Women with blood pressures over 160/110 mm Hg should receive antihypertensive therapy.[41] Options for parenteral treatment in the emergency department include labetalol, hydralazine, and the calcium channel blocker nicardipine. Patients with end-organ damage or evidence of preeclampsia need aggressive management, including magnesium therapy and, ultimately, delivery. For outpatient therapy, methyldopa, labetalol, amlodipine, and slow-release preparations of nifedipine have been shown to be safe and effective in pregnancy. ACE inhibitors, thiazide diuretics, and the beta-blocker atenolol should not be prescribed for pregnant women.

Arrhythmias

Cardiac conduction disorders can be exacerbated in pregnant women with established arrhythmias and structural heart disease, or they can occur de novo. The reason for the increase in arrhythmias during pregnancy is unknown. It is postulated to be related to the hormonal and physiologic cardiac changes that occur during pregnancy, such as atrial and ventricular stretch due to increased intravascular volume and heart rate.

TABLE 16-4.

Cardiac Medications That Are Contraindicated During Pregnancy

Amiodarone
Beta-blockers in the first trimester
Atenolol
Thiazide diuretics
Angiotensin-converting enzyme inhibitors

The complaint of palpitations is common among pregnant patients presenting to the emergency department. In most cases, there is no concomitant cardiac arrhythmia, suggesting that patients' perception of palpitations might be related to physiologic changes such as increased heart rate and cardiac output. One study that examined the incidence of arrhythmia in pregnant women without preexisting cardiac disease demonstrated a higher incidence of atrial and ventricular ectopic beats in patients presenting with symptoms of palpitations.[42] Twenty percent were found to have more than 10 premature ventricular contractions per hour. Six percent had more than 100 premature atrial contractions in 24 hours. The incidence of ectopic activity was significantly reduced during postpartum cardiac monitoring. The study further compared symptomatic patients with asymptomatic patients and found a higher incidence of ventricular ectopic beats in symptomatic patients. In patients with structurally normal hearts and mild symptoms, no treatment other than reassurance is required.[43] Patients should be advised to discontinue potential precipitants including stimulants, caffeine, alcohol, and smoking.

KEY POINT

Most pregnant women with palpitations have no concomitant cardiac arrhythmia or sequelae.

Research addressing the relationship between pregnancy and paroxysmal supraventricular tachycardia (PSVT) has demonstrated that first-onset PSVT during pregnancy is rare.[44] However, symptoms of PSVT are exacerbated during pregnancy in 22% of patients with the underlying condition. Overall, attacks of PSVT were not associated with any significant maternal or fetal hazard. The management of PSVT is unchanged in the setting of pregnancy. Beyond vagal maneuvers, intravenous adenosine has been safely used in pregnant women.[43] Beta-blockers may be used, but the American Heart Association recommends avoiding their use in the first trimester. Atenolol is the only beta-blocker that is absolutely contraindicated in pregnancy. It is designated as unsafe by the US Food and Drug Administration because of its association with intrauterine growth retardation, preterm delivery, and neonatal hypoglycemia. Catheter ablation is safe and recommended for treatment of poorly tolerated refractory supraventricular tachycardia.[43]

Atrial fibrillation and flutter are less common than PSVT but are more likely to occur in women with structural heart disease and cardiomyopathy. Furthermore, thyroid dysfunction is more common in pregnancy and should be investigated if these arrhythmias develop. Rate control is recommended with beta-blockers or digoxin. Amiodarone should be avoided because of its potential to cause fetal harm. Patients should have an echocardiogram to assess for structural heart disease. Anticoagulation should be deferred to obstetric and cardiology consultants. Electrical cardioversion can be performed at all stages of pregnancy and should be used in patients with hemodynamic compromise or medication-refractory tachyarrythmias.[38]

Cardiac Arrest

Cardiac arrest in pregnancy is an uncommon catastrophic

event, estimated to occur in 1 of 30,000 pregnancies in the United States.[38] The causes of cardiac arrest are varied but in general can be classified into three major categories: hypovolemia, pump failure, and obstruction. Hypovolemia can be caused by hemorrhage, trauma, sepsis, or aortic dissection. Pump failure can result from MI, cardiomyopathy, or unstable arrhythmias. Obstruction refers to pulmonary embolism, amniotic fluid embolism, or pericardial tamponade.

Several modifications to standard cardiopulmonary resuscitation are necessary in pregnant patients. The primary approach of addressing circulation with chest compressions followed by airway and then breathing and defibrillation (C-A-B-D) is unchanged. However, the physiologic changes of pregnancy cause several unique differences in cardiopulmonary resuscitation efforts. Compression of the inferior vena cava by a gravid uterus can result in decreased venous return and cardiac output. The traditional left lateral tilting of the patient with hypotension or fetal distress poses a challenge to the performance of effective chest compressions. Therefore, the recommended technique is to manually displace the uterus to the left, allowing the patient to remain in the supine position.[38]

KEY POINT

Manual displacement of the gravid uterus to the left is critical to successful resuscitation.

Venous access should be established above the diaphragm. Medications delivered via the femoral vein and other lower extremity access sites might not reach the maternal heart.[45] Chest compressions should be performed higher on the sternum to compensate for the displacement of the diaphragm by the gravid uterus.[38] Pregnancy requires no changes in the medications used in advanced cardiovascular life support. Perimortem cesarean delivery leads to decreased aorta and vena cava compression and can increase maternal cardiac output by 25%.[45] Optimal maternal and fetal outcomes are achieved if the procedure is performed within the first 5 minutes after arrest. Perimortem cesarean delivery is not indicated in women with a gestational age less than 20 weeks.[45] Cardiopulmonary resuscitation should not be interrupted during a perimortem cesarean delivery.

KEY POINT

Perimortem cesarean delivery should be performed within the first 5 minutes after arrest.

Cardiac Disease in Cancer Patients

Cardiac disease in patients with cancer has a multitude of causes. Since cancer more commonly occurs in older patients, preexisting risk factors such as smoking, hypertension, diabetes, and hyperlipidemia account for many cases of CAD and ACS among them. These factors are also associated with the development of heart failure and cardiomyopathy. However, chemotherapy, radiotherapy, and the immunosuppressive effects of cancer treatment can precipitate the development of cardiac disease, including cardiomyopathy, CAD, pericardial disease, and arrhythmias.

Heart Failure and Dilated Cardiomyopathy

Heart failure and left ventricular dysfunction can develop as side effects of chemotherapy. The highest rates of this complication are associated with the use of anthracyclines (doxorubicin, idarubicin, epirubicin, mitoxantrone), alkylating agents (cyclophosphamide), and the monoclonal antibody trastuzumab. These agents are used for a variety of cancers, including breast cancer and lymphoma.[46,47] Cancer patients presenting to the emergency department with signs and symptoms consistent with previously undiagnosed heart failure should be questioned regarding their current or previous exposure to the drugs listed above.

KEY POINT

Cancer patients on high doses of cardiotoxic chemotherapeutics, those with a history of mediastinal irradiation, and patients concurrently exposed to multiple cardiotoxic drugs are at increased risk for heart failure

Anthracycline-related cardiomyopathy has a reported incidence as high as 26% and can occur up to 20 years after exposure.[46] Late-onset, progressive cardiomyopathy, as it is known, occurs at least 1 year after completion of therapy, but clinical signs of heart failure might not develop until many years later. The mechanism of this effect is related to oxygen free-radical formation, causing apoptosis of myocardial cells and subsequent cell loss. Patients at increased risk for this side effect include those receiving higher doses of these agents, those with a history of mediastinal irradiation, and those concurrently exposed to other cardiotoxic chemotherapeutics.[46] In addition, patients at the extremes of age have a greater risk of cardiotoxicity. Clinically, patients can be asymptomatic for years but experience a slowly progressive subclinical decline in left ventricular ejection fraction. Patients at high risk for cardiomyopathy who are exposed to anthracyclines are typically monitored for this effect by their oncologists, who are likely to follow left ventricular ejection fraction measurements and possibly biomarkers such as troponin and BNP levels.[46,47] In the emergency department, such information can be helpful in gauging baseline cardiac function in a patient who has been exposed to anthracycline.

KEY POINT

Anthracycline-related cardiomyopathy is common and can occur up to 20 years after exposure.

Cyclophosphamide is an alkylating chemotherapeutic agent that is associated with cardiomyopathy in up to 28% of exposed patients.[46] Similar to that of anthracyclines, the effect of cyclophosphamide appears to be dose related, occurring predominantly in elderly patients and more likely in those with a history of mediastinal irradiation. Unlike patients who have taken anthracyclines, however, these patients present within 1 to 10 days after administration of their first dose.[46] Therefore, the link between exposure to cyclophosphamide and development of signs and symptoms of heart failure is not as difficult to recognize based on the history alone.

Patients exposed to the monoclonal antibody trastuzumab, used to treat breast cancer, have a higher incidence of cardiomyopathy when they have a history of exposure to an anthracycline or cyclophosphamide. The cardiotoxicity of trastuzumab is not dose related and is reversible upon its discontinuation.[47]

In all cases of chemotherapeutic-related cardiomyopathy and heart failure, patients should be treated based on current heart failure treatment standards. The initiation of ACE inhibitors, angiotensin II receptor blockers, or beta-blockers has been shown to improve the survival rate for these patients. In the case of trastuzumab, recognition of the relationship between this agent and the development of heart failure allows reversal of the effects with cessation of the drug.[46]

> **KEY POINT**
>
> ACE inhibitors, angiotensin II receptor blockers, and beta-blockers improve the survival rate for cancer patients with chemotherapy-induced cardiomyopathy.

Acute Coronary Syndrome and Myocardial Infarction

ACS and MI can occur in cancer patients as a result of preexisting CAD, chemotherapy, and radiation. The antimetabolite 5-fluorouracil (5-FU) has a reported cardiotoxicity of myocardial ischemia as high as 68%, resulting in a mortality rate of up to 13%.[47] This cardiotoxicity usually becomes clinically evident within 72 hours after the infusion but can occur any time from 2 to 5 days after the initiation of treatment. The mechanism of this effect is unknown, but theories have focused on vasospasm, coronary artery thrombosis, and arteritis.[46] Discontinuation of the agent for patients who develop chest pain is recommended, as the symptoms are usually reversible.[47]

In addition to chemotherapeutics, radiation therapy increases the risk of CAD and subsequent ACS. MI is one of the most common types of cardiovascular disease in survivors of Hodgkin lymphoma who received high-dose mediastinal radiation.[48] In addition, breast cancer survivors treated with left-sided chest radiation have a significantly increased rate of CAD and nonfatal MI, compared with those who received no radiation or only right-sided therapy.[48]

Cancer patients presenting with signs and symptoms consistent with ACS should be treated with conventional therapies, including antiplatelet agents, PCI, and fibrinolytics.[46] A thorough investigation for alternative diagnoses such as pulmonary embolus, pericarditis, and pleural effusion should be pursued, given the increased incidence of these diagnoses in this population. Factors that complicate fibrinolysis and intervention, such as thrombocytopenia and recent surgery, are more common in cancer patients. These factors should not exclude patients from treatment, however, as studies have shown improved survival for thrombocytopenic patients placed on aspirin without any increase in bleeding events.[46] Close consultation with a cardiologist as well as the patient's oncologist is recommended.

> **KEY POINT**
>
> Complicating factors such as thrombocytopenia and recent surgery should not exclude cancer patients with ACS from treatment with conventional therapies such as antiplatelet agents.

Pericardial Disease

Pericardial disease is a common complication of malignancy. Patients suffering from breast, lung, and hematologic cancers are most often affected. Almost 66% of cancer patients have some kind of pericardial effusion.[19] Up to 34% of these are malignant,[49] while the rest are related to radiation or opportunistic infection.[19] The risk of radiation pericarditis is dose related. It can occur up to 20 years after completion of therapy.[19] On the opposite end of the time spectrum, pericardial effusion and pericarditis are the initial presentation of cancer in 5% to 7% of patients. Further evaluation for a neoplastic cause should be pursued in patients who do not respond to therapy with nonsteroidal anti-inflammatory drugs, have a history of malignancy, or present with recurrent or incessant pericarditis.[50]

> **KEY POINT**
>
> Patients with pericarditis who have a history of malignancy, those who do not respond to nonsteroidal anti-inflammatory therapy, and those who experience recurrent pericarditis should be evaluated for a malignant effusion.

The likelihood of symptoms being caused by pericardial effusion varies with the rate of fluid accumulation. Most malignant effusions form slowly over time and therefore can be very large without significant hemodynamic compromise. Those that form rapidly can cause severe symptoms and tamponade physiology with only a small fluid accumulation.[49] Most malignant effusions are small and asymptomatic. Patients rarely present with the Beck triad of jugular venous distention, distant heart sounds, and hypotension. More commonly, patients present complaining of progressive dyspnea on exertion, chest pain, and fatigue.[49,51] Chest radiograph findings include an enlarged cardiac silhouette and increased transverse diameter, while the ECG might show characteristic low voltage with nonspecific ST-segment or T-wave changes. The diagnostic modality of choice is echocardiogram, which allows assessment of the size of the effusion as well as its hemodynamics. Initial support with intravenous fluids is recommended for patients who are hypovolemic but should be avoided in those who are euvolemic or hypervolemic. Given that up to 50% of malignant pericardial effusions recur, drain placement with pericardiocentesis is often recommended. In the emergency department, patients demonstrating cardiac tamponade physiology should undergo emergent pericardiocentesis with ultrasound guidance, if available, and the fluid that is drained should be sent for cytology and cultures.[49]

> **KEY POINT**
>
> Cancer patients with pericardial effusions tend to present to

the emergency department complaining of dyspnea, chest pain, and fatigue.

Arrhythmias

Bradycardia and QTc prolongation are the most common arrhythmias seen in cancer patients. Although bradycardia can be related to fibrosis of the conduction system as a result of radiation exposure, amyloidosis, or invasion by primary cardiac tumors, it is also a side effect of the chemotherapeutic agents paclitaxel and thalidomide. Paclitaxel-related bradycardia is a reversible phenomenon that is usually asymptomatic and occurs in up to 30% of exposed patients. Typical clinical symptoms include fatigue, decreased exercise tolerance, syncope, and dizziness. Patients who are taking paclitaxel and present with these symptoms should be evaluated with an ECG, electrolyte measurement, and thyroid studies. Discharge with a Holter monitor is also useful. In cases of progressive atrioventricular conduction disturbance or hemodynamic compromise, paclitaxel should be discontinued. Most cases are not this severe, so patients can continue their treatment with close oncologic followup.[46]

Bradycardia can also occur in patients treated with thalidomide, although the incidence appears to be lower than that associated with paclitaxel. In asymptomatic patients, close followup is recommended, as a reduction in the dose of thalidomide might assist with resolution. For symptomatic patients, the agent should be discontinued. Cases of third-degree atrioventricular block associated with thalidomide use requiring pacemaker placement have been reported. In addition, patients with multiple myeloma and no other chemotherapeutic options have had pacemakers placed to enable them to continue the thalidomide therapy without experiencing bradycardia.[46]

QTc prolongation can occur for a variety of reasons in cancer patients. Concurrent renal, hepatic, or cardiac disease increases the likelihood of QTc prolongation and torsade de pointes. Up to 36% of cancer patients have baseline ECG abnormalities.[46] Many cancer patients are exposed to QTc-prolonging medications, aside from their chemotherapeutic agents, such as antiemetics, antifungals, quinolone antibiotics, and methadone for pain control. Furthermore, cancer patients are more likely to experience electrolyte disturbances as a result of vomiting, diarrhea, or malnutrition, which can lead to QTc prolongation.[46]

The chemotherapeutic agent most likely to prolong the QTc interval is arsenic trioxide. QTc prolongation occurs in 40% to 100% of patients who are given this drug and can last up to 8 weeks after infusion.[47] Many patients exhibit QTc intervals above 500 msec, which greatly increases their risk of developing torsade de pointes and is an indication for discontinuation of therapy. Levels of potassium and magnesium should be monitored closely and rechecked in patients who are taking this therapeutic agent and present with any indication of cardiac or electrolyte problems. If torsade de pointes develops, conventional therapy with intravenous magnesium, defibrillation, and overdrive pacing are indicated as clinically necessary. QTc-prolonging medications should not be prescribed from the emergency department for patients who are receiving arsenic trioxide.[46,47]

KEY POINT

QTc prolongation longer than 500 msec or more than 60 msec above the patient's baseline interval greatly increases the risk of torsade de pointes and is an indication for discontinuation of therapy.

References

1. Mishra RK. Cardiac emergencies in patients with HIV. *Emerg Med Clin North Am*. 2010;28:273-282.
2. Boccara F, Mary-Krause M, Teiger E, et al. Acute coronary syndrome in human immunodeficiency virus-infected patients: characteristics and 1 year prognosis. *Eur Heart J*. 2011;32:41-50.
3. Deeks SG, Gandhi RT, Chae CU, Lewandrowski KB. Case records of the Massachusetts General Hospital. Case 30-2012. A 54-year-old woman with HIV infection, dyspnea, and chest pain. *N Engl J Med*. 2012;367:1246-1254.
4. DAD Study Group, Friis-Moller N, Reiss P, et al. Class of antiretroviral drugs and the risk of myocardial infarction. *N Engl J Med*. 2007;356:1723-1735.
5. Strategies for Management of Antiretroviral Therapy (SMART) Study Group, El-Sadr WM, Lundgren J, et al. CD4+ count-guided interruption of antiretroviral treatment. *N Engl J Med*. 2006;355:2283-2296.
6. Oliviero U, Bonadies G, Apuzzi V, et al. Human immunodeficiency virus per se exerts atherogenic effects. *Atherosclerosis*. 2009;204:586-589.
7. Shaikh S, Torres M. HIV emergencies. *Crit Decis Emerg Med*. 2011;25:14-18.
8. Pearce D, Ani C, Espinosa-Silva Y, et al. Comparison of in-hospital mortality from acute myocardial infarction in HIV sero-positive versus sero-negative individuals. *Am J Cardiol*. 2012;110:1078-1084.
9. Hunt K, Hughes CA, Hills-Nieminen C. Protease inhibitor-associated QT interval prolongation. *Ann Pharmacother*. 2011;45:1544-1550.
10. Singh M, Arora R, Jawad E. HIV protease inhibitors induced prolongation of the QT Interval: electrophysiology and clinical implications. *Am J Ther*. 2010;17:e193-e201.
11. Charbit B, Rosier A, Bollens D, et al. Relationship between HIV protease inhibitors and QTc interval duration in HIV-infected patients: a cross-sectional study. *Br J Clin Pharmacol*. 2009;67:76-82.
12. Soliman EZ, Lundgren JD, Roediger MP, et al. Boosted protease inhibitors and the electrocardiographic measures of QT and PR durations. *AIDS*. 2011;25:367-377.
13. Prendergast BD. HIV and cardiovascular medicine. *Heart*. 2003;89:793-800.
14. Barbaro G, Fisher SD, Giancaspro G, Lipshultz SE. HIV-associated cardiovascular complications: a new challenge for emergency physicians. *Am J Emerg Med*. 2001;19:566-574.
15. Heidenreich PA, Eisenberg MJ, Kee LL, et al. Pericardial effusion in AIDS: incidence and survival. *Circulation*. 1995;92:3229-3234.
16. Chen Y, Brennessel D, Walters J, et al. Human immunodeficiency virus-associated pericardial effusion: report of 40 cases and review of the literature. *Am Heart J*. 1999;137:516-521.
17. Mayosi BM. Contemporary trends in the epidemiology and management of cardiomyopathy and pericarditis in sub-Saharan Africa. *Heart*. 2007;93:1176-1183.
18. Ntsekhe M, Hakim J. Impact of human immunodeficiency virus infection on cardiovascular disease in Africa. *Circulation*. 2005;112:3602-3607.
19. Maisch B, Seferovic PM, Ristic AD, et al. Guidelines on the diagnosis and management of pericardial diseases executive summary: The Task Force on the Diagnosis and Management of Pericardial Diseases of the European Society of Cardiology. *Eur Heart J*. 2004;25:587-610.
20. Biondi-Zoccai G, D'Ascenzo F, Modena MG. Novel insights on HIV/AIDS and cardiac disease: shedding light on the HAART of Darkness. *Eur Heart J*. 2012;33:813-815.
21. Sliwa K, Carrington MJ, Becker A, et al. Contribution of the human immunodeficiency virus/acquired immunodeficiency syndrome epidemic to de novo presentations of heart disease in the Heart of Soweto Study cohort. *Eur Heart J*. 2012;33:866-874.
22. Barbaro G, Di Lorenzo G, Grisorio B, Barbarini G. Cardiac involvement in the acquired immunodeficiency syndrome: a multicenter clinical-pathological study. Gruppo Italiano per lo Studio Cardiologico dei pazienti affetti da AIDS Investigators. *AIDS Res Hum Retroviruses*. 1998;14:1071-1077.
23. Barbaro G, Di Lorenzo G, Grisorio B, Barbarini G. Incidence of dilated cardiomyopathy and detection of HIV in myocardial cells of HIV-positive patients. Gruppo Italiano per lo Studio Cardiologico dei Pazienti Affetti da AIDS. *N Engl J Med*. 1998;339:1093-1099.
24. Kuklina E, Callaghan W. Chronic heart disease and severe obstetric morbidity among hospitalisations for pregnancy in the USA: 1995-2006. *BJOG*. 2011;118:345-352.

25. Burlingame J, Horiuchi B, Ohana P, et al. The contribution of heart disease to pregnancy-related mortality according to the pregnancy mortality surveillance system. *J Perinatol*. 2012;32:163-169.
26. Simpson LL. Maternal cardiac disease: update for the clinician. *Obstet Gynecol*. 2012;119(2 Pt 1):345-359.
27. Ahmad WA, Khanom M, Yaakob ZH. Heart failure in pregnancy: an overview. *Int J Clin Pract*. 2011;65:848-851.
28. James AH, Jamison MG, Biswas MS, et al. Acute myocardial infarction in pregnancy: a United States population-based study. *Circulation*. 2006;113:1564-1571.
29. Roth A, Elkayam U. Acute myocardial infarction associated with pregnancy. *J Am Coll Cardiol*. 2008;52:171-180.
30. Shade GH Jr, Ross G, Bever FN, et al. Troponin I in the diagnosis of acute myocardial infarction in pregnancy, labor, and post partum. *Am J Obstet Gynecol*. 2002;187:1719-1720.
31. Sahni G. Chest pain syndromes in pregnancy. *Cardiol Clin*. 2012;30:343-367.
32. O'Gara PT, Kushner FG, Ascheim DD, et al. 2013 ACCF/AHA Guideline for the management of ST-elevation myocardial infarction: executive summary: a report of the American College of Cardiology Foundation/American Heart Association Task Force on Practice Guidelines. Available at: http://circ.ahajournals.org/content/early/2012/12/17/CIR.0b013e3182742c84.citation. Accessed April 15, 2014.
33. Siu SC, Sermer M, Colman JM, et al. Prospective multicenter study of pregnancy outcomes in women with heart disease. *Circulation*. 2001;104:515-521.
34. Hameed AB, Chan K, Ghamsary M, Elkayam U. Longitudinal changes in the B-type natriuretic peptide levels in normal pregnancy and postpartum. *Clin Cardiol*. 2009;32:E60-E62.
35. Hsu CH, Gomberg-Maitland M, Glassner C, Chen JH. The management of pregnancy and pregnancy-related medical conditions in pulmonary arterial hypertension patients. *Int J Clin Pract Suppl*. 2011;65(s172):6-14.
36. Hsich EM, Pina IL. Heart failure in women: a need for prospective data. *J Am Coll Cardiol*. 2009;54:491-498.
37. Phillips SD, Warnes CA: Peripartum cardiomyopathy: current therapeutic perspectives. *Curr Treat Options Cardiovasc Med*. 2004;6:481-488.
38. Vanden Hoek TL, Morrison LJ, Shuster M, et al. Part 12: cardiac arrest in special situations: 2010 American Heart Association Guidelines for Cardiopulmonary Resuscitation and Emergency Cardiovascular Care. *Circulation*. 2010;122(18 suppl 3):S829-S861.
39. Villar J, Carroli G, Wojdyla D, et al. Preeclampsia, gestational hypertension and intrauterine growth restriction, related or independent conditions? *Am J Obstet Gynecol*. 2006;194:921-931.
40. Vest AR, Cho LS. Hypertension in pregnancy. *Cardiol Clin*. 2012;30:407-423.
41. Vidaeff AC, Carroll MA, Ramin SM. Acute hypertensive emergencies in pregnancy. *Crit Care Med*. 2005;33(10 suppl):S307-S312.
42. Shotan A, Ostrzega E, Mehra A, Johnson JV, Elkayam U. Incidence of arrhythmias in normal pregnancy and relation to palpitations, dizziness, and syncope. *Am J Cardiol*. 1997;79:1061-1064.
43. Blomstrom-Lundqvist C, Scheinman MM, Aliot EM, et al. ACC/AHA/ESC guidelines for the management of patients with supraventricular arrhythmias--executive summary: a report of the American College of Cardiology/American Heart Association Task Force on Practice Guidelines and the European Society of Cardiology Committee for Practice Guidelines (Writing Committee to Develop Guidelines for the Management of Patients with Supraventricular Arrhythmias) developed in collaboration with NASPE-Heart Rhythm Society. *J Am Coll Cardiol*. 2003;42:1493-1531.
44. Lee SH, Chen SA, Wu TJ, et al. Effects of pregnancy on first onset and symptoms of paroxysmal supraventricular tachycardia. *Am J Cardiol*. 1995;76:675-678.
45. Farinelli CK, Hameed AB. Cardiopulmonary resuscitation in pregnancy. *Cardiol Clin*. 2012;30:453-461.
46. Yeh ET, Bickford CL. Cardiovascular complications of cancer therapy: incidence, pathogenesis, diagnosis, and management. *J Am Coll Cardiol*. 2009;53:2231-2247.
47. Youssef G, Links M. The prevention and management of cardiovascular complications of chemotherapy in patients with cancer. *Am J Cardiovasc Drugs*. 2005;5:233-243.
48. Travis LB, Ng AK, Allan JM, et al. Second malignant neoplasms and cardiovascular disease following radiotherapy. *J Natl Cancer Inst*. 2012;104:357-370.
49. McCurdy MT, Shanholtz CB. Oncologic emergencies. *Crit Care Med*. 2012;40:2212-2222.
50. Imazio M, Brucato A, Derosa FG, et al. Aetiological diagnosis in acute and recurrent pericarditis: when and how. *J Cardiovasc Med* (Hagerstown). 2009;10:217-230.
51. Behl D, Hendrickson AW, Moynihan TJ. Oncologic emergencies. *Crit Care Clin*. 2010;26:181-205.

CARDIOVASCULAR EMERGENCIES

CHAPTER 17

Special Populations: Pulmonary Hypertension and Cardiac Transplant

John C. Greenwood and Michael E. Winters

IN THIS CHAPTER

Pulmonary hypertension
Classification
Clinical presentation
Resuscitation of the critically ill patient
Mechanical circulatory support

Cardiac transplant
Immunosuppression
Acute rejection
Infection
Cardiac allograft vasculopathy

As the number of visits to emergency departments continues to rise, it is clear that emergency physicians are now caring for an increasing number of patients with complex health issues. Two such patient populations are those with pulmonary hypertension and those who have received a cardiac transplant. Both patient populations can present to the emergency department with myriad signs and symptoms. In addition, both patient populations can rapidly develop cardiovascular collapse. It is imperative that emergency physicians be knowledgeable regarding the emergency department management of acutely ill patients with pulmonary hypertension or a cardiac transplant. This chapter discusses critical aspects in the emergency department evaluation and management of these two complex patient populations.

Pulmonary Hypertension

The critically ill emergency department patient with pulmonary hypertension can be one of the most challenging patients for emergency physicians to manage. Many patients with pulmonary hypertension come to the emergency department with complex medication regimens; some are receiving a continuous infusion of a pulmonary vasodilator. Further complicating emergency department evaluation and management are difficulties in assessing intravascular volume status, the frequent need for inotropic support to augment right ventricular function, and the poor sensitivity and specificity of diagnostic tests to determine the cause of acute decompensation. In the first section of this chapter, we review the clinical presentation and diagnosis of patients in whom pulmonary hypertension is suspected and discuss the emergency department management of critically ill patients with pulmonary hypertension.

Epidemiology

The exact prevalence of pulmonary hypertension remains unknown. The estimated overall prevalence of pulmonary arterial hypertension ranges from 6 to 15 patients per million; however, pulmonary hypertension has been found in up to 50% of select patient populations.[1-3] The most common causes of pulmonary hypertension are parenchymal lung disease and left heart disease.[2] Although improved identification and treatment regimens have led to better outcomes, mortality rates for patients with pulmonary hypertension remain unacceptably high.

Definition

In 2008, the World Symposium on Pulmonary Hypertension defined pulmonary hypertension as a mean pulmonary artery pressure (PAP) greater than 25 mm Hg at rest.[4,5] The definition is further divided into precapillary and postcapillary forms, based on whether the mean pulmonary capillary wedge pressure (PCWP) is less than or greater than 15 mm Hg. Patients with pulmonary hypertension secondary to left heart disease have a PCWP higher than 15 mm Hg, whereas those with pulmonary hypertension stemming from other causes have a PCWP less than 15 mm Hg.[5] Although PAP can be estimated indirectly through a variety of radiologic studies, definitive diagnosis requires measurements made during right-heart catheterization.

Pathophysiology

Under normal conditions, the PAP is approximately 20% of the systemic pressure, with an upper limit of normal of 20 mm Hg. Pulmonary hypertension encompasses a spectrum of diseases that can affect the pulmonary arteries, the alveoli and capillary beds, or the pulmonary veins. Its exact pathophysiology remains incompletely described, but multiple pathogenic mechanisms have been proposed (Table 17-1). The net effect of these pathogenic processes is right ventricular remodeling and altered perfusion of the right coronary artery, which eventually lead to right ventricular dysfunction.

Anatomically, the right ventricle (RV) is a thin-walled, crescent-shaped structure that shares the interventricular septum with the left ventricle (LV). The free wall of the RV is highly distensible and readily responds to changes in preload. The RV, however, is unable to overcome large changes in pulmonary vascular resistance (PVR). In fact, the normal RV cannot tolerate acute increases in mean PAP greater than 40 mm Hg. Sudden increases in PAP can result in right ventricular dilation, increases in right ventricular oxygen consumption, reduced right ventricular contractility, and paradoxical movement of the intraventricular septum toward the LV, resulting in impairment of LV output. Chronic elevations in PVR cause the RV to undergo a process of adaptive hypertrophy. Sustained elevations in PAP cause a pressure-induced growth of right ventricular cardiomyocytes and proliferation of a collagen-based extracellular matrix.[6-8] Changes in the anatomic structure of the RV eventually result in systolic and diastolic dysfunction as well as increase the risk of arrhythmias related to abnormal conduction.[9]

KEY POINT

Right ventricular remodeling results in systolic and diastolic dysfunction, leading to reduced contractility and right ventricular output.

Perfusion of the right coronary artery is also severely reduced in patients with advanced pulmonary hypertension. The blood supply of the RV varies according to the anatomic dominance of the coronary system. In approximately 80% of people, the right coronary artery supplies blood to the RV.[10,11] Under normal circumstances, the right coronary artery is perfused during both systole and diastole.[12] As a result of elevations in right ventricular wall tension and transmural pressure, perfusion of the right coronary artery occurs almost exclusively during diastole in patients with advanced pulmonary hypertension.[13-15] Malp-

TABLE 17-1.

Proposed Pathogenic Mechanisms of Pulmonary Hypertension

Endothelial dysfunction
Earliest abnormality
Aggravated by hypoxia and acidosis
Vasoactive mediator imbalance
Impaired nitric oxide and prostacyclin production (vasodilators)
Increased endothelin 1 production (vasoconstrictor)
Altered lung permeability
Abnormal hypoxic vasoconstriction
Microvascular thrombosis
Vascular remodeling

TABLE 17-2.

WHO Classification of Pulmonary Hypertension[2]

1. Pulmonary arterial hypertension
Idiopathic
Familial
Associated with pulmonary arterial hypertension
Connective tissue disorders
Congenital systemic-to-pulmonary shunts
Portal hypertension
Human immunodeficiency virus
Drugs/toxins
Hemoglobinopathies
2. Pulmonary hypertension with left heart disease
Left atrial disease
Left ventricular disease
Valvular disease
3. Pulmonary hypertension associated with lung or hypoxemic disease
Chronic obstructive pulmonary disease
Interstitial lung disease
4. Pulmonary hypertension due to chronic thrombotic or thromboembolic disease
5. Miscellaneous
Sarcoidosis
Histiocytosis X
Extrinsic pulmonary vascular compression (eg, tumor, adenopathy)

erfusion of the right coronary artery leads to right ventricular ischemia, which can rapidly progress to right ventricular failure.

> **KEY POINTS**
>
> Right coronary artery perfusion occurs almost exclusively during diastole in patients with advanced pulmonary hypertension.
>
> Right ventricular failure is the hallmark of decompensated pulmonary hypertension.

Classification

The World Health Organization (WHO) classifies pulmonary hypertension into five groups based on precipitating cause and response to treatment (Table 17-2). WHO Group 1, with an estimated prevalence of 6 to 15 patients per million,[3,16] includes diseases that increase pressure within the smaller pulmonary arteries, resulting in an increase in PVR. Patients with WHO Group 1 pulmonary hypertension have an extremely high mortality rate: 1- and 5-year rates range from 7% to 32% and 40% to 79%, respectively.[16,17]

Clinical Presentation (Table 17-3)

Patients with diagnosed, or undiagnosed, pulmonary hypertension typically present with symptoms related to right-sided heart failure. Dyspnea at rest, or with exertion, is the most common symptom, followed by chest pain, fatigue, and syncope.[3,16] Patients might also report orthopnea, paroxysmal nocturnal dyspnea, early satiety, and anorexia, which are caused by elevated pulmonary pressures. Delays in diagnosis are common; the average duration of symptoms prior to confirmation of the diagnosis ranges from 12 to 24 months.[16]

Physical examination findings commonly associated with pulmonary hypertension include jugular venous distention, hepatomegaly, peripheral edema, ascites, digital clubbing, a holosystolic murmur of tricuspid regurgitation, and a palpable parasternal lift secondary to right ventricular hypertrophy. Cyanosis is seen in approximately 20% of these patients and suggests significant right-to-left shunting, reduced cardiac output, or marked impairment of pulmonary gas transfer.[18] Imminent cardiovascular collapse should be suspected in any pulmonary hypertension patient presenting with hypotension, diminished pulse pressure, and cool extremities.[19]

> **KEY POINT**
>
> Patients with pulmonary hypertension usually present to the emergency department with symptoms related to right-heart failure.

Diagnosis

When evaluating the emergency department patient with suspected pulmonary hypertension, a number of laboratory and radiologic studies can be performed. It is important to recognize the utility and limitations of each study in the management of these patients.

Laboratory Testing

The goals of laboratory testing in the symptomatic patient with pulmonary hypertension are to exclude cardiac ischemia, determine if end-organ dysfunction is present, and assess global perfusion. The emergency physician should order cardiac enzyme concentrations (ie, troponin I, creatine phosphokinase), a B-type natriuretic peptide (BNP) level, a complete metabolic panel, and measurement of the serum lactate concentration. In patients with pulmonary arterial hypertension, elevations in troponin I, BNP, and creatinine are associated with an increased mortality rate.[20-22]

Electrocardiogram

An electrocardiogram (ECG) should be obtained as soon as possible in the symptomatic patient with pulmonary hyperten-

TABLE 17-3.

Clinical Findings of Pulmonary Hypertension

Symptoms
Dyspnea
Chest pain
Syncope/near syncope
Fatigue
Orthopnea
Paroxysmal nocturnal dyspnea
Signs
Jugular venous distention
Hepatomegaly
Peripheral edema
Ascites
Digital clubbing
Cyanosis
Parasternal lift

TABLE 17-4.

ECG Findings Associated With Pulmonary Hypertension[19]

Right-axis deviation
Tall R wave and small S wave, with R/S ratio greater than 1 in V_1
qR complex or rSR′ pattern in V_1
T-wave inversions in the anteroseptal +/- inferior leads
Large S wave and small R wave, with R/S ratio less than 1 in V_5 or V_6
Right atrial enlargement in II, III, and aVF
$S_1Q_3T_3$

sion. Common ECG findings in patients with pulmonary hypertension are listed in Table 17-4. Right-axis deviation is seen in almost 80% of pulmonary hypertension patients.[18] Figure 17-1 illustrates common ECG findings in patients with pulmonary hypertension. The ECG should be scrutinized for signs of right ventricular ischemia and the presence of any arrhythmia. Supraventricular tachycardias (ie, atrial fibrillation, atrial flutter, and AV nodal reentrant tachycardia [AVNRT]) are the most common arrhythmias seen in these patients.[23] Atrial fibrillation is a particularly malignant arrhythmia in pulmonary hypertension patients and is associated with a mortality rate higher than 80%.[23]

KEY POINTS

Atrial fibrillation, atrial flutter, and AVNRT are the most common arrhythmias in patients with pulmonary hypertension.

Right ventricular hypertrophy and right-axis deviation are seen on the ECG in most patients with pulmonary hypertension.

Arrhythmias should be identified and treated rapidly in patients with pulmonary hypertension. Tachyarrhythmias can impair ventricular filling, decrease cardiac output, and lead to right ventricular failure with cardiovascular collapse.[24]

Chest Radiography

A chest radiograph should be obtained in any symptomatic patient with pulmonary hypertension. Common findings are an enlarged hilar pulmonary arterial shadow, pulmonary venous congestion, constricted peripheral arterial vasculature ("pruning"), prominent right heart border, right atrial enlargement, and obliteration of the retrosternal space, indicating right ventricular hypertrophy.[18,25] Depending on the cause of the pulmonary hypertension, additional findings can also include hyperinflation, pulmonary fibrosis, and interstitial lung disease.

Computed Tomography

Computed tomography of the chest can be helpful when evaluating the patient with suspected pulmonary hypertension. Right ventricular enlargement, right ventricular hypertrophy, and enlargement of the main pulmonary artery more than 30 mm are highly suggestive of pulmonary arterial hypertension. In fact, if the maximum transverse diameter of the main pulmonary artery is greater than the diameter of the proximal ascending thoracic aorta, there is a 96% positive predictive value for the diagnosis of pulmonary hypertension.[26] In the emergency department evaluation, computed tomography of the chest can be useful in evaluating causes of acute decompensation, such as acute pulmonary embolism.[25]

Echocardiography

Echocardiography is perhaps the most useful diagnostic tool to aid emergency physicians in evaluating patients with suspected pulmonary hypertension. Transthoracic echocardiography can be performed rapidly and provides a wealth of information regarding the systolic and diastolic function of both the RV and LV. Evaluation of the RV is the single most important component of the echocardiographic examination in patients with suspected pulmonary hypertension. Right atrial enlargement and

FIGURE 17-1.

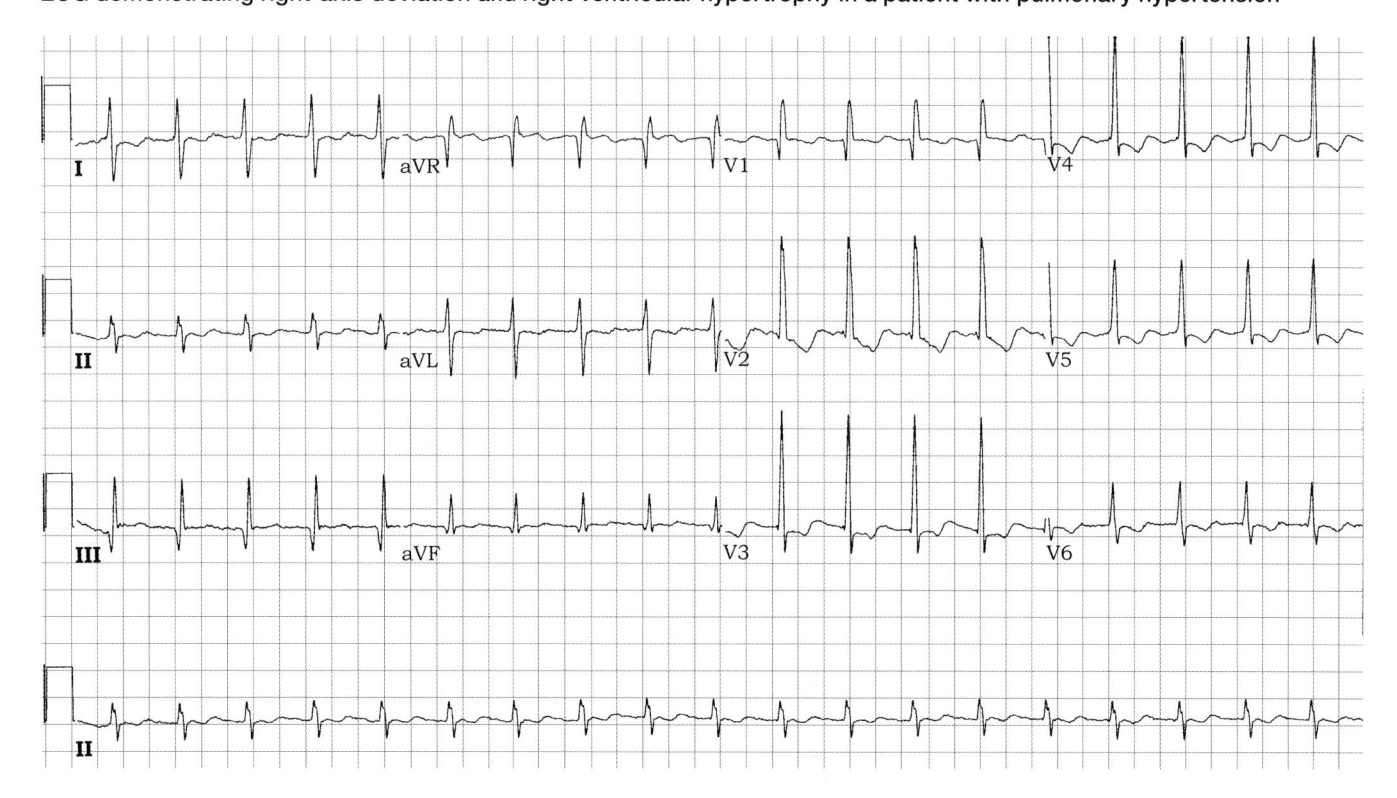

ECG demonstrating right-axis deviation and right ventricular hypertrophy in a patient with pulmonary hypertension

right ventricular dilation indicate elevated pulmonary arterial pressures.[5] In contrast to pulmonary hypertension secondary to acute PE, in which the RV is dilated and thin, the RV in most patients with pulmonary hypertension is thickened. Global right ventricular hypokinesis is also more likely to be seen, as opposed to the classically described McConnell sign of acute PE (hypokinesis of the free wall with normal apical contractility). Additional signs of right ventricular dysfunction include an RV-to-LV end diastolic diameter greater than 1 using the apical 4-chamber view, a right-ventricular end-diastolic diameter greater than 30 mm, or loss of inferior vena cava collapse with inspiration.[27] With advanced disease, the interventricular septum can paradoxically deviate toward the LV, creating a "D" appearance on a parasternal short-axis view (Figure 17-2). Pericardial effusion and septal displacement are considered late echocardiographic findings in severe pulmonary hypertension and indicate a poor prognosis.[28]

Emergency Department Resuscitation of the Critically Ill Pulmonary Hypertension Patient

Symptomatic pulmonary hypertension patients can progress rapidly to cardiovascular collapse. Causes of acute decompensation are listed in Table 17-5. The main tenets in treating the critically ill emergency department patient with pulmonary hypertension are listed in Table 17-6. These consist of optimizing intravascular volume, optimizing right ventricular systolic function, maintaining right coronary artery perfusion, and reducing right ventricular afterload. Importantly, evidence-based guidelines for the management of these patients have not been published. Most of the current published recommendations are based on expert opinion.

KEY POINT

Current recommendations on the management of critically ill patients with pulmonary hypertension are based predominantly on expert opinion.

Optimize Intravascular Volume

Intravascular volume assessment and fluid resuscitation can be challenging in the patient with pulmonary hypertension, because both hypovolemia and hypervolemia can be detrimental. The goal of fluid resuscitation in these patients is to ensure adequate, but not excessive, right ventricular preload. Unfortunately, traditional methods of evaluating intravascular volume status such as central venous pressure, pulse pressure variation, and stroke volume variation can be unreliable in patients with pulmonary hypertension. Most patients with pulmonary hypertension have an elevated central venous pressure at baseline yet can augment their cardiac output with additional fluid administration.[29] For the hypotensive patient, or one who appears to be hypovolemic, a 500-mL bolus of an isotonic crystalloid solution should be administered. Repeated fluid boluses may be administered, but patients require close monitoring to confirm a favorable hemodynamic response.[30] Continuous, unmonitored fluid administration is not recommended.

Right ventricular failure and hypotension are more often the result of increased right ventricular afterload and hypervolemia, rather than volume depletion.[31] Many unstable patients with pulmonary hypertension who are hypervolemic require early initiation of vasopressor and inotropic medications rather than repeated fluid boluses. Once they become hemodynamically stable, these patients require diuresis or initiation of ultrafiltration therapy.

KEY POINTS

Avoid unmonitored, continuous fluid administration to pulmonary hypertension patients.

Administer an initial 500-mL bolus of an isotonic crystalloid fluid to pulmonary hypertension patients. The decision to administer additional boluses must be based on meticulous monitoring of the patient's response.

FIGURE 17-2.

Echocardiographic findings in a patient with pulmonary hypertension. Left, Apical view demonstrating right ventricular hypertrophy, dilation, and right atrial dilation. Right, Parasternal short view demonstrating septal bowing and the "D" sign.

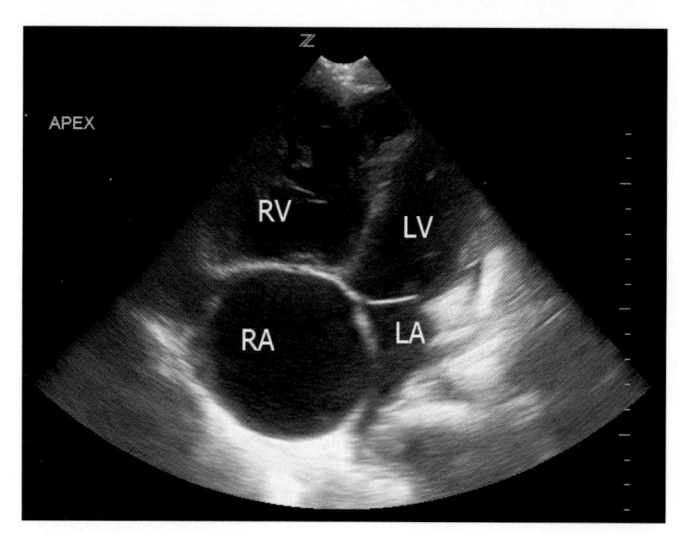

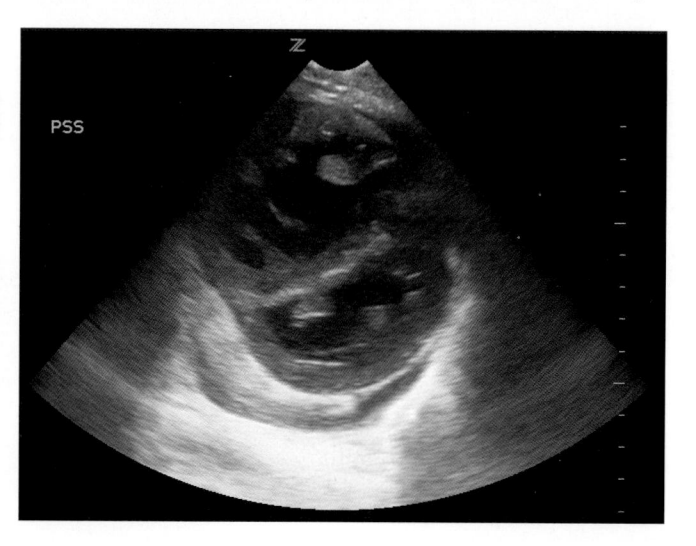

Optimize Right Ventricular Systolic Function

In addition to preload optimization, it is crucial to optimize right ventricular systolic function in the critically ill patient. This can be accomplished with the use of inotropic medications. The two most commonly used inotropic medications are dobutamine and milrinone. Dobutamine, the preferred inotropic agent, is a selective beta$_1$-agonist that increases myocardial contractility and reduces PVR and systemic vascular resistance.[32,33] In patients with pressure-induced right heart failure, dobutamine has been found to be superior to vasopressors (eg, norepinephrine) alone.[34] If there is evidence of right heart failure such as elevated BNP levels or signs of end-organ malperfusion, a dobutamine infusion should be initiated at 2 mcg/kg/min and titrated to a maximum of 10 mcg/kg/min, as long as the patient is not hypotensive and the mean arterial pressure is higher than 65 mm Hg. At doses higher than 10 mcg/kg/min, dobutamine has been shown to increase PVR and produce tachycardia and is associated with an increased mortality rate.[34,35] The use of dobutamine is limited by its beta$_2$ activity that can cause hypotension at higher doses.

Milrinone, a phosphodiesterase inhibitor, increases contractility by inhibiting phosphodiesterase-3, thus increasing cyclic AMP levels and the intracellular calcium concentration. Milrinone has been shown to increase right ventricular function and decrease PVR. A milrinone infusion should be started at 0.375 mcg/kg/min and titrated to a maximum of 0.75 mcg/kg/min. At higher doses, milrinone can cause systemic hypotension, necessitating the co-administration of a vasopressor medication.

In addition to administering inotropic medications, it is important to maintain sinus rhythm. As previously discussed, arrhythmias, such as atrial fibrillation and atrial flutter can impair right ventricular systolic function and have disastrous effects on the critically ill pulmonary hypertension patient.

KEY POINTS

Dobutamine is the preferred inotropic agent to augment right ventricular systolic function.

Initiate a dobutamine infusion at 2 mcg/kg/min and titrate to a maximum of 10 mcg/kg/min.

Dobutamine doses greater than 10 mcg/kg/min can be detrimental.

TABLE 17-5.

Causes of Acute Decompensation in Patients With Pulmonary Hypertension

Arrhythmias (atrial fibrillation, atrial flutter, AVNRT)
Catheter-related infection
Catheter occlusion or pump malfunction
Gastrointestinal hemorrhage
Pneumonia
Pulmonary embolism
Right ventricular ischemia

Maintain Right Coronary Artery Perfusion

To preserve right coronary artery blood flow and prevent right ventricular ischemia, it is critical to maintain the mean arterial blood pressure above the PAP. In critically ill patients, right coronary artery perfusion is preserved by augmenting aortic root pressure with vasopressor medications. Little has been published regarding the use of specific vasopressor medications in the setting of pulmonary hypertension. Nevertheless, for the hypotensive patient with a mean arterial pressure below 65 mm Hg, norepinephrine is the recommended vasopressor of choice, as it improves right ventricular function through increases in systemic vascular resistance and cardiac output. The initial dose of norepinephrine is 0.05 mcg/kg/min. Although there is no true maximum dose of norepinephrine, higher doses have been reported to cause pulmonary vasoconstriction, a detrimental effect for patients with impaired right ventricular function. Dopamine should be used with caution in these patients, because it has been associated with an increased incidence of tachyarrhythmias compared with other vasopressor agents.[36] Phenylephrine should be avoided, because it increases mean PAP and PVR, thereby worsening right ventricular systolic function.

KEY POINTS

Norepinephrine is the vasopressor of choice for the critically ill pulmonary hypertension patient.

Dopamine and phenylephrine should be avoided in the critically ill pulmonary hypertension patient.

Reduce Right Ventricular Afterload

The final tenet in managing the critically ill emergency department patient with pulmonary hypertension is reducing right ventricular afterload. This can be accomplished by ensuring adequate oxygenation, avoiding hypercapnia and acidosis, and administering pulmonary vasodilators. Prolonged hypoxemia and hypercapnia are common precipitants of increased PVR.[37-39] In emergency department patients with pulmonary hypertension,

TABLE 17-6.

Tenets of Emergency Department Management of Pulmonary Hypertension

Optimize intravascular volume status (right ventricular preload)
Optimize right ventricular systolic function
Inotropic medications
Maintain sinus rhythm
Maintain adequate right coronary artery perfusion
Vasopressor medications
Reduce right ventricular afterload
Maintain adequate oxygenation
Avoid hypercapnia and acidosis
Pulmonary vasodilator medications

supplemental oxygen should be applied to maintain the arterial oxygen saturation above 90%.[31,40] Every attempt should be made to avoid endotracheal intubation and mechanical ventilation. Initiation of positive-pressure ventilation in these patients can have negative hemodynamic effects by increasing PVR and reducing venous return. If mechanical ventilation is required, the use of lung protective ventilator settings (Table 17-7) is recommended to avoid lung injury and increases in PVR. Permissive hypercapnia should be avoided, because it can increase PVR by approximately 50% and mean PAP by approximately 30%.[41] Plateau pressures should be monitored frequently, the goal plateau pressure being less than 30 cm H_2O. Excessive plateau pressures can cause direct compression of the pulmonary vasculature, further increasing PVR.

KEY POINTS

Avoid permissive hypercapnia in the mechanically ventilated pulmonary hypertension patient.

Maintain plateau pressures of less than 30 cm H_2O in the mechanically ventilated pulmonary hypertension patient.

Pulmonary vasodilators are rarely administered to hemodynamically unstable patients with pulmonary hypertension in the emergency department. Nevertheless, given their frequent use in stable pulmonary hypertension patients, it is important for emergency physicians to be familiar with them. The pulmonary vasodilators that are commonly used in pulmonary hypertension are prostanoids, phosphodiesterase inhibitors, and endothelin receptor antagonists. For any patient with pulmonary hypertension presenting to the emergency department, it is critical to determine if any of these medications has been discontinued abruptly. If so, the medication must be reinitiated as soon as possible to prevent rebound pulmonary hypertension and cardiovascular collapse.[42,43] In all cases, these medications can be restarted through a peripheral intravenous catheter and do not require immediate central venous access.

Prostanoids. Most patients with advanced pulmonary hypertension are receiving prostanoid therapy. Prostanoids (epoprostenol, prostacyclin, iloprost, treprostinil) are potent systemic and pulmonary vasodilators that have both antiplatelet and antiproliferative effects. Epoprostenol was the first therapy approved for use in advanced pulmonary arterial hypertension and is classically used as the initial treatment of choice. Epoprostenol is administered continuously through a peripherally inserted central catheter. This drug has an extremely short half-life of just 2 to 5 minutes.[44,45] Treprostinil can be administered through a continuous intravenous infusion or subcutaneously. In contrast to epoprostenol, the half-life of treprostinil is approximately 4 to 5 hours, making it a more attractive alternative for outpatient management. The initial doses and half-lives of prostanoids are listed in Table 17-8. If pump malfunction or catheter occlusion occurs, both epoprostenol and treprostinil can be administered through a peripheral intravenous catheter. In the crashing patient, the benefits of administering a prostanoid to reduce right ventricular afterload must be weighed against the potential for systemic hypotension at higher doses.

Nitric Oxide. Inhaled nitric oxide is a potent pulmonary vasodilator that can be administered by face mask or during mechanical ventilation. Local effects of inhaled nitric oxide include a reduction in PAP and PVR, improved oxygenation, and reversal of hypoxic vasoconstriction without affecting systemic vascular resistance or cardiac output.[33,46] Inhaled nitric oxide therapy appears to have a short-term benefit in patients with acute right heart failure secondary to pulmonary hypertension but does not appear to provide an overall mortality benefit other than for patients with acute postoperative pulmonary hypertension.[47,48] In patients with acute right heart failure secondary to pulmonary arterial hypertension, inhaled nitric oxide therapy has been found to result in a 38% reduction in PVR, a 36% increase in cardiac output, and a 28% increase in Pao_2/Fio_2.[47] Abrupt discontinuation of inhaled nitric oxide therapy can result in rebound pulmonary hypertension and therefore should be avoided. Inhaled nitric oxide therapy has also been associated with methemoglobinemia. Serum concentrations of methemoglobin should be determined prior to initiation of therapy and monitored every 6 hours during treatment.[27]

Phosphodiesterase Inhibitors. Phosphodiesterase-5 (PDE-5) inhibitors (sildenafil) increase cyclic GMP signaling and can potentiate the effects of nitric oxide. PDE-5 inhibitors can reduce PVR acutely, increase cardiac output, and reduce PCWP. Although these agents can improve clinical end points in the stable patient with chronic pulmonary hypertension, their use has not been evaluated in the pulmonary hypertension patient with acute right ventricular failure. Thus, they are not recommended in this setting.[31,49]

KEY POINTS

Epoprostenol has a half-life of 2 to 5 minutes. If it is discontinued abruptly, it must be restarted ASAP and can be given through a peripheral intravenous line.

Abrupt discontinuation of inhaled nitric oxide causes rebound pulmonary hypertension and must be avoided.

PDE-5 inhibitors are not recommended for the acutely decompensated pulmonary hypertension patient with right ventricular failure.

Arrhythmias

As previously discussed, arrhythmias represent one of the most common precipitants of acute decompensation in the critically ill patient. Atrial fibrillation and atrial flutter are the

TABLE 17-7.

Initial Ventilator Settings for Patients With Pulmonary Hypertension[32]

Tidal volume: 6 to 8 mL/kg ideal body weight
Respiratory rate: set to approximate baseline minute ventilation; do not exceed 35 breaths/min; avoid hypercapnia
Positive end-expiratory pressure (PEEP): 3 to 8 cm H_2O
Fraction of inspired oxygen (Fio_2): minimal level to maintain arterial oxygen saturation (Spo_2) above 90%

most prevalent arrhythmias and are independent predictors of death.[50] In fact, more than 80% of patients with pulmonary hypertension presenting with atrial fibrillation or atrial flutter will experience hemodynamic compromise or acute right ventricular failure.[23,51] In general, all patients with atrial fibrillation or atrial flutter should be treated with electrical or chemical cardioversion to restore sinus rhythm.[23] Rate control with beta-adrenergic receptor antagonists or calcium channel blockers is not recommended because these medications can impair cardiac contractility and worsen PVR.

KEY POINT

Pulmonary hypertension patients with atrial fibrillation or atrial flutter should be treated with electrical or chemical cardioversion.

Mechanical Circulatory Support

The use of extracorporeal life support (ECLS) has been reported as salvage therapy for patients with pulmonary hypertension who present with refractory shock.[52,53] The goal of ECLS is to provide a bridge to heart or lung transplantation. ECLS has also been used as a bridge to pulmonary vasodilator therapy.[54] Percutaneous veno-arterial or veno-venous extracorporeal membrane oxygenation can be initiated rapidly at the bedside and provide up to 6 L/min of cardiac output. Once ECLS is initiated, many patients experience a rapid reversal of hemodynamics, a decrease in vasopressor dose and need for inotropic support, improved gas exchange, and improved end-organ perfusion.[55] The use of ECLS in the critically ill patient is extremely resource intensive and should be considered on a case-by-case basis.

Cardiac Transplant

Since the first successful cardiac transplant by Barnard in 1967, the annual number of heart transplant recipients has grown steadily. More than 5,000 cardiac transplants are now performed annually worldwide.[56] As a result of improvements in surgical techniques, immunosuppressive medication regimens, recognition of complications, and surveillance for and treatment of rejection, the half-life of a cardiac transplant rose from 5 years in the 1980s to more than 10 years in 2001.[57] The current median survival of a heart transplant patient ranges from 10 to 13 years.[56,58] More patients with cardiac transplant are living longer, but many develop complications of drug therapy, rejection, infection, and allograft vasculopathy. Acutely ill patients with cardiac transplant are often transported to emergency departments for evaluation, so it is critical for the emergency physician to be knowledgeable regarding the management of this special patient population. The following section focuses on the care of the patient who has had a cardiac transplant, with specific emphasis on immunosuppressive medications, infection, acute rejection, arrhythmias, and cardiac allograft vasculopathy.

Physiology

The transplanted heart is a denervated organ. At the time of transplantation, the sympathetic and parasympathetic nerves are severed. The loss of vagal tone results in a resting heart rate between 90 and 100 beats/min and predisposes these patients to higher rates of arrhythmias.[59,60] Denervation also results in a delayed response when increases in cardiac output are needed such as during exertion or stress. Although autonomic nerve innervation is lost, intrinsic cardiac function is preserved. The transplanted heart remains sensitive to changes in filling conditions.[60] In fact, preservation of the Frank-Starling volume-pressure relationship is critical to altering contractility.[60]

KEY POINTS

The resting heart rate of the transplanted heart ranges from 90 to 100 beats/min.

Due to the loss of autonomic nerve innervation, the patient with a cardiac transplant is predisposed to arrhythmias.

Surgical Procedures

The two most common surgical procedures for orthotopic cardiac transplantation are the biatrial and bicaval techniques. In both, the donor's left atrium is sutured to a remnant of the recipient's left atrium, which contains the pulmonary veins. In the biatrial technique, small cuffs of the recipient's right and left atria are sutured to the donor's right and left atria, with anastomoses at the aorta and pulmonary artery.[59] In the bicaval technique, the most common technique in the United States, the anastomoses are located at the left atrium, inferior vena cava, superior vena cava, aorta, and pulmonary artery. By preserving the donor's entire right atrium, the bicaval technique decreases the incidence of atrial arrhythmias, improves atrial function, and decreases the need for a permanent pacemaker.[61,62]

TABLE 17-8.

Prostanoid Infusions in Patients With Pulmonary Hypertension

Drug	Initial Dose	Target Dose	Half-Life	Steady State
Epoprostenol (intravenous)	2 mcg/kg/min	20 to 40 mcg/kg/min	2 to 5 min[a]	15 min
Treprostinil (subcutaneous)	1.25 mcg/kg/min	40 mcg/kg/min	4 to 5 hr	10 hr
Treprostinil (intravenous)	1.25 mcg/kg/min	40 mcg/kg/min	4 to 5 hr	10 hr

[a]At a temperature of 37°C and a pH of 7.4

Immunosuppression

To prevent, or limit, rejection of the transplanted heart, patients are placed on complex immunosuppressive medication regimens. These regimens are divided into three categories: induction, maintenance, and rejection therapy. It is unlikely that an emergency physician will encounter a patient receiving induction medications, because these drugs are administered preoperatively and in the immediate postoperative period prior to hospital discharge. However, acutely ill patients presenting to the emergency department should be receiving maintenance immunosuppressive medications. These maintenance regimens typically consist of a corticosteroid, a calcineurin inhibitor, and an antiproliferative agent. Corticosteroids cause lymphocyte depletion, whereas calcineurin inhibitors block the action of calcineurin, a key participant in T-cell activation. The two most common calcineurin inhibitors used in clinical practice are cyclosporine and tacrolimus. Because of its lower incidence of side effects, tacrolimus is the preferred calcineurin inhibitor. Antiproliferative agents inhibit the proliferation of activated T or B cells. The most common antiproliferative agent used in maintenance regimens is mycophenolate mofetil. This compound is hydrolyzed to mycophenolic acid, which blocks purine

TABLE 17-9.

Adverse Effects of Maintenance Immunosuppressive Medications[59]

Medication	Class	Adverse Effects
Tacrolimus	Calcineurin inhibitor	Nephrotoxicity
		Neuropathy
		Hyperglycemia
		Hypertension
		Hyperlipidemia
		Hyperkalemia
		Hypomagnesemia
		Thrombocytopenia
Mycophenolate mofetil	Antiproliferative	Diarrhea
		Vomiting
		Leukopenia
		Thrombocytopenia
		Hypertension
Prednisone/methylprednisolone	Corticosteroid	Hypertension
		Hyperlipidemia
		Pancreatitis
		Peptic ulcer formation
		Cataract formation
		Adrenal suppression
		Psychosis
Sirolimus		Hyperlipidemia
		Thrombocytopenia
		Leucopenia
		Hypertension
		Peripheral edema
		Insomnia
		Impaired wound healing

synthesis and prevents proliferation of T and B cells. Sirolimus is a newer immunosuppressive medication that inhibits the activation of T cells after stimulation by interleukin 2. Sirolimus has been used in maintenance regimens to reduce the dose of a tacrolimus or cyclosporine when nephrotoxicity has developed.

Emergency physicians must be able to recognize the adverse effects of these medications (Table 17-9). It is equally important to know which commonly used emergency department medications affect the level of immunosuppression (Table 17-10).

KEY POINTS

The most common maintenance immunosuppressive medication regimen comprises tacrolimus, mycophenolate mofetil, and prednisone.

The most common adverse effect of tacrolimus is nephrotoxicity.

The most common adverse effects of mycophenolate mofetil are vomiting and diarrhea.

Acute Rejection

Acute rejection occurs in up to 40% of patients during the first year after surgery and is a leading cause of death.[59,63] Episodes of acute rejection are classified as either cellular or humoral. Acute cellular rejection, the more common form, is T-cell mediated.[57] It typically occurs within the first few weeks to months following surgery and is asymptomatic in some patients. Acute humoral rejection occurs within the first several months after surgery and is mediated by antibodies directed

TABLE 17-10.
Common Medications That Adversely Affect Immunosuppression. Adapted from: Constanzo MR, Dipchand A, Starling R, et al. The International Society of Heart and Lung Transplant guidelines for the care of heart transplant patients. *J Heart Lung Transplant.* 2010;29:927. Used with permission.

Medications that increase immunosuppression levels	Medications that decrease immunosuppression levels
Antiepileptics	Antimicrobials
Phenytoin	Erythromycin
Fosphenytoin	Clarithromycin
Carbamazepine	Metronidazole
Phenobarbital	Levofloxacin
Antimicrobials	Antifungals
Nafcillin	Ketoconazole
Rifampin	Fluconazole
Caspofungin	Voriconazole
Antiretrovirals	Clotrimazole
Efavirenz	Itraconazole
Nevirapine	Cardiovascular
Etravirine	Diltiazem
	Amiodarone
	Verapamil
	Endocrine
	Glyburide
	Glipizide
	Antiretrovirals
	Protease inhibitors
	Indinavir
	Nelfinavir
	Ritonavir

against donor HLA antigens.[57] Essentially, antibody complexes deposit on the vascular endothelium of the transplanted heart, causing vessel injury and thrombosis.[59] Although humoral rejection accounts for less than 20% of cases, it carries a much higher risk of graft failure and death compared with cellular rejection.[64]

The clinical presentation of acute rejection can range from no symptoms to sudden death. Initial symptoms are often nonspecific and include fever, myalgias, nausea, vomiting, dyspnea, weight gain, and peripheral edema.[60,65] Patients can also present with bradycardia, atrial fibrillation, or atrial flutter.[60] In fact, the emergency physician should suspect acute rejection in any transplant patient with atrial fibrillation or atrial flutter.[59] In rare cases, patients present with hypotension, cardiogenic shock, or sudden death. These dramatic presentations are seen more often with acute humoral rejection.[57]

Right ventricular endomyocardial biopsy remains the gold standard for the diagnosis of acute rejection. Laboratory testing to determine concentrations of BNP, troponin I, troponin T, and C-reactive protein is unreliable and therefore not useful in the evaluation of patients with suspected acute rejection.[66] Transthoracic echocardiography can be helpful in certain patients by demonstrating systolic or diastolic dysfunction. Unfortunately, these findings are insensitive and nonspecific. Therefore, the use of echocardiography is not recommended for the diagnosis of acute rejection.[66]

Treatment of the patient with acute rejection depends on whether the episode is cellularly or humorally mediated. Symptomatic patients with acute cellular rejection should receive high-dose corticosteroid therapy.[66] Either methylprednisolone (250 to 1,000 mg/day) or prednisone (1 to 3 mg/kg/day) may be administered.[66] Hemodynamically compromised patients with acute cellular rejection may be given antithymocyte antibodies (but this therapy is rarely, if ever, initiated in the emergency department).[66] Symptomatic patients with acute humoral rejection are also treated with high-dose corticosteroids. Additional therapies for patients with humoral rejection include plasmapheresis and intravenous immunoglobulin.[66]

KEY POINTS

Suspect acute rejection in any patient with atrial fibrillation or atrial flutter after cardiac transplant.

BNP, troponin I, and C-reactive protein concentrations are unreliable in the diagnosis of acute rejection.

Endomyocardial biopsy is the gold standard for diagnosing rejection.

Patients with suspected acute rejection should receive high-dose corticosteroids.

Infection

Infections remain a significant cause of morbidity and mortality in patients after cardiac transplant. In fact, infections are the most common cause of death after the first year following transplantation. Infections can be grouped according to the time from transplantation. Those that occur within the first month following transplantation are usually caused by nosocomial organisms that become established at surgical sites, in indwelling catheters, or in association with mechanical ventilation. The organisms most commonly responsible for these early infections are *Staphylococcus aureus*, *Pseudomonas aeruginosa*, and members of the Enterobacteriaceae family.

Infections that occur 1 to 6 months after transplantation are typically caused by opportunistic organisms such as cytomegalovirus (CMV), herpes simplex virus, *Pneumocystis jirovecii*, *Listeria*, *Nocardia*, *Toxoplasma gondii*, *Candida* species, *Cryptococcus*, and *Aspergillus*. Of these organisms, CMV remains a significant cause of morbidity and mortality among these patients.[64] It is critical to maintain a high degree of suspicion for CMV infection in any patient seen in an emergency department within the first few months after cardiac transplant. The clinical manifestations of CMV infection range from mild signs and symptoms (ie, fever, myalgia, and malaise) to life-threatening respiratory failure (ie, pneumonitis). Additional signs of CMV infection include hepatitis, leukopenia, and thrombocytopenia.[59]

Infections that emerge more than 6 months after transplantation are usually pneumonia and urinary tract infections caused by community-acquired organisms.

KEY POINTS

Infections within the first month after transplantation are usually caused by nosocomial organisms.

Infections that occur 1 to 6 months after surgery are generally caused by opportunistic organisms.

Maintain a high degree of suspicion for CMV infection in any cardiac transplant patient who seeks treatment in the emergency department within the first few months after transplantation.

Infections after the first 6 months are more likely to be pneumonia or urinary tract infections caused by community-acquired organisms.

Arrhythmias

Bradycardia

Most clinicians define bradycardia in this special group of patients as a heart rate less than 80 beats/min.[57] Up to 40% of these patients experience bradyarrhythmia.[57] Sinus node dysfunction is the most common cause of bradycardia in the cardiac transplant patient, followed by junctional bradycardia and atrioventricular blocks.[57] Since the transplanted heart is a denervated organ, atropine is ineffective in augmenting heart rate.[57] For the transplant patient who is hemodynamically unstable secondary to bradycardia, isoproterenol may be administered while preparations are made to initiate pacing.[57] Most of these patients will require a permanent pacemaker.[57] Any patient presenting with a bradyarrhythmia more than 2 weeks after surgery requires a biopsy to assess for acute rejection.

Atrial Fibrillation and Atrial Flutter

Both atrial fibrillation and atrial flutter are associated with acute rejection and require prompt treatment.[57,67,68] As in the management of nontransplant patients, hemodynamically unstable patients with a cardiac transplant who develop atrial fibrillation or atrial flutter should undergo electrical cardioversion. For stable patients, rate control can be attempted with beta-blockers, calcium channel blockers, or amiodarone.[57] Of these, beta-blockers are preferred because of the transplanted heart's increased sensitivity to adrenergic agents.[57] Diltiazem and verapamil, common medications used for rate control in the nontransplant patient, should be used with caution in patients with a cardiac transplant because these medications can interact with immunosuppressive medications and affect the level of immunosuppression.[57]

AV Nodal Reentrant Tachycardia

These patients are at risk for AVNRT. Hemodynamically unstable patients with AVNRT should be treated with electrical cardioversion. For stable patients, adenosine remains the drug of choice; however, it should be administered at half the dose given to nontransplant patients[57] because of the transplanted heart's increased sensitivity to adenosine.[57] Digoxin and vagal maneuvers are ineffective for treating AVRNT in a transplanted (denervated) heart, so their use is not recommended.

Ventricular Tachycardia and Ventricular Fibrillation

Thankfully, the incidence of malignant ventricular arrhythmias in patients with transplanted hearts has decreased in recent years.[57,69] Treatment of ventricular tachycardia or ventricular fibrillation in these patients remains the same as in nontransplant patients—defibrillation, cardioversion, and antiarrhythmic medication. Both procainamide and amiodarone can be administered safely to the transplant recipient.

KEY POINTS

Atropine is ineffective in the transplanted heart.

Any patient presenting with bradycardia more than 2 weeks after cardiac transplant surgery requires a biopsy to assess for acute rejection.

Diltiazem should be used with caution for rate control of atrial fibrillation or atrial flutter.

The dose of adenosine should be decreased in these patients when they develop AVNRT.

TABLE 17-11.
Risk Factors for the Cardiac Allograft Vasculopathy

Antecedent coronary artery disease
Cellular rejection
Diabetes
Hyperlipidemia
Hypertension
Obesity
Smoking

Cardiac Allograft Vasculopathy

Cardiac allograft vasculopathy (CAV) is a rapidly progressive atherosclerosis that is the most common cause of late transplant dysfunction.[57,70] CAV can occur as early as 3 months after transplant and is found in up to one third of patients by 5 years.[57,71] CAV is caused by a variety of immunologic and nonimmunologic mechanisms that ultimately result in generalized intimal proliferation of the graft vascular endothelium.[59] Risk factors for CAV are listed in Table 17-11.[72,73] In contrast to the discrete, eccentric lesions of traditional atherosclerotic disease, CAV causes a generalized, concentric narrowing along the entire length of the coronary vessel. As a result, traditional coronary angiography typically underestimates the extent of disease.[57] Given its ability to detect concentric disease, intravascular ultrasonography is currently the recommended imaging modality for the diagnosis of CAV.[57,66] For centers that do not have the capability to perform intravascular ultrasonography, dobutamine stress echocardiography might be useful and is recommended as a sensitive, noninvasive test to detect CAV.[66] For the few patients who have CAV and amenable lesions, percutaneous coronary angiography with stent placement or coronary artery bypass grafting could be beneficial. For most patients, however, these therapies are ineffective, so treatment consists primarily of strict risk factor control.

KEY POINTS

CAV causes a concentric narrowing along the entire length of the coronary vessel.

Traditional angiography is insensitive in the diagnosis of CAV.

Intravascular ultrasonography is the recommended imaging modality for diagnosing CAV.

Conclusion

Patients who have received a cardiac transplant and those with pulmonary hypertension are some of the most challenging patient populations an emergency physician will encounter. Both patient populations have altered physiology, are on complex medication regimens, and can rapidly deteriorate during the course of an emergency department evaluation. With knowledge of the key points highlighted in this chapter, emergency physicians can effectively and confidently care for the acutely ill patient with pulmonary hypertension or a cardiac transplant.

References

1. Tapson VF, Humbert M. Incidence and prevalence of chronic thromboembolic pulmonary hypertension: from acute to chronic pulmonary embolism. *Proc Am Thorac Soc.* 2006;3:564-567.
2. Simonneau G, Robbins IM, Beghetti M, et al. Updated clinical classification of pulmonary hypertension. *J Am Coll Cardiol.* 2009;54(1 suppl):S43-S54.
3. Humbert M, Sitbon O, Chaouat A, et al. Pulmonary arterial hypertension in France: results from a national registry. *Am J Respir Crit Care Med.* 2006;173:1023-1030.
4. Badesch DB, Champion HC, Sanchez MA, et al. Diagnosis and assessment of pulmonary arterial hypertension. *J Am Coll Cardiol.* 2009;54(1 suppl):S55-S66.

5. Galie N, Hoeper MM, Humbert M, et al. Guidelines for the diagnosis and treatment of pulmonary hypertension: the Task Force for the Diagnosis and Treatment of Pulmonary Hypertension of the European Society of Cardiology (ESC) and the European Respiratory Society (ERS), endorsed by the International Society of Heart and Lung Transplantation (ISHLT). *Eur Heart J.* 2009;30:2493-2537.

6. Bogaard HJ, Abe K, Vonk Noordegraaf A, Voelkel NF. The right ventricle under pressure: cellular and molecular mechanisms of right-heart failure in pulmonary hypertension. *Chest.* 2009;135:794-804.

7. Janicki JS, Brower GL, Gardner JD, et al. Cardiac mast cell regulation of matrix metalloproteinase-related ventricular remodeling in chronic pressure or volume overload. *Cardiovasc Res.* 2006;69:657-665.

8. Baicu CF, Stroud JD, Livesay VA, et al. Changes in extracellular collagen matrix alter myocardial systolic performance. *Am J Physiol Heart Circ Physiol.* 2003;284:H122-H132.

9. Khan R, Sheppard R. Fibrosis in heart disease: understanding the role of transforming growth factor-beta in cardiomyopathy, valvular disease and arrhythmia. *Immunology.* 2006;118:10-24.

10. Farrer-Brown G. Vascular pattern of myocardium of right ventricle of human heart. *Br Heart J.* 1968;30:679-686.

11. Dell'Italia LJ. The right ventricle: anatomy, physiology, and clinical importance. *Curr Probl Cardiol.* 1991;16:653-720.

12. Haupt HM, Hutchins GM, Moore GW. Right ventricular infarction: role of the moderator band artery in determining infarct size. *Circulation.* 1983;67:1268-1272.

13. Nootens M, Wolfkiel CJ, Chomka EV, Rich S. Understanding right and left ventricular systolic function and interactions at rest and with exercise in primary pulmonary hypertension. *Am J Cardiol.* 1995;75:374-377.

14. van Wolferen SA, Marcus JT, Westerhof N, et al. Right coronary artery flow impairment in patients with pulmonary hypertension. *Eur Heart J.* 2008;29:120-127.

15. Gibbons Kroeker CA, Adeeb S, Shrive NG, Tyberg JV. Compression induced by RV pressure overload decreases regional coronary blood flow in anesthetized dogs. *Am J Physiol Heart Circ Physiol.* 2006;290:H2432-H2438.

16. Ling Y, Johnson MK, Kiely DG, et al. Changing demographics, epidemiology, and survival of incident pulmonary arterial hypertension: results from the pulmonary hypertension registry of the United Kingdom and Ireland. *Am J Respir Crit Care Med.* 2012;186:790-796.

17. Jing ZC, Xu XQ, Han ZY, et al. Registry and survival study in chinese patients with idiopathic and familial pulmonary arterial hypertension. *Chest.* 2007;132:373-379.

18. Rich S, Dantzker DR, Ayres SM, et al. Primary pulmonary hypertension: a national prospective study. *Ann Intern Med.* 1987;107:216-223.

19. McGoon M, Gutterman D, Steen V, et al. Screening, early detection, and diagnosis of pulmonary arterial hypertension: ACCP evidence-based clinical practice guidelines. *Chest.* 2004;126(1 suppl):14S-34S.

20. Heresi GA, Tang WH, Aytekin M, et al. Sensitive cardiac troponin I predicts poor outcomes in pulmonary arterial hypertension. *Eur Respir J.* 2012;39(4):939-944.

21. Benza RL, Miller DP, Gomberg-Maitland M, et al. Predicting survival in pulmonary arterial hypertension: insights from the Registry to Evaluate Early and Long-Term Pulmonary Arterial Hypertension Disease Management (REVEAL). *Circulation.* 2010;122:164-172.

22. Nagaya N, Nishikimi T, Okano Y, et al. Plasma brain natriuretic peptide levels increase in proportion to the extent of right ventricular dysfunction in pulmonary hypertension. *J Am Coll Cardiol.* 1998;31:202-208.

23. Tongers J, Schwerdtfeger B, Klein G, et al. Incidence and clinical relevance of supraventricular tachyarrhythmias in pulmonary hypertension. *Am Heart J.* 2007;153:127-132.

24. Rajdev A, Garan H, Biviano A. Arrhythmias in pulmonary arterial hypertension. *Prog Cardiovasc Dis.* 2012;55:180-186.

25. Barbosa EJ Jr, Gupta NK, Torigian DA, et al. Current role of imaging in the diagnosis and management of pulmonary hypertension. *AJR Am J Roentgenol.* 2012;198:1320-1331.

26. Tan RT, Kuzo R, Goodman LR, Siegel R, et al. Utility of CT scan evaluation for predicting pulmonary hypertension in patients with parenchymal lung disease. Medical College of Wisconsin Lung Transplant Group. *Chest.* 1998;113:1250-1256.

27. Matthews JC, McLaughlin V. Acute right ventricular failure in the setting of acute pulmonary embolism or chronic pulmonary hypertension: a detailed review of the pathophysiology, diagnosis, and management. *Curr Cardiol Rev.* 2008;4:49-59.

28. Raymond RJ, Hinderliter AL, Willis PW, et al. Echocardiographic predictors of adverse outcomes in primary pulmonary hypertension. *J Am Coll Cardiol.* 2002;39:1214-1219.

29. Price LC, Wort SJ, Finney SJ, et al. Pulmonary vascular and right ventricular dysfunction in adult critical care: current and emerging options for management: a systematic literature review. *Crit Care.* 2010;14(5):R169.

30. Haddad F, Doyle R, Murphy DJ, et al. Right ventricular function in cardiovascular disease, part II: pathophysiology, clinical importance, and management of right ventricular failure. *Circulation.* 2008;117:1717-1731.

31. Hoeper MM, Granton J. Intensive care unit management of patients with severe pulmonary hypertension and right heart failure. *Am J Respir Crit Care Med.* 15;184:1114-1124.

32. Zamanian RT, Haddad F, Doyle RL, et al. Management strategies for patients with pulmonary hypertension in the intensive care unit. *Crit Care Med.* 2007;35:2037-2050.

33. Vizza CD, Rocca GD, Roma AD, et al. Acute hemodynamic effects of inhaled nitric oxide, dobutamine and a combination of the two in patients with mild to moderate secondary pulmonary hypertension. *Crit Care.* 2001;5:355-361.

34. Kerbaul F, Rondelet B, Motte S, et al. Effects of norepinephrine and dobutamine on pressure load-induced right ventricular failure. *Crit Care Med.* 2004;32:1035-1040.

35. Sztrymf B, Souza R, Bertoletti L, et al. Prognostic factors of acute heart failure in patients with pulmonary arterial hypertension. *Eur Respir J.* 2010;35:1286-1293.

36. De Backer D, Biston P, Devriendt J, et al. Comparison of dopamine and norepinephrine in the treatment of shock. *N Engl J Med.* 2010;362:779-789.

37. Moudgil R, Michelakis ED, Archer SL. Hypoxic pulmonary vasoconstriction. *J Appl Physiol.* 2005;98:390-403.

38. Balanos GM, Talbot NP, Dorrington KL, et al. Human pulmonary vascular response to 4 h of hypercapnia and hypocapnia measured using Doppler echocardiography. *J Appl Physiol.* 2003;94:1543-1551.

39. Mekontso Dessap A, Charron C, et al. Impact of acute hypercapnia and augmented positive end-expiratory pressure on right ventricle function in severe acute respiratory distress syndrome. *Intensive Care Med.* 2009;35:1850-1858.

40. McLaughlin VV, Archer SL, Badesch DB, et al. ACCF/AHA 2009 expert consensus document on pulmonary hypertension: a report of the American College of Cardiology Foundation Task Force on Expert Consensus Documents and the American Heart Association: developed in collaboration with the American College of Chest Physicians, American Thoracic Society, Inc., and the Pulmonary Hypertension Association. *Circulation.* 2009;119:2250-2294.

41. Viitanen A, Salmenpera M, Heinonen J. Right ventricular response to hypercarbia after cardiac surgery. *Anesthesiology.* 1990;73:393-400.

42. Shapiro S, Hill NS. Transition from IV to subcutaneous prostacyclin: premature withdrawal? *Chest.* 2007;132:741-743.

43. Barst RJ, Rubin LJ, Long WA, et al. A comparison of continuous intravenous epoprostenol (prostacyclin) with conventional therapy for primary pulmonary hypertension. *N Engl J Med.* 1996;334:296-301.

44. Anderson JR, Nawarskas JJ. Pharmacotherapeutic management of pulmonary arterial hypertension. *Cardiol Rev.* 2010;18:148-162.

45. Safdar Z. Treatment of pulmonary arterial hypertension: the role of prostacyclin and prostaglandin analogs. *Respir Med.* 2011;105:818-827.

46. Cockrill BA, Kacmarek RM, Fifer MA, et al. Comparison of the effects of nitric oxide, nitroprusside, and nifedipine on hemodynamics and right ventricular contractility in patients with chronic pulmonary hypertension. *Chest.* 2001;119:128-136.

47. Bhorade S, Christenson J, O'Connor M, et al. Response to inhaled nitric oxide in patients with acute right heart syndrome. *Am J Respir Crit Care Med.* 1999;159:571-579.

48. George I, Xydas S, Topkara VK, et al. Clinical indication for use and outcomes after inhaled nitric oxide therapy. *Ann Thorac Surg.* 2006;82:2161-2169.

49. Barst RJ, Gibbs JS, Ghofrani HA, et al. Updated evidence-based treatment algorithm in pulmonary arterial hypertension. *J Am Coll Cardiol.* 2009;54(1 suppl):S78-S84.

50. Olsson KM, Nickel NP, Tongers J, et al. Atrial flutter and fibrillation in patients with pulmonary hypertension. *Int J Cardiol.* 2012 June 22 [Epub ahead of print].

51. Delcroix M, Naeije R. Optimising the management of pulmonary arterial hypertension patients: emergency treatments. *Eur Respir Rev.* 2010;19:204-211.

52. Olsson KM, Simon A, Strueber M, et al. Extracorporeal membrane oxygenation in nonintubated patients as bridge to lung transplantation. *Am J Transplant.* 2010;10:2173-2178.

53. de Perrot M, Granton JT, McRae K, et al. Impact of extracorporeal life support on outcome in patients with idiopathic pulmonary arterial hypertension awaiting lung transplantation. *J Heart Lung Transplant.* 2011;30:997-1002.

54. Srivastava MC, Ramani GV, Garcia JP, et al. Veno-venous extracorporeal membrane oxygenation bridging to pharmacotherapy in pulmonary arterial hypertensive crisis. *J Heart Lung Transplant.* 2010;29:811-813.

55. Sayer GT, Baker JN, Parks KA. Heart rescue: the role of mechanical circulatory support in the management of severe refractory cardiogenic shock. *Curr Opin Crit Care.* 2012;18:409-416.

56. Crespo-Leiro MG, Barge-Caballero E, Marzoa-Rivas R, et al. Heart transplantation. *Curr Opin Organ Transplant.* 2010;15:633-638.

57. Chacko P, Philip S. Emergency department presentation of heart transplant recipients with acute heart failure. *Heart Fail Clin.* 2009;5:129-143.

58. Taylor DO, Stehlik J, Edwards LB, et al. Registry of the International Society for Heart and Lung Transplantation: Twenty-sixth Official Adult Heart Transplant Report-2009. *J Heart Lung Transplant.* 2009;28:1007-1022.
59. Klein DG. Current trends in cardiac transplantation. *Crit Care Nurs Clin North Am.* 2007;19:445-460.
60. Blasco LM, Parameshwar J, Vuylsteke A. Anaesthesia for noncardiac surgery in the heart transplant recipient. *Curr Opin Anaesthesiol.* 2009;22:109-113.
61. Brandt M, Harringer W, Hirt SW, et al. Influence of bicaval anastomoses on late occurrence of atrial arrhythmia after heart transplantation. *Ann Thorac Surg.* 1997;64:70-72.
62. Beniaminovitz A, Savoia MT, Oz M, et al. Improved atrial function in bicaval versus standard orthotopic techniques in cardiac transplantation. *Am J Cardiol.* 1997;80:1631-1635.
63. Taylor DO, Edwards LB, Boucek MM, et al. Registry of the International Society for Heart and Lung Transplantation: twenty-third official adult heart transplantation report—2006. *J Heart Lung Transplant.* 2006;25:869-879.
64. Haddad H, Isaac D, Legare JF, et al. Canadian Cardiovascular Society Consensus Conference update on cardiac transplantation 2008: Executive Summary. *Can J Cardiol.* 2009;25:197-205.
65. Woods WA, McCulloch MA. Care of the acutely ill pediatric heart transplant recipient. *Pediatr Emerg Care.* 2007;23:721-724.
66. Costanzo MR, Dipchand A, Starling R, et al. The International Society of Heart and Lung Transplantation Guidelines for the care of heart transplant recipients. *J Heart Lung Transplant.* 2010;29:914-956.
67. Ahmari SA, Bunch TJ, Chandra A, et al. Prevalence, pathophysiology, and clinical significance of post-heart transplant atrial fibrillation and atrial flutter. *J Heart Lung Transplant.* 2006;25:53-60.
68. Cui G, Tung T, Kobashigawa J, et al. Increased incidence of atrial flutter associated with the rejection of heart transplantation. *Am J Cardiol.* 2001;88:280-284.
69. Tagusari O, Kormos RL, Kawai A, et al. Native heart complications after heterotopic heart transplantation: insight into the potential risk of left ventricular assist device. *J Heart Lung Transplant.* 1999;18:1111-1119.
70. Stehlik J, Edwards LB, Kucheryavaya AY, et al. The Registry of the International Society for Heart and Lung Transplantation: twenty-seventh official adult heart transplant report—2010. *J Heart Lung Transplant.* 2010;29:1089-1103.
71. Taylor DO, Edwards LB, Boucek MM, et al. Registry of the International Society for Heart and Lung Transplantation: twenty-fourth official adult heart transplant report—2007. *J Heart Lung Transplant.* 2007;26:769-781.
72. Jimenez J, Kapadia SR, Yamani MH, et al. Cellular rejection and rate of progression of transplant vasculopathy: a 3-year serial intravascular ultrasound study. *J Heart Lung Transplant.* 2001;20:393-398.
73. Valantine H. Cardiac allograft vasculopathy after heart transplantation: risk factors and management. *J Heart Lung Transplant.* 2004;23(5 suppl):S187-S193.

CHAPTER 18

Pharmacologic Approach to Cardiac Emergencies

Matthew Salzman

IN THIS CHAPTER

Mechanisms of action
Commonly used antihypertensive and antiarrhythmic medications
Specific treatment modalities
Management of cardioactive medication toxicities

Emergency physicians have a tremendous arsenal of pharmacotherapeutic agents at their disposal for managing cardiovascular emergencies such as acute coronary syndromes, congestive heart failure, arrhythmias, and cardiogenic shock, as well as hypertensive emergencies. This chapter reviews commonly available cardiovascular agents, their mechanisms of action, and their indications and contraindications. Additionally, this chapter reviews complications associated with these medications in overdose and their management.

Antihypertensive Medications

Multiple agents can be used in the setting of hypertensive emergencies to reduce blood pressure and heart rate slowly and effectively. Many of these medications can be given intravenously and subsequently titrated to the desired effect. Categories of medications that are effective in the emergent setting are beta-adrenergic antagonists, calcium channel antagonists, nitrates, and imidazoline or centrally acting alpha-receptor agonists.

CASE ONE

A 46-year-old man presents to the emergency department with the chief complaint of chest pain, which he describes as "tearing" and radiating from the substernal region straight back to between his scapulae. On presentation, his heart rate is 96 beats/min, the blood pressure in his right arm is 260/120 mm Hg, and his pulse oximetry reading is 96%. An electrocardiogram (ECG) reveals no evidence of acute ischemia or infarct. An upright chest radiograph shows a widened mediastinum. With a presumed diagnosis of thoracic aortic dissection, the goal of therapy is to reduce the patient's heart rate and blood pressure to reduce shearing forces on the aorta.

Beta-Adrenergic Antagonists

Three subtypes of beta-adrenergic antagonists are currently used: nonselective, selective, and those with alpha-adrenergic blockade properties. These medications predominantly antagonize beta-adrenergic receptors in a competitive and reversible fashion. Nonselective beta-blockers such as propranolol and sotalol antagonize both $beta_1$- and $beta_2$-receptors, whereas selective beta-blockers such as metoprolol and esmolol antagonize $beta_1$-receptors with much greater affinity than $beta_2$-receptors. Labetalol and carvedilol belong in a third category, as these medications also antagonize peripheral alpha-adrenergic receptors.[1] The commonly used beta-adrenergic antagonists, along with their recommended dosing, are listed in Table 18-1.

Three subtypes of beta-adrenergic receptors have been identified in the human body: $beta_1$, $beta_2$, and $beta_3$. These receptors are, in general, agonized by circulating catecholamines such as epinephrine and norepinephrine. In the heart, beta$_1$- and beta$_2$-receptors are found on the sinuatrial (SA) node, on the atrioventricular (AV) node, on the conducting pathways, and on myocytes. Direct beta$_1$- and beta$_2$-agonism initiate a complex second messenger system, ultimately resulting in increased heart rate (chronotropy), conduction velocity (dromotropy), and contractility (inotropy). In the periphery, beta$_2$-agonism in arteries and veins results in vasodilation by the same second messenger system as in the heart, whereas beta$_1$-agonism in the kidney causes increased renin release, resulting in vasoconstriction as well as sodium retention and increased intravascular volume.[1] The beta$_3$-receptor function is less well understood but is not believed to play a role in hemodynamic regulation.[2]

Beta-adrenergic antagonists directly inhibit the effects of circulating catecholamines such as norepinephrine and epinephrine, the concentrations of which are increased in excitatory states. In the heart, beta$_1$-receptors predominate in the SA node, AV node, and myocytes. Cardiac beta-receptor antagonism results in slower heart rate as well as decreased contractility, relaxation rate, and conduction velocity. This sympatholytic activity decreases myocardial oxygen demand and increases oxygen delivery, as the myocardium is perfused predominantly during diastole. In the periphery, beta-adrenergic antagonism can cause a small increase in vasomotor tone through vasoconstriction in vascular beds. This effect is believed to be minor and to be offset by decreased renin synthesis, resulting in vasodilation as well as decreased sodium retention and intravascular volume.[1]

Beta-adrenergic antagonists have a crucial role in the management of patients experiencing cardiac emergencies such as ST-elevation myocardial infarction (STEMI) and non-STEMI, aortic dissection, and ascending aortic aneurysm. It is important to note, however, that, although beta-blockers have an important role in chronic heart failure management, no evidence exists to support beta-adrenergic blockade in patients with acute decompensated heart failure.[3] These medications can be administered either orally or intravenously, although intravenous administration is preferred in patients with acute illness. Contraindications to beta-blocker therapy include previous hypersensitivity reactions, active asthma or chronic obstructive pulmonary disease exacerbations, and recent cocaine use. However, highly selective beta-adrenergic agents can be used safely in patients with underlying pulmonary disease.[1]

KEY POINT

Beta-blockers are most effective when treating hypertensive emergencies that require heart rate and blood pressure control. Esmolol, because of its high affinity for beta$_1$-receptors, does not decrease blood pressure to the same degree that it lowers heart rate. Therefore, an additional agent, such as nitroglycerin, might be necessary to achieve hemodynamic control. Addition of alpha-adrenergic blockade, as induced by labetalol, might obviate the need for multiple pharmacologic agents.

Calcium Channel Blockers

Five subtypes of calcium channel blockers have been described. However, it is simpler and still clinically relevant to consider calcium channel blockers as belonging to one of two categories: dihydropyridine or nondihydropyridine calcium channel antagonists. The nondihydropyridine agents, including verapamil and diltiazem, antagonize cardiac and peripheral vascular calcium channels (discussed elsewhere in this chapter). Dihydropyridine calcium channel blockers antagonize L-type calcium channels in vascular smooth muscle. By inhibiting intracellular calcium influx, they also inhibit calcium release from the sarcoplasmic reticulum, ultimately resulting in vascular relaxation and a decrease in systemic vascular resistance. Nicardipine is a dihydropyridine calcium channel blocker that is administered at 5 mg/hour and titrated to the desired hemodynamic effect, with a maximum dose of 15 mg/hour. It reduces myocardial and cerebral ischemia and increases coronary blood flow and stroke volume, making it a desirable agent for patients with hypertensive emergencies such as stroke and decompensated heart failure. Its onset of action is believed to be within 5 to 15 minutes after initiation of therapy.[4] Perhaps the biggest concern with nicardipine therapy is that it may cause excessive and rapid reductions in blood pressure; therefore, invasive arterial monitoring of the blood pressure is recommended. Additionally, because nicardipine acts peripherally, reflex tachycardia can occur.

KEY POINT

Dihydropyridine calcium channel blockers such as nicardipine are useful in decreasing systemic vascular resistance. They should be considered when blood pressure control is necessary but the heart rate is normal or low, as seen in patients with decompensated congestive heart failure and hemorrhagic stroke.

TABLE 18-1.

Beta-adrenergic Antagonists and Their Recommended Dosing

Medication	Loading Dose	Repeat Dose/Infusion
Metoprolol	2.5 to 5 mg IV	Repeat dose every 15 minutes
Esmolol	500 mcg/kg IV bolus	150 mcg/kg infusion, titrated to desired heart rate
Labetalol	10- to 20-mg IV bolus; may double loading dose in 10 min	2 mg/min infusion, titrated to blood pressure and heart rate

Alpha-Adrenergic and Imidazoline Receptor–Specific Medications

Alpha-adrenergic receptors are divided into two main subtypes, alpha$_1$ and alpha$_2$, both of which are further subdivided into multiple subtypes. These receptors are found throughout the body and are agonized by circulating catecholamines. Alpha-receptors are coupled to G proteins, and their agonism triggers a complex intracellular cascade that leads to vascular smooth muscle effects. Alpha$_1$-receptors in the peripheral vascular system are located postsynaptically, whereas alpha$_2$-receptors are located both presynaptically and postsynaptically. Alpha$_1$- and postsynaptic alpha$_2$-agonism result in vasoconstriction, whereas presynaptic alpha$_2$-agonism causes negative feedback, resulting in decreased norepinephrine release and vascular smooth muscle relaxation. In the central nervous system, postsynaptic alpha$_2$-agonism decreases excitatory neurotransmitter release, resulting in vasodilation and bradycardia.[5]

Imidazoline receptors are also divided into two subtypes: I$_1$ and I$_2$. These receptors are located predominantly in the ventrolateral medulla and, similar to the alpha-adrenergic receptors, are coupled to G proteins. Imidazoline receptor activation triggers an intracellular cascade that has not been elucidated completely. Further, it is believed that the imidazoline receptors are linked to the central alpha$_2$-receptors and that medications that agonize central alpha$_2$-receptors also stimulate the imidazoline receptors, resulting in decreased catecholamine release, with subsequent decreases in both heart rate and blood pressure.[6]

Clonidine is an imidazoline that agonizes central alpha$_2$-receptors and imidazoline receptors, decreasing sympathetic tone. A decreased level of circulating catecholamines lowers heart rate and blood pressure. Clonidine is available in tablet, transdermal patch, and intravenous formulations; in the United States, it is not approved for intravenous administration for hemodynamic control. In the outpatient setting, it is used widely in both oral and patch form to treat hypertension. In the emergency department, oral administration is used to control the ventricular response rate in patients with atrial fibrillation.[7] However, because of its slow onset of action and unpredictable effects, clonidine, in either oral or transdermal form, plays little role in the management of patients experiencing acute cardiovascular emergencies. Further, abrupt cessation of clonidine can result in an abrupt increase in circulating catecholamines, possibly precipitating a hypertensive emergency.

Phentolamine is not used commonly, but it can be particularly useful in hyperexcitatory states that result in an excess of circulating catecholamines such as cocaine-induced hypertensive emergencies, pheochromocytoma, and clonidine withdrawal. It is a nonselective alpha$_1$- and alpha$_2$-adrenergic antagonist. It antagonizes peripheral alpha-adrenergic receptors, resulting in arterial and venous smooth muscle relaxation. It also stimulates beta-adrenergic receptors, resulting in increased inotropy and chronotropy.[8] It can be given intravenously, at a standard dose of 1 to 5 mg IV in an adult. It has a rapid onset of action and short half-life (approximately 19 minutes). Repeat doses may be administered as needed.[4]

KEY POINTS

Patients who are experiencing cardiac emergencies such as stroke, acute myocardial infarction, or decompensated diastolic heart failure and who require rapid and controlled reduction in blood pressure should be given medications intravenously, because their effects and onset of action are more predictable. Oral agents such as clonidine are best reserved for outpatient management of hypertension.

Beta-adrenergic antagonists should not be administered to patients with acute cocaine toxicity because they might worsen hypertension as a result of unopposed alpha-adrenergic agonism. Labetalol should also be avoided, as its alpha-adrenergic effects are outweighed by its beta-adrenergic effects. Alternative agents such as phentolamine, nicardipine, and nitroglycerin should be considered.

Nitrates

Nitrates, most notably nitroglycerin and sodium nitroprusside, are vascular smooth muscle relaxers capable of preload and afterload reduction. Nitroglycerin can be administered in the form of 400-mcg sublingual tablets or as a titratable intravenous infusion. Each nitroglycerin molecule contains three NO$_2$ groups that, when adsorbed by the vascular endothelium, are metabolized to nitric oxide. Within these cells, nitric oxide stimulates guanosine 3′,5′-monophosphate synthesis, ultimately resulting in vasodilation.[9] At lower doses, nitroglycerin predominantly affects the venous system, resulting in decreased venous return and preload reduction. At higher doses, usually 100 mcg/min or more IV, nitroglycerin causes arteriolar vasodilation as well as reduction in central venous pressure and capillary wedge pressure, ultimately decreasing myocardial oxygen demand and optimizing myocardial contractility. Because of erratic absorption leading to uncontrolled dosing, use of nitroglycerin paste is not recommended in patients with acute cardiac conditions.

Nitroglycerin has a rapid onset of action and short half-life, generally believed to be between 1 and 4 minutes, making it ideal for titration. Nitroglycerin can cause abrupt drops in blood pressure, thereby reducing cerebral perfusion. This effect is generally short-lived and corrected by titrating therapy. Further, as a result of vasodilatory effects, the heart rate might increase slightly, increasing myocardial oxygen demand. Co-administration with a beta-blocker offsets this effect and should be considered when using nitroglycerin for acute coronary syndromes.

Sodium nitroprusside does not require vascular endothelial cell uptake to act as a nitric oxide donor. In the blood, nitroprusside is reduced and directly releases nitric oxide, which, similar to nitroglycerin, stimulates guanosine 3′,5′-monophosphate synthesis, ultimately resulting in vasodilation. Nitroprusside has a more pronounced effect on the arteriolar circulation, decreasing blood pressure and pulmonary vascular resistance. The net effect is an increase in heart rate and cardiac output.[9]

Nitroprusside also has a rapid onset of action and short half-life, making it an easily titratable drug. Beta-adrenergic blockers are generally co-administered with nitroprusside to attenuate the reflex tachycardia it produces. Nitroprusside administration can result in rapid lowering of blood pressure, also decreasing cerebral perfusion. Further, nitroprusside is metabolized to cyanide and thiocyanate. These metabolites can accumulate, resulting in oxidative phosphorylation inhibition and cellular asphyxia, with metabolism shunting from aerobic to anaerobic and, ultimately, lactic acidosis, hypotension, and death.[9] Co-administration with hydroxocobalamin, a newer antidote for cyanide poisoning, attenuates this effect greatly and should be considered in patients receiving nitroprusside therapy for more than 23 hours.

KEY POINT

Nitroprusside has been the gold standard medication when acute blood pressure control is needed. Over recent years, medications with improved safety profiles such as labetalol and nicardipine have been used with increasing frequency. When using nitrates, co-administration of a selective beta-blocker should be considered to offset the reflex tachycardia caused by these medications.

Therapeutic Decision Making

Ultimately, the goal of therapy for patients with hypertensive emergencies is a smooth and gradual decrease in heart rate and mean arterial pressure. Abrupt changes in vasomotor tone increase the risk of decreased cerebral perfusion pressure and subsequent stroke. Medications that can be given intravenously and have a rapid onset of action and short half-lives are preferable, as they can be titrated to the desired effect. Oral medications should be avoided because their absorption and effect can be unpredictable as well as irreversible. Beta-blockers should be avoided in patients who develop hypertensive emergencies as a result of cocaine or similar sympathomimetics because unopposed the alpha activity could exacerbate the hypertension. Table 18-2 provides a summary of antihypertensive agents and their indications.

KEY POINTS

Whenever possible, patients with hypertensive emergencies should be treated with intravenous medications that gradually decrease blood pressure. Patients with elevated heart rate and blood pressure can be given a single medication with both alpha- and beta-antagonistic properties (eg, labetalol). Alternatively, a vasodilator, such as nitroglycerin, may be used in combination with a highly selective beta-blocker, such as esmolol. If the patient's heart rate is normal or low, a peripherally acting calcium channel blocker such as nicardipine may be used. Phentolamine, the only imidazoline available for intravenous administration, should be reserved for patients with sympathomimetic-induced hypertensive emergencies and pheochromocytoma.

The best therapeutic choices for patients with suspected aortic dissection are those that slow the heart rate with beta-blockade and peripheral vascular dilatation. Combination therapy such as metoprolol and nitroprusside or a single agent such as labetalol would be effective choices. Labetalol, a peripheral alpha-receptor and cardiac beta-receptor antagonist, is effective at decreasing both heart rate and blood pressure, ultimately decreasing shearing forces on the aorta.

Antiarrhythmics

Tachyarrhythmias arise from three basic mechanisms: enhanced automaticity, reentry, and triggered activity. All tachyarrhythmias, regardless of site of origin, can arise from one of these mechanisms. Specifically, atrial, junctional, and ventricular tachycardias can be caused by any of these mechanisms, and clues to the cause are based largely on medical history and ECG interpretation. The choice of pharmacologic therapy depends on the underlying mechanism.

The Vaughn Williams system (Table 18-3) classifies medications according to the ion channel or receptor on which they primarily act and their subsequent transmembrane potential effects. This system has limitations in that many medications have pharmacologic effects beyond those described in this system. Additionally, it fails to include some medications used as antiarrhythmics, including digoxin, adenosine, and magnesium. A more advanced classification system, the Sicilian Gambit, was created to overcome the limitations of the Vaughn Williams system as electrophysiologic understanding evolved.[10] Unfortunately, its complexity limits its clinical utility.[11] Therefore, the Vaughn Williams system remains more widely used.

TABLE 18-2.

Antihypertensive Agents and Their Suggegsted Indications

Clinical scenario	Therapeutic goal	First choice	Second choice	Third choice
Aortic dissection, thoracic aneurysm	Decrease shearing forces on the aorta	Labetalol	Esmolol	Nitroprusside and metoprolol
Decompensated heart failure: diastolic dysfunction	Reduce preload and afterload with subsequent diuresis	Nitroglycerin followed by furosemide	Nicardipine followed by furosemide	Nitroprusside
Acute coronary syndrome/STEMI	Decrease myocardial oxygen demand	Nitroglycerin with or without the addition of metoprolol	Esmolol or labetalol	Nitroprusside and metoprolol
Hypertensive crisis	Decrease systemic vascular resistance and circulating catecholamines	Nicardipine	Labetalol	Phentolamine

Class I medications act predominantly on channels that regulate rapid sodium influx into the cell. This category is further subdivided into types a, b, and c, according to affinity for the sodium channel. Class Ia medications such as procainamide exhibit moderate sodium channel blockade effect, thereby slowing cardiac conduction and prolonging repolarization.[12] Class Ib antiarrhythmics such as lidocaine are weak sodium channel blockers and have little effect on normally functioning sodium channels. However, these medications exert their action on damaged or abnormal fibers, as seen in myocardial ischemia or infarct. These agents shorten repolarization and are useful in terminating ventricular arrhythmias in the setting of myocardial ischemia. Class Ic medications such as flecainide are strong sodium channel blockers and have little role in managing patients with acute cardiac conditions, as they can precipitate arrhythmias and other adverse cardiovascular events. In general, these medications are used in consultation with a cardiologist or electrophysiologist.

Class II medications are beta-adrenergic antagonists (discussed in depth earlier in this chapter). Class III medications such as amiodarone predominantly antagonize the potassium channels responsible for potassium efflux and repolarization. These medications are particularly useful for reentrant tachyarrhythmias, including supraventricular and ventricular arrhythmias. By prolonging the effective refractory period, normal cells are less likely to be activated by a premature depolarization, directing conduction via the normal pathways, thereby preventing and suppressing tachyarrhythmias.[12] Class IV medications are calcium channel antagonists and are discussed separately in this chapter.

Wide Complex Tachycardias: Class Ia, Ib and III Antiarrhythmics

CASE TWO

A 17-year-old boy presents to the emergency department with a chief complaint of palpitations and dizziness. His vital signs are as follows: heart rate, 180 beats/min; blood pressure, 115/60 mm Hg; respiratory rate, 22 breaths/min; and oxygen saturation, 99%. He is diaphoretic and uncomfortable. His ECG demonstrates a wide-complex tachycardia (Figure 18-1A). He is given procainamide at 50 mg/min. Shortly thereafter, his heart rate decreases to 76 beats/min (Figure 18-1B). He is admitted to the cardiac care unit with a diagnosis of atrial fibrillation with Wolff-Parkinson-White syndrome and scheduled for an electrophysiology study with possible ablation.

Procainamide, a class Ia antiarrhythmic, is particularly useful and may even be considered first-line therapy for patients with aberrant conduction pathways, such as Wolff-Parkinson-White syndrome. Because procainamide slows conduction through the AV node as well as accessory pathways, it is considered safe to use in wide complex tachycardias of unclear etiology, including supraventricular tachycardia with aberrancy, atrial fibrillation with rapid ventricular response, and ventricular tachycardia and fibrillation.[13] Procainamide is converted to an active metabolite, N-acetylprocainamide, which has a direct potassium blockade effect and, as such, is a class III antiarrhythmic (see below). Procainamide can initially increase the heart rate as a result of anticholinergic effect and, with continued infusion, this can lead to QRS widening and hypotension.[11] Prolonged procainamide administration has been associated with bone marrow suppression, fatal agranulocytosis, and a lupus-like syndrome. However, these effects are not relevant in the acute setting of the emergency department.

Procainamide should be given intravenously at 20 to 50 mg/min until arrhythmia suppression is achieved or to a maximum dose of 20 mg/kg. Alternatively, a bolus of 100 mg IV may be administered every 5 minutes until the arrhythmia is suppressed. If intravenous access has not been established, procainamide may be given intramuscularly, although this is not the preferred route because its absorption and onset of action are variable. The intramuscular dosage is 50 mg/kg/day, administered in divided doses every 3 to 6 hours.[11]

TABLE 18-3.

The Vaughn Williams Classification of Antiarrhythmics

Class	Examples	Mechanism of Action	Typical Indications
Ia	Quinidine, procainamide, disopyramide	Intermediate-strength sodium channel inhibition	Ventricular tachyarrhythmias and wide complex tachycardias of unclear etiology
Ib	Lidocaine, tocainide, mexiletine	Weak/fast sodium channel inhibition	Ventricular arrhythmias as a result of acute myocardial ischemia
Ic	Flecainide, propafenone	Strong/slow sodium channel inhibition	In consultation with cardiology consultant
II	Propranolol, metoprolol, esmolol	Beta-adrenergic antagonism	Narrow complex tachycardias requiring AV nodal suppression (eg, atrial fibrillation)
III	Amiodarone, ibutilide	Potassium channel blockade	Unstable patients with refractory ventricular arrhythmias
IV	Verapamil, diltiazem	Calcium channel blockade	Narrow complex tachycardias requiring AV nodal suppression (eg, atrial fibrillation)

CASE THREE

A 76-year-old woman with a history of hypertension and coronary artery disease presents to the emergency department complaining of chest pain. Her heart rate is 56 beats/min, her blood pressure is 80/40 mm Hg, her respiratory rate is 16 breaths/min, and her pulse oximetry reading is 99% on 2 liters of oxygen via nasal cannula. An ECG shows an acute ST-segment elevation in the inferior leads. Shortly after her arrival, she becomes unresponsive, and the cardiac monitor shows a wide complex tachycardia (Figure 18-2). She receives immediate direct electrocardioversion, with return of mentation and sinus rhythm. While awaiting transport to the cardiac catheterization lab, she continues to have intermittent episodes of wide complex tachycardia. She receives a loading dose of amiodarone, 150 mg IV, after which she has no further episodes of wide complex tachycardia.

Amiodarone is a class III antiarrhythmic agent that antagonizes potassium channels as well as beta-adrenergic receptors and calcium channels. These broad antagonistic effects result in a prolonged effective refractory period for all cardiac conduction cells, suppressing nodal as well as aberrantly conducted signals. Amiodarone has emerged as a popular choice for wide complex tachycardias, especially stable ventricular tachycardia. However, it is important to note that, according to the American College of Cardiology/American Heart Association/European Society of Cardiology guidelines, procainamide, sotalol, and lidocaine may also be used in this circumstance; amiodarone is best reserved for patients with poor left ventricular function or signs of heart failure.[13] Amiodarone has a long half-life, perhaps as long as 25 days.[14]

According to the advanced cardiovascular life support guidelines for pulseless ventricular tachycardia and ventricular fibrillation, amiodarone should be administered intravenously or intraosseously as a bolus dose of 300 mg. If the patient does not convert to a perfusing rhythm, an additional bolus of 150 mg may be administered.[14] Subsequently, an infusion of 60 mg/hour may then be initiated for 6 hours. Prolonged therapy with amiodarone can lead to a number of complications, including pulmonary fibrosis, thyroid dysfunction, corneal deposits, liver injury, and epididymo-orchitis. However, these effects are generally seen with long-term therapy and should not dissuade the physician from using amiodarone as indicated under urgent conditions.

Lidocaine, a class Ib antiarrhythmic, may also be considered for patients with wide complex tachycardias secondary to myocardial ischemia or infarction.[15] Lidocaine is administered as a bolus dose of 1 to 1.5 mg/kg. If arrhythmias persist or recur, additional boluses of 0.5 mg/kg may be administered. The maximum dose is a total of 3 mg/kg. Lidocaine is metabolized in the liver to active metabolites that also have sodium channel blockade effects. Patients with underlying liver disease are at risk for lidocaine toxicity, which can result in dizziness, altered mental status, and dysarthria, progressing further to seizures and, ultimately, respiratory depression. Additionally, because lidocaine is metabolized by the cytochrome P450 system in the liver, patients who take medications such as cimetidine and

FIGURE 18-1A.

Atrial fibrillation and WPW syndrome. This ECG shows an irregular wide complex rhythm with extremely rapid rates (>200-250 beats/min) in some areas. The QRS complexes do not have a typical bundle-branch block morphology and they vary on a beat-to-beat basis. These characteristics are indicative of the presence of a bypass tract.

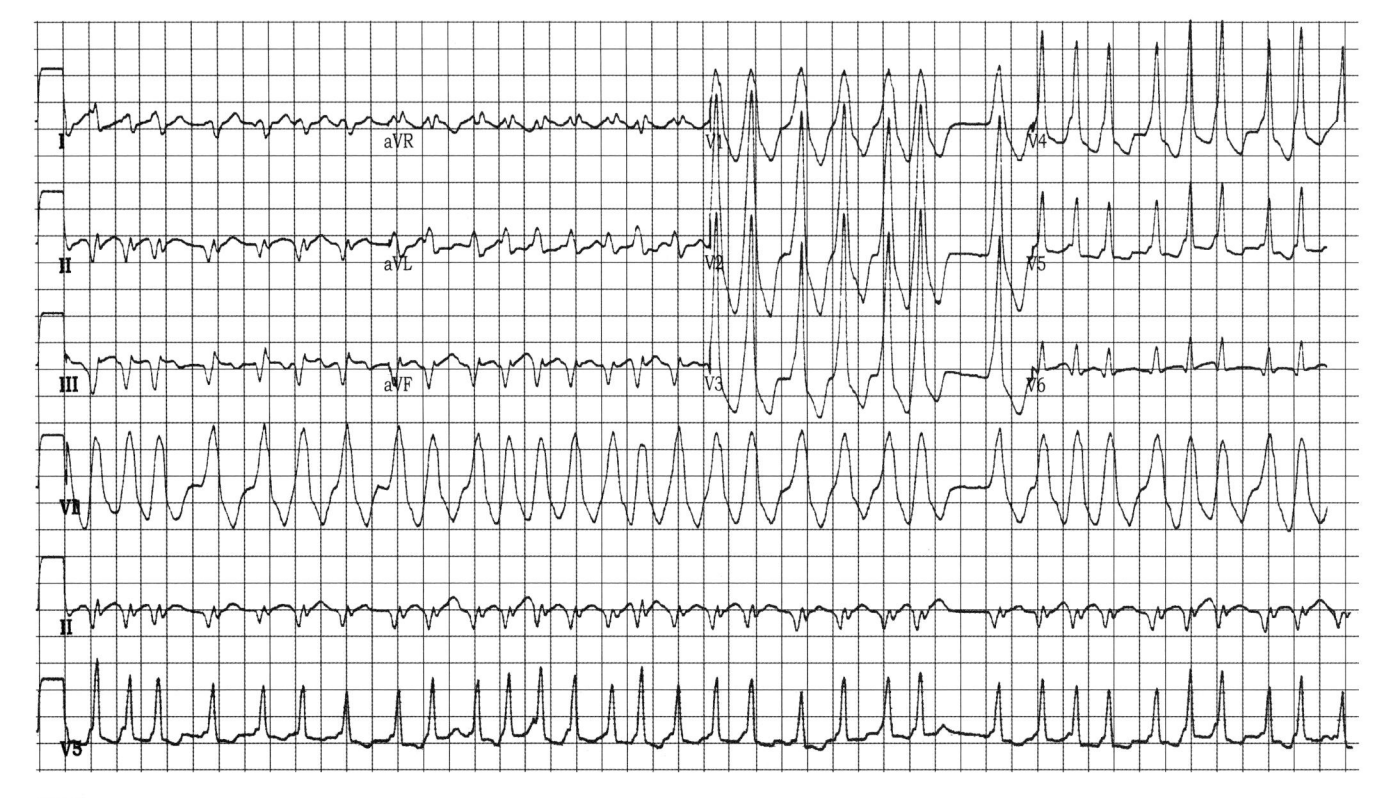

phenytoin, which inhibit P450 enzymes, are at risk for lidocaine toxicity even at therapeutic doses. Therefore, lidocaine should be used cautiously in these patients.[11]

Therapeutic Decision Making

Commonly available pharmacologic agents for wide complex tachycardias include procainamide, lidocaine, and amiodarone. Lidocaine should be administered to patients who have acute myocardial ischemia or infarct and in whom monomorphic ventricular tachycardia develops. Procainamide administration is preferred for patients with stable, sustained monomorphic ventricular tachycardia. Amiodarone is best used in patients who are unstable and refractory to shock or procainamide.[15]

KEY POINTS

Stable patients who can receive intravenous pharmacotherapy should have their ECGs assessed carefully to determine whether the rhythm involves a bypass tract. A bypass tract in itself does not generate a rhythm but has the potential to conduct very rapid rhythms to the ventricle.

Medications that affect the AV node alone, including beta-adrenergic antagonists and calcium channel antagonists, should be avoided because they can enhance conduction through the aberrant pathway, ultimately leading to cardiovascular collapse.

Narrow Complex Tachycardias: Adenosine and Class II and IV Antiarrhythmic Medications

The differential diagnosis behind any regular, narrow complex tachycardia includes AV node reentry and atrial flutter. Regardless of the primary rhythm, the fact that the QRS complex is narrow indicates that the rhythm uses the AV node to conduct antegrade to the ventricle. The initial focus of therapy in stable patients with non-sinus, narrow complex tachyarrhythmias is to slow conduction through the AV node, followed by sinus rhythm restoration. Agents that slow conduction through the AV node are adenosine, nondihydropyridine calcium channel blocking agents (Class IV), beta-blockers (Class II), as well as other agents that include AV node blockade as part of their pharmacology such as amiodarone and digoxin. Digoxin is not commonly used, however, because it has a delayed onset of action, taking up to 4 hours to slow the ventricular response; therefore, this medication is not discussed in this section.

CASE FOUR

A 57-year-old woman presents with the sensation of a rapid heart rate. She says that the sensation started spontaneously approximately 1 hour before her arrival. Her medical history is significant only for hypertension, for which she takes hydrochlorothiazide daily. She is in no distress and has a heart rate of 140 beats/min, which is irregular, a blood pressure of 160/80 mm Hg, and a normal pulse oximetry reading. An ECG reveals atrial fibrillation with rapid ventricular response (Figure

FIGURE 18-1B.
Followup ECG from the patient in Figure 18-1A after administration of procainamide, showing a slowed ventricular response rate and evidence of blocked conduction through the bypass tract (narrow QRS complexes). The rhythm converted back to normal sinus rhythm soon after this ECG was obtained.

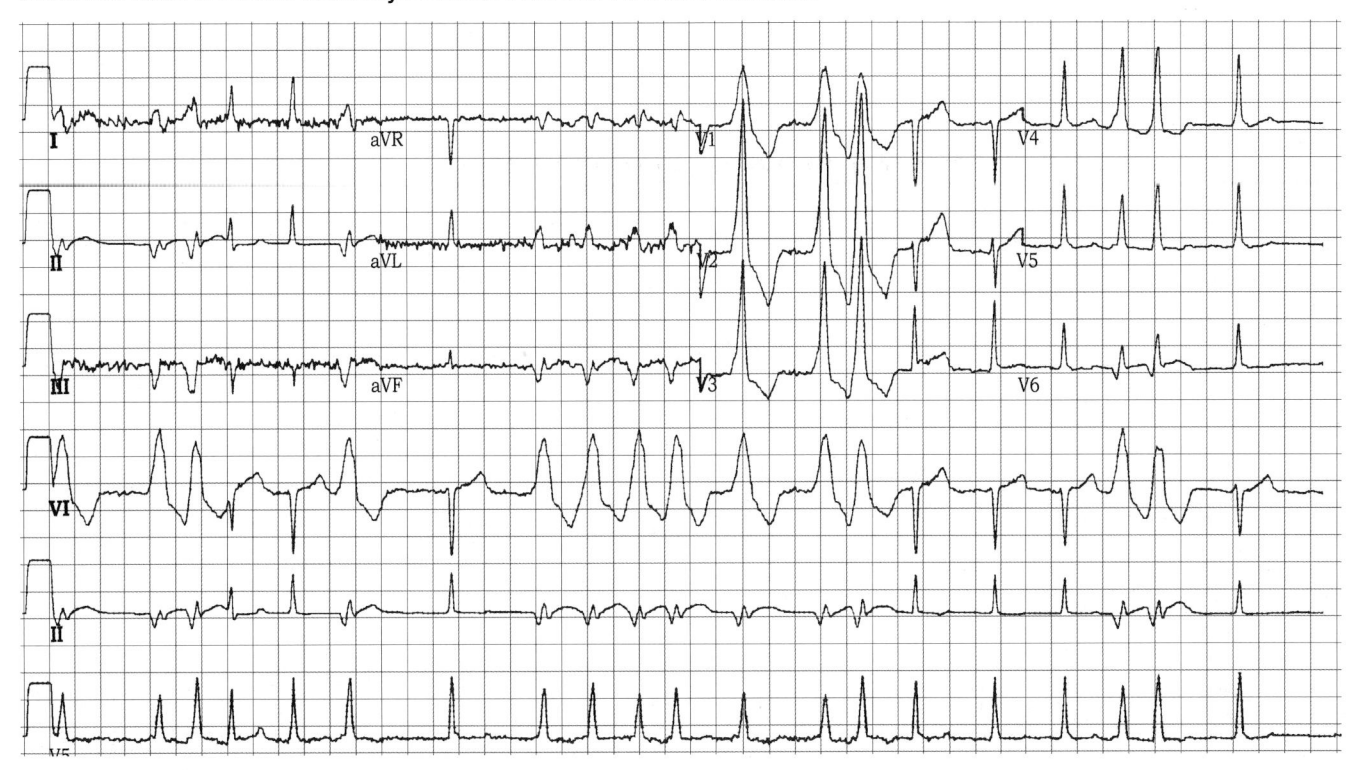

18-3). After peripheral vascular access is established and blood specimens are obtained for laboratory testing, diltiazem is administered as a bolus dose of 0.25 mg/kg. Her ventricular rate decreases to 70 beats/min and her blood pressure decreases to 130/60 mm Hg.

Class IV antiarrhythmic agents include the centrally acting or nondihydropyridine calcium channel blockers (eg, diltiazem and verapamil). These medications antagonize L-type calcium channels in the SA and AV nodes as well as the cardiac conduction cells. The nondihydropyridine calcium channel blockers are more selective for the cardiac calcium channels than the peripheral vascular smooth muscle calcium channels, but they do block these channels as well. Calcium influx inhibition slows AV nodal conduction, resulting in a decreased ventricular rate for patients with tachyarrhythmias that originate above the AV node, including atrial fibrillation, atrial flutter, and AV nodal reentrant tachycardia.[12]

Diltiazem should be administered intravenously at an initial dose of 0.25 mg/kg. A subsequent bolus of 0.35 mg/kg may be administered 15 minutes later if the initial dose fails to achieve adequate ventricular slowing. Subsequently, a continuous, titratable infusion should be started at a dose of 5 to 15 mg/hour.[11] Diltiazem has a rapid onset of action, usually within 4 minutes after administration, and a long half-life of approximately 3 hours.[11] For patients with atrial fibrillation or flutter, the goal of therapy with diltiazem is ventricular rate control, not cardioversion to sinus rhythm. Diltiazem alone generally will not convert these arrhythmias to sinus rhythm. Because diltiazem antagonizes calcium channels both in the heart and the vascular smooth muscle, it can cause hypotension. Additionally, because of its negative inotropic effects, diltiazem should be avoided in patients with acute decompensated heart failure. Finally, diltiazem is generally contraindicated in patients with wide complex tachyarrhythmias, because AV nodal suppression can enhance accessory pathway conduction, resulting in worsening hemodynamics, including cardiovascular collapse and death.[13]

Hemodynamically stable patients with atrial fibrillation or atrial flutter can be candidates for electrical or chemical cardioversion in the emergency department. However, the decision to use this intervention should be made in consultation with a cardiologist or electrophysiologist. Medications used for chemical cardioversion include amiodarone, ibutilide, procainamide, flecainide, propafenone, dronedarone, and sotalol. Amiodarone is the preferred drug for patients with an ejection fraction less than 35%.

Therapeutic Decision Making

The initial approach to treating hemodynamically stable patients in need of rate control should be either a calcium channel blocker or selective beta-blocker. There is no clear consensus as to which medication should be used first. Selective beta-adrenergic antagonists such as metoprolol and esmolol, discussed in detail elsewhere in this chapter, should be considered in patients with suspected coronary artery disease or evidence of acute ischemia on their ECG. Nondihydropyridine calcium channel blockers such as diltiazem as well as beta-blockers are effective in patients without clinical evidence of congestive heart failure, acute ischemia, or infarct on an ECG. Recent literature suggests

FIGURE 18-2.
This ECG shows a regular wide complex tachycardia with a single fusion beat, consistent with ventricular tachycardia.

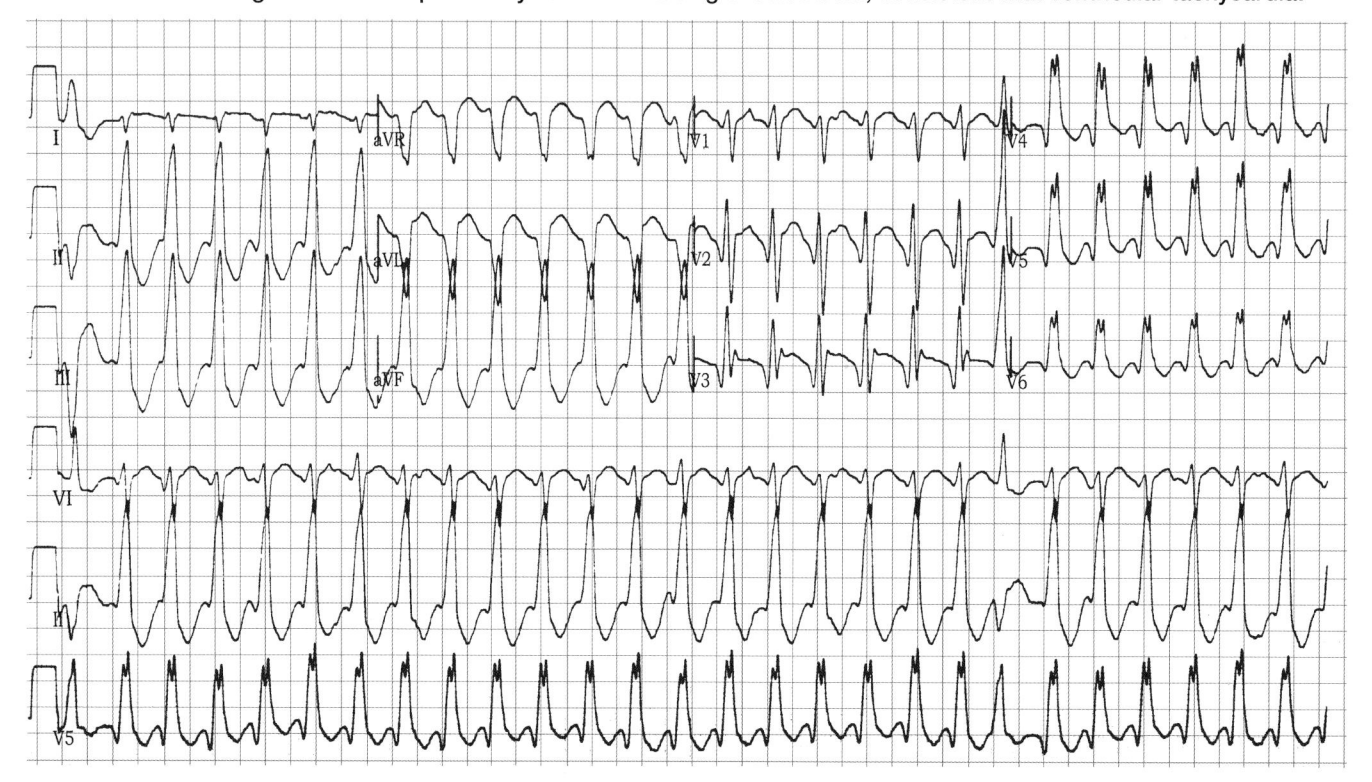

Pharmacologic Approach to Cardiac Emergencies

that, for patients in atrial fibrillation without underlying illness, beta-blockers and calcium channel blockers are equally safe and effective for ventricular rate control.[16]

KEY POINT

Occasionally, the initial therapeutic choice for ventricular rate control will be ineffective, suggesting the need for an alternative therapy. There is concern that administration of both intravenous calcium channel blockers and beta-blockers can cause AV dissociation. However, little evidence exists to support this fear, and administration of one class of medications does not contraindicate use of the other. Indeed, many patients are on long-term beta-blocker and calcium channel blocker medications and do not develop complete heart block.

CASE FIVE

A 27-year-old man without a relevant medical history presents complaining of palpitations. He is awake and alert with a blood pressure of 120/60 mm Hg and a heart rate of 180 beats/min. An ECG shows narrow complex tachycardia (Figure 18-4). Peripheral intravenous access is established and 6 mg of adenosine is administered via rapid intravenous push. After a brief period of asystole, normal sinus rhythm returns, with a heart rate of 60 beats/min.

Adenosine is a naturally occurring purine found throughout the body. Adenosine receptors are found throughout the heart as well as in the vascular smooth muscle. These receptors are coupled to G proteins, which, when agonized, further propagate a complex intracellular signaling pathway. In the vasculature, adenosine receptor agonism triggers smooth muscle relaxation with subsequent vasodilation. However, in the conduction system, adenosine receptor agonism inhibits the electrical impulse through the AV node. Adenosine has a rapid onset of action, usually within 10 to 15 seconds after administration. It also has a short half-life of approximately 10 seconds. It can be used therapeutically to terminate supraventricular tachycardias as well as diagnostically to distinguish among various types of narrow complex tachyarrhythmias.[13] It is generally given as a 6-mg IV push. Two subsequent doses of 12 mg each may be administered if the initial dose fails. It is important to note that, because of its very short half-life, adenosine should ideally be infused and flushed as rapidly as possible and through a proximal intravenous site. If given into the arm or hand, some clinicians advocate raising the extremity after administration to expedite delivery to the heart. Patients should be warned that, shortly after adenosine administration, they might feel unpleasant sensations such as nausea, warmth and diaphoresis, or generalized malaise.

Adenosine is generally considered safe in patients with wide complex tachyarrhythmias and has both diagnostic and therapeutic value in this scenario.[17] However, patients with tachyarrhythmias as a result of toxicity from methylxanthines (eg, caffeine, theophylline) are often refractory to adenosine, as these medications are adenosine receptor antagonists. Alterna-

FIGURE 18-3.

This ECG shows an irregular narrow complex tachycardia consistent with atrial fibrillation with a rapid ventricular response rate of approximately 170 beats/min.

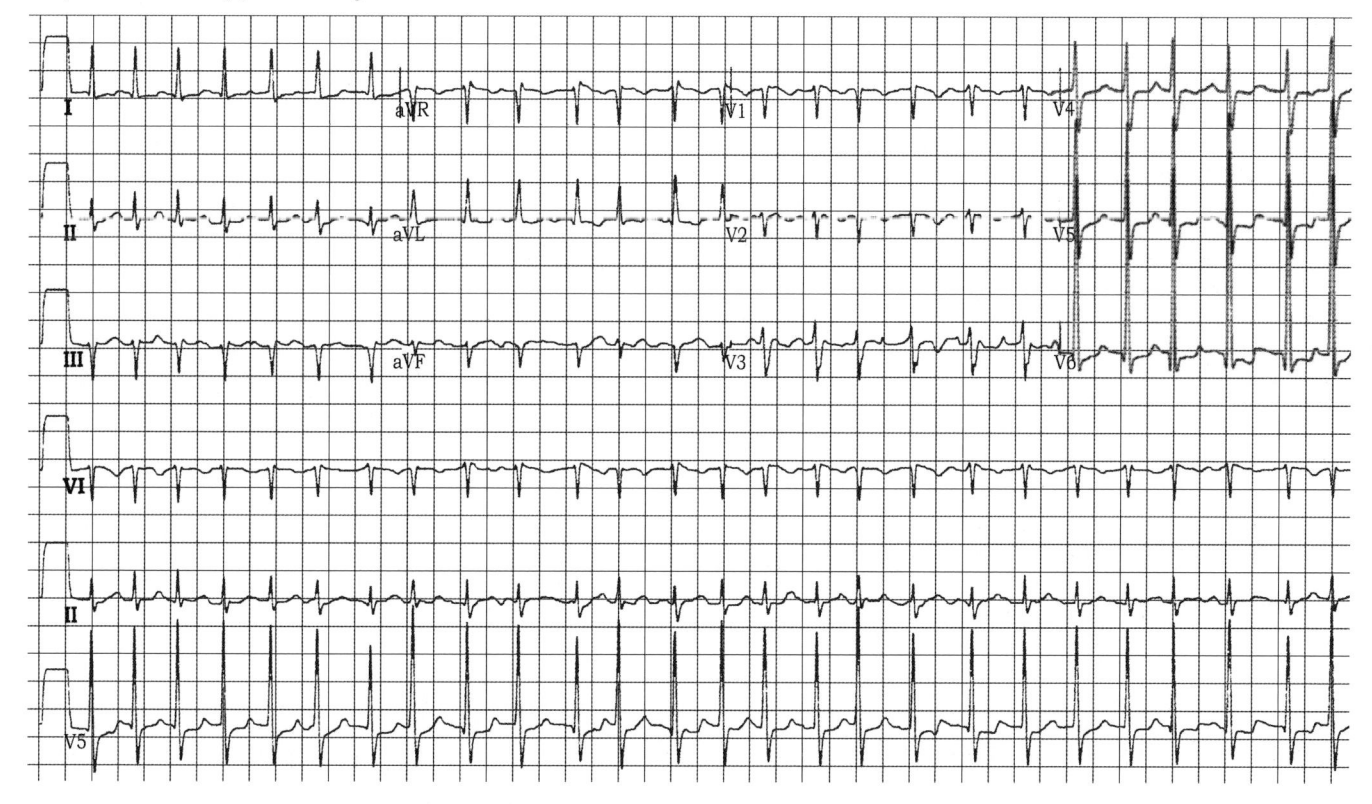

tive agents such as selective beta-adrenergic antagonists should be considered.

KEY POINTS

Narrow complex tachycardias can be treated with medications that block or slow conduction through the AV node. Adenosine is generally considered safe for wide and narrow complex tachycardias. Selective beta-adrenergic antagonists should be considered first-line therapy if there is concern about myocardial ischemia or hypotension. Nondihydropyridine calcium channel antagonists can be used to slow conduction if there is no evidence of myocardial ischemia. However, because these agents cause vasodilation in addition to nodal suppression, they should be avoided in hypotensive patients.

Congestive Heart Failure: ACE Inhibitors, Loop Diuretics

Initial management of acute exacerbations of heart failure usually focuses on optimizing blood pressure, preload and afterload reduction, and diuresis. The relative importance of each of these interventions depends on whether the underlying cause of failure is predominantly diastolic or systolic dysfunction.

CASE SIX

A 63-year-old man with a history of hypertension, non-ischemic dilated cardiomyopathy, and diabetes presents complaining of shortness of breath. His vital signs are as follows: blood pressure, 220/140 mm Hg; heart rate, 110 beats/min; respiratory rate, 22 breaths/min; and oxygen saturation, 86% on 6 L/min of oxygen via nasal cannula. He is diaphoretic and in moderate respiratory distress. He has marked pedal edema, jugular venous distention, and rales throughout his lung fields. An ECG shows no evidence of acute ischemia or infarct. He is started on noninvasive positive-pressure ventilation. A peripheral intravenous line is established, and he is started on a nitroglycerin infusion at 100 mcg/min. Once his hemodynamic parameters and clinical status have improved, he is given 40 mg of furosemide IV. After being weaned off ventilation, he is given 20 mg of lisinopril orally, and his nitroglycerin infusion is titrated down.

Pharmacologic Management of Congestive Heart Failure

Nitroglycerin is the mainstay of initial management of the hypertensive patient with acute decompensated congestive heart failure, as it can lower both preload and afterload, thereby improving myocardial performance. Nitroglycerin can be administered as a 400-mcg sublingual tablet while intravenous access is being established and an infusion is being prepared. The specific pharmacology of nitroglycerin is reviewed elsewhere in this chapter.

Angiotensin-converting enzyme (ACE) inhibitors are among the mainstays of chronic therapy for heart failure patients and are potentially beneficial in acutely decompensated heart failure. They competitively inhibit angiotensin-converting enzymes, which are responsible for, among other things, converting angiotensin I to angiotensin II. Angiotensin II acts on multiple organ systems throughout the body. It contributes to peripheral

FIGURE 18-4.
This ECG shows a regular narrow complex tachycardia, consistent with AV nodal reentrant tachycardia.

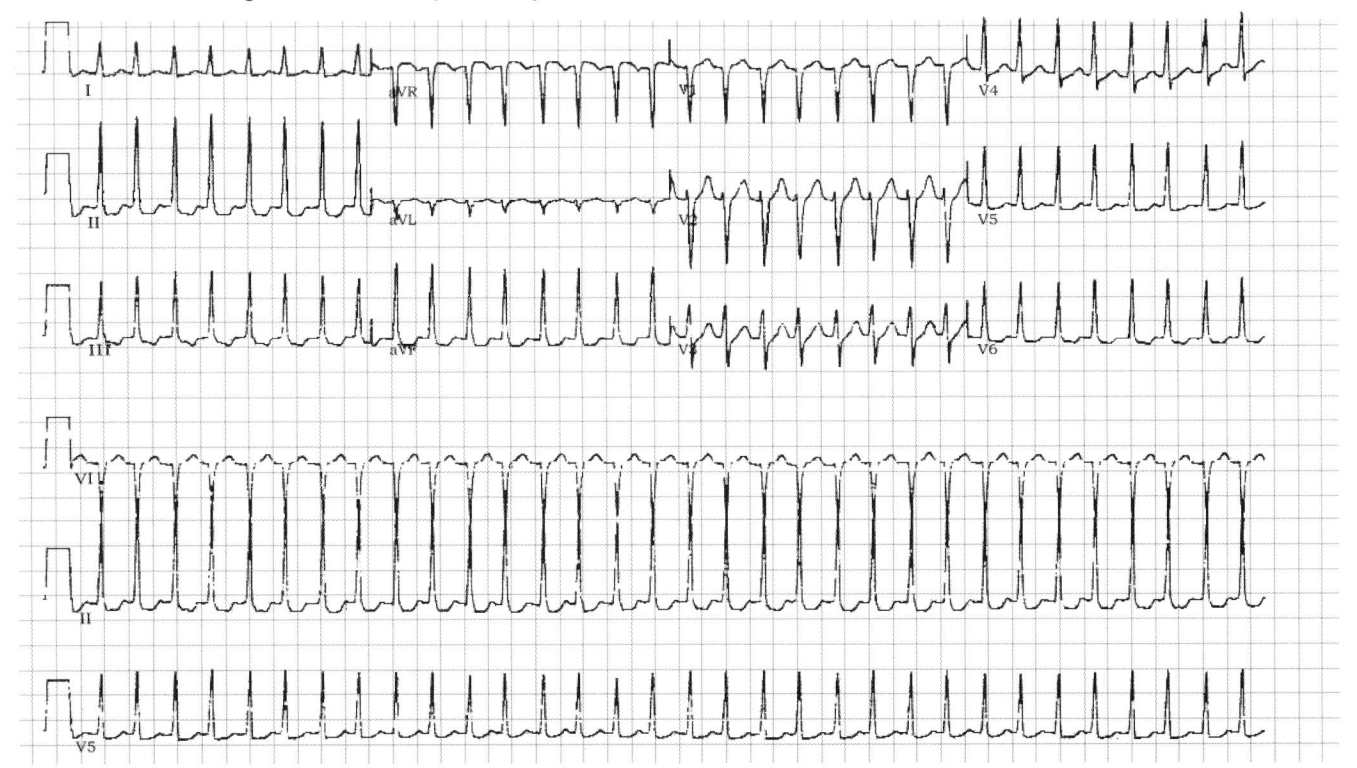

vascular vasoconstriction, both directly and indirectly through increased catecholamine release, coronary vasoconstriction, renal arteriolar vasoconstriction, and sodium reabsorption in the proximal tubules. ACE inhibitors, by decreasing levels of angiotensin II and other actions, reduce sympathetic tone, decrease vasopressin and aldosterone secretion, and promote natriuresis. These effects result in decreased intravascular volume as well as venous and arteriolar dilation, achieving both preload and afterload reduction without a change in heart rate.[18]

Enalaprilat is the only ACE inhibitor available for intravenous administration. It can be given in increments of 0.625 mg, up to a total dose of 5 mg IV.[18] Its onset of action is rapid, with blood pressure reduction achieved generally within 15 minutes after administration. As discussed in Chapter 7, however, the literature on the use of ACE inhibitors in the acute resuscitation of patients with decompensated heart failure is not abundant. Therefore, the ideal patient and optimal timing for the use of ACE inhibitors for this condition are not addressed well in most national guidelines. ACE inhibitors should be used cautiously, if at all, in patients with a borderline blood pressure. Further, ACE inhibitor administration is contraindicated in pregnant women, in patients with bilateral renal artery stenosis, and in those with a history of allergy or angioneurotic edema.

KEY POINTS

Patients with elevated blood pressure and decompensated heart failure need rapid reduction in systemic vascular resistance to maximize cardiac output. Nitrates can be administered sublingually, pending establishment of intravenous access.

Diuresis

Loop diuretics were once the primary therapy for patients in acute decompensated heart failure. Current recommendations include loop diuretics, but generally in combination with nitrates to achieve preload and afterload reduction. Furosemide is the most commonly administered loop diuretic; bumetanide and torsemide are also available. These medications inhibit sodium reabsorption in the loop of Henle and both the proximal and distal renal tubules, ultimately leading to decreased intravascular volume and subsequent preload reduction. However, patients with acute heart failure typically have poor renal perfusion because of increased afterload, and so the diuretic effect is often markedly delayed. The administration of high doses of loop diuretics such as 1 mg/kg of furosemide in patients with acute decompensated heart failure is associated with initial adverse hemodynamic effects, including elevations of mean arterial pressure, left and right heart filling pressures (preload), and systemic vascular resistance (afterload). The adverse effects are thought to be due to initial vasoconstriction and might worsen clinical symptoms. For this reason, there is no role for high doses of loop diuretics in the management of decompensated heart failure.[3]

Therapeutic Decision Making

Managing acute congestive heart failure is more complex than simple diuresis. It is more appropriate to conceptualize cardiogenic pulmonary edema as multifactorial pump failure. As such, the treatment is also multifactorial, including positive-pressure ventilation, preload and afterload reduction, and diuresis. Aggressive treatment with a multimodal approach frequently prevents the need for endotracheal intubation and mechanical ventilation and the associated complications. Pharmacologic mainstays in the initial management of the patient with decompensated heart failure with adequate or elevated blood pressure include sublingual nitroglycerin followed by a drip, low-dose diuresis, and further afterload reduction if needed with ACE inhibitors.

Cardiogenic Shock: Norepinephrine, Dobutamine, Dopamine

Cardiogenic shock, defined as hypotension with end-organ hypoperfusion as a result of pump failure, is challenging to treat and carries a mortality rate of approximately 50%.[19] Most commonly, cardiogenic shock is a result of acute myocardial infarction. Other causes include myocarditis, myocardial contusion, and ingestion of cardioactive medications, including beta-adrenergic antagonists, calcium channel blockers, and cardiac glycosides.[19]

CASE SEVEN

A 45-year-old man presents to the emergency department after a syncopal event. He is complaining of crushing substernal chest pressure that started while he was playing tennis, just prior to his arrival. His vital signs are as follows: heart rate, 54 beats/min; blood pressure, 76/40 mm Hg; respiratory rate, 24 breaths/min; pulse oximetry, 88% on 6 L/min oxygen via nasal cannula. An ECG shows ST-segment elevations in the precordial leads with reciprocal changes (Figure 18-5). His lung examination is remarkable for rales throughout. The cardiac catheterization lab is notified. Prior to transport to the catheterization lab, he undergoes rapid sequence intubation to maximize oxygenation and is started on an infusion of norepinephrine and dobutamine to keep his systolic blood pressure above 90 mm Hg.

Drugs that are effective in the management of cardiogenic shock include dopamine, dobutamine, and norepinephrine. Each has a unique mechanism of action. Understanding the different mechanisms will guide the physician in selecting the most appropriate medication for the patient in cardiogenic shock, pending definitive interventional therapy (percutaneous transluminal coronary angioplasty, coronary artery bypass grafting, or intra-aortic balloon pump).

Dopamine is a beta- and alpha-adrenergic agonist with effects that change as dosage increases. Beta-adrenergic agonism is achieved initially at doses between 5 and 10 mcg/kg/min. As doses increase above 10 mcg/kg/min, alpha-adrenergic agonism occurs. Lower doses of dopamine raise heart rate and stroke volume, while higher doses increase systemic vascular resistance and blood pressure.[20] Dopamine has traditionally been recommended as the initial vasopressor for patients with profound hypotension and cardiogenic shock. However, this medication is associated with more tachyarrhythmias and higher mortality rates than norepinephrine therapy.[21]

Norepinephrine is a potent, nonselective alpha- and beta-adrenergic agonist. Direct adrenergic agonism in the vascular smooth muscle results in peripheral vasoconstriction and a subsequent increase in blood pressure. Norepinephrine also agonizes myocardial beta-receptors, thereby increasing heart rate and cardiac output. It should be started at the lowest possible dose, usually 0.05 to 0.2 mcg/kg/min, and titrated to reach a systolic blood pressure of 90 mm Hg or a mean arterial pressure of 60 mm Hg. Vasopressors can increase myocardial oxygen demand, potentially worsening failing areas of the heart; however, they should not be withheld from patients with evidence of end-organ hypoperfusion.[22]

Dobutamine is an inotrope that agonizes myocardial $beta_1$- and $beta_2$-receptors, thereby increasing stroke volume and cardiac output. Dobutamine also agonizes peripheral beta- and alpha-receptors. Because of equal agonism of these receptors in the periphery, the vasoactive effects are generally offset without a subsequent change in blood pressure. Dobutamine can improve systemic perfusion if the blood pressure is above 90 mm Hg. It can be started at an infusion of 3 to 15 mcg/kg/min. If the patient's systolic blood pressure is less than 90 mm Hg, a vasopressor such as norepinephrine should be initiated first, with the subsequent addition of dobutamine, if the blood pressure reaches or exceeds 90 mm Hg. Alternative treatments for patients with refractory cardiogenic shock, including vasopressin and levosimendan, are still under investigation. Their administration may be considered after consultation with a cardiologist.[22]

Therapeutic Decision Making

Cardiogenic shock is a feared complication in patients with acute myocardial infarction. The goal of therapy remains revascularization. The pharmacologic treatments discussed above are bridging therapies to invasive techniques that go beyond the scope of this chapter (percutaneous transluminal coronary angioplasty, coronary artery bypass grafting,, and intra-aortic balloon pump). Pharmacologic therapy initiation should not delay potentially curative intervention in the cardiac catheterization lab. Initial pharmacologic therapy should include either dopamine or norepinephrine for patients with clinically significant hypotension. For patients whose blood pressure is not critically low, dobutamine should be the initial therapy, with dopamine or norepinephrine as back up in the case of worsening hypotension.

Cardioactive Agent Toxicity—Calcium Channel Blockers, Beta-Blockers, Digoxin

The clinical findings of hypotension and bradycardia without evidence of myocardial infarct or ischemia should lead the physician to consider beta-blocker, calcium channel blocker, or cardiac glycoside overdose. Cardiac toxicity as a result of cardioactive agent ingestion or overdose is less likely to respond to conventional treatments for hypotension and bradycardia, specifically pressors and atropine. Familiarity with novel treatments for beta-blocker and calcium channel blocker overdoses as well as cardiac glycoside toxicity can reduce the risk of death in patients with hemodynamic compromise after overdose.

FIGURE 18-5.

STEMI. This ECG shows normal sinus rhythm with anterolateral ST-segment elevations and reciprocal ST-segment depressions in the inferior leads.

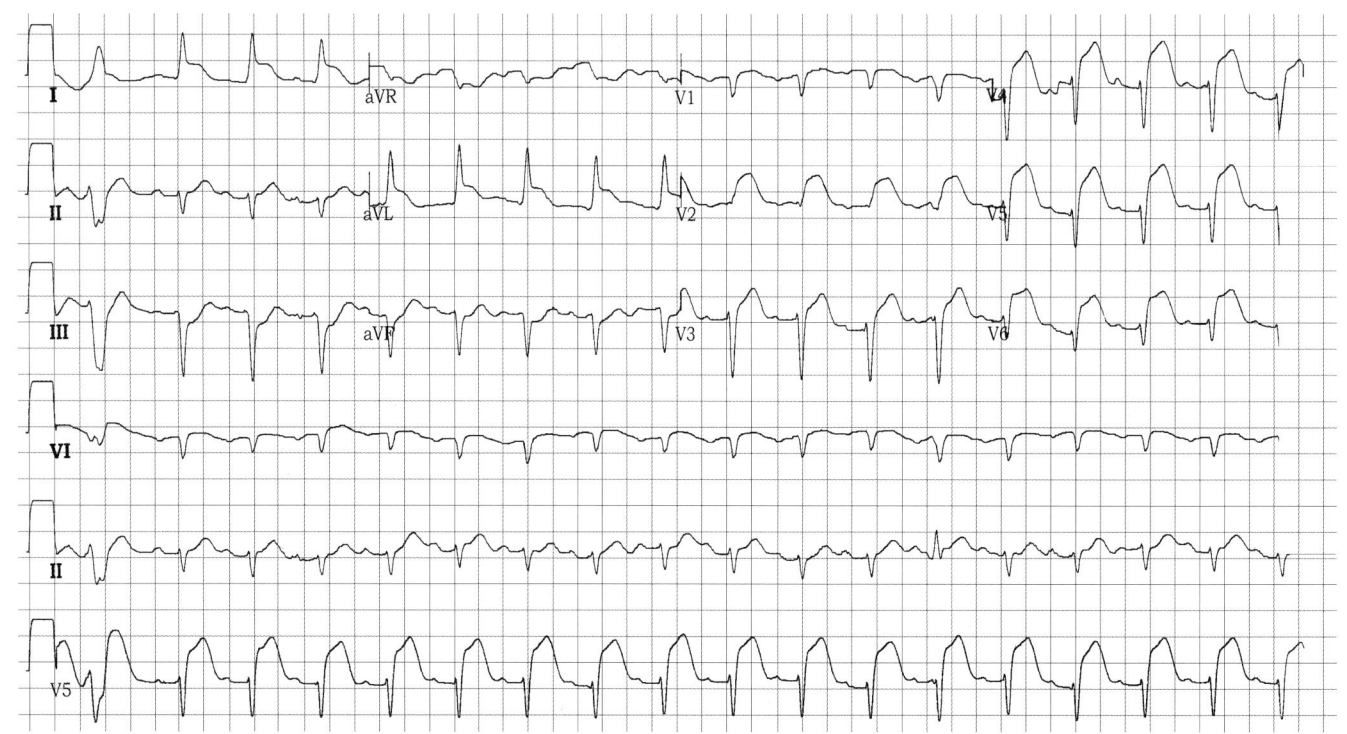

CASE EIGHT

A 32-year-old woman presents with altered mental status, a heart rate of 32 beats/min, a blood pressure of 64/38 mm Hg, and a pulse oximetry reading of 88% on room air. A bedside glucose measurement is 42 mg/dL, and an ECG shows sinus bradycardia without ST elevations or depressions. She is given intravenous dextrose and a normal saline bolus and is placed on a cardiac monitor. Shortly after her arrival, the patient's mother arrives with an empty bottle of 50-mg metoprolol tablets. A dose of glucagon, 10 mg IV, is administered, which improves the patient's heart rate, blood pressure, and mentation.

Patients suspected of beta-blocker or calcium channel blocker overdose with persistent hemodynamic instability despite conventional aggressive resuscitation therapy should be considered candidates for glucagon or hyperinsulinemic euglycemic therapy. Glucagon directly agonizes a specific glucagon receptor adjacent to the beta-adrenergic receptor on the cardiac myocyte. Direct glucagon receptor agonism increases intracellular concentrations of cyclic AMP as well as arachidonic acid, thereby increasing heart rate, stroke volume, and cardiac output. Glucagon may also be administered to hypotensive and bradycardic patients who have overdosed on calcium channel blockers, although the mechanism by which these patients receive benefit is not well understood. Glucagon should be administered as a bolus dose of 3 to 5 mg; higher doses might be required to achieve hemodynamic improvement. A continuous infusion may be started at 3 to 10 mg/hour and titrated to the effective dose, generally not to exceed 10 to 12 mg/hour.[23] This dosing regimen could exceed the hospital's supply of glucagon, in which case alternative therapies need to be considered.

Hyperinsulinemic euglycemic therapy can be useful for both beta-blocker and calcium channel blocker overdose. High-dose insulin therapy increases myocardial glucose uptake, thereby improving aerobic metabolism and subsequently increasing inotropy and chronotropy. Serum glucose levels should be checked prior to initiating therapy, because beta-blocker overdose is often associated with hypoglycemia and calcium channel blocker overdose can cause hyperglycemia. Patients with a serum glucose concentration less than 200 mg/dL should receive a bolus of intravenous dextrose of 0.5 to 1 g/kg prior to initiation of hyperinsulinemic therapy. After a dextrose load, an insulin bolus of 0.5 units/kg should be given intravenously, followed by a continuous infusion of 0.5 to 1 units/kg/hour along with a dextrose infusion to maintain euglycemia. Serum glucose levels should be monitored every 20 minutes for the first hour, then hourly while hyperinsulinemic euglycemic therapy continues. The insulin infusion should be titrated until a systolic pressure of 100 mm Hg and a heart rate of 50 beats/min or more are achieved. The dextrose infusion might need to be titrated to maintain euglycemia. Serum potassium levels also should be monitored every hour, as hyperinsulinemic euglycemic therapy can result in hypokalemia that needs correction.[24]

KEY POINTS

Calcium channel blocker and beta-blocker overdose might require a multifaceted approach, including vasopressors, intravenous fluids, glucagon, hyperinsulinemic euglycemic therapy, or a combination of these. Early consultation with a clinical toxicologist or regional poison control center will help with the selection of the best therapeutic options for these patients to maximize hemodynamic improvement.

CASE NINE

A 76-year-old woman presents with new onset of confusion, after 2 days of vomiting and diarrhea. Her medical history is notable for atrial fibrillation, heart failure, and hypertension, for which she takes digoxin, spironolactone, and amlodipine. Her heart rate is 52 beats/min and irregular and her blood pressure is 98/52 mm Hg. She is in no apparent distress, but she is confused and appears dry. An ECG demonstrates atrial fibrillation with a slow ventricular rate, and laboratory testing reveals a serum digoxin level of 2.3 ng/mL and new renal insufficiency (creatinine level, 3.0 mg/dL). She is given gentle intravenous rehydration and admitted to the telemetry unit for ongoing cardiac monitoring as well as serial measurement of her digoxin levels and chemistry panels, including BUN and creatinine levels.

Digoxin toxicity is uncommon but does occur occasionally in the United States. Nonpharmaceutical cardiac glycoside intoxication (with lily of the valley, yellow oleander, or foxglove) is even rarer in the United States but is a common poisoning in developing nations. Cardiac glycosides are sodium-potassium ATPase poisons that ultimately result in increased intracellular calcium concentrations, ultimately increasing inotropy and automaticity. Additionally, cardiac glycosides enhance vagal tone, resulting in decreased chronotropy.[25]

Cardiac glycoside toxicity is often described as either acute or chronic. After a single, large ingestion of a cardiac glycoside, patients can be asymptomatic initially but then abruptly decompensate, with altered mental status, gastrointestinal symptoms, tachyarrhythmias or bradyarrhythmias, and hypotension. Patients with chronic digoxin poisoning are likely to present with gastrointestinal complaints and confusion. Tachyarrhythmia caused by enhanced automaticity of non-sinus cells predominates in acute poisoning, whereas bradyarrhythmia due to enhanced AV nodal blockade is more likely in chronic poisoning. Virtually any arrhythmia is possible after cardiac glycoside overdose, while bidirectional ventricular tachycardia is virtually pathognomonic for cardiac glycoside poisoning. Historically, elevated serum potassium levels predicted mortality after cardiac glycoside overdose; however, the availability of Fab fragments for digoxin overdose has limited the prognostic value of hyperkalemia in this setting.

Patients with cardiac glycoside poisoning need continuous cardiac monitoring, and their serum digoxin and electrolyte levels should be checked. Acute, large digoxin ingestions or any nonpharmaceutical cardiac glycoside ingestion should prompt treatment with digoxin Fab fragments (Digibind, DigiFab), even in the absence of symptoms or hemodynamic compromise. These patients should be given between 10 and 20 vials initially and might require additional doses. Patients with chronic di-

goxin toxicity may not need Fab fragments and might respond to supportive measures such as intravenous hydration and electrolyte correction. However, if arrhythmias occur and raise concern, patients may be given 3 to 6 vials empirically. Alternatively, if a serum digoxin level has been obtained, the number of vials given can be calculated using the following formula[25]:
Number of vials = (serum digoxin level × weight in kg) ÷ 100.

KEY POINTS

Cardiac glycoside poisoning can present with a variety of clinical findings, including gastrointestinal symptoms, altered sensorium, and a wide range of arrhythmias. Electrolyte abnormalities are also often present. Hyperkalemia induces concern and, if untreated, is a marker for an increased mortality rate. Fab fragments have reduced the mortality rate associated with this disease, and hyperkalemia is an indication for Fab treatment.

The formula for Fab fragment dosing with a known serum digoxin level is (serum digoxin level × weight in kg) ÷ 100. If a large ingestion or nonpharmaceutical cardiac glycoside ingestion is suspected, 10 to 20 vials of Fab fragments should be given empirically.

Conclusion

A wide variety of pharmacologic options are available for treatment of the patient with an acute cardiac condition. Too often, the therapeutic choice is based on algorithms that do not apply to every patient. Familiarity with these medications and their mechanisms of action will enable treating physicians to tailor specific therapy for their patients, based on the underlying pathophysiologic process. Patients with cardioactive medication toxicity might not respond to conventional treatments, so the emergency care provider must be familiar with novel treatments for these conditions.

References

1. López-Sendón J, Swedberg K, McMurray J, et al. Expert consensus document on beta-adrenergic receptor blockers. *Eur Heart J.* 2004;25(15):1341-1362.
2. Brubacher J. B-Adrenergic antagonists. In: Flomenbaum N, Howland MA, Goldfrank LR, eds. *Goldfrank's Toxicologic Emergencies.* New York: McGraw-Hill; 2006:924-941.
3. Nieminen MS, Böhm M, Cowie MR, et al. Executive summary of the guidelines on the diagnosis and treatment of acute heart failure: the Task Force on Acute Heart Failure of the European Society of Cardiology. *Eur Heart J.* 2005;26(4):384-416.
4. Marik PE, Varon J. Hypertensive crises: challenges and management. *Chest.* 2007;131(6):1949-1962.
5. Khan ZP, Ferguson CN, Jones RM. alpha-2 and imidazoline receptor agonists. Their pharmacology and therapeutic role. *Anaesthesia.* 1999;54(2):146-165.
6. Curry S, Mills KC, Ruha AM. Neurotransmitters and neuromodulators. In: Flomenbaum N, Howland MA, Goldfrank LR, eds. *Goldfrank's Toxicologic Emergencies.* New York: McGraw-Hill; 2006:214-248.
7. Simpson CS, Ghali WA, Sanfilippo AJ, et al. Clinical assessment of clonidine in the treatment of new-onset rapid atrial fibrillation: a prospective, randomized clinical trial. *Am Heart J.* 2001;142(2):E3.
8. National Center for Biotechnology Information, US National Library of Medicine. Phentolamine - compound summary. Available at: http://pubchem.ncbi.nlm.nih.gov/summary/summary.cgi?cid=5775#x94. Accessed on August 12, 2013.
9. Sanders DB, Kelley T, Larson D. The role of nitric oxide synthase/nitric oxide in vascular smooth muscle control. *Perfusion.* 2000;15(2):97-104.
10. The Sicilian gambit. A new approach to the classification of antiarrhythmic drugs based on their actions on arrhythmogenic mechanisms. Task Force of the Working Group on Arrhythmias of the European Society of Cardiology. *Circulation.* 1991;84(4):1831-1851.
11. Fulton S, Jackimczyk KC. Antidysrhythmics. Emergent. *Emerg Med Clin North Am.* 2000;18(4):655-669.
12. Klabunde RE. *Cardiovascular Pharmacology Concepts* [e-book]. Available at: www.cvpharmacology.com/index.html. Accessed on August 12, 2013.
13. Blomström-Lundqvist C, Scheinman MM, Aliot EM, et al. ACC/AHA/ESC guidelines for the management of patients with supraventricular arrhythmias--executive summary: a report of the American College of Cardiology/American Heart Association Task Force on Practice Guidelines and the European Society of Cardiology Committee for Practice Guidelines (Writing Committee to Develop Guidelines for the Management of Patients With Supraventricular Arrhythmias). *Circulation.* 2003;108(15):1871-1909.
14. Amiodarone - Compound Summary (CID 2157). Bethesda, Maryland: National Center for Biotechnology Information. Available at: http://pubchem.ncbi.nlm.nih.gov/summary/summary.cgi?cid=2157&loc=ec_rcs#x9. Accessed on August 19, 2013.
15. European Heart Rhythm Association; Heart Rhythm Society, Zipes DP, Camm AJ, Borggrefe M, et al. ACC/AHA/ESC 2006 guidelines for management of patients with ventricular arrhythmias and the prevention of sudden cardiac death: a report of the American College of Cardiology/American Heart Association Task Force and the European Society of Cardiology Committee for Practice Guidelines (Writing Committee to Develop Guidelines for Management of Patients With Ventricular Arrhythmias and the Prevention of Sudden Cardiac Death). *J Am Coll Cardiol.* 2006;48(5):e247-e346.
16. Scheuermeyer FX, Grafstein E, Stenstrom R, et al. Safety and efficiency of calcium channel blockers versus beta-blockers for rate control in patients with atrial fibrillation and no acute underlying medical illness. *Acad Emerg Med.* 2013;20(3):222-230.
17. Marill KA, Wolfram S, Desouza IS, et al. Adenosine for wide-complex tachycardia: efficacy and safety. *Crit Care Med.* 2009;37(9):2512-2518.
18. López-Sendón J, Swedberg K, McMurray J, et al. Expert consensus document on angiotensin converting enzyme inhibitors in cardiovascular disease. The Task Force on ACE-inhibitors of the European Society of Cardiology. *Eur Heart J.* 2004;25(16):1454-1470.
19. Meer J, Mattu A. Cardiogenic shock. In: Winters M, DeBlieux P, Marcolini E, et al, eds. *Emergency Department Resuscitation of the Critically Ill.* Dallas, TX: American College of Emergency Physicians; 2011:69-76.
20. Hollenberg SM. Vasoactive drugs in circulatory shock. *Am J Respir Crit Care Med.* 2010;183(7):847-855.
21. De Backer D, Biston P, Devriendt J, et al. Comparison of dopamine and norepinephrine in the treatment of shock. *N Engl J Med.* 2010;362(9):779-789.
22. Reynolds HR, Hochman JS. Cardiogenic shock: current concepts and improving outcomes. *Circulation.* 2008;117(5):686-697.
23. Howland M. Glucagon. In: Flomenbaum N, Howland MA, Goldfrank LR, et al, eds. *Goldfrank's Toxicologic Emergencies.* New York: McGraw Hill; 2006:942-945.
24. Shepherd G, Klein-Schwartz W. High-dose insulin therapy for calcium-channel blocker overdose. *Ann Pharmacother.* 2005;39(5):923-930.
25. Hack J, Lewin NA. Cardioactive steroids. In: Flomenbaum N, Howland MA, Goldfrank LR, et al, eds. *Goldfrank's Toxicologic Emergencies.* New York: McGraw-Hill; 2006:971-982.

CHAPTER 19

Complications of Implanted Cardiac Devices

Vaishal M. Tolia and Theodore C. Chan

IN THIS CHAPTER

Pacemakers

Implantable cardioverter-defibrillators

Left ventricular assist device

Albert Hyman introduced the term *artificial pacemaker* in 1932. Since then, implanted cardiac devices such as pacemakers and defibrillators have become commonplace (Figure 19-1).[1] With advances in technology and the aging population, emergency physicians are more likely than ever to encounter patients with complications of these devices. This chapter provides a framework for managing the various unique complications associated with pacemakers, implantable cardioverter-defibrillators (ICDs), and ventricular assist devices (VADs). Pacemakers and ICDs can develop complications related to the procedure of implantation and or to actual device function. Emergency physicians are more likely to see device malfunction complications, often after much time has elapsed since the device was implanted. Unfortunately, there is no registry or reporting mechanism to determine the annual incidence of pacemaker malfunction. The US Food and Drug Administration (FDA) reported that, from 1993 to 2002, the rate of malfunction declined from 0.9% to 0.14%. A limitation of this information is that the definition of true malfunction has not been delineated or agreed on by major societies.[2] Emergency physicians have to prepare for the increasing population of patients with VADs (in some patients as they await cardiac transplantation). This chapter reviews common complications related to VADs as well as key points to remember when dealing with these complex patients.

Complications of Pacemaker Implantation

Procedure-related problems can occur at three main sites: the generator implant site, also known as the "pocket"; the site of transvenous lead placement; and the electrode-myocardium interface.[3]

Pocket Complications

The pulse generator of a pacemaker is commonly implanted surgically into the subcutaneous or submuscular pectoralis region of the chest wall. Procedural complications include hematoma formation, wound dehiscence, device migration and/or erosion, and infection.[4]

The development of a hematoma might be related to residual bleeding from creating the pocket or to venous injury from advancing the lead. More serious cases can be caused by arterial injury leading to blood dissecting the tissue planes of the chest wall. Decompression through needle aspiration can temporarily decrease the size and pressure from the hematoma but risks damage to components. Emergency physicians might be required to correct coagulopathy if the bleeding cannot be controlled with conservative measures. Ultimately, surgical evaluation and exploration will likely be required to assess the underlying cause.[3]

On rare occasions, insufficient pocket size for the pulse generator can lead to suture damage and wound breakdown. Trauma and infection (discussed below) can have similar results. Consultation is required to replant the device into a more appropriately formed pocket or change the site of implantation.[4]

Device migration refers to movement of the pacemaker from the original site through the surrounding tissue slowly, over time. The vast majority of patients do not experience complications and do not require intervention as long as function and comfort are preserved. However, if migration leads to erosion of the pocket wall and local tissue injury, the generator and other components can become exposed, leading to device malfunction and failure.[5] Débridement of the site and relocation of the pacemaker are necessary. Often with exposed hardware, infection has to be managed before considering replantation, which might require percutaneous temporary pacing.[6]

Pocket infection continues to be a serious, potentially life-threatening problem. Device infections are characterized as either superficial or deep. Superficial infections induce localized inflammation involving the skin; they are related to the incision but do not involve the pocket or hardware. Often, these infections can be treated successfully with oral antibiotics. However, it can be extremely difficult to distinguish a superficial from a deep infection, so any superficial infection should be assumed to be deep until it is evaluated by a specialist. Deep infections can be acute or chronic/progressive and involve the pocket and its components, often with an associated bacteremia. Deep infections almost always require removal of the device and intravenous administration of broad-spectrum antibiotics.

Pacemaker endocarditis has also been described.[7] The most common symptoms are fever and chills, and the common laboratory features are elevated erythrocyte sedimentation rate, leukocytosis, microscopic hematuria, and anemia.[8] Early or acute infections are usually caused by *Staphylococcus aureus*, which tends to be more aggressive and associated with sepsis. Late infections that present with a more indolent course are often attributed to *Staphylococcus epidermidis*.[3] Other bacterial species have also been implicated in pacemaker infections (Table 19-1).[9]

Treatment of pocket infections usually requires surgical intervention with a period of decontamination before replantation of hardware. Attempts at salvaging the implant site are usually futile.[10] The vast majority of infections are caused by gram-positive organisms, and initial treatment with intravenous vancomycin is recommended after obtaining at least two sets of blood cultures. Some surgeons or electrophysiologists ask for cultures from the pocket itself. Specimens for these cultures can be obtained by creating a sterile field, inserting a saline-filled syringe into the pocket space (immediately around the pulse generator), and then irrigating and aspirating the wound. A discussion with the specialist is warranted before obtaining a pocket aspirate. Assessing for other sources or sequelae of infection, such as septic emboli, is important as well. In addition to basic laboratory analysis (complete blood count, chemistry, coagulation measurements), a two-view chest radiograph, urinalysis, and blood and urine cultures should also be obtained. Communicate with the surgeon or electrophysiologist to arrange hospital admission. Figure 19-2 presents an algorithm for management of patients with infected implanted cardiac devices.

KEY POINTS

When assessing a patient with pocket-related pacemaker complications:

- Have a high suspicion for infection.
- Thoroughly evaluate the pocket of the device along with its function.
- Communicate with the specialist.
- Request laboratory tests, an electrocardiogram (ECG), and a chest radiograph.

Pacemaker Lead Complications

The electrical leads of a pacemaker usually traverse the venous system into the right atrium or right ventricle (or both, in the case of the dual-chambered variety). Biventricular pacemakers involve the right ventricle as well as the coronary sinus to reach the left ventricle. Complications associated with placing these leads into their appropriate location include pneumothorax/hemothorax, venous thrombosis, lead infection, implant pericarditis, exit block, and perforation.

Pneumothorax and hemothorax are known complications of central venous access via the internal jugular or subclavian venous system (Figure 19-3). Despite the reduction in complica-

FIGURE 19-1.

Albert Hyman's artificial pacemaker. From: Aquilina O. A brief history of cardiac pacing. *Images Paediatr Cardiol.* 2006;8:17-81. Used with permission.

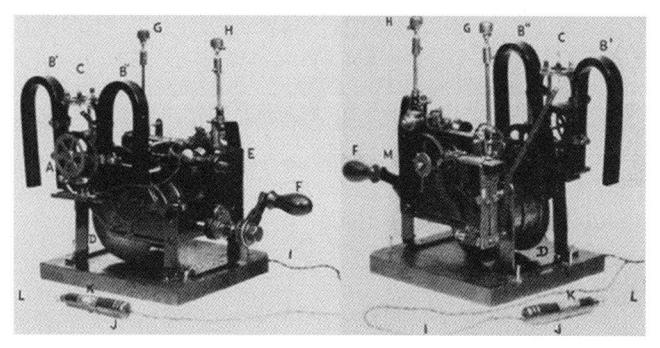

TABLE 19-1.

Microbiology of Permanent Pacemaker/ICD Infections[9]

Coagulase-negative staphylococci	42%
Methicillin-sensitive *S. aureus*	25%
Methicillin-resistant *S. aureus*	4%
Other gram-positive cocci	4%
Gram-negative bacilli	9%
Polymicrobial	7%
Fungal	2%
Culture negative	7%

tions that has been achieved with ultrasound and fluoroscopy, there is still a risk of pleural or venous injury resulting in the collection of air or blood in the pleural space. Small injuries are often not immediately apparent and can produce delayed symptoms 24 to 48 hours after the procedure.[11] Pneumothorax can lead to subcutaneous emphysema and dissection of air through tissue and fascial planes. This air insulation of the pacemaker leads can cause device malfunction and subsequent hypotension or syncope in addition to respiratory distress.[12] Chest tube placement is required in 1% to 2% of patients who receive implanted cardiac devices and should be considered for any pneumothorax or hemothorax that is significantly symptomatic or occupies more than 1 cm between the lung margin and chest wall on chest radiograph. There have been no publications on the use of mobile chest drainage devices for use in pacemaker-associated pneumothorax other than one describing a case series on submammary device implantation in women.[13] Most of these complications require intervention and admission to the hospital.

Damage to the venous endothelium during lead placement can also contribute to the development of venous thrombosis. This complication occurs in almost half of patients undergoing pacemaker placement, most of who remain asymptomatic.[7] Acute thrombosis occurs in 1% to 3% of patients and can present with pain and swelling on the side ipsilateral to the device or procedure.[7] Duplex ultrasonography has overtaken venography as the diagnostic study of choice for detecting deep venous thrombosis, particularly for emergency department patients.

Superior vena cava syndrome is a rare complication of upper extremity venous thrombosis and can lead to hemodynamic compromise and dyspnea due to the interruption of venous return. Slowly developing thrombi that occur more chronically

FIGURE 19-2.

Mayo Clinic algorithm of cardiac device infection management. A, Treatment algorithm based on blood and generator pocket cultures. This algorithm applies only to patients with complete explanation of the implanted system. B, Algorithm for reimplantation of new pulse generator. From: Sohail MR, Uslan DZ, Khan AH, et al. Management and outcome of permanent pacemaker and implanted cardioverter-defibrillator infections. *J Am Coll Cardiol.* 2007;49:1851-1859. Open archive.

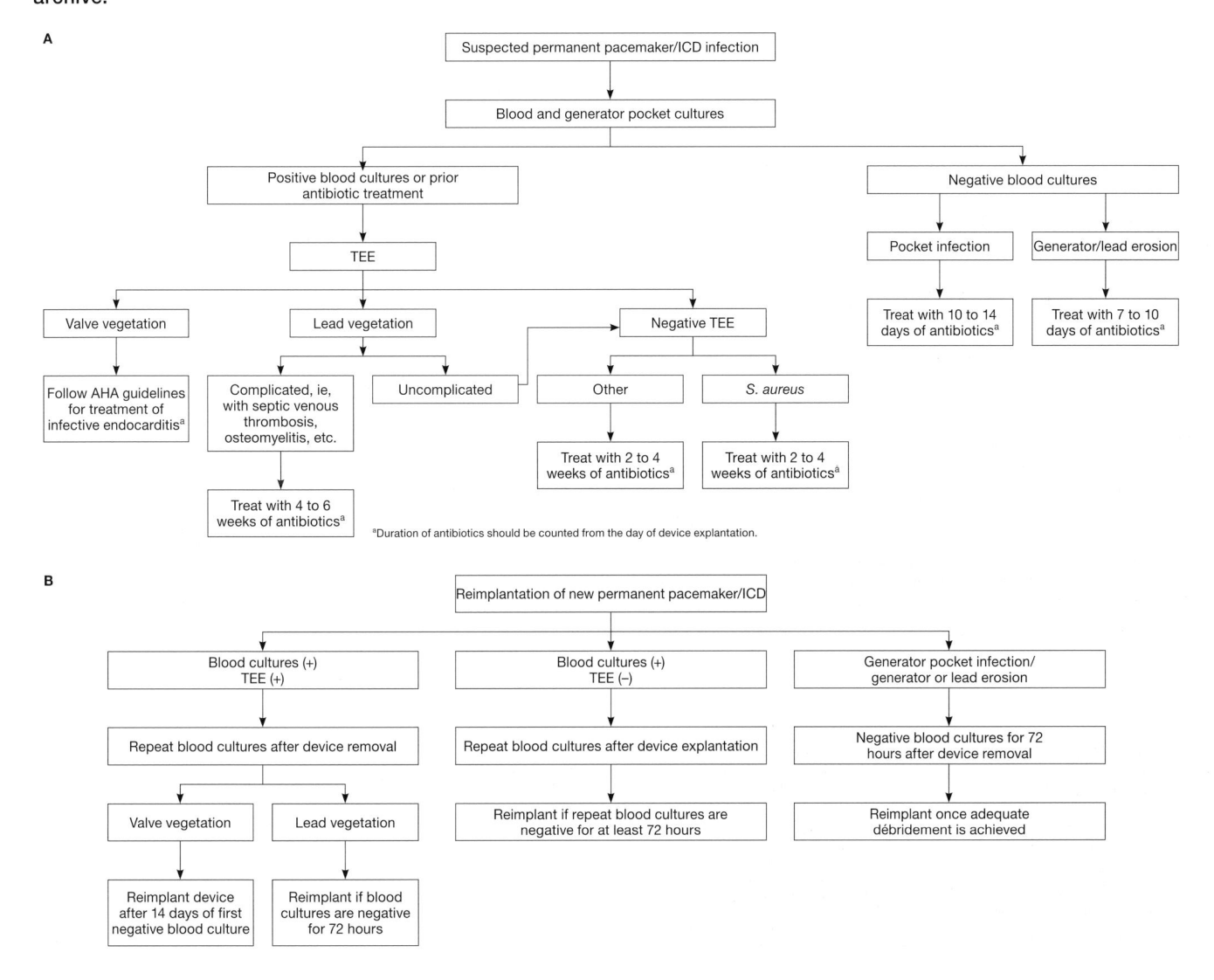

allow time for collaterals to develop and are often found incidentally.[3] Treatment for venous thrombosis is the same as for other deep vein thromboses. Lead removal is usually not necessary. Depending on the location of the thrombosis and the patient's symptoms, fibrinolytic therapy is being used increasingly as a treatment modality.[14] Patients are usually bridged with heparin or a low-molecular-weight heparin product and started on warfarin.[15,16]

Lead infection is less common than pocket infection, but the mortality rate can be as high as 27%, even with lead removal and broad-spectrum antibiotics.[17] As with pocket infections, staphylococci are the predominant culprits. Most patients require transesophageal echocardiography for evaluation of the nature and location of the vegetation. Infection is an absolute indication for lead removal, often requiring open-heart surgery.[17] Patients come to the emergency department with fever, chills, and signs of sepsis. A complete workup, including empiric antibiotics, fluid resuscitation, and subspecialist consultation for removal of the hardware, should be undertaken urgently.

Pericarditis and perforation constitute a rare but potentially serious complication of lead placement. This problem is more common with fixation leads that are screwed into the myocardium, particularly into the thin-walled atria. Inflammation from deep implantation can lead to pericarditis.[18] Patients with this type of pericarditis usually present to the emergency department with chest pain, sometimes pleuritic in nature. Treatment is similar to pericarditis from other causes, with nonsteroidal anti-inflammatory medications or steroids as the initial treatment of choice. Patients with post-pacemaker pericarditis should be followed closely for the development of cardiac tamponade. Emergency physicians should evaluate patients who present with pericarditis symptoms using bedside cardiac ultrasound, particularly if symptomatic pericardial effusion is suspected. Perforation or symptomatic effusion/tamponade requires immediate treatment and lead repositioning.[7]

A patient with lead dislodgement without perforation might present with pacemaker dysfunction. This is usually evident on an ECG or a chest radiograph. Atrial leads can usually be found in the right atrial appendage, whereas right ventricular leads can be located at the apex of the right ventricle. Emergency physicians might have to institute temporary pacing if the dislodgement causes malfunction in a patient who is pacemaker dependent.[3] Finally, exit block occurs when a local inflammatory reaction related to lead placement causes electrode-myocardium interference. This can result in undersensing, in which electric activity within the chamber goes undetected, usually requiring repositioning or replacement of the leads. Patients often present with extracardiac stimulation and symptoms such as intractable hiccups.[3] Modern leads are steroid eluting, reducing the risk of this inflammation-mediated complication.

KEY POINTS

Review lead positioning carefully on a chest radiograph.

Have a low threshold for emergency bedside cardiac ultrasound.

Treat uncomplicated venous thrombosis the same as other deep vein thromboses.

Communicate with the subspecialist early in the course, especially if lead replacement or repositioning is needed.

FIGURE 19-3.

Chest CT showing large hemothorax, pneumothorax, and pneumopericardium. From Enes EG, Kayrak M. Common pacemaker problems: lead and pocket complications. In: Das MR, ed. *Modern Pacemakers—Present and Future*. 2011. Available from www.intechopen.com/download/get/type/pdfs/id/13786. Open access.

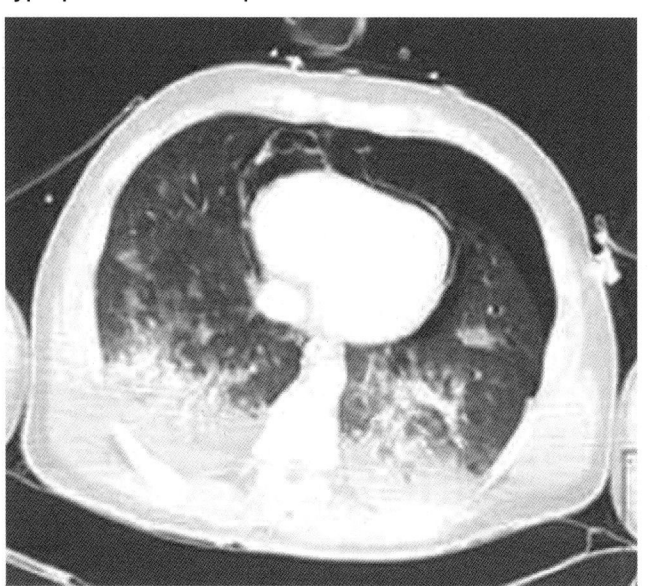

TABLE 19-2.

Causes of Failure to Pace

Oversensing (skeletal myopotentials, connection problems, normal cardiac rhythm sensing)
Lead fracture or dislodgement
Electromagnetic interference
Battery failure or component failure (primary or from trauma)
Pseudomalfunction
Hysteresis (normal pacemaker programming)

TABLE 19-3.

Causes of Failure to Capture

Lead damage or dislodgement
Exit block
Long QT syndrome
Battery depletion
Elevated pacing threshold (acute myocardial infarction, electrolyte abnormality, medications, defibrillation)

Pacemaker Malfunction

This section focuses on the diagnosis and management of pacemaker device malfunction, including failure to pace, failure to capture, undersensing, pacemaker-mediated arrhythmias, and twiddler's syndrome. Overall failure rates seem to have fallen over the past decade as a result of improvements in technology and operator skills.[2] One of the central solutions to pacemaker function issues is the application of a magnet over the pulse generator box. This reverts the pacemaker to an asynchronous mode of pacing (such as AOO, VOO, or DOO) by eliminating sensing. This process can evaluate battery life, assess capture, and treat certain arrhythmias. Removal of the magnet will put the pacemaker back into its last programmed mode.[3]

Failure to Pace

The basic premise of this malfunction is that the pacemaker fails to deliver a stimulus to the myocardium. Patients can present with a variety of symptoms, depending on the health of their underlying native rhythm, anywhere from near syncope to severe bradycardia and hypoperfusion. Absence of pacing artifact on an ECG is an initial clue. Oversensing (inappropriate inhibition caused by detection of electrical activity other than R waves) is one of the more common causes of output failure, particularly in unipolar lead settings. The source of the oversensing is usually pectoralis skeletal muscle myopotentials, which can be reproduced by having patients move their arms or by stimulating the muscle near the lead.[19] Depending on the type of implanted device, placing a magnet over a pacemaker can turn off the sensing function and help diagnose oversensing as a cause of malfunction. Other causes of pacing failure are listed in Table 19-2.[20]

Trauma, damage to leads, and component or battery failure all require repair or replacement of necessary components. Hysteresis is a normal programming function in which the escape rate is lower than the base rate and thus is often misinterpreted as pacemaker failure. This setting is ideal for patients who need only intermittent pacing support and can otherwise function on their native rhythm at lower rates. This programming mode can be determined through interrogation.[21]

Failure to Capture

This condition occurs when the delivered pacemaker stimulus fails to cause appropriate myocardial depolarization and contraction. Table 19-3 lists some common causes of failure to capture[20] (Figure 19-4).

Low current from battery failure or lead problems can result in a pacing artifact on the ECG but a stimulus that is too weak to create myocardial depolarization. Exit block, often related to the post-implantation inflammatory changes that prevent myocardial depolarization following a pacer stimulus, is now rare, owing to steroid-eluting leads.[4] Ischemic myocardium and metabolic derangements such as hypothyroidism, acidemia, and electrolyte abnormalities can elevate the pacing threshold and cause failure to capture.[22-25] Some antiarrhythmic agents can also elevate the pacing threshold, usually at supratherapeutic levels. Flecainide, a class IC agent, can do the same at therapeutic levels. If failure to capture should occur as a result of these medications, isoproterenol has been described as a therapeutic option.[11,26] In pacemaker patients with ventricular arrhythmias who receive defibrillation, about half suffer from failure to cap-

FIGURE 19-4.

Patient with intermittent loss of capture (arrows), leading to junctional escape beat (J). Safety pacing (S) ensues, narrowing the AV interval to prevent the stimulus from falling on the T wave.

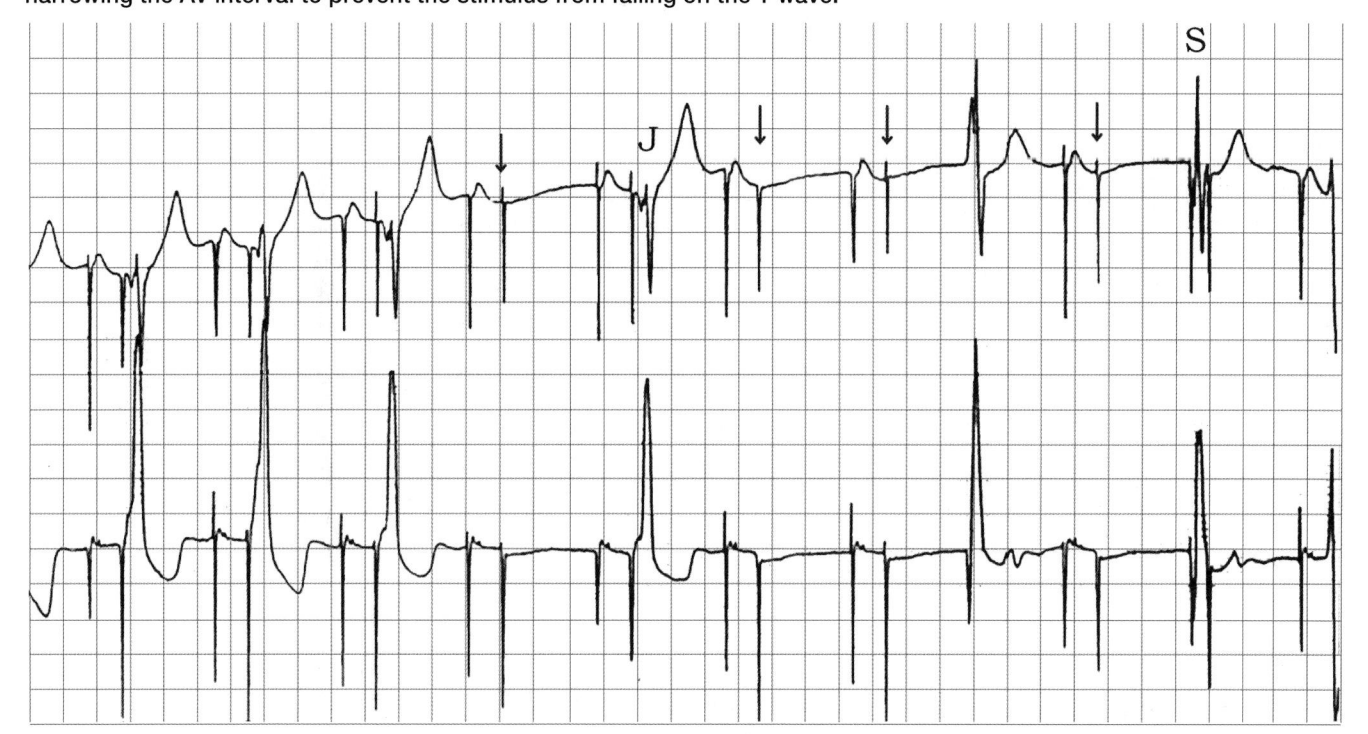

ture in the post-shock period, likely due to tissue damage from the shock.[27]

Undersensing

An important function of a pacemaker is to detect and analyze innate cardiac activity native to the patient. Programming of particular amplitude and frequencies of leads at the time of implantation allows this sensing to occur. Undersensing occurs when a pacemaker fails to recognize intrinsic depolarization, resulting in failure to inhibit pacing activity. Obvious findings might not be evident on telemetry monitoring or a 12-lead ECG.[20] Undersensing has multiple causes such as new arrhythmias, bundle-branch blocks, and myocardial infarction, as well as mechanical lead abnormalities. Treatment can be based on reprogramming (in the case of a nonmechanical cause) to a higher sensitivity or treatment of the underlying disorder.[28] In

FIGURE 19-5.

Undersensing. Pacemaker fails to detect cardiac activity and delivers inappropriate pacing output on a T wave, leading to ventricular fibrillation.

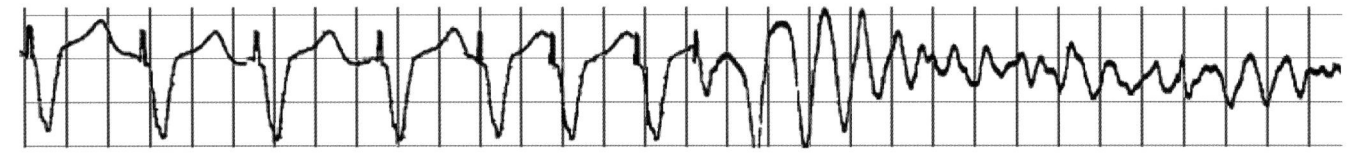

FIGURE 19-6.

Pacemaker-mediated tachycardia. A premature ventricular contraction initiates a run of pacemaker-mediated tachycardia (arrow). A retrograde P wave is buried in the following T wave, and the pacemaker paces the ventricle, setting up a reentry tachycardia. Application of a magnetic field will terminate this process.

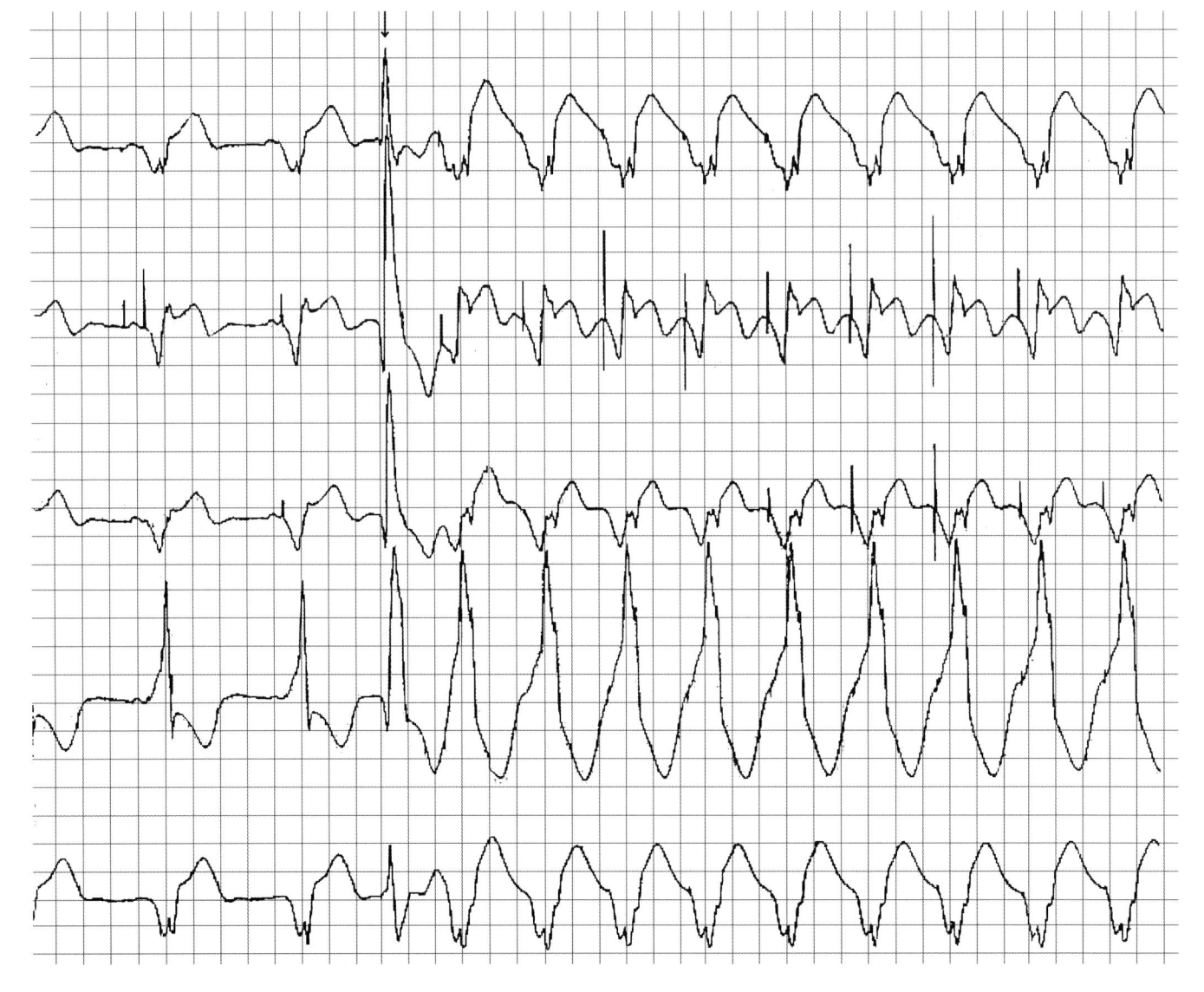

unstable patients, restoring hemodynamic parameters should be the priority, followed by electrophysiology consultation to identify the cause of the undersensing (Figure 19-5).

Pacemaker-Mediated Arrhythmias

The pacemaker itself can occasionally act as a source of arrhythmia in situations such as pacemaker-mediated tachycardia, runaway pacemaker, lead dislodgement arrhythmia, and sensor-induced tachycardia.

Pacemaker mediated tachycardia is a reentry arrhythmia that can occur in dual-chambered devices in which the pacemaker itself acts as part of the reentry circuit. If a premature ventricular contraction conducts retrograde to cause an atrial depolarization that arrives after the atrial refractory period, it will be sensed, resulting in a ventricular paced beat. If this paced beat also conducts retrograde to cause an atrial depolarization that arrives after the atrial refractory period, a recurrent circuit will occur, resulting in pacemaker-mediated tachycardia. The upper limit of the tachycardia is the programmed upper pacemaker threshold. In the emergency department, application of a magnet should remove the sensing function, interrupting the reentry circuit and resulting in a return to synchronous pacing[29] (Figure 19-6). Adenosine, carotid massage, transcutaneous pacing, and, rarely, chest wall thump may all be used if a magnet is not available, particularly for unstable patients.[30]

Runaway pacemaker and lead dislodgement arrhythmia occur when the pacemaker fires rapid, inappropriate discharges, leading to malignant ventricular arrhythmias such as ventricular tachycardia or fibrillation. This is a true pacemaker malfunction and a medical emergency. Reprogramming, magnet application, and occasionally surgical lead interruption could all be necessary. Modern pacemakers have a set upper limit that prevents this life-threatening occurrence.[31] Another cause of ventricular arrhythmias is lead dislodgement, in which the tip of the lead bounces off the ventricular wall, causing arrhythmia. Surgical correction is its main treatment.

Electromagnetic interference, loud noises and vibration, and even seizures have been known to stimulate vibration-based sensors, leading to increased pacemaker activity.[32-35] Some pacemakers have temperature sensors, which can be activated in febrile patients. Other forms include minute ventilation-based sensors, which can malfunction in response to hyperventilation, arm movement, or electrocautery. Magnet application is reliable in terminating this tachyarrhythmia.[36,37]

Twiddler's Syndrome

First described in 1968, twiddler's syndrome refers to pacemaker malfunction caused by intentional or unintentional mechanical disturbance, or "twiddling," of the pacemaker leads by the patient. Patients with this condition usually come to the emergency department with pacemaker failure. Children are more susceptible to "twiddling" because of their propensity to touch their devices. The emergency physician can palpate the pocket and/or leads to evaluate for loosening or excessive mobility. The ECG will show failure to capture. A chest radiograph might confirm the diagnosis. Surgical correction and revision are ultimately required.[38-40]

KEY POINTS

An ECG and chest radiograph can be helpful in identifying the cause of pacemaker malfunction.

Magnet application and interrogation can be both diagnostic and therapeutic.

Early specialty consultation will likely be needed.

Misinterpretation of appropriate function often leads to the conclusion that a pacemaker is malfunctioning.

Implantable Cardioverter-Defibrillator Complications

Life-threatening ventricular arrhythmias can be terminated effectively with an ICD, thus preventing sudden cardiac death. ICD implantation has become much more common, as it has been shown to improve survival, particularly in patients with advanced cardiomyopathy. Complications of ICDs mirror those of pacemakers, with issues arising from procedural problems, infection, lead complications and failure, and ICD-induced arrhythmias (often from inappropriate shocks).

Inappropriate Shocks

Approximately one fourth of patients with an ICD will, at some point, experience an inappropriate shock, usually caused by a supraventricular arrhythmia. Firing of the ICD in such circumstances does not correlate with worsening cardiac function and increased risk of death in the same way that shocks triggered by ventricular arrhythmias do.[41]

Electrical Storm

Atrial fibrillation with rapid ventricular response can induce recurrent shocks in a short time or inappropriate shocks (as described above). Frequent recurrence of ventricular fibrillation/tachycardia, usually at least 3 episodes in a 24-hour period, can be caused by electrolyte imbalance, drug toxicity, myocardial infarction, or stress. Patients often present with syncope and/or weakness. Treatment is based mainly on the underlying cause, and amiodarone is often used as an antiarrhythmic agent.[42]

KEY POINTS

ICD complications are very similar to those of pacemakers.

Interrogation is often necessary to evaluate the reason for inappropriate shocks.

Always evaluate for secondary causes of ICD discharge.

Implantable Assisted Circulation Device Complications

The number of people with advanced heart failure is increasing. Heart transplantation is often the optimal therapy for those with severe disease but is a highly limited resource, contributing to a mortality rate of close to 80%.[43] VADs function as a bridge to transplant or, for some, destination therapy, with evidence of significant survival benefit.[44] With the increased use of such devices, emergency physicians need to become familiar with the complications associated with them. Some emergency departments and hospitals have on-call coordinators and a specific protocol and process for dealing with patients with VADs. Training and strong communication links between the cardiology team and emergency physicians and nurses are essential for handling these complex patients and their complications.

The two basic types of VADs are the older pulsatile-flow and the newer continuous-flow devices (axial or centrifugal flow). Continuous-flow VADs maintain continuous circulation and have fewer complications related to the device, yielding similar quality-of-life improvement compared with volume displacement models.[45] Patients with continuous-flow VADs have no palpable pulse, and an automated blood pressure cuff might not record a blood pressure. Examination should include listening over the heart to determine if the motor is functioning; assessing signs of perfusion, including mental status, mean arterial pressure via manual Doppler, and skin color/temperature; and performing bedside echocardiography.

Emergency physicians should not attempt to manipulate any wires or the drive-line, because of the risk of damage and disconnection. Several models of VADs are available. It is important for emergency physicians to be very familiar with the normal function and troubleshooting of the devices used at their institution or within the community they serve. Each device has specific management characteristics.

Bleeding and thrombosis are frequently encountered complications.[46] Hypotension can occur from bleeding, mechanical failure, infection, or dehydration. Ongoing low-flow states should be prevented and any infection needs to be managed swiftly and expeditiously. Crystalloid fluid resuscitation is important to ensure proper volume and perfusion. Patients are prone to ventricular arrhythmias, which is usually the reason for the ICD. In general, these arrhythmias, along with acute coronary syndromes, should be treated similarly to those in patients without VADs.

Pump thrombosis can cause the drive to become hot in response to a high rate of revolutions and low flow. Dilated chambers can be seen on bedside echocardiography. Treatment consists of administration of heparin or even fibrinolytics in

FIGURE 19-7.

Alarm panel on Heartmate II. Image courtesy of Cassia Chevillon, BSN, RN, CCRN.

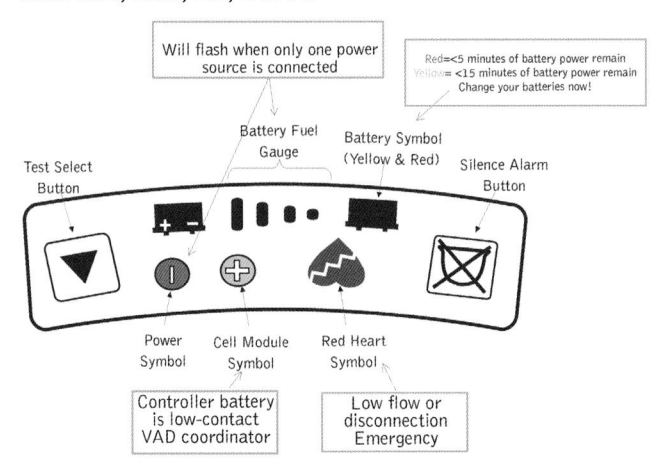

FIGURE 19-8.

Algorithm for the emergent management of a patient with a VAD. Courtesy of Dr. George Higgins from Maine Medical Center.

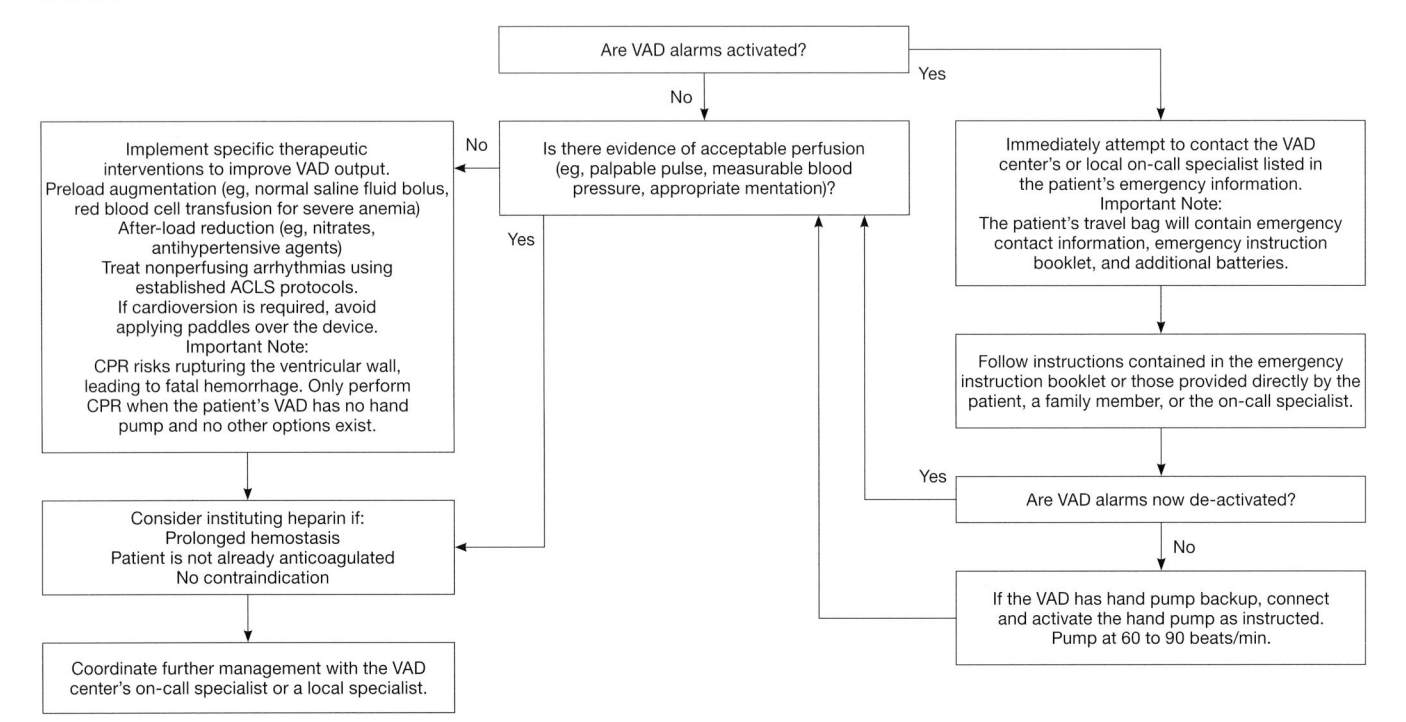

This guideline was ratified by the emergency department faculty at Maine Medical Center in May 2010. It reflects our expert opinion and is not necessarily applicable to all institutions.
It is intended to be a reference for clinicians caring for patients and is not intended to replace providers' clinical judgment. Produced by George Higgins, MD

the near-arresting patient. If a patient does arrest, chest compressions should be avoided avoided unless it can be determined that the pump is not working, in which case it might be helpful.[47] Regardless, getting the pump to function again should be the primary goal.

Finally, knowing the significance of various alarms is of paramount importance (Figure 19-7). In general, continue troubleshooting until you see a green light. Close consultation with a VAD specialist should be initiated immediately in almost all cases. Knowing the technical aspects of the VAD that is used in your institution is of utmost importance (Figure 19-8).

KEY POINTS

Know the technical aspects and complications of the types of VADs used in the institution where you practice.

Be aware of what the alarms mean.

Know how to access equipment and contact coordinators and specialists immediately.

Avoid dehydration and low-flow states.

Maintain a high suspicion for infection and treat aggressively.

Ensure electrolyte levels are stable.

References

1. Aquilina O. A brief history of cardiac pacing. *Images Paediatr Cardiol.* 2006;27:17-81.
2. Maisel WH. Pacemaker and ICD generator reliability: meta-analysis of device registries. *JAMA.* 2006;295:1929-1934.
3. Cardall TY, Chan TC. Permanent cardiac pacemakers: issues relevant to the emergency physician, Part I. *J Emerg Med.* 1999;3:479-489.
4. Byrd CL. Management of implant complications. In: Ellenbogen KA, Kay GN, Wilkoff BL, eds. *Clinical Cardiac Pacing.* Philadelphia: WB Saunders; 1995:491-522.
5. Binder T, Domanovits H, Berr T, Laggner A. Complete generator extrusion as a cause of pacemaker dysfunction [letter]. *Am J Emerg Med.* 1995;13:670-671.
6. Har-Shai Y, Amikam S, Bolous M, Peled IJ. The management of soft tissue complications related to pacemaker implantations. *J Cardiovasc Surg.* 1994;35(suppl 1):211-217.
7. Enes EG, Kayrak M. Common pacemaker problems: lead and pocket complications. In: Das MR, ed. *Modern Pacemakers - Present and Future.* 2011. Available at: http://www.intechopen.com/download/get/type/pdfs/id/13786. Accessed on January 17, 2014.
8. Arber N, Pras E, Copperman Y, et al. Pacemaker endocarditis: report of 44 cases and review of the literature. *Medicine.* 1994;73:299-305.
9. Sohail MR, Uslan DZ, Khan AH, et al. Management and outcome of permanent pacemaker and implantable cardioverter-defibrillator infections. *J Am Coll Cardiol.* 2007;49:1851-1859.
10. Molina JE. Undertreatment and overtreatment of patients with infected antiarrhythmic implantable devices. *Ann Thorac Surg.* 1997;63:504-509.
11. Atlee JL. Management of patients with pacemakers or ICD devices. In: Atlee JL, ed. *Arrhythmias and Pacemakers: Practical Management for Anesthesia and Critical Care Medicine.* Philadelphia: WB Saunders; 1996:295-329.
12. Aggarwal RK, Connelly DT, Ray SG, et al. Early complications of permanent pacemaker implantation: no difference between dual- and single-chamber systems. *Br Heart J.* 1995;73:571-575.
13. Giudici MC, Meierbachtol CJ, Paul DL, et al. Submammary device implantation in women: a step-by-step approach. *J Cardiovasc Electrophysiol.* 2013;24:1-4.
14. Beygui RE, Olcott C 4th, Dalman RL. Subclavian vein thrombosis: outcome analysis based on etiology and modality of treatment. *Ann Vasc Surg.* 1997;11:247-255.
15. Blom JW, Doggen CJ, Osanto S, Rosendaal FR. Old and new risk factors for upper extremity deep venous thrombosis. *J Thromb Haemost.* 2005;3:2471-2478.
16. Rooden CJ, Tesselaar ME, Osanto S, et al. Deep vein thrombosis associated with central venous catheters-a review. *J Thromb Haemost.* 2005;3:2409-2419.
17. Klug D, Lacroix D, Savoye C, et al. Systemic infection related to endocarditis on pacemaker leads: clinical presentation and management. *Circulation.* 1997;95:2098-2107.
18. Sivakumaran S, Irwin ME, Gulamhusein SS, Senaratne PJ. Postpacemaker implant pericarditis: incidence and outcome with active-fixation leads. *PACE.* 2002;25:833-837.
19. Gross JN, Platt S, Ritacco R, et al. The clinical relevance of electromyopotential oversensing in current unipolar devices. *Pacing Clin Electrophysiol.* 1992;15:2023-2027.
20. Cardall TY, Brady WJ, Chan TC, et al. Permanent cardiac pacemakers: issues relevant to the emergency physician, Part II. *J Emerg Med.* 1999;4: 697-709.
21. Papa LA, Abkar KB, Chung EK. Pacemaker hysteresis. *Heart Lung.* 1974;3;982-984.
22. Dohrmann ML, Goldschlager NF. Myocardial stimulation threshold in patients with cardiac pacemakers: effect of physiologic variables, pharmacologic agents, and lead electrodes. *Cardiol Clin.* 1985;3:527-537.
23. Hughes JC Jr, Tyers GFO, Torman HA. Effects of acid-base imbalance on myocardial pacing thresholds. *J Thorac Cardiovasc Surg.* 1975;69:743-746.
24. Schlesinger Z, Rosenberg T, Stryjer D, et al. Exit block in myxedema, treated effectively with thyroid hormone therapy. *Pacing Clin Electrophysiol.* 1980;3:737-739.
25. Barold SS, Falkoff MD, Ong LS, Heinle RA. Hyperkalemia induced failure of atrial capture during dual-chamber cardiac pacing. *J Am Coll Cardiol.* 1987;10:467-469.
26. Hellestrand KJ, Burnett PJ, Milne JR, et al. Effect of the antiarrhythmic agent flecainide acetate on acute and chronic pacing thresholds. *Pacing Clin Electrophysiol.* 1983;6:892-899.
27. Altamura G, Bianconi L, Lo Bianco F, et al. Transthoracic DC shock may represent a serious hazard in pacemaker-dependent patients. *Pacing Clin Electrophysiol.* 1995;18:194-198.
28. Love CJ, Hayes DL. Evaluation of pacemaker malfunction. In: Ellenbogen KA, Kay GN, Wilkoff BL, eds. *Clinical Cardiac Pacing.* Philadelphia: WB Saunders; 1995:656-683.
29. Oseran D, Ausubel K, Klementowicz PT, Furman S. Spontaneous endless loop tachycardia. *Pacing Clin Electrophysiol.* 1986;9:379-386.
30. Barold SS, Falkoff MD, Ong LS, Heinle RA. Pacemaker endless loop tachycardia: termination by simple techniques other than magnet application. *Am J Med.* 1988;85:817-822.
31. Mickley H, Andersen C, Nielsen LH. Runaway pacemaker: a still-existing complication and therapeutic guidelines. *Clin Cardiol.* 1989;12:412-414.
32. Snoeck J, Beerkhof M, Claeys M, et al. External vibration interference of activity-based rate-responsive pacemakers. *Pacing Clin Electrophysiol.* 1992;15:1841-1845.
33. Gordon RS, O'Dell KB, Low RB, Blumen IJ. Activity-sensing permanent internal pacemaker dysfunction during helicopter aeromedical transport. *Ann Emerg Med.* 1990;19:1260-1263.
34. French RS, Tillman JG. Pacemaker function during helicopter transport. *Ann Emerg Med.* 1989;18:305-307.
35. Fromm RE Jr, Taylor DH, Cronin L, et al. The incidence of pacemaker dysfunction during helicopter air medical transport. *Am J Emerg Med.* 1992;10:333-335.
36. Vanderheyden M, Timmermans W, Goethals M. Inappropriate rate response in a VVI-R pacemaker. *Acta Cardiol.* 1996;51:545-550.
37. Seeger W, Kleinert M. An unexpected rate response of a minute-ventilation dependent pacemaker [letter]. *Pacing Clin Electrophysiol.* 1989;12:1707.
38. Newland GM, Janz TG. Pacemaker-twiddler's syndrome: a rare cause of lead displacement and pacemaker malfunction. *Ann Emerg Med.* 1994;23:136-138.
39. Ellis GL. Pacemaker twiddler's syndrome: a case report. *Am J Emerg Med.* 1990;8:48-50.
40. Abrams S, Peart I. Twiddler's syndrome in children: an unusual cause of pacemaker failure. *Br Heart J.* 1995;73:190-192.
41. Rosenqvist M, Beyer T, Block M, et al. Adverse events with transvenous implantable cardioverter-defibrillators: a prospective multicenter study. European 7219 Jewel ICD investigators. *Circulation.* 1998;98:663-670.
42. Credner SC, Klingenheben T, Mauss O, et al. Electrical storm in patients with transvenous implantable cardioverter-defibrillators: incidence, management and prognostic implications. *J Am Coll Cardiol.* 1998;32:1909-1915.
43. Rogers JG, Butler J, Lansman SL, et al. Chronic mechanical circulatory support for inotrope-dependent heart failure patients who are not transplant candidates: results of the INTrEPID Trial. *J Am Coll Cardiol.* 2007;50:741-747.
44. Rose EA, Gelijns AC, Moskowitz AJ, et al, Randomized Evaluation of Mechanical Assistance for the Treatment of Congestive Heart Failure (REMATCH) Study Group. Long-term use of a left ventricular assist device for end-stage heart failure. *N Engl J Med.* 2001;345:1435-1443.
45. Slaughter MS, Rogers JG, Milano CA, et al. Advanced heart failure treated with continuous-flow left ventricular assist device. *N Engl J Med.* 2009;361:2241-2251.

46. Sun BC, Catanese KA, Spanier TB, et al. 100 long-term implantable left ventricular assist devices: the Columbia Presbyterian interim experience. *Ann Thorac Surg.* 1999;68:688-694.
47. Weingart S. Left Ventricular Assist Devices (LVADS). *EMCrit Blog – A Discussion of the Practice of ED Critical Care*, July 2012. Available at http://emcrit.org/wee/left-ventricular-assist-devices-lvads. Accessed on January 17, 2014.

CHAPTER 20

Use of Emergency Department Observation Units for Cardiac Patients

Christopher W. Baugh and J. Stephen Bohan

IN THIS CHAPTER

Observation unit logistics

Observation units and specific cardiac conditions

Protocols of care for cardiac patients

The role of observation in medicine is as ancient as Hippocrates, to whom the following quotation is attributed: "A great part, I believe, of the Art is to be able to observe."[1] The modern concept of observation units emerged in the early 1970s but did not gain widespread recognition until a decade later, when the first chest pain units were established.[2] Indeed, chest pain has historically been the complaint most commonly managed in observation units and best studied in the medical literature.[3]

Observation as a disposition option after emergency department evaluation provides a third destination for patients who do not fit neatly into a "discharge home or admit to inpatient" dichotomy. Payer guidelines in the United States specify that observation should typically last up to 24 hours but not more than 48 hours. Most emergency department observation units self-impose a 24-hour maximum to maintain patient throughput. The purpose of an observation evaluation is to provide additional time for diagnostics and treatments to determine if a patient needs inpatient admission. Despite the passive connotation of the term "observation," it is intended to be a very active and continuous evaluation.[4]

About a third of all emergency departments in the United States have a dedicated observation unit.[5] Those without a dedicated space for observation can still provide this service, but patients are managed in acute care emergency department beds or inpatient care areas. The act of observation has always been distinct from a specific location within the emergency department or hospital; however, all of the studies that show the many benefits of observation care (eg, greater efficiency, shorter length of stay, lower cost, greater patient satisfaction) were conducted in dedicated observation units.[6]

To achieve maximum efficiency, an evidence-based approach to managing specific conditions is essential. A successful observation unit will employ condition-specific protocols of care that explicitly detail the inclusion and exclusion criteria for observation unit care, the available diagnostic and treatment options, and the end points of the observation visit, with time limitations and specific criteria to trigger discharge home or further hospitalization. These protocols are informed by the scientific literature and institution-specific resources and should be formulated by the emergency department staff in conjunction with the specialty relevant to the particular complaint.[4]

KEY POINTS

Observation provides an additional 24 to 48 hours for further diagnostics and treatment to determine if inpatient admission is necessary.

Observation is a status, not a specific location.

Condition-specific protocols are essential to achieve efficient patient selection and management in an observation unit.

Observation Unit Logistics

The ideal location for an observation unit is within or contiguous to the main emergency department. This proximity minimizes patient transport times and allows efficient coverage arrangements. In addition, this arrangement facilitates rapid response for a patient who is clinically deteriorating; in fact, Medicare policy states that the clinician responsible for an observation patient must be "immediately available" to respond.[7] However, because emergency department crowding is a pervasive problem, it might not be possible to reallocate valuable acute care beds to create an observation unit within an existing department's footprint. As a result, many institutions find space as close as possible to the emergency department to fill this need.

Most observation units are staffed by emergency physicians and have about 10 beds.[6] About 80% of observation patients are discharged home after their observation stay; the remainder requires hospitalization.[8] Close relationships with consulting services such as cardiology are an important resource for observation patients and help to avoid unnecessary hospitalizations. Observation patients typically have high priority for diagnostic tests, such as cardiac stress tests and echocardiography because delays in such testing could result in exclusion from observation unit care due to logistics alone. For example, if a stress test is not available for 2 days because of a holiday and cannot be obtained on an outpatient basis, the patient would not be a candidate for management in the observation unit and would need to be hospitalized in an inpatient area.

KEY POINTS

The ideal location for an observation unit is contiguous with the emergency department.

Close relationships with consulting services reduce the number of unnecessary hospitalizations.

Observation unit patients should have high priority for diagnostic tests.

Specific Conditions

Chest Pain

Chest pain is the most common complaint managed in an observation unit, accounting for nearly one in five visits.[9] This finding is not surprising for several reasons: chest pain units were the forerunner of modern observation units, chest pain is the most widely studied observation condition, chest pain is a common emergency department complaint (the reason for 5% to 7% of all visits), and the diagnostic pathway to perform risk stratification for acute coronary syndrome (ACS) can be reasonably completed within the confines of the typical resources and timeframe of an observation unit visit.[10]

The emergency department evaluation of chest pain patients has evolved over the years since chest pain units first appeared in the early 1980s. In the 1990s, the introduction of sensitive biomarkers for myocardial death in the form of conventional troponin assays was a tremendous leap forward in the evaluation of these patients.[11] In addition, other factors such as improved training and understanding of the pathophysiology of ischemic heart disease and the increasing availability and modalities of cardiac stress tests increased both the skill and diagnostics available to effectively "rule out" myocardial ischemia as the underlying cause of chest pain.

The objective of observation unit evaluation for a patient who has chest pain and is suspected of having ACS is to determine if inpatient admission is needed. ACS can be divided into three discrete categories: ST-elevation myocardial infarction (STEMI), non-STEMI (NSTEMI), and unstable angina (UA). A STEMI patient is not a candidate for care in an observation unit. Observation is intended to identify subtle or evolving presentations of NSTEMI or UA. An algorithm for identifying chest pain patients most appropriate for management in an observation unit is presented as Figure 20-1. Ideal candidates should be at low and intermediate risk for ACS, with uncertainty about the necessity for inpatient admission and without a safe plan for discharge to home after the initial emergency department evaluation.

By definition, a patient with NSTEMI has a positive troponin test.[12] As a result, one of the key components of a chest pain observation stay is serial troponin testing. As cardiac biomarkers evolve, the trend of achieving very sensitive results at ever decreasing intervals between assays has emerged. The timing between sets of conventional troponin assays has decreased from 12 hours to 6 hours at most institutions, and emerging data for "highly sensitive" troponin assays currently available in Europe are building a case for a 3-hour interval.[13,14] If the troponin value remains negative or undetectable after sufficient time has elapsed, NSTEMI is excluded from the differential diagnosis. Patients with chronic troponin elevations, often those with comorbidities such as kidney disease and peripheral vascular disease, represent a greater challenge, as the magnitude and change in troponin over time must be factored into the medical decision making; a positive troponin result alone does not necessarily represent an acute cardiac event that requires intervention.

Patients with serial troponin assays that are normal or unchanged usually require further evaluation for new-onset angina, especially UA. UA is more prevalent in women and the elderly, often with an atypical presentation that is difficult to confirm based on history alone.[10] ECG changes are often present, including dynamic changes over time. As a result, repeat evaluations, including ECGs, are an essential component of observation for the chest pain patient. For patients categorized as low risk for ACS, the absence of obstructive coronary artery disease on coronary computed tomography angiography can be diagnostic in ruling out ACS as the origin of chest pain.[15] However, the actual utility of the test remains uncertain; some authors have argued that this test might be unnecessary in a low-risk population, given the potential harms of ionizing radiation, contrast media, and indeterminate findings that require further testing.[16,17] Conventional stress testing such as the exercise tolerance test with or without myocardial perfusion imaging from the observation unit has traditionally been a key component of the evaluation for patients with a concern for UA as the origin of their chest pain. It has a strong negative predictive value for major adverse cardiac events.[18] In addition, one study suggested that positive stress tests are missed when patients are discharged home with plans for followup stress testing (suggesting that the positive result would have been detected if the test had been performed before discharge).[19]

Multiple high-quality studies have described improved outcomes for patients with chest pain managed in observation units compared with usual inpatient care. For example, four prospective randomized studies concluded that observation chest pain protocols are associated with lower cost, shorter length of stay, and improved resource utilization.[20-23] Two population studies of the outcomes of patients with chest pain after the implementation of an emergency department observation unit found a significant reduction in both cost and inpatient admission, including a reduced rate of missed myocardial infarction.[23,24] Improved patient satisfaction and even quality of life have been reported after observation care rather than inpatient care, without any increase in adverse outcomes.[25]

Looking ahead, as further evidence clarifies the optimal testing interval for sensitive troponin tests, the role of an observation evaluation in truly low-risk patients, as defined by any one of the validated risk stratification tools, becomes less apparent. As a result, the future will likely see fewer low-risk chest pain patients in observation units, creating capacity to manage other patients—perhaps higher-risk chest pain patients or patients with entirely different complaints.

KEY POINTS

Chest pain is the most common condition currently managed in observation units.

The observation evaluation provides risk stratification for ACS, allowing more patients with disease to be detected and appropriately managed and more patients without disease to be sent home without unnecessary and potentially harmful diagnostics and exposure to the hazards of hospitalization.

Future protocols for cardiac marker testing that allow more rapid assessment of low-risk patients with ACS may reduce the need for observation unit stays.

Syncope

In the United States, 3% to 5% of emergency department visits are for syncope, which is one of the top three observation unit diagnoses.[9,26] Patients presenting to the emergency department with syncope and a high risk for serious cardiac events such as ventricular arrhythmias warrant inpatient admission for

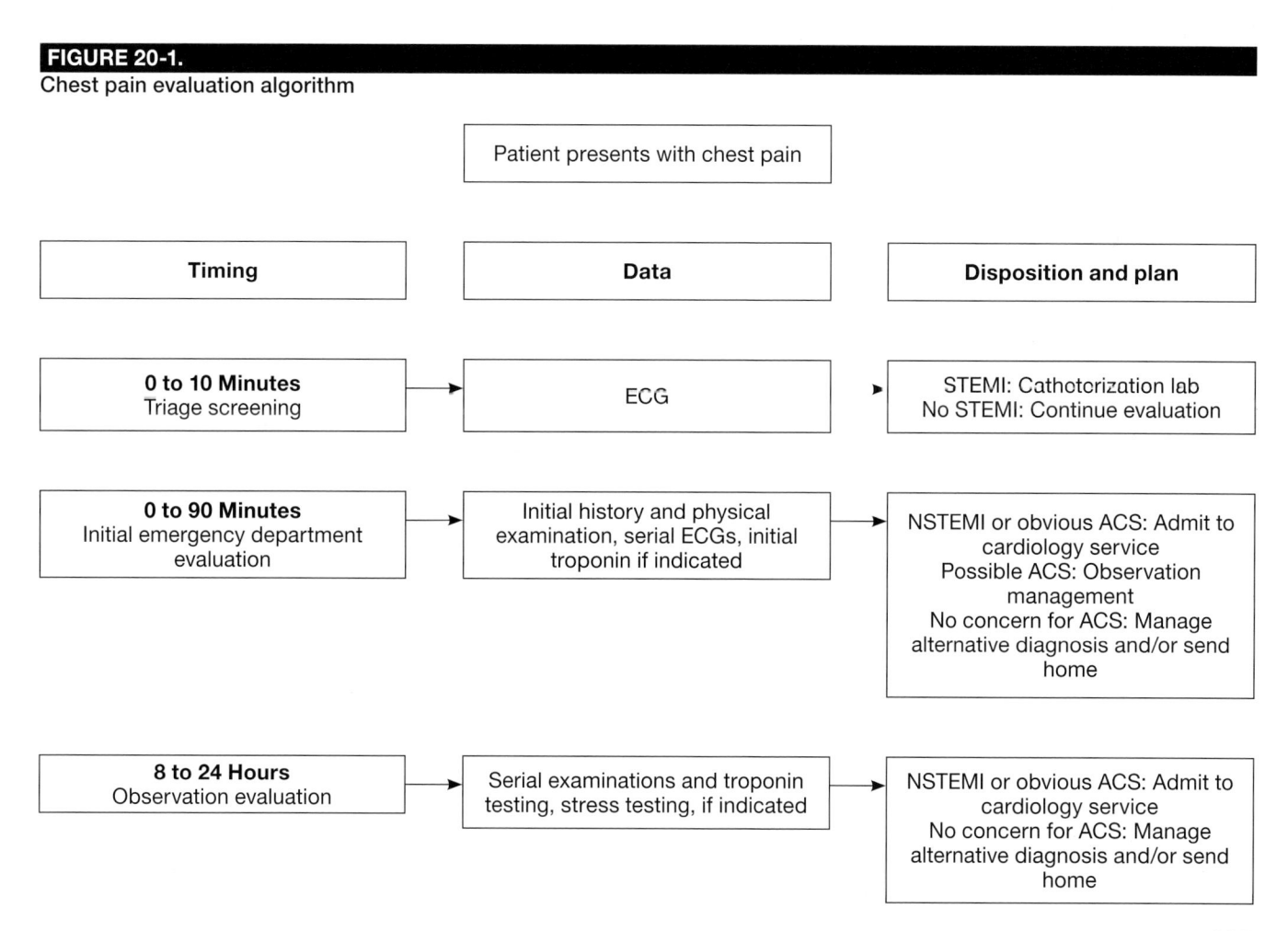

FIGURE 20-1.
Chest pain evaluation algorithm

Timing	Data	Disposition and plan
Patient presents with chest pain		
0 to 10 Minutes — Triage screening	ECG	STEMI: Catheterization lab / No STEMI: Continue evaluation
0 to 90 Minutes — Initial emergency department evaluation	Initial history and physical examination, serial ECGs, initial troponin if indicated	NSTEMI or obvious ACS: Admit to cardiology service / Possible ACS: Observation management / No concern for ACS: Manage alternative diagnosis and/or send home
8 to 24 Hours — Observation evaluation	Serial examinations and troponin testing, stress testing, if indicated	NSTEMI or obvious ACS: Admit to cardiology service / No concern for ACS: Manage alternative diagnosis and/or send home

workup and treatment of the underlying disease processes. On the other hand, patients at very low risk for serious causes of syncope such as those with a clear vasovagal episode and normal emergency department evaluation do not require any further hospital evaluation and can be discharged home safely. Patients who lack high-risk features such as known critical aortic stenosis or a severely depressed ventricular ejection fraction and who do not have a clear vasovagal cause or an obvious disposition option can be classified as intermediate risk. These patients are ideal for an observation evaluation, so that diagnostics such as extended cardiac telemetry, echocardiogram, and serial examinations can exclude dangerous causes of syncope and facilitate a safe discharge to home. Table 20-1 lists risk stratification criteria that can be used to identify the intermediate-risk syncope patients best suited for an observation unit.[26]

Many tests conducted on patients during an inpatient admission for syncope have low diagnostic yield.[27] For example, among patients studied by Mendu and colleagues, cardiac enzymes, computed tomography scanning, echocardiography, carotid ultrasonography, and electroencephalography affected diagnosis or management in less than 5% of cases and confirmed the cause of syncope in less than 2% of cases.[27] Such literature suggests that standardized observation unit protocol can increase efficiency by lowering health care costs and hospital length of stay by eliminating unnecessary testing.

Without an observation unit option, many emergency physicians default to a higher level of care; thus, it is not surprising that Quinn and associates reported that 30% of syncope patients admitted by emergency physicians have an estimated risk of serious outcomes of less than 2%.[28] In one prospective study, patients at intermediate risk for syncope were randomized to an observation unit or inpatient admission after initial emergency department management. The observation protocol included serial vital signs and continuous cardiac monitoring for up to 6 hours. When clinically indicated, further testing such as an ECG or tilt-table testing was performed. Forty-three percent of the observation unit patients required subsequent hospitalization compared with 98% of patients randomized to standard care. Two-year clinical outcomes, including all-cause mortality and recurrent syncope, were similar between observation patients and inpatient controls groups.[26]

KEY POINTS

Observation is an ideal strategy for syncope patients at intermediate risk for adverse outcomes.

Typical observation unit interventions for syncope patients include cardiac telemetry, serial examinations, and additional testing as indicated (eg, echocardiography).

Measurement of orthostatic vital signs is an inexpensive test that has a high diagnostic yield compared with other diagnostics usually associated with a syncope evaluation.

Congestive Heart Failure

Emergency department visits for acute decompensated heart failure (ADHF) represent almost 20% of the total heart failure-specific ambulatory care delivered each year, and most of these visits lead to hospitalization.[29] Evidence suggests that observation unit management of heart failure can be safe and cost effective when patients are selected carefully.[30,31] Visits for ADHF represent the seventh most common diagnosis for observation unit patients.[9] One study found that the introduction of an observation protocol for heart failure led to a 56% reduction in the 90-day emergency department revisit rate for heart failure and a 64% reduction in the 90-day rehospitalization rate. In addition, there was a trend toward a reduction in the 90-day mortality rate, from 4% to 1%.[32]

Because patients presenting to the emergency department with ADHF tend to be medically complicated, with other comorbidities and on multiple medications, careful selection of patients likely to do well in an observation unit setting is critical. Additionally, even with very selective criteria, these patients tend to require subsequent inpatient hospitalization at a higher rate than other observation unit patients with unrelated

TABLE 20-1.

Syncope Risk Stratification. Adapted from: Shen WK, Decker WW, Smars PA, et al. Syncope Evaluation in the Emergency Department Study (SEEDS): a multidisciplinary approach to syncope management. *Circulation*. 2004;110:3636-3645. Used with permission from Wolters Kluwer.

High Risk	Intermediate Risk	Low Risk
Chest pain and/or ECG suggesting ACS	Presentation not consistent with a vasovagal or orthostatic cause	History consistent with a vasovagal or orthostatic cause
Signs of CHF on examination	Lack of high-risk features	Normal ECG and cardiac examination
Moderate to severe valvular disease		Lack of high-risk features
History of ventricular arrhythmias		
Persistent sinus bradycardia		
Prolonged QTc (>500 msec)		
Low ejection fraction (<40%)		
Cardiac devices with dysfunction		

complaints. Typically, one expects about 20% of observation patients to stay in the hospital; this rate can approach 30% or higher for ADHF patients.[33,34] This higher rate can be acceptable as long as it is appropriately anticipated.

Another unique aspect of this population is that observation unit nurses tend to focus on tasks more commonly practiced on inpatient floors than in the emergency department. Strict measurement of input and output, taking accurate weights, and adherence to fluid restrictions and low-sodium diets are essential components of treating this patient population. As a result, before implementing an observation protocol for ADHF, inservice training with an ongoing educational program will be helpful in ensuring that these tasks are completed accurately, which ultimately will allow more patients to be managed successfully in the observation unit.

This higher inpatient hospitalization rate emphasizes the importance of a close working relationship between the observation team and the patient's cardiologist. This collaboration facilitates transition of care to an inpatient team as well as outpatient followup for patients after management in the observation unit. These patients are at risk for future episodes of decompensation for many reasons. One goal of the observation unit stay is to exclude dangerous causes of exacerbation such as acute myocardial infarction while performing sufficient diuresis to allow the patient to be safely discharged home. Close communication with outpatient care providers to get treatment recommendations augments the observation unit team's ability to care for these patients. Close followup with outpatient care providers, ideally with an appointment already scheduled at the time of discharge from the observation unit, is essential to help the patient to do well at home.

The structured care delivered with standardized protocols improves efficiency, often allowing similar care to that of the inpatient setting in a shorter amount of time. Appropriate patient selection is a key initial component of a heart failure observation protocol (Table 20-2). For example, Diercks et al reported that heart failure patients with a systolic blood pressure above 160 mm Hg on emergency department presentation and a normal initial cardiac troponin I level were significantly more likely to be discharged from observation and not experience a 30-day adverse event (death, readmission, myocardial infarction, arrhythmia).[30] Another study found that a blood urea nitrogen level below 30 mg/dL significantly predicted successful observation unit management resulting in discharge home.[33]

KEY POINTS

Careful selection of emergency department patients for observation care maximizes successful management. Factors associated with discharge home include a blood urea nitrogen level below 30 mg/dL, systolic blood pressure above 160 mm Hg, and a normal troponin I value.

A close relationship with inpatient cardiologists and the patient's outpatient care providers is essential to successful management.

ADHF patients require hospitalization after an observation unit stay at a higher rate than patients with other conditions.

Atrial Fibrillation

Atrial fibrillation is the most common sustained cardiac arrhythmia in adults and, not surprisingly, the most common arrhythmia managed in the emergency department.[35] The incidence of atrial fibrillation increases with age, to almost 5% among people over 69 years of age.[36] Given the projected aging of the US population in the coming years, the number of emergency department visits for atrial fibrillation is expected to rise. Hospitalizations for atrial fibrillation have increased by 66% over the past 20 years.[37] Strategies to identify treatments that safely restore sinus rhythm in patients with acute-onset atrial fibrillation from the emergency department, often involving the use of an observation unit, are of great interest and will gain importance as this disease becomes more common.

According to current guidelines from the American College of Cardiology/American Heart Association (ACC/AHA) and recent studies, patients presenting to the emergency department with a clear onset of atrial fibrillation within the past 48 hours are candidates for expedited cardioversion; in this case, observation unit management is likely to avoid inpatient hospitalization.[36,38,39] There are conflicting recommendations around the role of anticoagulation in these patients if they lack risk factors for stroke. Some society guidelines recommend routine anticoagulation during cardioversion,[40] while others, including those from the ACC/AHA, do not.[41] Ross reported that, with a protocolized observation unit approach, 82% of this subset may be discharged home in an average of 11.8 ± 7 hours.[42] Kim et al reported that an atrial fibrillation observation protocol showed a favorable trend toward mean cost reduction ($1,706 compared to $879).[43] Decker et al reported the results of a randomized trial that compared protocolized care in an observation setting with routine hospitalization in patients with acute-onset uncomplicated atrial fibrillation. Their protocol started with pharmacologic heart rate control using a calcium channel blocker or a beta-blocker. All patients received continuous cardiac monitoring and were reassessed after 6 hours. Those still in atrial fibrillation were sedated and received electrical cardioversion followed by observation for at least 2 more hours. Those in sinus rhythm after the 2-hour observation period were discharged home with cardiology followup. Patients in the observation unit group had substantially shorter hospitalizations, with a median length of stay of 10.1 versus 25.2 hours and were 12% more likely to be discharged home in sinus rhythm. There were no significant differences between the groups in terms of their frequency of recurrent atrial fibrillation, rehospitalization, number of tests or procedures, or adverse events during their 6-month followup.[36]

Stiell et al showed that 95% of patients with acute-onset atrial fibrillation could be discharged home using an emergency department protocol of chemical cardioversion followed by electrical cardioversion if the chemical attempt was unsuccessful. Ninety percent of the 660 patients who underwent the protocol regained normal sinus rhythm.[39] Another therapeutic option for some patients could be the act of observation with continuous cardiac telemetry alone; up to 50% of these patients spontaneously convert to normal sinus rhythm within 24 hours after rate control alone.[36] When patients present early within the 48-hour window of onset, the observation approach might work well, especially when other management options are contraindicated. An observation unit pathway for managing patients with atrial fibrillation of recent onset is presented in Figure 20-2. Chemical and electrical cardioversion have unique advantages and disadvantages. For example, success rates are higher for electrical cardioversion, but not all eligible candidates are ideal for the required procedural sedation, which also consumes more nursing resources.

After cardioversion, the decision to start anticoagulation, with options ranging from aspirin to warfarin or other agents, can be informed by calculation of the patient's $CHADS_2$ score and discussions with outpatient care providers. Very often, this decision can be delayed for outpatient followup if it can be arranged quickly following the observation unit stay.[44]

KEY POINTS

Patients presenting with uncomplicated atrial fibrillation and a clear onset within 48 hours or less are candidates for an

TABLE 20-2.

Inclusion and Exclusion Criteria for Observation Unit Management of Acute Decompensated Heart Failure. From: Storrow AB, Collins SP, Lyons MS, et al. Emergency department observation of heart failure: preliminary analysis of safety and cost. *Congest Heart Fail.* 2005;11:68-72. Used with permission from John Wiley and Sons.

Inclusion criteria	
Two from the left column *or* one from the left column plus two from the right column	
Paroxysmal nocturnal dyspnea	Extremity edema
Neck vein distention	Night cough
Pulmonary edema (on chest radiograph)	Dyspnea on exertion
Rales	Hepatomegaly
Cardiomegaly	Pleural effusion
S_3 gallop	Tachycardia (≥130 bpm)
Jugular venous distention	
	and
B-type natriuretic peptide level higher than 100 pg/mL	
Designated for admission by the emergency physician	
Provided informed consent	
Exclusion criteria	
Alternative diagnosis explaining acute clinical presentation	
Hypoxia (oxygen saturation <90% on room air)	
Severe respiratory distress	
Hypotension (systolic blood pressure <90 mm Hg)	
Temperature >100°F	
Syncope	
Requirement of intravenous infusion to treat hypo/hypertension	
ECG with ischemic changes not known to be old	
Serum markers indicative of myocardial necrosis	
New-onset heart failure	
Severe electrolyte imbalances	
Currently receiving dialysis	
Failure to provide informed consent	
Younger than 18 years old	

observation protocol.

For patients who do not cardiovert spontaneously, either chemical or electrical cardioversion is a good option to establish normal sinus rhythm.

A precise time of onset of atrial fibrillation can be difficult to elicit and is a key component of safe observation unit cardioversion.

Conclusion

The emergency department observation unit is an important resource that enables clinicians to provide efficient evaluation and treatment of a wide range of patients presenting with common cardiac complaints. Over time, this role will evolve as more evidence contributes to the development of new standards of care. The inherent flexibility and efficiency of the observation unit will ensure this setting will continue to be a valuable disposition strategy in the future.

References

1. Lyons AS. Hippocrates. Available at: www.healthguidance.org/entry/6338/1/Hippocrates.html. Accessed on January 15, 2014.
2. Gururaj VJ, Allen JE, Russo RM. Short stay in an outpatient department: an alternative to hospitalization. *Am J Dis Child.* 1972;123:128-132.
3. Ross MA, Aurora T, Graff L, et al. State of the art: emergency department observation units. *Crit Pathw Cardiol.* 2012;11:128-138.
4. Graff LG. *Observation Medicine: The Healthcare System's Tincture of Time.* American College of Emergency Physicians online content. Available at: http://www.acep.org/Physician-Resources/Practice-Resources/Administration/Observation-Medicine/. Accessed January 15, 2014.
5. Niska R, Bhuiya F, Xu J. National Hospital Ambulatory Medical Care Survey: 2007 Emergency Department Summary. National Health Statistics Reports, No. 26. Hyattsville, MD: US Department of Health and Human Services, August 6, 2010.
6. Baugh CW, Venkatesh AK, Hilton JA, et al. Making greater use of dedicated hospital observation units for many short-stay patients could save $3.1 billion a year. *Health Aff (Millwood).* 2012;31:2314-2323.
7. *Medicare Claims Processing Manual.* Publication 100-04. Centers for Medicare & Medicaid Services. Transmittal 1466, 2008. Available at: http://www.cms.gov/Regulations-and-Guidance/Guidance/Manuals/Internet-Only-Manuals-IOMs-Items/CMS018912.html. Accessed on January 15, 2014.
8. Baugh CW, Venkatesh AK, Bohan JS. Emergency department observation units: a clinical and financial benefit for hospitals. *Health Care Manage Rev.* 2011;36:28-37.
9. Venkatesh AK, Geisler BP, Gibson Chambers JJ, et al. Use of observation care in US emergency departments, 2001 to 2008. *PLoS ONE.* 2011;6:e24326.
10. Mehta RH, Eagle KA. Missed diagnoses of acute coronary syndromes in the emergency room—continuing challenges. *N Engl J Med.* 2000;342:1207-1210.
11. Panteghini M. Acute coronary syndrome: biochemical strategies in the troponin era. *Chest.* 2002;122:1428-1435.
12. Anderson JL, Adams CD, Antman EM, et al. ACC/AHA 2007 guidelines for the management of patients with unstable angina/non ST-elevation myocardial infarction: a report of the American College of Cardiology/American Heart Association Task Force on Practice Guidelines (Writing Committee to Revise the 2002 Guidelines for the Management of Patients With Unstable Angina/Non ST-Elevation Myocardial Infarction): developed in collaboration with the American College of Emergency Physicians, the Society for Cardiovascular Angiography and Interventions, and the Society of Thoracic Surgeons: endorsed by the American Association of Cardiovascular and Pulmonary Rehabilitation and the Society for Academic Emergency Medicine. *Circulation.* 2007;116:e148-e304.
13. Keller T, Zeller T, Ojeda F, et al. Serial changes in highly sensitive troponin I assay and early diagnosis of myocardial infarction. *JAMA.* 2011;306:2684-2693.
14. Reichlin T, Irfan A, Twerenbold R, et al. Utility of absolute and relative changes in cardiac troponin concentrations in the early diagnosis of acute myocardial infarction. *Circulation.* 2011;124:136-145.
15. Antman EM, Cohen M, Bernink PJ, et al. The TIMI risk score for unstable angina/non-ST elevation MI: a method for prognostication and therapeutic decision making. *JAMA.* 2000;284:835-842.
16. Litt HI, Gatsonis C, Snyder B, et al. CT angiography for safe discharge of patients with possible acute coronary syndromes. *N Engl J Med.* 2012;366:1393-1403.
17. Prasad V, Cheung M, Cifu A. Chest pain in the emergency department: the case against our current practice of routine noninvasive testing. *Arch Intern Med.* 2012;172:1506-1509.
18. Manini AF, McAfee AT, Noble VE, Bohan JS. Prognostic value of the Duke treadmill score for emergency department patients with chest pain. *J Emerg Med.* 2010;39:135-143.
19. Madsen T, Mallin M, Bledsoe J, et al. Utility of the emergency department observation unit in ensuring stress testing in low-risk chest pain patients. *Crit Pathw Cardiol.* 2009;8:122-124.
20. Roberts RR, Zalenski RJ, Mensah EK, et al. Costs of an emergency department-based accelerated diagnostic protocol vs hospitalization in patients with chest pain: a randomized controlled trial. *JAMA.* 1997;278:1670-1676.
21. Farkouh ME, Smars PA, Reeder GS, et al. A clinical trial of a chest-pain observation unit for patients with unstable angina. Chest Pain Evaluation in the Emergency Room (CHEER) Investigators. *N Engl J Med.* 1998;339:1882-1888.
22. Gomez MA, Anderson JL, Karagounis LA, et al. An emergency department-based protocol for rapidly ruling out myocardial ischemia reduces hospital time and expense: results of a randomized study (ROMIO). *J Am Coll Cardiol.* 1996;28:25-33.
23. Goodacre S, Nicholl J, Dixon S, et al. Randomised controlled trial and economic evaluation of a chest pain observation unit compared with routine care. *BMJ.* 2004;328:254.
24. Graff LG, Dallara J, Ross MA, et al. Impact on the care of the emergency department chest pain patient from the chest pain evaluation registry (CHEPER) study. *Am J Cardiol.* 1997;80:563-568.
25. Rydman RJ, Zalenski RJ, Roberts RR, et al. Patient satisfaction with an emergency department chest pain observation unit. *Ann Emerg Med.* 1997;29:109-115.
26. Shen WK, Decker WW, Smars PA, et al. Syncope Evaluation in the Emergency Department Study (SEEDS): a multidisciplinary approach to syncope management. *Circulation.* 2004;110:3636-3645.

FIGURE 20-2.

Observation pathway for atrial fibrillation of recent onset

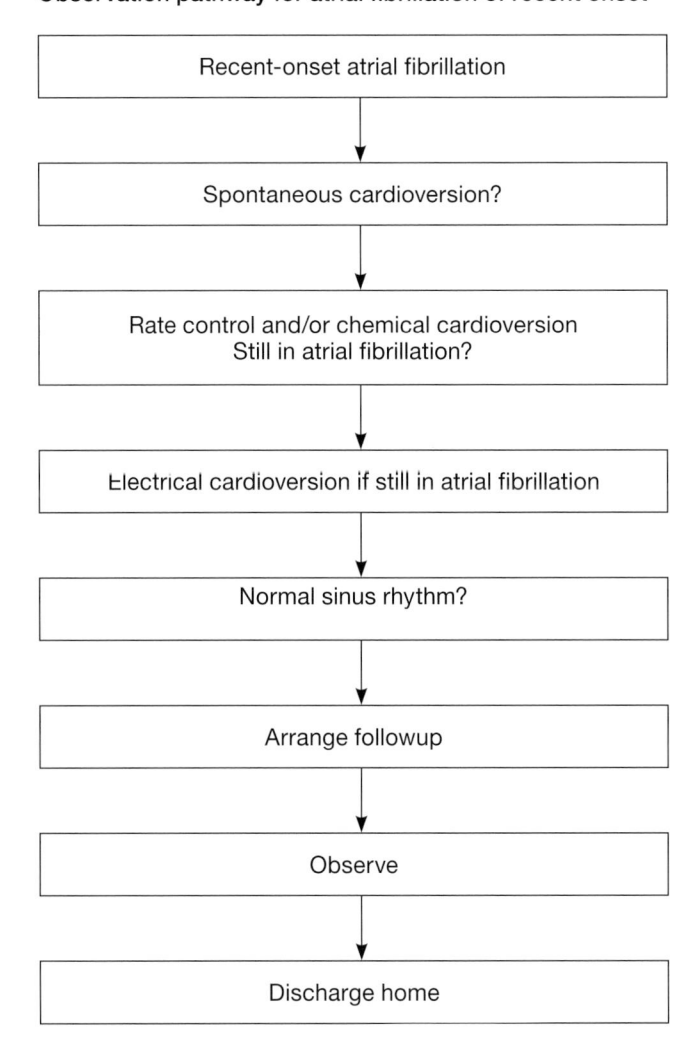

Recent-onset atrial fibrillation
↓
Spontaneous cardioversion?
↓
Rate control and/or chemical cardioversion
Still in atrial fibrillation?
↓
Electrical cardioversion if still in atrial fibrillation
↓
Normal sinus rhythm?
↓
Arrange followup
↓
Observe
↓
Discharge home

27. Mendu ML, McAvay G, Lampert R, et al. Yield of diagnostic tests in evaluating syncopal episodes in older patients. *Arch Intern Med.* 2009;169:1299-1305.
28. Quinn JV, Stiell IG, McDermott DA, et al. The San Francisco Syncope Rule vs physician judgment and decision making. *Am J Emerg Med.* 2005;23:782-786.
29. Schappert SM, Rechtsteiner EA. Ambulatory medical care utilization estimates for 2006. *Natl Health Stat Report.* 2008;(8):1-29.
30. Diercks DB, Peacock WF, Kirk JD, Weber JE. ED patients with heart failure: identification of an observational unit-appropriate cohort. *Am J Emerg Med.* 2006;24:319-324.
31. Peacock WF 4th, Young J, Collins S, et al. Heart failure observation units: optimizing care. *Ann Emerg Med.* 2006;47:22-33.
32. Peacock WF 4th, Remer EE, Aponte J, et al. Effective observation unit treatment of decompensated heart failure. *Congest Heart Fail.* 2002;8:68-73.
33. Burkhardt J, Peacock WF, Emerman CL. Predictors of emergency department observation unit outcomes. *Acad Emerg Med.* 2005;12:869-874.
34. Storrow AB, Collins SP, Lyons MS, et al. Emergency department observation of heart failure: preliminary analysis of safety and cost. *Congest Heart Fail.* 2005;11:68-72.
35. Cristoni L, Tampieri A, Mucci F, et al. Cardioversion of acute atrial fibrillation in the short observation unit: comparison of a protocol focused on electrical cardioversion with simple antiarrhythmic treatment. *Emerg Med J.* 2011;28:932-937.
36. Decker WW, Smars PA, Vaidyanathan L, et al. A prospective, randomized trial of an emergency department observation unit for acute onset atrial fibrillation. *Ann Emerg Med.* 2008;52:322-328.
37. Friberg J, Buch P, Scharling H, et al. Rising rates of hospital admissions for atrial fibrillation. *Epidemiology.* 2003;14:666-672.
38. Wann LS, Curtis AB, January CT, et al. 2011 ACCF/AHA/HRS Focused Update on the Management of Patients With Atrial Fibrillation (Updating the 2006 Guideline): A Report of the American College of Cardiology Foundation/American Heart Association Task Force on Practice Guidelines. *Circulation.* 2011;123:104-123.
39. Stiell IG, Clement CM, Perry JJ, et al. Association of the Ottawa Aggressive Protocol with rapid discharge of emergency department patients with recent-onset atrial fibrillation or flutter. *CJEM.* 2010;12:181-191.
40. Camm AJ, Kirchhof P, Lip GY, et al. Guidelines for the management of atrial fibrillation: the Task Force for the Management of Atrial Fibrillation of the European Society of Cardiology (ESC). *Eur Heart J.* 2010;31:2369-2429.
41. Fuster V, Ryden LE, Cannom DS, et al. ACC/AHA/ESC 2006 guidelines for the management of patients with atrial fibrillation: a report of the American College of Cardiology/American Heart Association Task Force on practice guidelines and the European Society of Cardiology Committee for Practice Guidelines developed in collaboration with the European Heart Rhythm Association and the Heart Rhythm Society. *Circulation.* 2006;114:e257-e354.
42. Ross MA, Davis B, Dresselhouse A. The role of an emergency department observation unit in a clinical pathway for atrial fibrillation. *Crit Pathw Cardiol.* 2004;3:8-12.
43. Kim MH, Morady F, Conlon B, et al. A prospective, randomized, controlled trial of an emergency department-based atrial fibrillation treatment strategy with low-molecular-weight heparin. *Ann Emerg Med.* 2002;40:187-192.
44. Singer DE, Albers GW, Dalen JE, et al. Antithrombotic therapy in atrial fibrillation: American College of Chest Physicians Evidence-Based Clinical Practice Guidelines (8th edition). *Chest.* 2008;133:546S-592S.

CHAPTER 21

Reducing the Risk of Malpractice

Michael Jay Bresler

IN THIS CHAPTER

The scope of the problem

The medical history

Examination

Electrocardiogram

Cardiac markers

Differential diagnosis

Treatment

Documentation and communication

The Scope of the Problem

Malpractice: a word that provokes a visceral response in all physicians. Unfortunately, our society is litigious. Many of us will be sued at least once in our careers. But, contrary to common belief, emergency medicine is not one of the specialties at greatest risk. Although we do not generally have an established relationship with our patients, and although we practice in an exceedingly chaotic environment with critically ill patients, our liability falls approximately in the middle of the various specialties.[1] However, within our specialty, myocardial infarction (MI) and chest pain are two of the most frequent sources of medicolegal liability.[1]

According to a recent unscientific survey conducted by the American Medical Association, 5% of responding physicians had faced a malpractice claim during the previous year.[2,3] A more thorough study analyzed claims reported by a large insurance company, involving 25 specialties from 1991 through 2003.[2] In any given year, 7.4% of all physicians were dealing with a malpractice claim, and 1.6% of claims finalized that year resulted in a payment. However, 78% of all finalized claims between 1991 and 2003 did not result in payment. It was estimated that 75% of physicians in low-risk specialties and 99% of those in high-risk specialties had been sued by age 65. Although the source of these data was a single insurance company, the carrier is quite large, with clients in all 50 states.[2] The data probably reflect the national average. Another study suggested that 40% of lawsuits were not associated with medical error. Twenty-eight percent of these cases resulted in payment, compared with 73% when medical error was judged to have occurred.[4]

KEY POINT

Although many physicians will eventually be sued, most lawsuits do not result in payment of claims.

The Physician Insurers Association of America (PIAA) has compiled data specific to emergency medicine litigation. The full survey includes 22 insurance companies representing 30 major medical and dental specialties in over 255,000 closed claims and lawsuits between 1985 and 2010.[1] Emergency medicine ranks 15th of 28 specialties in the number of closed claims during that period. The percentage of paid claims to closed claims was 26%, the lowest of all medical specialties. The total indemnity paid on behalf of emergency physicians was $271 million. However, this amount ranked only 16th of the 28 specialties in dollars paid and was 1.3% less than the average.[1] The most common "misadventure" among emergency physicians was "diagnostic error," accounting for 46% of all claims. For claims involving diagnostic error, "acute myocardial infarction" was the most common condition.[1]

> **KEY POINTS**
>
> Emergency physicians rank approximately in the middle of specialties in terms of frequency of lawsuits and indemnity dollars paid. However, the percentage of cases in which a claim was rewarded was the lowest of all the specialties.[1]
>
> Diagnostic error accounts for nearly half of all malpractice claims against emergency physicians. Within this category, acute myocardial infarction was the most common condition.[1]

Overall, "myocardial infarction, acute" accounted for 18% of claims filed, and "chest pain, not otherwise defined" accounted for an additional 13%, the total of the two representing 31% of all malpractice claims against emergency physicians. Another 6.5% of cases involved "aortic aneurysm." (It is not clear whether this entity includes both thoracic aortic dissection and abdominal aortic aneurysm, since the terms are often confused in medical records.) Fifty-three percent of claims involving myocardial infarction resulted in payment.[1]

> **KEY POINT**
>
> Acute MI and chest pain account for 31% of all malpractice claims against emergency physicians. Fifty-three percent of claims involving MI resulted in payment.[1]

The PIAA data from 1985 through 2007 were also analyzed for claims arising from an event originating in the emergency department but not necessarily involving emergency physicians.[5] Patients younger than 18 years were excluded. Interestingly, only 19% of these suits involved an emergency physician. Error in diagnosis was the most common claim, and the most frequent diagnoses resulting in payment were "myocardial infarction, acute" and "chest pain, not otherwise defined." Of patients who died, these two conditions ranked first and second, with "aortic aneurysm" third.[5]

Only 7% of the claims involving an event that originated in the emergency department progressed to trial, and of these, only 15% resulted in a verdict for the plaintiff. Settlement without trial was the result in 29% of cases, and the remaining 64% were withdrawn, dropped, or dismissed.[5]

> **KEY POINT**
>
> Most lawsuits involving care originating in the emergency department do not result in payment and do not involve an emergency physician.[5]

What we can learn from these data is that cardiovascular disorders are the major source of litigation, not only for emergency physicians but also for others treating patients in the emergency department. This chapter discusses ways in which we can lower the risk of litigation. The best way to do that is to provide quality medical care, establish a good rapport with our patients and their families, and document well. In this discussion of providing quality medical care for our cardiovascular patients, we will necessarily review some of the same material presented in more detail earlier in this book, but with a specific emphasis on avoiding error in diagnosis and treatment. This chapter may thus serve to reinforce some of the important points made in prior discussions.

The Medical History

Because the electrocardiogram (ECG) and cardiac markers may be unremarkable during the early phase of an acute myocardial infarction (AMI)—and may well remain unremarkable during the entire course of an acute coronary syndrome (ACS)—gathering a meticulous history of the present illness is often the most crucial part of the evaluation of patients with potential acute cardiovascular disorders.

> **KEY POINT**
>
> A meticulous history of the present illness is crucial.

Presenting Complaint

Although a complaint of chest pain certainly raises concern for AMI or ACS, many patients with these emergency conditions do not complain of chest pain. Nonspecific symptoms such as dizziness, weakness, and dyspnea could be the result of an acute cardiac event. This presentation is more common with women and the elderly. The pain may be limited to the epigastrium, arm, or jaw. And, of course, chest pain can be caused by a myriad of other disorders such as acute aortic dissection, pulmonary embolus, pneumonia, esophagitis, or gastrointestinal disorders.

Language

A frequent challenge that emergency physicians face is a language barrier. The physician and patient might speak different languages. But even when they can communicate in a common language, if their native languages are different, important nuance can be lost. Even when the patient and physician speak the same native language, another problem often arises.

Doctor: I understand you've been weak and dizzy. Have you had any chest pain?

Patient: No.

Beyond the obvious difference in technical terminology, patients just do not speak like doctors. To us, "chest pain" includes pressure, aching, burning, and any abnormal chest symptom. But patients who feel burning or pressure might not describe it as "pain" or might actually deny having chest pain when asked. A better approach is to inquire about "chest discomfort or symptoms."

> **KEY POINT**
>
> Beware of language barriers—both inadequate English and nonmedical terminology.

Duration of Symptoms

Doctor: How long have you had pain?

Patient: For the past 24 hours.

Do not confuse duration of an entire set of symptoms with duration of each episode. Continuous chest symptoms for 24 hours with nondiagnostic ECG findings and cardiac markers are not likely to be of cardiac origin. However, chest symptoms occurring intermittently for 24 hours, with each episode lasting 20 minutes, could well be cardiac.

Remember that nondiagnostic ECG findings and cardiac markers do not rule out unstable angina (UA). In fact, they are the hallmark of UA. Missing an ST-elevation MI (STEMI) is not likely. But missing UA is a definite danger if the history is not assessed accurately. The pain might have resolved, and the "diagnostic" studies are nondiagnostic. Failure to diagnose UA, resulting in a bad patient outcome, is a common cause of litigation in emergency medicine.

KEY POINT

Crucial questions that may be helpful regarding duration of symptoms:
- When did the pain begin?
- When did the entire set of symptoms begin?
- When did this specific episode begin?
- When was last time you had *no* symptoms?
- How long was the longest episode?
- How short was the shortest episode?

Quality of the Pain

Chest "pain" might be described as pressure, burning, sharp, dull, or pleuritic. Or, as discussed above, the patient might deny having "pain" but not volunteer another description of the type of chest discomfort.

Exacerbating Factors

Exertional pain raises a concern for cardiac ischemia. If the pain is worse when the patient is lying down or bending over, it could be esophageal. If it is worse when the patient is lying down, better when sitting up and better when bending over, it could be due to pericarditis. But any of these patterns could be indicative of cardiac ischemia.

Pleuritic Chest Pain

A complaint of pain with breathing is a frequent factor in cases leading to litigation. Pleuritic chest pain does not exclude AMI. Cardiac pain, especially infarction, can be worse with breathing. But, in contrast to pulmonary etiologies, non–pleural-based processes such as AMI also cause pain *between breaths*.

KEY POINT

In patients with pleuritic chest pain, always ask if the pain is present between breaths. If it is, think cardiac.

Radiation of Pain

Cardiac pain can be substernal, epigastric, or right sided. It can radiate to either or both arms, the neck, the jaw, the face, or the back. It may thus mimic acute aortic dissection (see discussion below).

Associated Symptoms

Cardiac pain can be associated with dizziness, nausea, dyspnea, palpitations, and especially diaphoresis.

KEY POINT

Diaphoresis accompanying chest pain is particularly suggestive of an acute cardiac event.

Risk Factors

Cardiac risk factors include a history of cardiac pathology, smoking, hypertension, diabetes, hyperlipidemia, obesity, inactivity, age, and family history of early MI. Cocaine use, either acute or chronic, is also a risk factor.

Examination

Tenderness on palpation is a common misleading factor when the diagnosis of ACS or MI is missed, especially in frail, elderly patients, who may find it painful when a clinician presses on the rib cage. Another factor to be considered is whether chest or arm pain with truncal or arm movement *exactly* reproduces the symptoms. This suggests, but does not necessarily prove, a noncardiac etiology.

Electrocardiogram

The ECG is discussed in detail elsewhere in this book. In this section, we briefly summarize some of the issues regarding the ECG that can lead to incorrect diagnosis resulting in litigation.

Doctor: Your ECG shows no abnormalities, so we know you're not having a heart attack.

When the initial ECG is nondiagnostic, comparison of previous or successive ECGs can be crucial to proper diagnosis. A change from earlier ECGs or a change in serial studies during the emergency department course often leads to a diagnosis that might otherwise have been missed from a single ECG. This is particularly important in the presence of left bundle-branch block (LBBB) or a pacemaker, both of which can obscure the signs of AMI, as well as for patients with continuing or recurrent chest pain, in whom the ST changes of AMI can evolve and become apparent only over time. For patients with continuing chest pain, serial ECGs obtained during the first hour are advised if there is any question of AMI. In such patients, if the pain resolves but later recurs, a repeat ECG is indicated.

Left Bundle-Branch Block

A right bundle-branch block (RBBB) will not obscure the signs of AMI, but an LBBB can lead to misdiagnosis. Many analytic criteria have been suggested for diagnosing AMI in the presence of LBBB, the most well-known of which are those of Sgarbossa[6] (see Chapter 2). These criteria, although poorly sensitive, are very specific. In an effort to improve sensitivity, many modifications of the Sgarbossa criteria have been published, but they are often difficult to apply in clinical practice.[7]

What is very important, therefore, is comparison of ECGs. As with any case of suspected AMI or ACS, comparison with previous ECGs and with successive serial ECGs may reveal the acute cardiac event in patients with LBBB.

KEY POINTS

Indicators of AMI in the presence of LBBB according to the Sgarbossa criteria[6]:

- Paradoxic ST-segment concordance with QRS larger than 1 mm
- Exaggerated ST-segment discordance with QRS larger than 5 mm
- ST segment depression of more than 1 mm in leads V_1, V_2, or V_3

Serial ECGs and comparison with previous studies can be crucial to diagnosing AMI in patients with nondiagnostic studies. This is particularly important in patients with continuing symptoms, recurrent symptoms, LBBB, or a pacemaker.

Early Repolarization

The ST-segment elevation of early repolarization (addressed in Chapter 2) might be misdiagnosed as AMI or, alternatively, an AMI might be misdiagnosed as early repolarization. In early repolarization, the elevated ST segments are usually found in the precordial leads. If they also appear in the limb leads, there is no correlation with an anatomic vessel. This is in contrast to AMI, in which the ST elevation usually reflects a specific vascular pattern such as anterior or inferior wall MI.

With early repolarization, the ST segment appears normal; it just "takes off" at a higher place, that is, the J point is elevated. The ST segment of early repolarization is usually concave upward. With AMI, however, the ST segment usually looks abnormal. It might be concave upward but more commonly is convex upward. And, importantly, in contrast to AMI, there are no reciprocal changes in early repolarization.

KEY POINT

Clues to differentiating early repolarization from AMI:

- ST elevation corresponding to an anatomic vessel in AMI
- Reciprocal changes reflecting AMI
- An abnormal appearance of the elevated ST segment in AMI
- Prior ECGs show similar ST segments with early repolarization

Pericarditis

As with early repolarization, acute pericarditis can be confused with AMI and vice versa. Pericarditis is characterized by diffuse ST elevation not corresponding to anatomic vessels. Another finding of acute pericarditis may be PR depression, particularly in the inferior limb leads and the lateral precordial leads V_5 and V_6. Although often not present, PR depression, when present, is a strong indicator of pericarditis.

PR elevation and ST depression can be seen in lead aVR. These findings are also suggestive of pericarditis, although they are not specific.

Over time, T waves in pericarditis may invert, but only *after* the elevated ST segments have returned to baseline. In contrast,

FIGURE 21-1.

Pulmonary embolus. $S_1Q_3T_3$ and T-wave inversion in precordial and inferior leads plus an incomplete RBBB pattern. This combination strongly suggests right heart strain from a large pulmonary embolus.

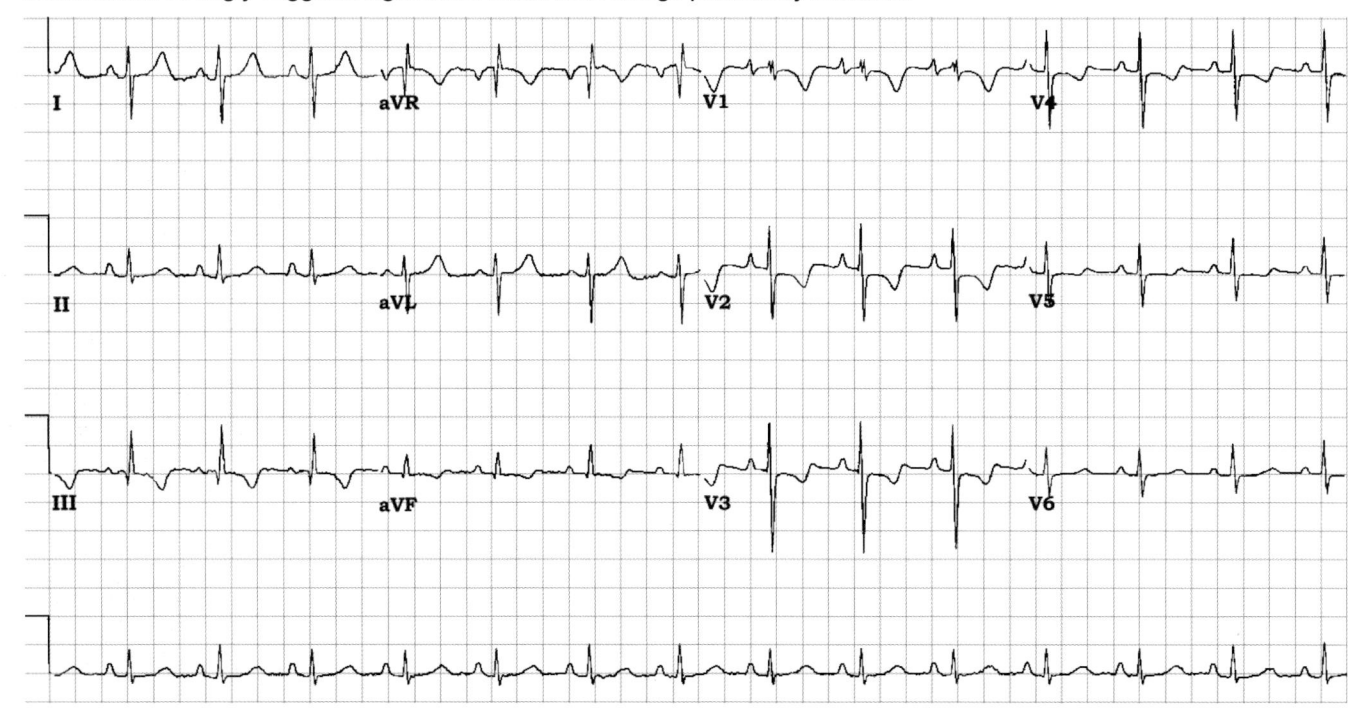

with AMI, the T waves begin to invert *while* the ST segments are still elevated. Pericarditis is discussed in more detail in Chapter 14.

KEY POINT

To distinguish pericarditis from MI, look for the following:

ST elevation that corresponds to an anatomic vascular distribution. If present, think AMI.

PR depression, which strongly suggests pericarditis.

T-wave inversion in the presence of ST elevation. This is not pericarditis: think AMI.

Posterior Wall MI

Although the ECG findings of acute posterior wall MI (see Chapter 2) are often not recognized, it is fortunate that most posterior wall MIs accompany the more obvious signs of inferior MI. They are sometimes present with lateral MI. However, up to 4% to 5% of cases of acute MI present as isolated posterior wall infarcts,[8] and this can easily be missed.

In most ECGs, the R wave in leads V_1 to V_3 is smaller than the S wave. However, an R wave larger than the S is suggestive of posterior MI. ST depression in the same leads is also an indicator, which can easily be misdiagnosed as septal ischemia. This error can be prevented by obtaining posterior leads V_8 and V_9, which will reveal the ST elevation of MI.

KEY POINT

R larger than S with ST depression in V_1 to V_3 is highly suggestive of acute posterior wall MI.

Pulmonary Embolus (Figure 21-1)

The classic ECG findings that suggest pulmonary embolus are a new S wave in lead I and a new Q and an inverted T wave in lead III ($S_1Q_3T_3$). However, although these findings are "classic," they actually are neither sensitive nor specific. They could reflect a previous inferior MI. They can also be seen with other causes of right ventricular strain such as pulmonary hypertension, pneumothorax, and bronchospasm.

A significant shift of the QRS axis toward the right compared with previous ECGs might suggest acute right heart strain, possibly due to pulmonary embolus. A tall R wave in lead V_1, or an incomplete right bundle-branch pattern, is another finding that suggests right heart strain.

Another sign of pulmonary embolus is T-wave inversion, which may be found especially in cases of large pulmonary emboli. T-wave inversion tends to occur most commonly in the right precordial leads but can appear in the inferior leads as well (Figure 21-1).

Prolonged QT Interval

This discussion of ECGs so far has dealt with diagnosing AMI and pulmonary embolus. Other ECG patterns can reflect potentially serious disorders that, if missed, could be deleterious to our patients and lead to litigation.

Prolonged QT interval is one of these patterns. The QTc (c = corrected for heart rate) is normally less than 450 msec. Patients with intervals larger than 500 msec are at significantly increased risk for sudden polymorphic ventricular tachycardia (torsade de pointes), which can deteriorate to ventricular fibrillation. Arrhythmia can be precipitated by exercise or by a long list of medications that can prolong the QT interval. That list is nearly endless and will not be delineated here. It includes a number of antibiotics (particularly macrolides and quinolones) and many antipsychotic medications. Electrolyte disorders can also prolong the QTc, as can a few other less common causes.

Torsade de pointes typically produces sudden death if not recognized and treated immediately. If the arrhythmia resolves spontaneously, patients might present simply complaining of an episode of lightheadedness, palpitations, or syncope, or they might even report a seizure. When these patients come to the emergency department for care, an ECG typically demonstrates the prolonged QTc. If the diagnosis is missed, the patient could go on to experience sudden death. Patients who present with syncope or near-syncope and who have a prolonged QTc should be admitted for a workup of the underlying cause (see Chapter 11). If a reversible cause is not found, implantation of a defibrillator should be considered.

KEY POINTS

In patients with syncope or near-syncope, particularly during exertion:

Check the ECG for a prolonged QTc interval.

Evaluate their medications for those that might prolong the QTc interval.

Check their electrolytes and correct them as needed.

If the ECG reveals a prolonged QTc interval in any patient, try to avoid prescribing medications that could exacerbate this problem.

In syncope associated with exercise, consider the following:

Myocardial ischemia

Arrhythmia

Prolonged QTc interval

Hypertrophic cardiomyopathy, especially in young patients

Brugada Syndrome

Another condition that has recently gained increased attention from the emergency medicine community is Brugada syndrome. A congenital abnormality, it can lead to sudden ventricular tachycardia and fibrillation. Patients can present with syncope or sudden death. In contrast to syncope in patients with prolonged QTc, which can be precipitated by exertion, arrhythmia in people with Brugada syndrome often occurs at rest.

In this condition, the ECG is characterized by RBBB or an incomplete RBBB pattern with ST elevation in leads V_1 to V_2 but without the typical S wave in V_6 that would normally be present with RBBB. Brugada syndrome and other potential deadly conditions identifiable on the ECG are discussed further in Chapter 11.

> **KEY POINT**
>
> In patients with sudden syncope, particularly at rest, evaluate the ECG for signs of Brugada syndrome: RBBB or incomplete RBBB pattern with ST elevation in leads V_1 to V_2 without a wide S wave in V_6.

Cardiac Markers

Doctor: Your blood test for heart attack is normal and you've had pain for 6 hours, so we know you're not having a heart attack.

Cardiac makers are discussed at length in Chapter 3. The important medicolegal issue regarding markers is that they remain normal in UA, and they could be normal early in the course of an AMI. As with the ECG, serial marker studies are indicated if there is a question of AMI and the initial value is normal.

> **KEY POINTS**
>
> Cardiac markers remain normal with UA.
>
> Cardiac markers might be normal during the first hours of AMI, whether STEMI or NSTEMI.
>
> If MI is suspected, obtain serial marker measurements.
>
> Look for abnormal values as well as rising values within the normal range.

Differential Diagnosis

STEMI, NSTEMI, and UA

As discussed above, undiagnosed UA leading to MI and/or sudden death is a major cause of litigation in emergency medicine.[1] The pain has resolved and both serial markers and serial ECGs remain nondiagnostic. But even if the diagnosis of an acute cardiac event is established, it is important to differentiate between STEMI, NSTEMI, and UA. Table 21-1 summarizes the differences between these three entities.

The differential diagnosis of chest pain includes a number of potentially serious, as well as less serious, disorders in addition to acute cardiac events. Misdiagnosis can be in either direction (Table 21-2).

Aortic Dissection

Treatment of ACS typically involves antiplatelet and anticoagulant medications and, in the case of STEMI, a fibrinolytic agent as well. These medications can be disastrous if the true diagnosis is acute aortic dissection. A more common cause of litigation, however, is missing the diagnosis of aortic dissection after a negative workup for AMI or ACS.[1] It is thus critical to distinguish acute cardiac from acute aortic pathology and to make the correct diagnosis if either is present.

The symptoms accompanying dissection can be extremely variable.[9-11] Chest pain radiating to the back is often considered a hallmark of thoracic aortic dissection. But according to the *International Registry* of *Acute Aortic Dissection*, "back pain" was reported as a symptom in only 53% of cases, and "posterior chest pain" in only 36%.[9] (It is not clear how much overlap existed between the two patient populations.)

> **KEY POINT**
>
> Although chest pain radiating to the back suggests aortic dissection, the absence of back pain does not rule it out.

Other evidence of dissection might include differential pulses between the right arm and the other extremities, because most dissections begin in the aortic arch distal to the origin of the blood supply to the right arm (the brachiocephalic artery and its subdivision, the right subclavian artery). Neurologic signs and symptoms might reflect impaired cerebral or spinal circulation. The chest film might reveal a widened mediastinum, left pleural effusion, or other signs of dissection. A new aortic insufficiency murmur is strongly suggestive of dissection. An echocardiogram can reveal a pericardial effusion. And, of course, a computed tomography angiogram (CTA) is usually diagnostic[12] (Table 21-3).

Pulmonary Embolus

This potentially fatal condition can be missed easily in patients evaluated for a cardiac event. Indicators of pulmonary embolism (PE) include dyspnea, hypoxia, recent surgery or in-

TABLE 21-1.

ECG Findings and Cardiac Markers in STEMI, NSTEMI, and UA

STEMI
Elevated ST segments in anatomic leads
Elevated markers
Both can be nondiagnostic early in the course
NSTEMI
Nondiagnostic ECG
Elevated markers
UA
Nondiagnostic ECG
Normal markers

TABLE 21-2.

Differential Diagnosis (partial) of Chest Pain

Aortic dissection
Pulmonary embolus
Chest wall tenderness
Gastrointestinal
Gastrointestinal gas
Esophagitis
Esophageal spasm

activity, limb immobilization, pleuritic chest pain with minimal, if any, pain between breaths, normal breath sounds or sometimes wheezing, unexplained tachycardia, an ECG with $S_1Q_3T_3$ and/or inverted precordial T waves, an elevated D-dimer level, and findings of deep vein thrombosis either clinically or by ultrasonography. Ventilation-perfusion scanning of the lungs or CTA may reveal the diagnosis (Table 21-4).

Gastrointestinal Symptoms

Gastrointestinal symptoms often mimic acute cardiac ischemia. The patient might have a history of esophageal reflux disease. Gastrointestinal symptoms are generally caused by one or more of the following entities: gastrointestinal gas, esophagitis, or esophageal spasm.

Gastrointestinal Gas

Gastrointestinal gas can cause epigastric pain or chest pain. The pain can be pleuritic and either present or absent between breaths.

Esophagitis

Esophagitis generally causes a burning substernal pain, which may be worse if the patient is lying down or bending over. It might be exacerbated by eating and relieved by antacids.

A "GI cocktail" containing antacids is often used to distinguish esophagitis from cardiac ischemia. Countless lawsuits have been based on false conclusions from this "test." Cardiac pain can be experienced as burning. Both UA and esophageal "heartburn" can be intermittent. If the symptoms resolve following the antacid, there might or might not be a causal relationship. If the symptoms are not relieved within a minute or two after swallowing the antacid, the test is probably worthless. And even if there is a close temporal relationship, a conclusion of gastrointestinal etiology might not be accurate.

KEY POINT

Many lawsuits result from misdiagnosis based on resolution of pain following a "GI cocktail."

Esophageal Spasm

Esophageal spasm typically causes a pressure-type substernal pain. It may even radiate down the left arm. It is often not relieved by antacid. Like angina, it might be abolished by nitroglycerin, a smooth-muscle relaxant. Many patients admitted to the hospital or observation unit to rule out MI have esophageal spasm. But because the symptoms of esophageal spasm and MI are so similar, it is best to consider such symptoms as cardiac until it is proved otherwise (Table 21-5).

Pneumonia versus Heart Failure

In addition to patients with chest pain, dyspneic patients also present a potential medicolegal risk for emergency physicians.

Acute heart failure and pneumonia can be difficult to distinguish. Sudden onset is more typical of acute pulmonary edema, but pneumonia can also present acutely. Both generally cause rales on lung auscultation. The rales of mild heart failure can be more prominent over the inferior lung fields. The rales of pneumonia can be unilateral or more localized than those of heart failure. However, the two entities can be difficult to distinguish based on lung auscultation alone.

The neck veins might be distended in patients with heart failure. B-type natriuretic peptide (BNP) or N-terminal pro-BNP levels are elevated in patients with heart failure but do not distinguish acute from chronic. The white blood cell count and lactate level might be elevated in pneumonia. A history of heart failure as well as the patient's medication list may point in one direction or the other (Table 21-6).

Treatment

Most lawsuits involving cardiovascular problems in emergency medicine involve failure to diagnose.[1] Much less common is litigation based on treatment decisions. A few potential areas of concern are discussed here.

Time to treatment of acute MI is occasionally a factor in litigation. As discussed in Chapter 5, rapid treatment of AMI with either a lytic agent or percutaneous coronary intervention saves

TABLE 21-3.

Factors That Can Help in Diagnosing Acute Aortic Dissection

Sudden onset of extreme chest or upper back pain
Pulse deficits
Neurologic signs and symptoms
Chest radiograph
Echocardiogram
CTA

TABLE 21-4.

Factors That Can Help in Diagnosing Pulmonary Embolus

Dyspnea
Hypoxia
Recent surgery or inactivity
Limb immobilization
Pleuritic chest pain with little, if any, pain between breaths
Normal breath sounds or sometimes wheezing
Unexplained tachycardia
ECG with $S_1Q_3T_3$ and/or inverted precordial T waves
Elevated D-dimer
Deep vein thrombosis, either clinically or by ultrasonography
Ventilation/perfusion scan
CTA

CARDIOVASCULAR EMERGENCIES

cardiac muscle. Although logistics often preclude strict compliance with published guidelines, every attempt should be made to minimize time to treatment.

Another potential area of concern is the *treatment of wide complex tachycardias*. These can be associated with an underlying preexcitation syndrome such as Wolff-Parkinson-White (WPW). (Differentiation of ventricular tachycardia from supraventricular tachycardia with aberration is discussed in Chapter 10.)

In the presence of an underlying preexcitation syndrome such as WPW, drugs that slow conduction through the AV node can shift conduction to an accessory pathway, leading to a more rapid and potentially lethal tachycardia. Therefore, drugs to be avoided in the treatment of wide complex tachycardia include beta-blockers, calcium channel blockers, and digoxin. Appropriate treatment depends on the type of rhythm, but, in general, safe choices for treating wide complex tachycardias include procainamide, magnesium, lidocaine, and cardioversion. Amiodarone is a reasonable option as well if atrial fibrillation with WPW syndrome is not a concern.

KEY POINTS

With wide complex tachycardias, avoid beta-blockers, calcium channel blockers, and digoxin.

Depending on the specific rhythm, safe treatment choices can include:

- Amiodarone
- Procainamide
- Magnesium
- Lidocaine
- Cardioversion

TABLE 21-5.

Gastrointestinal Causes of Chest Pain

Gastrointestinal gas
Epigastric or chest pain
May be pleuritic
May be present or absent between breaths
Esophagitis
Usually a burning substernal pain
May be worse supine or bending over
May be exacerbated by eating and relieved by antacids
Esophageal spasm
Substernal pain, often pressure
May radiate down left arm
Often not relieved by antacid
May be relieved by nitroglycerin

Documentation and Communication

A few final comments are relevant to all emergency department patients.

Be sure to review the paramedic notes if they are available. If they are not, it is advisable to document that fact.

Nursing notes are also important. Be aware that many are written during the course of the patient's emergency department stay—and often after the patient has been discharged.

The patient's medication list provides a rapid clue to the medical history and perhaps to the cause of the current problem.

KEY POINT

Paramedic notes, nursing notes, and medication lists are important. Read them. Be aware that such notes might be entered into the medical record after you have completed your charting.

If confidentiality is not an issue, engage the patient's family in discussion. Remember that if the patient dies, it is the family who will sue. Also important is that many cardiac patients, especially men, are in denial. Many of them come to the hospital only at the insistence of their family. The family might provide crucial information omitted by the patient.

KEY POINTS

Family members are important.
- They can provide crucial information.
- They can help the patient understand the situation and the after-care instructions.
- In many ways, they are your patients also. They might need to be comforted.
- If the patient dies, they are the ones who might sue.

As stated previously, most lawsuits against emergency physicians treating cardiovascular patients involve misdiagnosis.[1] Most of these patients have been discharged from the emergency department. If there is litigation, an unanticipated bad outcome has usually occurred. The diagnostic modalities currently available to us are not perfect. It is inevitable that some patients with UA will be discharged. But even those for whom discharge was appropriate can meet an unfortunate outcome. Therefore, communication and documentation are absolutely crucial.

It is advisable to never tell a patient that his or her symptoms are not cardiac in origin or that a cardiac condition has been "ruled out." We really cannot absolutely rule out a cardiac event

TABLE 21-6.

Common Causes of Acute Dyspnea

Bronchospasm
Heart failure
Pneumonia
Pulmonary embolus

in the emergency department. What we should tell the patient and the family is that our evaluation finds no evidence of an acute cardiac event, but that there are no 100% guarantees. The importance of close followup should be stressed, along with information regarding symptoms that would warrant immediate return to the emergency department. If appropriate, followup evaluation should be arranged. This discussion should be documented, including the presence of relevant family members.

If the patient refuses admission and leaves against medical advice, explain the potential consequences, arrange for appropriate followup if possible, and encourage the patient to return if he or she has a change of mind. Document all of this as well as the presence of those who witnessed the conversation.

The medical record is absolutely critical, not only to winning a malpractice lawsuit but also to avoiding a suit in the first place. Assuming your care was appropriate, your record should provide such a thorough explanation of the rationale for your decisions that any subsequent reading by an attorney or an expert witness should preclude litigation. You should not have to explain in front of a jury years later why you sent that patient with chest pain home. Your record should explain your thought process sufficiently, so that the prospective plaintiff's attorney and the physician expert reviewer will conclude that your care met the standard expected.

KEY POINT

Your chart should explain the rationale for your decisions so well that review years later will prevent litigation.

If you are sued, remember that you are not alone. Most physicians face litigation during our careers. It is important not to allow the emotional stress of a lawsuit to invade either your own sense of well-being or that of your family. Many local medical societies can provide resources to assist you. The American College of Emergency Physicians has a number of resources available to its members, including a panel to evaluate unscientific testimony as well as resources for emotional support.[13]

Finally, the best way to avoid being sued is to provide the best emergency medical care that you can. Keep an open mind, consider all possibilities, and be ready to question your initial assumptions. Never forget the importance of good communication with the patient and the family. And remember to *document well*.

References

1. Risk Management Review. *Emergency Medicine, January 1, 1985–December 31, 2010*. Rockville, MD: Physician Insurers Association of America; 2011.
2. Jena AB, Seabury S, Lakdawalla D, Chandra A. Malpractice risk according to physician specialty. *N Engl J Med*. 2011;365(7):629-636.
3. Kane D. Policy Research Perspectives – Medical Liability Claims Frequency: A 2007–2008 Snapshot of Physicians. Chicago, Illinois: American Medical Association; 2010:1-7.
4. Studdert DM, Mello MM, Gawande AA, et al. Claims, errors, and compensation payments in medical malpractice litigation. *N Engl J Med*. 2006;354(19):2024-2033.
5. Brown TW, McCarthy ML, Kelen GD, Levy F. An epidemiologic study of closed emergency department malpractice claims in a national database of physician malpractice insurers. *Acad Emerg Med*. 2010;17(5):553-560.
6. Sgarbossa EB, Pinski SL, Barbagelata A, et al. Electrocardiographic diagnosis of evolving acute myocardial infarction in the presence of left bundle-branch block. *N Engl J Med*. 1996;334(8):481-487.
7. Smith SW, Dodd KW, Henry TD, et al. Diagnosis of ST-elevation myocardial infarction in the presence of left bundle-branch block with the ST-elevation to S-wave ratio in a modified Sgarbossa rule. *Ann Emerg Med*. 2012;60(6):766-776.
8. Anderson JL, Adams CD, Antman EM, et al. ACC/AHA 2007 guidelines for the management of patients with unstable angina/non-ST-elevation myocardial infarction. *Circulation*. 2007;116(7):e148-e304.
9. Hagan PG, Nienaber CA, Isselbacher EM, et al. The International Registry of Acute Aortic Dissection (IRAD): new insights into an old disease. *JAMA*. 2000;283(7):897-903.
10. Harris KM, Strauss CE, Eagle KA, et al. Correlates of delayed recognition and treatment of acute type A aortic dissection. The International Registry of Acute Aortic Dissection (IRAD). *Circulation*. 2011;124(18):1911-1918.
11. Miller DC, Stinson EB, Oyer PE, et al. Operative treatment of aortic dissections. Experience with 125 patients over a sixteen-year period. *J Thorac Cardiovasc Surg*. 1979;78(3):365-382.
12. Hiratzka LF, Bakris GL, Beckman JA, et al. 2010 ACCF/AHA/AATS/ACR/ASA/SCA/SCAI/SIR/STS/SVM guidelines for the diagnosis and management of patients with thoracic aortic disease. *Circulation*. 2010;121(13):e266-e369.
13. Andrew L. We are not malpractice magnets! *ACEP News*. November 2012:19.

CARDIOVASCULAR EMERGENCIES

Index

A

abdominal aorta, emergencies, 86f
abdominal aortic aneurysms (AAAs), ultrasound, 86f
accelerated diagnostic protocol (ADP), 43-44
acetazolamide, 234
ACUITY trial, 99
action potentials, creation of, 131
acute aortic dissection, 236, 307t
acute chest pain, approach to, 1-10
acute coronary syndrome (ACS), 1-2
    adjunctive therapy, 96-100
    biomarkers, 37-51
    bradyarrhythmias related to, 138-139
    in cancer patients, 251
    causes of, 1
    "classic" presentation, 1-2
    clinical decision rules, 7-8
    ECG abnormalities predictive of, 21-22
    electrocardiogram in, 11-35, 11t
    HIV and, 243
    imaging, 37-51
    initial diagnostic testing, 40f
    myocardial infarction and, 243-244
    myocardial ischemia and, 37-38
    risk stratification, 45
    symptom evaluation, 38t
    T-wave inversion in, 16f
acute decompensated heart failure (ADHF)
    emergency department visits for, 296-297
    observation unit criteria, 298f
acute heart failure (AHF), 111-127, 237. see also heart failure
    ancillary tests, 113-117
    clinical presentation, 113
    definition of, 111-112
    diagnosis, 113
    hypertensive, 119-121, 121f
    hypotensive, 122-124, 123f
    initial management, 117-119, 119t
    management, 120f, 121f
    normotensive, 121-122, 122f
    pathophysiology, 112-113
    patient characteristics, 114t-115t
    prognostic factors, 118t
acute kidney injury, 202
acute myocardial infarction (AMI). see also myocardial infarction (MI)
    cardiogenic shock and, 103
    definition of, 5
    medical history, 302
    posterior, 23f
acute myocarditis, 34
acute myopericarditis, 34
acute renal failure, 237
adenosine
    in AV nodal blockade, 157
    cardiac stress use, 48t
    mechanism of action, 277
    in pregnancy, 249
    in PVST, 156
adjunctive therapy, ACS, 96-100
AED
    geographic mapping of, 194
airway adjuncts, 190
airways, advanced, 190
albumin, cardiac, 43
alkylating agents, cardiomyopathy and, 250
alpha-adrenergic agonists, 235
alpha-adrenergic blockers, 235
alpha-adrenergic receptors, 271
alpha methyldopa, 235
American College of Cardiology, 40, 42
American College of Emergency Physicians (ACEP), 54t
amlodipine, 233
amiodarone, 145-146
    contraindications, 249t
    CPR and, 191-192
    indications, 273t
    IV, 175
    mechanism of action, 274
    in pregnancy, 249
    for PVST, 153-154
AMIS plus registry, 106
amphetamine toxicity, 237
analgesics, 93-94
angiotensin-converting enzyme (ACE) inhibitors, 93
    afterload reduction and, 121
    in congestive heart failure, 278
    contraindications, 249t
    for hypertension, 233-234
    teratogenicity, 248
angiotensin II, 232f, 233t
angiotensin II receptor blockers (ARBs), 234
anterior STEMI
    description of, 19
    ST-segment elevation, 19f
anterolateral STEMI, 20f
anthracyclines, cardiomyopathy and, 250
antiarrhythmic drugs
    CPR and, 191-192
    mechanisms of action, 272-273
    for narrow complex tachycardias, 275
    for wide complex tachycardias, 274-275
anticoagulant therapy, 99
antidromic conduction, 163
antihypertensive agents, 238t
    case studies, 269
    indications, 272t
    during pregnancy, 249

antiretroviral (ARV) therapies, 243-244
aortic aneurysms, malpractice cases, 302
aortic dissection, 3
   acute, 236
   computed tomography angiography, 6
   differential diagnosis, 306
   echocardiography, 57
   ultrasound, 86f
aortic valve, echocardiography, 64f
apical views
   5-chamber, 67f
   anatomic correlation, 61, 66f
   echocardiography, 66f
   probe position, 59f, 61, 66f
   pulmonary emboli, 79, 81
ARMYDA 6 trial, 97
arrhythmias. *see also* specific arrhythmias
   in cancer patients, 252
   cardiac transplants and, 265-266
   pacemaker-mediated, 289
   during pregnancy, 249
   in pulmonary hypertension, 261-262
arsenic trioxide, 252
ascites, pericardial fluid versus, 67, 76f
Aspergillus infection, 265
aspirin
   adjunctive therapy using, 96
   in pericarditis, 215
   safety in pregnancy, 248
assisted circulation devices, complications, 289-291
atenolol, 249, 249t
atherosclerotic plaques, 37
atorvastatin, 80
atrial fibrillation (AF)
   cardiac transplants and, 265-266
   cardioversion, 147
   emergency department observation, 297-299
   electrocardiogram, 274f
   MAT with, 159f
   mechanism of, 146
   NCT and, 144f, 145
   observation pathway, 299f
   in pregnancy, 249
   with rapid ventricular response, 146f
   wide QRS complexes with, 166f
atrial flutter
   atrial fibrillation and, 146
   cardiac transplants and, 265-266
   NCT focus, 146f
   in pregnancy, 249
   with variable conduction, 151f
   ventricular rate of 150 bpm, 151f
atrioventricular (AV) block
   beta receptors, 270
   case studies, 134-140
   first-degree, 133, 134, 134f
   Mobitz I, 135, 135f
   Mobitz II, 135, 136f
   second-degree, 133-135
   third-degree, 133, 136-137, 137f, 138f
atrioventricular (AV) node, 133
atropine
   CPR and, 191
   hemodynamic compromise and, 132
   SA nodal discharge and, 138
AV block, 130
AV nodal reciprocating tachycardia (AVNRT), 158f, 266
AV node blocking agents, 145
AV reentrant tachycardia (AVRT), 156f
   AVNRT compared with, 158f

B

B-mode ultrasound, 53
B-type natriuretic peptide (BNP), 43, 116, 181, 307
"bangungut," 168
Beck triad, 4
bedside echocardiography, 116
bedside ultrasound, 53-89, 106
benzodiazepines, 237
beta-adrenergic antagonists, 269-270
   in AV nodal blockade, 157
   contraindications, 121, 249t
   dosages, 270t
   for hypertension, 233, 234t
   in NCTs, 145
   nonselective, 269
   in pregnancy, 249
   for PVST, 153-154
   selective, 269
   subtypes of, 269-270
   toxicity, 140, 280-282
beta-blockers. *see* beta-adrenergic antagonists
beta-receptor antagonists, 92-93
bilevel positive airway pressure (BiPAP), 118
biomarkers
   chest pain evaluation, 6
   kinetics of elevation, 41f
   myocardial infarction, 39-40
   summary, 43
bivalirudin, 99
blood pressure. *see also* hypertension; hypotension
   asymptomatic markedly elevated, 238
   autoregulation, 230-231, 231f
   emergency department management, 230t
   hypertensive emergencies, 227-241
blood urea nitrogen (BUN), 116-117
bradyarrhythmias, 129-141
   in cancer patients, 252
   diagnosis, 131-140
   exogenous causes, 139-140
   initial management, 129-130
   mechanisms, 131
   metabolic causes, 139
   neurologic causes, 139-140
   toxins and, 140
   treatment, 131-140
bradycardia
   cardiac transplants and, 265
   causes of, 131t
brain stem reflexes, impaired, 203
brainstem ischemia, 179
Brugada syndrome, 168, 174
   arrhythmias and, 178

assessment of, 305-306
electrocardiogram, 182f
syncope in, 181
bundle-branch block (BBB). *see also* left bundle-branch block (LBBB); right bundle-branch block (RBBB)
rate-related, 163
ventricular paced rhythms and, 28f

C

C-reactive protein (CRP), 43
calcium channel blockers (CCBs), 93, 270
categories, 270
contraindications, 121
for hypertension, 233, 234t
in NCT, 145
overdoses, 140
for PVST, 153-154
toxicity, 280-282
calcium sorting computed tomography, 38-39, 44t
calcium sorting coronary computed tomography, 46-47
cancer patients
acute coronary syndrome in, 251
arrhythmias in, 252
cardiac disease in, 250-252
myocardial infarction in, 251
pericardial disease in, 251-252
Candida infections, 265
CAPTIM trial, 94
carbonic anhydrase inhibitors, 234
cardiac allograft vasculopathy (CAV), 266
cardiac arrest
causes of, 250
focused echocardiography, 86-87
modern management of, 187-199
in pregnancy, 249-250
cardiac catheterization, diagnostic, 47-48
cardiac cells, types of, 131
cardiac conduction, normal, 130
cardiac imaging, 45
cardiac magnetic resonance imaging (CMR), 48-49, 215
cardiac markers, 306
cardiac power, concept of, 104
cardiac syncope, 178-179
cardiac tamponade
chest pain in, 3-4
echocardiogram, 58f, 69-73
right atrial collapse and, 77f
right ventricular collapse, 78f
cardiac toxidromes, 140
cardiac transplants, 262-266
acute rejection, 264-265
immunosuppression in, 263-264
infections, 265
physiology of, 262-264
cardiac wheezing, 113
cardiogenic shock, 103-110
assessments, 105-106
case study, 279
causes of, 104t
epidemiology, 103
etiology, 104

hemodynamic monitoring, 106
management algorithm, 105
medical management, 106-107
metoprolol and, 92
pathophysiology, 105
pharmacologic management, 279-280
postresuscitation, 202
prediction scores, 104-105, 104t
presentation, 105-106
reperfusion, 106
resuscitation, 105-106
risk factors, 93, 104-105
RUSH protocol, 87t
stabilization, 106
therapeutic decision making, 280
cardiomyopathy, 179
antiretroviral therapy and, 257
in cancer patients, 250-251
cyclophosphamide and, 250-251
dilated, 250-251
postpartum, 248
in pregnancy, 248
cardiopulmonary resuscitation (CPR)
bystander, 187
evidence-based care, 194f
feedback devices, 188
future directions, 194-195
pharmacology, 191-192
during pregnancy, 250
recommendations versus actual performance, 188
regionalization of care, 192-193, 193t
ventilation during, 191
cardioversion
electrical, 147
in pregnancy, 249
synchronized direct-current (DC), 147
carotid sinus hypersensitivity, 179
carvedilol, mechanism of, 269
central venous pressure (CVP), 72f
cerebral edema, ICP and, 201
chaotic atrial rhythm. see multifocal atrial tachycardia
chaotic atrial tachycardia. *see* multifocal atrial tachycardia
chest compressions, 188-189, 188f, 192
chest pain
causes of, 2t
differential diagnosis, 306t
emergency department observation units, 294-295
evaluation algorithm, 295f
gastrointestinal causes of, 308t
pleuritic, 303
chest radiographs (CXR)
in acute heart failure, 113-114
chest pain evaluation, 4-5
pulmonary capillary wedge pressure and, 116t
in pulmonary hypertension, 258
chlorthalidone, 234
chronic renal failure, 228
circulatory support, 188
circulatory support devices, 107-108
CK-MB, elevation, 41f
clevidipine, 233, 234, 236
clonidine, 235, 271

clopidogrel, 96-97
cocaine
 sinus tachycardia and, 147f
 toxicity of, 237
colchicine, 215
coma, 203
COMMIT trial, 92
communication, malpractice-related to, 308-309
complete heart block. *see* atrioventricular (AV) block, third-degree
compression-to-ventilation ratios, 188
computed tomography (CT)
 calcium-sorting, 44t
 in pulmonary hypertension, 258
computed tomography angiography (CTA), 6
concealed accessory tracts, 163
congestive heart failure (CHF)
 case study, 278
 emergency department observation, 296-297
 management of, 278-279
 therapeutic decision making, 279
coronary anatomy, 18f, 19
coronary arteries
 dissection, 247
 occlusion, 45-46, 95
coronary artery bypass grafting (CABG), 106
coronary artery disease (CAD)
 ACS and, 37
 ACS evaluation, 44t
 HIV and, 243
 nonobstructive, 37-38
 obstructive, 37-38
coronary atherosclerosis, 37
coronary computed tomography angiography (CCTA), 6-7
 in ACS evaluation, 44t
 coronary artery disease and, 47
 post-contrast, 47f
corticosteroids, adverse effects of, 263
creatine kinase (CK), 41f
creatine phosphokinase (CPK), 41f
CREDO trial, 97
cricoid pressure, 190
CRUSADE trial, 93
Cryptococcus infection, 265
cyclophosphamide, cardiomyopathy and, 250-251
cyclosporine, adverse effects of, 263
cytomegalovirus (CMV), 265

D

D-dimer assays, 6
DAVIT (Danish Verapamil Infarction Trial), 93
DeBakey classification, 3
defibrillation, 189-190
defibrillators
 energy type, 189
 timing of, 189
 type, 189
diastolic heart failure, 73
digoxin
 bradycardia and, 131
 in pregnancy, 249
 safety in pregnancy, 248

toxicity, 280-282
dilated cardiomyopathy, 250-251
diltiazem, 233
 in AV nodal blockade, 157
 for hypertension, 234
 indications, 273t
 mechanism of action, 276
 for PVST, 153
dipyridamole, 48t
disopyramide, indications, 273t
distributive shock, RUSH protocol, 87t
diuresis, 122, 279
diuretics, 234-235
dobutamine
 cardiac stress use, 48t
 for cardiogenic shock, 280
 dosing, 124t
 in hypotensive AHF, 123, 124
 indications, 107
 mechanism of action, 107t, 124t
 in pulmonary hypertension, 260
documentation, malpractice-related to, 308-309
dofetilide, 165f
dopamine
 for cardiogenic shock, 279-280
 characteristics, 130t
 dosing, 124t
 in hypotensive AHF, 123, 124
 indications, 107
 mechanism of action, 107t, 124t
 in sinus bradycardia, 132
Doppler ultrasound
 aorta view, 69f
 color-flow, 53, 71
 echocardiography and, 53
 inferior vena cava view, 69f
 pulsed-wave, 53, 71
DOSE trial, 122
doxazosin, 235
doxorubicin, cardiomyopathy and, 250
DuraHeart, 108
dyspnea, causes of, 308t

E

E-point septal separation (EPSS), 57f, 75
early repolarization, misdiagnosis, 304
echocardiography
 anatomic correlation, 55-57
 apical four-chambered view, 45f
 apical window, 61
 B-mode ultrasound, 53
 basic concepts, 53-55
 bedside, 116
 in cardiac arrest, 86-87
 cardiac preset, 53
 Doppler ultrasound, 53
 inferior vena cava, 61, 63
 M-mode ultrasound, 53
 parasternal long-axis view, 55, 58f
 probe position, 55
 probe selection, 53

proximal aortic aneurysm, 62f
in pulmonary hypertension, 258-259, 259f
sonographic windows, 55-61
standard windows, 59f
stress, 48
subxiphoid window, 59
echocardiography, resting, 44t, 45-46
echocardiography, stress, 44t
eclampsia, 237
ectopic beats, in pregnancy, 249
Ehlers-Danlos syndrome, 3
ejection fraction (EF), 77, 80f
elastin, atrial wall, 228
electrical alternans, 217, 218f
electrical cardioversion, 249
electrocardiogram (ECG)
  12-lead, 11-12
  15-lead, 22-24, 24t
  15-lead, placement of, 28f
  80-lead, 24
  in acute coronary syndrome, 11-35, 11t
  in acute heart failure, 114-115
  additional leads in ACS, 22-24
  in atrial fibrillation, 149-150
  in atrial flutter, 150
  body mapping, 24
  in cardiogenic shock, 106t
  causes of ST elevation, 4t
  chest pain evaluation, 4
  confounding patterns, 26-32
  predictive features, 22
  in pulmonary hypertension, 257-258, 257t, 258f
  regional correlations, 19t
  in risk management, 303-306
  serial monitoring, 24-25
  in sinus tachycardia, 149
  in syncope, 181
electrolytes
  abnormalities in AHF, 116
  TMM and, 205-206
electrophysiology, basics of, 130-131
emergency department
  languages, 302
  observation units, 293-300
  presenting complaints, 302
emergency medicine, ultrasound, 54-55
enalaprilat, 279
encephalopathy, hypertensive, 235-236
end-tidal CO_2 monitoring, 191
endocarditis, 209-226
  case studies, 219, 222, 223
  infective, 219-224
  noninfective, 224
  pacemaker-related, 283
  presentation, 220-221
  right-sided native-valve infective, 222
  treatment
endothelial dysfunction, 230
enoxaparin, 99
epinephrine, 107t, 130t
epirubicin, cardiomyopathy and, 250
epoprostenol, 261, 262t

esmolol, 145
  in AV nodal blockade, 157
  dosage, 270t
  for hypertension, 234
  indications, 273t
  mechanism of, 269
  for PVST, 153-154
esophageal perforations, 2
esophageal rupture, 2-3
esophagitis, differential diagnosis, 307
European Science Council, 42
European Society of Cardiology, 40, 42
exercise treadmill testing
  characteristics, 44t
  lead placement, 48
  patient selection, 48
extracorporeal life support (ECLS), 195, 262
extracorporeal membrane oxygenation (ECMO), 108

F

factor Xa inhibitors, 99
felodipine, 233
fenoldopam, 232, 237
fibrinolytic therapy
  during cardiac arrest resuscitation, 192
  contraindications, 95t
  coronary patency rates, 98t
  dosage, 98t
  in STEMI, 94-95
fibrinolytics, function of, 94
flecainide, indications, 273t
fluid resuscitation, 259
5-fluorouracil (5-FU), 251
Focused Assessment with Sonography for Trauma (FAST), 54-55
fondaparinux, 99
fractional shortening, 75
Framingham Heart Study, 177, 227-228
Frank-Starling volume-pressure relationship, 262
furosemide, 248, 279

G

gastrointestinal gas, 307
gastrointestinal symptoms, 307
Geneva scores, revised, 7t, 8
glomerular filtration rates (GFR), 116-117
glucagon therapy, 140
glycoprotein IIb-IIIa receptor antagonists, 98-99
glycoside poisoning, 281-282
GUSTO-I trial, 104
GUSTO-II trial, 104, 105

H

heart, normal conduction, 130
heart failure (HF). *see also* acute heart failure (AHF)
  all-cause mortality, 112f
  in cancer patients, 250-251
  cyclophosphamide and, 250-251
  diastolic, 73
  differential diagnosis, 307

hospital admissions, 124-125
in pregnancy, 248
HEART pathway, 44
HEART score, 8
HeartMate, 108
HeartMate II alarm panel, 290f
HeartWare, 108
hemorrhagic stroke, 236
hemothorax, 284-285, 286f
heparins
    low-molecular-weight (LMWHs), 99
    safety in pregnancy, 248
    unfractionated (UFH), 99
hepatojugular reflux, 113
herpes simplex virus, 265
highly active antiretroviral therapy (HAART)
    cardiac disease and, 243
    dilated cardiomyopathy and, 257
    myocardial disease and, 257
    pericardial disease and, 255
His-Purkinje system, 130, 131
HIV infection
    cardiac disease and, 243-247
    inflammation and, 244
    pericardial disease and, 245-246
    QTc prolongation and, 244-245
HMG-CoA reductase inhibitors, 93
holiday heart syndrome, 146
HORIZONS-AMI trial, 97, 99
hydralazine, 121, 235, 248
hydrochlorothiazide, 234
Hyman, Albert, 283, 283f
hyperacute T waves, 12-13, 12f, 13f
hyperglycemia, TMM and, 205-206
hyperinsulinemic euglycemic therapy, 281
hyperkalemia, 130-131, 139, 161
hypertension
    in acute heart failure, 118, 119-121
    in CPR patients, 201
    management of, 228-229
    pathophysiology, 229-232
    during pregnancy, 248-249
    pregnant patients in the emergency department, 249
    therapeutic decision making, 272
    treatment modalities, 232-235
hypertensive emergencies, 227-241
    case studies, 227, 239
    emergency department management, 235t
    treatment recommendations, 238t
hypertensive encephalopathy, 235-236
hypertropic cardiomyopathy, 181
    characteristics, 179
    electrocardiogram, 183f
hyperventilation, avoidance of, 201
hyponatremia, AHF prognosis and, 116
hypoperfusion, patients with, 132
hypotension, TMM and, 205-206
hypothyroidism, in bradyarrhythmia, 139
hypovolemia, cardiac arrest and, 250
hypovolemic shock, RUSH protocol, 87t

I

ibuprofen, in pericarditis, 215
ibutilide, indications, 273t
ice water face immersion, 157
idarubicin, cardiomyopathy and, 250
imidazoline receptors, 271
immunosuppression
    in cardiac transplants, 263-264
    drug interactions, 264t
    maintenance medications for, 263t
implantable assisted circulation device complications, 289-291
implantable cardioverter-defibrillators (ICDs), 283
    complications, 289
    infections related to, 285f
implanted cardiac devices, complications of, 283-292
impulse conduction disorders, 133
impulse generation disorders, 131-133
indapamide, 234
indomethacin, 215
infections
    cardiac device-related, 285f
    cardiac transplants and, 265
inferior STEMI, 21f
    early warning, 26f
    with posterior AMI, 23f
    with RV infarction, 22f
inferior vena cava (IVC)
    collapsibility, 73
    echocardiography, 61, 63
    high CVP, 73f
    inspiratory collapse, 72f
    long axis view, 70f
    subxiphoid 2-chamber view, 68f
    volume status, 63, 65
inotropes
    for cardiogenic shock, 107, 107t
    in pulmonary hypertension, 260
internal jugular veins (IJV)
    echocardiography, 65, 71-73
    evaluation of, 65, 71-73, 72f
    probe placement, 73f
International Liaison Committee on Resuscitation, 188
International Registry of Acute Aortic Dissection, 3
intraaortic balloon pump (IABP), 107
intracranial pressure, increased, 201
    bradyarrhythmias and, 139-140
intravenous fluids, CPR and, 192. *see also* fluid resuscitation
ischemia, on echocardiograms, 45-46
ischemia-modified albumin, 43
ischemia-reperfusion injury, 202f
ischemic stroke, 236
ISIS-1 trial, 92
isoproterenol, 130t

J

Janeway lesions, 220
Jarvik device, 108
jugular venous distention (JVD), 113

K
Kerley B lines, 113

L
labetalol, 235, 236
    dosage, 270t
    for hypertension, 234
    mechanism of, 269
"laitai," 168
language barriers, 302
lateral STEMI, 20f
left anterior descending artery (LAD)
    anatomy, 17-18
    branches, 19
    occlusion, 19
    unobstructed, 47f
left bundle-branch block (LBBB), 26-29, 170, 303-304
    Sgarbossa clinical prediction rules, 29
    ST-segment abnormalities and, 28f
left circumflex coronary artery (LCX), 19
left main coronary artery (LMCA), 17, 25f
left ventricle
    contractility, 79f
    M-mode ultrasound, 56f
    poor contractility, 80f
    subxiphoid 2-chamber view, 68f
    systolic contractility, 73
left ventricular aneurysms (LVA), 34, 34f
left ventricular assist devices (LVADs), 108
left ventricular hypertrophy (LVH), 31-32, 32f, 220f
levosimendan, 107t
lidocaine
    CPR and, 191-192
    indications, 273t
    mechanism of action, 274-275
lipid emulsion therapy, 140
lipid-lowering agents, 93
Listeria infection, 265
loop diuretics
    in congestive heart failure, 278, 279
    for hypertension, 234
    in normotensive AHF, 122
Lund University Cardiac Arrest System (LUCAS), 192
lung ultrasonography
    in acute heart failure, 115-116
    in pulmonary edema, 117f

M
M-mode ultrasound, 53
    assessment of contractility, 75
    E-point septal separation, 57f
    left ventricle, 56f
Mackler triad, esophageal rupture, 2
malpractice
    communication-related, 308-309
    documentation-related, 308-309
    reducing the risk of, 301-309
    scope of the problem, 301-302
    treatment-related, 307-308

Marfan syndrome, aortic dissection and, 3
mass effect, bradyarrhythmias and, 139-140
McConnell sign, 259
mean platelet volume, 6
mean pulmonary artery pressure (PAP), 255-256
medical histories
    duration of symptoms, 302-303
    exacerbating factors, 303
    language issues, 302
    pleuritic chest pain, 303
    presenting complaints, 302
    quality of pain, 303
    reduction of malpractice risk, 302-303
methicillin-resistant *Staphylococcus aureus* (MRSA), 222
methoxyisobutyl isonitrile SPECT (rNIP), 44t
methylprednisone, adverse effects of, 263t
metoprolol, 145
    in AV nodal blockade, 157
    dosage, 270t
    for hypertension, 234
    indications, 273t
    IV, 92
    mechanism of, 269
    for PVST, 153
    study of toxicity, 281
mexiletine, indications, 273t
milrinone
    dosing, 124t
    in hypotensive AHF, 123, 124
    indications, 107
    mechanism of action, 107t, 124t
    in pulmonary hypertension, 260
mitoxantrone, cardiomyopathy and, 250
mitral regurgitation, papillary muscle rupture and, 104
mitral valve, TEE, 224f
morphine
    in hypotensive AHF, 124
    for pain relief, 93-94
multifocal atrial tachycardia (MAT), 158-159, 158f, 159f
    atrial fibrillation in, 159f
    WPW and, 144f
mycophenolate mofetil, adverse effects of, 263, 263t
myocardial infarction (MI)
    acute coronary syndrome and, 243-244
    anterolateral, 214f
    biomarkers, 39-40
    in cancer patients, 251
    in pregnancy, 247-248
    Q waves after, 17
    risk factors in pregnancy, 247t
    STEMI versus NSTEMI, 38
    symptoms, 45
myocardial injury, biomarkers, 42t
myocardial ischemia
    acute coronary syndrome and, 37-38
    identification of, 38-39
myocardial stunning, 202
myocarditis, 209-226
    acute, 34
    antiretroviral therapy and, 257
    causes of, 213t
    complications of, 218-219

description of, 212
management, 215-216
presentation, 212-215
myocardium
blood supply, 17
healthy, 216f
myoglobin, elevation, 41f

N

N-terminal pro-B type natriuretic peptide (NT-proBNP), 6, 43
narrow complex tachycardias (NCTs), 143-160
approach to, 143-148
assessment algorithm, 145f
case study, 275-276, 277
diagnosis algorithm, 145f
differential considerations, 144f
electrocardiogram, 277f, 278f
medications, 275-278
MI with, 167f
rhythms, 148-155
therapeutic decision making, 276-278
natriuretic peptide testing, 116
nesiritide, in acute heart failure, 119-120
neurologic syncope, 179
neuroprognostication, 206
nicardipine, 233, 236, 237
for hypertension, 234
mechanism of, 270
nifedipine, 233
contraindications, 93
nitrates
anti-ischemic therapy, 91-92
contraindications, 91-92
mechanism of action, 271-272
safety in pregnancy, 248
nitric oxide, in pulmonary hypertension, 261
nitroglycerin therapy, 91-92, 232
in acute heart failure, 119
in congestive heart failure, 278-279
mechanism of action, 271
safety in pregnancy, 248
nitroprusside, 232, 237
mechanism of action, 271-272
Nocardia infection, 265
non–ST-elevation myocardial infarction (NSTEMI), 1, 237
differential diagnosis, 306, 306t
modern treatment of, 91-100
observation unit evaluation, 294
T-wave inversion, 15-17
noninvasive ventilation (NIV), 118
norepinephrine
for cardiogenic shock, 280
characteristics, 130t
in hypotensive AHF, 123
indications, 107
mechanism of action, 107t
in pulmonary hypertension, 260
North American Chest Pain Rule (NACPR), 8, 44
NT-proB-NP, 116

O

OASIS trial, 99
obesity, high blood pressure and, 228
observation units
emergency department, 293-300
logistics, 294
patient selection, 297
obstructive shock, RUSH protocol, 87t
omeprazole, 97
orthodromic depolarization, 163
orthodromic tachycardia, 144f
Osborne waves, 139
out-of-hospital cardiac arrest (OHCA), 187
oxygen therapy, 93
in cardiogenic shock, 106
oxygenation, 190-191

P

P waves
morphology, 160f
retrograde, 154f, 288f
sinuatrial (SA) block and, 132
pacemaker-mediated tachycardia, 288t
pacemakers
arrhythmias mediated by, 289
causes of failure to capture, 286t, 287-288, 287f
causes of failure to pace, 286t, 287
device migration, 283
electromagnetic interference, 289
endocarditis, 283
history of, 283f
infections, 284t
lead complications, 284-286
malfunction, 287-291
pocket infections, 283
runaway, 289
undersensing, 288-289
pacer wires, subxiphoid view, 82f
pain
assessment of, 303
radiation of, 303
palpitations
in the emergency department, 249
in pregnancy, 249
papillary muscle rupture, 104
parasternal long-axis view, 55, 58f
anatomy correlation, 60f, 61f, 63f
aortic valve, 64f
pericardial effusion, 67
probe position, 59f, 60f
paroxysmal nocturnal dyspnea (PND), 113
paroxysmal supraventricular tachycardia (PVST), 143, 155-159
electrocardiogram, 152f, 153f, 155
focus of, 152f
management, 155-156
NCT and, 144f
in pregnancy, 249
with retrograde P waves, 154f
with ST-segment depression, 154f
PERC (pulmonary embolism rule-out criteria) Rule, 7t
percutaneous coronary intervention (PCI), 94-95, 192-193

safety in pregnancy, 248
survival benefits, 106
pericardial disease, cancer patients, 251-252
pericardial effusions
   B-mode ultrasound, 55f
   clotted, 74f
   D-dimer assays, 6
   echocardiographic image, 5, 5f
   echocardiographic windows, 67, 69
   electrical alternans, 217, 218f
   fresh, 74f
   grading scale, 75t
   HAART and, 255
   location of effusions, 69
   pathophysiology, 67
   sonography appearance, 67
   subxiphoid view, 219f
pericardial fat pads, subxiphoid view, 76f
pericardial fluid
   ascites versus, 67, 76f
   location of, 67
   pleural fluid versus, 67
pericardial tamponade, 217
pericardiocentesis, ultrasound-guided, 71, 78f
pericarditis, 209-226
   case study, 209, 212, 219
   causes of, 213t, 246t
   complications of, 216
   ECG, 210f-212f
   echocardiography in, 217
   electrocardiogram, 214f
   HAART and, 255
   management, 215-216
   misdiagnosis, 304-305
   presentation, 212-215
   ST-segment abnormalities in, 33f
   treatment of, 217t
   tuberculosis-related, 246
peripheral arterial cannulation, 108
peripheral vascular resistance (PVR), increased, 260-261
peripheral vasodilators, 233t
perivascular cuffing, 113-114
phenoxybenzamine, 235
phentolamine, mechanism of action, 271
phenylephrine, mechanism of action, 107t
pheochromocytoma, 237
phosphodiesterase inhibitors, 261
Physician Insurers Association of America (PIAA), 301-302
platelets, aggregation, 96-97
pleural effusion, parasternal long axis view, 74f
pleural fluid, pericardial fluid versus, 67
Pneumocystis jirovecii infection, 265
pneumonia, differential diagnosis, 307
pneumopericardium, chest CT image, 286f
pneumothorax
   chest CT image, 286f
   echocardiography of, 5
   pacemaker leads and, 284-285
"pokkuri," 168
polymorphic ventricular tachycardia, 166-168
positive airway pressure (CPAP), 118
post-cardiac arrest syndrome (PCAS), 201-207
   clinical features, 201-202
   evaluation, 201-206
   ischemia-reperfusion injury in, 202f
   pathophysiology, 201
   treatment, 201-206
posterior descending artery, 19
posterior wall AMI
   ECG findings suggestive of, 25t
   ECG recognition, 305
postresuscitation cardiogenic shock, 202
postresuscitation neurologic injury, 203
potassium-sparing diuretics, 234
prasugrel, 97-98
prazosin, 235
prednisone, adverse effects of, 263t
preeclampsia, 237, 249
pregnancy
   acute myocardial infarction in, 247-248
   arrhythmias during, 249
   cardiac arrest during, 249-250
   cardiac disease in, 247-250
   CPR during, 250
   hypertension during, 248-249
preload optimization, 259
premature ventricular contractions (PVCs), 167f
   pacemaker-mediated tachycardia, 288t
   in pregnancy, 249
primary percutaneous coronary intervention (pPCI)
   in STEMI, 95-96
procainamide, 147, 175
   in AV nodal blockade, 157
   bradycardia and, 131
   CPR and, 191-192
   indications, 273, 273t
   mechanism of action, 275f
propafenone, indications, 273t
propranolol
   indications, 273t
   mechanism of, 269
prostanoids
   infusions, 262t
   in pulmonary hypertension, 261
protease inhibitors, 243-244
proton-pump inhibitors (PPIs), 97
provocative testing, 48
proximal aortic aneurysm, 62f
Pseudomonas aeruginosa infection, 265
pulmonary artery catheter insertion, 106
pulmonary capillary wedge pressure
   radiologic findings and, 116t
pulmonary edema, 237
   lung ultrasound, 84f
pulmonary emboli (PE)
   acute chest pain in, 2
   assessment of, 305
   computed tomography angiography, 6
   diagnosis of, 307t
   differential diagnosis, 306-307
   echocardiography for, 77-81
   electrocardiogram, 304f
   hemodynamically significant, 79-81
   risk factors, 2

risk stratification, 7t
pulmonary embolism rule-out criteria (PERC) rule, 7t
pulmonary hypertension, 255-262
    causes of acute decompression in, 260t
    clinical presentation, 257, 257t
    definition, 255-256
    diagnosis, 257-259
    ECG findings, 257t
    echocardiogram, 259f
    emergency department resuscitation in, 259-262
    emergency department management of, 260t
    epidemiology of, 255
    mechanisms of, 256t
    pathophysiology, 256-257
    in pregnancy, 248
    ventilator settings in, 261t
    WHO classification system, 256t, 257
pulse generators, implantation, 283-284
pump failure, cardiac arrest and, 250
pump thrombosis, 290-291
$P2Y_{12}$ ADP inhibitors, 96-97

Q

Q waves, 17
    completed infarction, 12f
    established AMI, 18f
QRS complexes
    sinuatrial (SA) block and, 132
    wide, 174f
QT intervals
    long, 167f, 168
    prolonged, 182f
QTc prolongation
    assessment of, 305
    in cancer patients, 252
    HIV infection and, 244-245, 245t
quinidine
    bradycardia and, 131
    indications, 273t

R

radiation therapy
    coronary artery disease and, 251
    pericarditis related to, 251
radionucleotide perfusion imaging
    ischemic heart, 46f
    normal heart, 46f
    resting, 46
Rapid Ultrasound in SHock (RUSH), 83-85, 84f, 85f
rapid ventricular response (RVR), 146f
reentrant atrioventricular tachycardia, 174-175
regadenoson (Lexiscan/RapiScan), 48t
rejection, acute, 264-265
renal artery stenosis, 228
renin-angiotensin-aldosterone system (RAAS), 231-232
renin-angiotensin-aldosterone system (RAAS) inhibitors, 93
renin inhibitors, 234
reperfusion, cardiogenic shock prevention, 106
reserpine, 235
resting radionucleotide perfusion imaging, 46

resuscitation ultrasound protocols, 81, 83-85, 83t
return of spontaneous circulation (ROSC), 187
revascularization, early, 103
right atrial collapse, 77f
right atrium, thrombus, 82f
right bundle-branch block (RBBB), 170
right coronary artery (RCA)
    anatomy, 17, 19
    maintenance of perfusion, 260
    occluded, 96f
    unobstructed, 47f
right ventricle
    dilated, 4f
    optimization of systolic function, 260
    reduction of afterload, 260-261
    strain, 81f
    subxiphoid 2-chamber view, 68f
    thrombus entering, 82f
right ventricular failure, 104
right ventricular myocardial infarction (RVMI)
    description, 19
    ECG findings, 24t
    inferior wall STEMI and, 23
right ventricular pacemaker, 29-31, 31f
rule out myocardial ischemia (ROMI), 38-39
    case studies, 38, 39, 39f, 45, 49

S

San Francisco Syncope Rule, 183, 184t
seizures, syncope differentiated from, 180t
Seldinger technique, 108
Sgarbossa clinical prediction rule, 29, 30f, 303-304
shock
    causes of, 85
    types of, 87t
SHOCK registry, 104-105
SHOCK trial, 104, 106
SHOCKD mnemonic, 105t
Sicilian Gambit system, 272
sildenafil, in pulmonary hypertension, 261
Simpson's modified rule, 77, 80f
single-photon emission CT (SPECT), 48
sinuatrial (SA) node, 130
    beta receptors, 270
    block, 132
sinus arrest, 132, 133f
sinus bradycardia, 132-133
sinus exit block, 132
sinus node dysfunction, 131-132
sinus tachycardia, 148-159
    cocaine use and, 147f
    in NCT, 147f
    NCT and, 144f, 145
    ST-segment changes and, 4
    T-wave changes and, 4
sirolimus, adverse effects of, 263t, 264
SOAP-2 trial, 107
sodium ion channels, 262
sodium nitroprusside
    in acute heart failure, 120-121
    mechanism of action, 271

sonographic windows, 55-61
sonospirometry, 63
spironolactone, 234
spontaneous pneumothorax, classes of, 3
ST-elevation myocardial infarction (STEMI), 237
    benign early repolarization, 32f, 33-34
    complications, 96
    diagnosis of, 1
    differential diagnosis, 306, 306t
    diffuse, 4
    early, 13f
    ECG progression, 12f
    emergency department management of, 97t
    electrocardiogram, 280f
    elevated ST segment, 12f
    fibrinolytics in treatment of, 94-95
    inferior, 4
    management overview, 94f
    mimic patterns, 33-34, 33t
    modern treatment of, 91-100
    observation unit evaluation, 294
    primary percutaneous coronary intervention, 95-96
    revascularization therapy, 94-96
ST-segment depression, 14-15, 15f
    ACS-related presentations, 15
    lead aVL, 26f
    lead aVR, 24f
    nonischemic causes of, 15
    reciprocal, 21-22
ST-segment elevation, 13-14
    anterior STEMI, 19f
    established STEMI, 14f, 15f
    lead aVR, 21
    in left ventricular aneurysms, 34f
    right ventricular pacemaker and, 31f
Stanford classification, aortic dissection, 3
Staphylococcus aureus infection, 221, 265, 283
Staphylococcus epidermidis, 283
statins
    benefits of, 106
    use in the emergency department, 93
Strategies for Management of Antiretroviral Therapy (SMART) study, 244
Streptococcus viridans infection, 222
stress echocardiography, 48, 48t
stress radionucleotide perfusion imaging, 48
stress testing, 45
stroke, bradyarrhythmias and, 139-140
subarachnoid hemorrhage, 179
subxiphoid window, 59
    2-chamber view, 68f
    anatomic correlation, 59, 64f, 65f
    probe position, 59f
    pulmonary emboli, 79, 81
superior vena cava syndrome, 285-286
supraventricular tachycardia (SVT), 161t, 163, 169-171
Swedish Registry of Cardiac Intensive Care, 94
syncope, 177-186, 178-179
    causes of, 177-180, 178t
    disposition, 183-185
    emergency department disposition algorithm, 184f
    electrocardiograms, 181
    followup, 183-185
    inpatient evaluation, 184-185
    observation unit evaluation, 295-206
    outpatient evaluation, 185
    pathophysiology, 177
    patient evaluation, 180-183
    physical examination, 181
    risk stratification, 296f
    seizures differentiated from, 180t
    symptoms associated with, 180
    unexplained, 183-184
systolic contractility, left ventricle, 73

T

T-wave inversion, 12f, 15-17
    in acute coronary syndrome (ACS), 16f
    causes of, 16t
    normalization, 15-16
    pseudonormalization, 16
T waves
    hyperacute, 12-13, 12f
    too tall, 27f
tachyarrhythmias
    pacemaker-associated, 174
    troponin release, 5
tachycardia-bradycardia syndrome, 131
tachycardias
    narrow complex, 143-160
    pacemaker-mediated, 162
tacrolimus, adverse effects of, 263, 263t
targeted temperature management (TTM), 202, 203-206
    criteria, 204t
    induction, 204-205, 205t
    maintenance, 205
    patient populations, 206
    pediatric populations, 206
    phases of, 204f
    physiologic effects, 205-206
    potential adverse events, 205t
    practice guidelines, 206
    prehospital cooling, 206
    rewarming, 205
tension pneumothorax, 3
terazosin, 235
termination-of-resuscitation, 193
    prehospital, 193t
thalidomide, for bradycardia, 252
therapeutic hypothermia, 108, 139
thiazide diuretics, 234, 249t
thrombolysis in myocardial infarction (TIMI) risk score, 8, 8t
ticagrelor, 98
tilt-table testing, 185
tissue perfusion testing, 48
tocainide, indications, 273t
tongue biting, 181
torsade de pointes (TdP), 144-145, 168, 173, 305
Toxoplasma gondii infection, 265
transcutaneous pacing, 130
transthoracic echocardiography, 45-46, 224f
transvenous pacemaker placement, 81
trastuzumab, cardiomyopathy and, 250, 251

treatment effects, 92t
treprostinil infusions, 262t
triamterene, for hypertension, 234
trimethaphan, 235
TRITON-TIMI 38 trial, 97, 98
troponin I (TnI), 42
troponin T (TnT), 42
troponins, cardiac, 39, 41-42
    in acute heart failure, 116
    kinetics of elevation, 41f
    multi-marker approach, 43
    in myocardial injury, 5
tuberculosis, pericarditis, 246
Twiddler's syndrome, 289

U

ultrasonography
    abdominal aortic aneurysm, 86f
    aortic dissection, 86f
    B-mode, 53
    bedside, 5
    bedside emergent, 53-89
    chest pain evaluation, 5
    consensus guidelines, 54t
    functional categories, 54t
    lung, in AHF, 115-116, 117f
    M-mode, 53
    probe orientation, 54-55
    resuscitation, 81-86
    transvenous pacemaker placement, 81
universal termination-of-resuscitation rule, 193
unstable angina (UA), 237
    differential diagnosis, 306, 306t
    observation unit evaluation, 294
    TIMI risk scores and, 8
USIC trial, 94

V

vagal maneuvers, 145, 157
    in pregnancy, 249
vagolysis, therapeutic, 130
valsalva, 157
Vancouver Chest Pain Rule, 44
vasoactive medications, 130t
vasoconstriction, causes of, 230
vasodilation, causes of, 230
vasodilators, peripheral, 233t
vasopressin, in vasodilatory shock, 108
vasopressors
    for cardiogenic shock, 107, 107t
    CPR and, 191
vasovagal syncope, 179
Vaughn Williams classification system, 162, 272, 273t
venous cannulation, 108
ventilation, during CPR, 191
ventricular assist devices (VADs), 283
    emergent management, 290f
    function of, 289
    types of, 290
ventricular fibrillation (VF), 168f, 266

ventricular free wall rupture, 104
ventricular septal defect (VSD), 58f
ventricular septal rupture (VSR), 104
ventricular tachycardia (VT), 163-166
    cardiac transplants and, 266
    polymorphic, 166-168
    pulseless, 173
    stable, 173
    supraventricular tachycardia differentiated from, 169-171
    SVT differentiated from, 161t
verapamil, 233, 234, 273t

W

Wellens syndrome, 16, 17f
Wells scores, 7t, 8
Wenckebach block, 130, 134-135, 135f, 221
WEST trial, 94
wheezing, coarse, 113
wide complex tachycardia (WCT), 161-175
    case study, 273-275
    diagnosis, 174
    differential diagnosis, 161-163, 170t
    electrocardiogram, 175f, 276f
    normal axis, 164f
    prognosis, 174
    therapeutic decision making, 275
    treatment, 171-174
    treatment algorithm, 173f
Wolff-Parkinson-White (WPW) syndrome, 143, 156-158, 156f
    characteristics of, 163
    electrocardiogram, 274f
    electrocardiography, 156f, 157f
    management, 157-158
    NCT and, 144f
    syncope in, 181
World Health Organization, 42